Biological Potential and Medical Use of Secondary Metabolites

Biological Potential and Medical Use of Secondary Metabolites

Special Issue Editors

Ana M. L. Seca
Diana Pinto

MDPI • Basel • Beijing • Wuhan • Barcelona • Belgrade

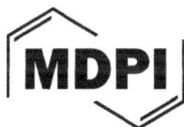

MDPI

Special Issue Editors
Ana M. L. Seca
University of the Azores,
Portugal

Diana Pinto
Universidade de Aveiro,
Portugal

Editorial Office
MDPI
St. Alban-Anlage 66
4052 Basel, Switzerland

This is a reprint of articles from the Special Issue published online in the open access journal *Medicines* (ISSN 2305-6320) from 2018 to 2019 (available at: https://www.mdpi.com/journal/medicines/special_issues/secondary_metabolites)

For citation purposes, cite each article independently as indicated on the article page online and as indicated below:

LastName, A.A.; LastName, B.B.; LastName, C.C. Article Title. *Journal Name* **Year**, *Article Number*, Page Range.

ISBN 978-3-03921-187-6 (Pbk)
ISBN 978-3-03921-188-3 (PDF)

Cover image courtesy of Ana M. L. Seca and Diana Pinto.

Contents

About the Special Issue Editors

Ana M. L. Seca was born in Aveiro at 1969. She has a degree in Chemistry and a Ms in Science and Technology of Paper and Forest Products, both obtained from the University of Aveiro, Portugal, where she also received her Ph.D. in Chemistry in 2000. Since then she has been Assistant Professor at the University of Azores (Portugal), and since 2016 she has been a member of the Center for Ecology, Evolution, and Environmental Changes-cE3c (ABG). Her current research interests comprise the isolation and identification of secondary metabolites with potential pharmacological applications and the synthesis of pharmaceutically relevant natural compound derivatives using the microwave irradiation. She has supervised more than 15 students and published more than 40 SCI papers and 8 book chapters.

Diana Pinto studied chemistry at the University of Aveiro (Portugal), where she graduated in analytical chemistry in 1991. In 1996, she received her Ph.D. in chemistry at Aveiro University. She then joined the Department of Chemistry at Aveiro University, where she is currently Assistant Professor of Organic Chemistry. Diana is an expert in organic synthesis, including the development of new strategies towards the synthesis of nitrogen and oxygen heterocyclic compounds that can be used as new drugs. Over the years, her research has also been focused on the application of environmental friendly methodologies in organic synthesis, with an emphasis on the application of microwave irradiation. Besides her strong interest in organic synthesis, Diana is also developing active research in the isolation and characterization of natural products, focusing on medicinal plants. Currently, she is the author and co-author of 120 SCI papers and 18 book chapters. She has supervised more than 27 Ph.D. and M.Sc. students, and she has also participated in financed Portuguese and European projects.

medicines

MDPI

Editorial

Biological Potential and Medical Use of Secondary Metabolites

Ana M. L. Seca [1,2,*] and Diana C. G. A. Pinto [2,*]

1   cE3c-Centre for Ecology, Evolution and Environmental Changes/Azorean Biodiversity Group, University of Azores, Rua Mãe de Deus, 9501-801 Ponta Delgada, Portugal
2   QOPNA & LAQV-REQUIMTE, University of Aveiro, 3810-193 Aveiro, Portugal
*   Correspondence: ana.ml.seca@uac.pt (A.M.L.S.); diana@ua.pt (D.C.G.A.P.);
    Tel.: +351-296-650-174 (A.M.L.S.); +351-234-401-407 (D.C.G.A.P.)

Received: 5 June 2019; Accepted: 5 June 2019; Published: 12 June 2019

Abstract: This *Medicines* special issue focuses on the great potential of secondary metabolites for therapeutic applications. The special issue contains 16 articles reporting relevant experimental results and overviews of bioactive secondary metabolites. Their biological effects and new methodologies that improve the lead compounds' synthesis were also discussed. We would like to thank all 83 authors, from all over the world, for their valuable contributions to this special issue.

Keywords: secondary metabolites; biological activities; medicinal applications; plants; seaweeds

---

This editorial is an introduction to the special issue "Biological Potential and Medical Use of Secondary Metabolites" and contains an overview on the role of secondary metabolites as medicines. In fact, secondary metabolites, used as a single compound or as a mixture, are medicines that can be effective and safe even when synthetic drugs fail. They may even potentiate or synergize the effects of other compounds in the medicine. The research and review articles published in this special issue highlight the secondary metabolites with greater potential for therapeutic application as well as new sources of secondary metabolites well known for their therapeutic properties. The manuscripts published in this special issue are also a showcase of the different methodologies and approaches that researchers use to evaluate, demonstrate, and enhance the properties of secondary metabolites extracted from natural sources including terrestrial plants, marine species, and fungi species such as mushrooms.

Ocimum sanctum L. (according to the "The Plant List" database, this name is a synonym of *Ocimum tenuiflorum* L.), is an Ayurvedic herb of Southeast Asia with a long history of traditional use to treat cough, respiratory disorders, poisoning, impotence, and arthritis [1] and with great chemopreventive and therapeutic potential. Flegkas et al. [2] isolate several secondary metabolites from different classes (four terpenoids, four phenolic derivatives, three flavonoids, two lignans, and one sterol) using chromatographic techniques and elucidate their structures using spectroscopic methods. They also report the interesting proapoptotic and selective activity displayed using (-)-rabdosiin, a tetramer composed of a lignan skeleton connected to two caffeic acids, against MCF-7, SKBR3, and HCT-116 cancer cell lines [2], suggesting this secondary metabolite to be a leading central structure in the development of anticancer drugs.

Malaria continues to be a disease without much effective treatment because of the appearance of mechanisms of resistance to current drugs, so the development of new antimalarial drugs is an important area of research. Based on previous knowledge about antiplasmodial activity against a chloroquinone-sensitive strain of *Plasmodium falciparum* of sargahydroquinoic acid, the main metabolite of brown alga *Sargassum incisifolium* (Turner) C. Aggard, Munedzimwe et al. [3] converted this meroditerpene into several derivatives using semi-synthesis to look for more active derivatives.

Ten sargahydroquinoic acid derivatives were assessed regarding their antiplasmodial activity and to explore some structure–activity relationships. The results show that sarganaphthoquinoic acid and sargaquinoic acid are the most promising selective antiplasmodial derivatives. Additionally, the presence of a quinone and carboxylic acid were important for selective activity against the chloroquine-resistant Gambian FCR-3 strain of *P. falciparum* [3].

Several secondary metabolites isolated from the same seaweed, *Sargassum incisifolium*, and some semisynthetic derivatives were tested to evaluate their potential as modulators of inflammatory bowel diseases, such as Crohn's disease and ulcerate colitis, using various in vitro assays [4]. In fact, inflammatory bowel diseases have become a global health challenge since conventional treatments exhibit moderate efficacy and have significant side effects. The natural compound sargahydroquinoic acid was identified as a promising lead compound due to its effects on various therapeutic targets relevant to inflammatory bowel diseases treatment. Conversion of sargahydroquinoic acid to sarganaphthoquinoic acid greatly improved the peroxisome proliferator activated receptor gamma (PPAR-γ) activity, but this structural modification significantly decreased its antioxidant activity and had a minimal effect on cytotoxicity against a HeLa cancer cell line [4].

Artemisinin is a sesquiterpene lactone compound with a unique chemical structure derived from the sweet wormwood plant, *Artemisia annua* L. It is a very successful clinical drug used in the treatment of malaria [5], and now has a second life as an antitumor agent [6]. Therefore, there is a great demand for new sources of artemisinin, in particular among another *Artemisia* species. Furthermore, since the biotransformation and accumulation of artemisinin depends on the natural conditions, such as light intensity, Numonov et al. [7] evaluated the content of the artemisinin in eight *Artemisia* species collected in Tajikistan, a country with a relatively large number of sunny days per year. The artemisinin content on *Artemisia* hexane extracts, prepared using ultrasound-assisted extraction, was determinate using HPLC. The highest content found, in this study, was in *Artemisia vachanica* Krasch. ex Poljakov (0.34% of dried plant), a new source of artemisinin, and the species with the second-highest content after *Artemisia annua* (0.45 %), while *Artemisia leucotricha* Krasch. ex Ladygina (according to the "The Plant List" database, this name is a synonym of *Seriphidium leucotrichum* (Krasch.) Y.R.Ling.) was the only one in which no artemisinin was detected. The same work shows that the treatment of *Artemisia annua* hexane extract with silica gel as an adsorbent resulted in the enrichment of artemisinin [7].

Pristimerin and tingenone belong to the class of quinonemethide triterpenoids, known as celastroloids, a relatively small class of compounds that exhibit interesting biological activities, such as cytotoxicity and anti-inflammatory, antimicrobial, and antioxidant properties, and accumulate mainly in the root of *Celastraceae* species. Taking into account the chemotaxonomic and therapeutic relevance of quinonemethide triterpenoids like pristimerin and tingenone, Taddeo et al. [8] developed an analytical method for its identification and quantification in the root of species of *Maytenus chiapensis* Lundell. These authors suggest the use of RP HPLC-PDA for the analysis of n-hexane-Et_2O extract (1:1), the ideal solvent for extraction of these two bioactive secondary metabolites. The proposed method is useful in the analysis of other species of *Celastraceae* and in the analysis of commercial samples [8].

The *Boswellia* sp. are resiniferous trees and shrubs that produce oleo-gum resin, well known as frankincense [9], a natural product of high commercial value used in traditional medicine, religious ceremonies, and cosmetic and perfumery products [10]. Byler and Setzer [11] identified the biomolecular targets docked by some frankincense secondary metabolites using reverse docking analysis, showing that some diterpenes exhibited selective docking to bacterial protein targets and to acetylcholinesterase, while some triterpenoids targeted specific antineoplastic molecular targets, diabetes-relevant targets, and protein targets involved in inflammatory processes. Several medicinal properties of frankincense were corroborated by the molecular docking properties of their di- and triterpenoids. This study opens the way for further investigations of the biomolecular targets identified in this work regarding the improvement of new inhibitors to be used in the treatment of bacterial infections, and inflammatory, diabetes, and Alzheimer's diseases.

Quy and Xuan [12] used a more traditional approach to suggest cordycepin identified in the mushroom *Cordyceps militaris* (L.) Link ethyl acetate extract as the responsible agent for the extract´s xanthine oxidase inhibitory activity. Using the bio-guided assays approach, they identified the constituents of the most active fractions using GC-MS. They revealed that the fungus *Cordyceps militaris*, used in traditional medicine, is a potential source of cordycepin, the largest constituent of the fraction exhibiting the highest anti-xanthine oxidase effect. Thus, the *Cordyceps militaris* fractions and/or its constituent cordycepin could be beneficial for hyperuricemia treatment. However, more in depth studies and in vivo trials on compounds purified from this medicinal fungus are needed.

Polyphenols are a vast and heterogeneous set of secondary metabolites that include flavonoids, stilbenes, lignans, benzoic acid derivatives, and cinnamic acids, among others, which have in common at least one hydroxylated aromatic ring. They are the subject of vast research as they possess biological properties relevant to well-being and improved health [13–15]. In fact, it is known that the consumption of specific types of food (e.g., fruits) rich in polyphenols exerts a positive effect on health, improving, for example, the antioxidant and anti-inflammatory responses of the organism and helps fight cardiovascular and cancer diseases [13,16]. The antioxidant potential and total polyphenols content in most of the 17 ancient regional varieties of apples from the province of Siena in Tuscany are remarkably higher when compared with two commercial varieties, being in some cases about 8 times higher. In addition, older varieties showed lower glucose contents and higher contents of xylitol and pectins, which are also relevant factors for considering older varieties with the highest potential as nutraceuticals [17].

The polar extracts of *Glycyrrhiza glabra* L., *Paeonia lactiflora* Pall., and *Eriobotrya japonica* (Thunb.) Lindl., three known species frequently used in traditional Chinese medicine, were analysed using LC-MS and their total phenolic contents, and antioxidant, antimicrobial, and cytotoxic activities, were evaluated [18]. The terpenoid glycosides was the most abundant class in all three species. Glycyrrhizic acid and (iso)liquiritin apioside isomers were the most abundant secondary metabolites in the *Glycyrrhiza glabra*, while in the *Paeonia lactiflora*, the most abundant were paeoniflorin derivatives, and in *Eriobotrya japonica*, the most abundant were the nerolidol derivatives. The *Paeonia lactiflora* extract was the most antioxidant one, which was more active than the (-)-epigallocatechin gallate positive control [18].

The defensins are a family of cysteine-rich peptides with ≈29–42 amino acids, that play a very important role in the defense system of plants, insects, animals, and humans against invasion by microorganisms. Many of these peptides have been proposed as novel natural antibiotics with great potential for application toward human health and agriculture [19,20]. In fact, due to the increase in the phenomena of resistance to conventional antibiotics, the development of new classes of drugs to combat infections by microorganisms has intensified, with defensins being one of those classes that has gained prominence. Ishaq et al. [21] present the most current overview of the plant defensins applications in the treatment of human infections by viruses, bacteria, and fungi; treatment of hemorrhoids, liver disorders, and cancer; and its use in agriculture as a way to increase agricultural production using natural compounds as phytosanitary agents.

Cannabis species contain more than 545 secondary metabolites of different classes but they are chiefly known to possess a great structural diversity of non-nitrogen compounds capable of interfering with the central nervous system, known as cannabinoids, which also exhibit very interesting pharmaceutical properties [22]. The increasing interest of patients regarding the medicinal use of *Cannabis* has been accompanied by a renewed interest of scientists in the potential medical use of various constituents of this plant [22,23]. The review of the literature on cannabinoids identified in *Cannabis* and their application for therapeutic purposes, on the evaluation of its toxicological effects, and the development and improvement of new methodologies for its detection and quantification presented by Gonçalves et al. [24] is of great interest. It opens new lines of research in order to increasingly distinguish the recreational use of the medicinal use of both herbal products derived from *Cannabis* and its secondary metabolites.

Like *Cannabis*, kratom (*Mitragyna speciosa* (Korth.) Havil.) is a species that is also used for medical purposes as an analgesic, and for social and recreational use, being a source of psychoactive agents, mainly alkaloids, and a cheap alternative to opiate-rich substances [25]. The most recent review of the literature on *Mitragyna speciosa* [26] presents the state of the art for its major secondary metabolites, the potential beneficial and toxicological effects derived from its use, and the methodologies for its detection in plant and biological samples. It is concluded that the use of kratom or its metabolites may cause dependence; increase blood pressure; cause liver, renal, and neuronal toxicity; emphysema; excess alveoli inflammation; and even death. On the other hand, kratom has interesting effects, namely antinociceptive, anti-inflammatory, gastrointestinal, antidepressant, antioxidant, and antibacterial properties [26]. However, further studies are required to support the use of the species or its secondary metabolites for clinical purposes.

Tavares and Seca [27] demonstrate how *Juniperus* species are a good bet as a source of secondary metabolites by presenting a review about diterpenes, flavonoids, and one lignan identified in *Juniperus* as having a high potential for the development of new antitumor, antibacterial, and antiviral drugs. Deoxypodophyllotoxin appears to be the most promising lead compound since it has reported antitumor effects against breast cancer acquired resistant cells (MCF-7/A), with a very interesting IC_{50} value in the nanomolar level. The dehydroabietic acid methyl ester derivative, with the substituent (2-(4-(3-(*tert*-butoxycarbonylamino)phenyl)-1*H*-1,2,3-triazol-1-yl)acetamido) at C-14, also seems to be an excellent leader compound since it has shown IC_{50} values between 0.7–1.2 µM against PC-3, SK-OV-3, MCF-7, and MDA-MB-231 tumour cell lines, which is an activity higher than the one exhibited by the anticancer agent 5-FU used clinically.

The *Scabiosa* genus, despite the great controversy regarding the taxonomic classification of its species, is widely considered to be valuable in traditional medicine and the biological potential of its secondary metabolites as effective agents in the treatment of various diseases is well known [28]. Pinto et al. [28] present an update on the information about flavonoids, iridoids, and saponins from *Scabiosa* species that can be highlighted both from the point of view of their biological properties and from the in vivo assays already performed. In fact, these secondary metabolites exhibit interesting effects, such as anti-inflammatory and antitumoral activities, effects that validate and extend some traditional uses of *Scabiosa* species, as well as inspire the development of new drugs based on extracts or pure secondary metabolites. On the other hand, this review also demonstrates that the phytochemistry of several *Scabiosa* species has been neglected. These findings should encourage further studies that can reveal the medicinal potential of this species.

An essential oil is a complex mixture of volatile compounds that exhibit the ability to control the infectious/parasitic diseases, which is a great continuing challenge for global health. In fact, essential oils could exhibit a dual role, being able to control vectors, important in the cycle of disease transmission, and they exhibit relevant activity against the pathogens [29]. However, the solubility and stability of essential oils poses significant problems in the formulation of new products for both vector and parasite control. Echeverría and Albuquerque [30] review several studies related to the development of nanoemulsions containing essential oils as effective formulations to control diseases in humans and animals, since they have lower cost and ecological toxicity. The authors emphasize these formulations as water-soluble and stable alternatives, able to act as larvicides, insecticides, repellents, and acaricides, as well as having antiparasitic properties, such that they have proved to be very efficient in the treatment and prevention of infectious and parasitic diseases. In addition, the nanoemulsion formulation of essential oils makes this pesticide more environmentally friendly [30].

The use of bioinformatics and omic workflow is a very recent approach in the effort to discover natural products in various environments, such as soils, aquatic environments, and microbial communities. Chen et al. [31] present a literature review highlighting several methods, mainly bioinformatics, used to identify biosynthetic gene clusters that encode the biosynthesis of secondary metabolites in the environment, especially in environments where microorganisms are rarely cultivated.

There are also several examples of how recent studies have explored the genetic basis for the synthesis of new natural products that have broad medical and industrial applications [31].

By considering all the information given in this special issue, one can confirm the importance of plants in the development of new medicines. They are an important source of bioactive or inspiring molecules. Skepticism can arise from the use of pure isolated compounds if we consider that plants have a mixture of several bioactive molecules that can synergize the biological effects. However, mixtures can also be developed, and the knowledge of their composition will allow for the optimization of its effect, not only against the disease but also on the patient. The authors of the current editorial hope that this special issue stimulates further research, in particular, research involving clinical trials.

Author Contributions: A.M.L.S. and D.C.G.A.P. conceived, designed, and wrote the editorial.

Funding: Funded by FCT—Fundação para a Ciência e a Tecnologia, the European Union, QREN, FEDER, COMPETE, by funding the cE3c Centre (FCT Unit funding (Ref. UID/BIA/00329/2013, 2015–2018) and UID/BIA/00329/2019) and the QOPNA research unit (project FCT UID/QUI/00062/2019).

Conflicts of Interest: The authors declare no conflict of interest.

References

1. Singh, D.; Chaudhuri, P.K. A review on phytochemical and pharmacological properties of Holy basil (*Ocimum sanctum* L.). *Ind. Crops Prod.* **2018**, *118*, 367–382. [CrossRef]
2. Flegkas, A.; Ifantis, T.M.; Barda, C.; Samara, P.; Tsitsilonis, O.; Skaltsa, H. Antiproliferative activity of (-)-rabdosiin isolated from *Ocimum sanctum* L. *Medicines* **2019**, *6*, 37. [CrossRef] [PubMed]
3. Munedzimwe, T.C.; van Zyl, R.L.; Heslop, D.C.; Edkins, A.L.; Beukes, D.R. Semi-synthesis and evaluation of sargahydroquinoic acid derivatives as potential antimalarial agents. *Medicines* **2019**, *6*, 47. [CrossRef] [PubMed]
4. Nyambe, M.N.; Koekemoer, T.C.; van de Venter, M.; Goosen, E.D.; Beukes, D.R. In vitro evaluation of the phytopharmacological potential of *Sargassum incisifolium* for the treatment of inflammatory bowel diseases. *Medicines* **2019**, *6*, 49. [CrossRef] [PubMed]
5. Wang, J.G.; Xu, C.C.; Wong, Y.K.; Li, Y.J.; Liao, F.L.; Jiang, T.L.; Tu, Y.Y. Artemisinin, the magic drug discovered from traditional Chinese medicine. *Engineering* **2019**, *5*, 32–39. [CrossRef]
6. Efferth, T. Artemisinin–second career as anticancer drug? *World J. Tradit. Chin. Med.* **2015**, *1*, 2–25. [CrossRef]
7. Numonov, S.; Sharopov, F.; Salimov, A.; Sukhrobov, P.; Atolikshoeva, S.; Safarzoda, R.; Habasi, M.; Aisa, H.A. Assessment of artemisinin contents in selected *Artemisia* species from Tajikistan (central Asia). *Medicines* **2019**, *6*, 23. [CrossRef]
8. Taddeo, V.A.; Castillo, U.G.; Martínez, M.L.; Menjivar, J.; Jiménez, I.A.; Núñez, M.J.; Bazzocchi, I.L. Development and validation of an HPLC-PDA method for biologically active quinonemethide triterpenoids isolated from *Maytenus chiapensis*. *Medicines* **2019**, *6*, 36. [CrossRef] [PubMed]
9. Moussaieff, A.; Mechoulam, R. *Boswellia* resin: From religious ceremonies to medical uses; A review of in-vitro, in-vivo and clinical trials. *J. Pharm. Pharmacol.* **2009**, *61*, 1281–1293. [CrossRef] [PubMed]
10. Brendler, T.; Brinckmann, J.A.; Schippmann, U. Sustainable supply, a foundation for natural product development: The case of Indian frankincense (*Boswellia serrata* Roxb. ex Colebr.). *J. Ethnopharmacol.* **2018**, *225*, 279–286. [CrossRef] [PubMed]
11. Byler, K.B.; Setzer, W. Protein targets of frankincense: A reverse docking analysis of terpenoids from *Boswellia* oleo-gum resins. *Medicines* **2018**, *5*, 96. [CrossRef] [PubMed]
12. Quy, T.N.; Xuan, T.D. Xanthine oxidase inhibitory potential, antioxidant and antibacterial activities of *Cordyceps militaris* (L.) Link fruiting body. *Medicines* **2019**, *6*, 20. [CrossRef] [PubMed]
13. Tangney, C.; Rasmussen, H.E. Polyphenols, inflammation, and cardiovascular disease. *Curr. Atheroscler. Rep.* **2013**, *15*, 324. [CrossRef] [PubMed]
14. Ganesan, K.; Xu, B. A critical review on polyphenols and health benefits of black soybeans. *Nutrients* **2017**, *9*, 455. [CrossRef] [PubMed]
15. Cory, H.; Passarelli, S.; Szeto, J.; Tamez, M.; Mattei, J. The role of polyphenols in human health and food systems: A mini-review. *Front. Nutr.* **2018**, *5*, 87. [CrossRef] [PubMed]

16. Mileo, A.M.; Nisticò, P.; Miccadei, S. Polyphenols: Immunomodulatory and therapeutic implication in colorectal cancer. *Front. Immunol.* **2019**, *10*, 729. [CrossRef] [PubMed]

17. Berni, R.; Cantini, C.; Guarnieri, M.; Nepi, M.; Hausman, J.F.; Guerriero, G.; Romi, M.; Cai, G. Nutraceutical characteristics of ancient *Malus* × *domestica* Borkh. fruits recovered across Siena in Tuscany. *Medicines* **2019**, *6*, 27. [CrossRef] [PubMed]

18. Zhou, J.-X.; Braun, M.S.; Wetterauer, P.; Wetterauer, B.; Wink, M. Antioxidant, cytotoxic, and antimicrobial activities of *Glycyrrhiza glabra* L., *Paeonia lactiflora* Pall., and *Eriobotrya japonica* (Thunb.) Lindl. extracts. *Medicines* **2019**, *6*, 43. [CrossRef] [PubMed]

19. Dong, H.; Lv, Y.; Zhao, D.; Barrow, P.; Zhou, X. Defensins: The case for their use against mycobacterial infections. *J. Immunol. Res.* **2016**, *2016*, 7515687. [CrossRef]

20. Shafee, T.M.; Lay, F.T.; Phan, T.K.; Anderson, M.A.; Hulett, M.D. Convergent evolution of defensin sequence, structure and function. *Cell. Mol. Life Sci.* **2017**, *74*, 663–682. [CrossRef]

21. Ishaq, N.; Bilal, M.; Iqbal, H.M.N. Medicinal potentialities of plant defensins: A review with applied perspectives. *Medicines* **2019**, *6*, 29. [CrossRef] [PubMed]

22. Richins, R.D.; Rodriguez-Uribe, L.; Lowe, K.; Ferral, R.; O'Connell, M.A. Accumulation of bioactive metabolites in cultivated medical *Cannabis*. *PLoS ONE* **2018**, *13*, e0201119. [CrossRef] [PubMed]

23. Cohen, K.; Weizman, A.; Weinstein, A. Positive and negative effects of *Cannabis* and cannabinoids on health. *Clin. Pharmacol. Ther.* **2019**, *105*, 1139–1147. [CrossRef] [PubMed]

24. Gonçalves, J.; Rosado, T.; Soares, S.; Simão, A.Y.; Caramelo, D.; Luís, Â.; Fernández, N.; Barroso, M.; Gallardo, E.; Duarte, A.P. *Cannabis* and its secondary metabolites: Their use as therapeutic drugs, toxicological aspects, and analytical determination. *Medicines* **2019**, *6*, 31. [CrossRef] [PubMed]

25. Adkins, J.E.; Boyer, E.W.; McCurdy, C.R. *Mitragyna speciosa*, a psychoactive tree from Southeast Asia with opioid activity. *Curr. Top. Med. Chem.* **2011**, *11*, 1165–1175. [CrossRef] [PubMed]

26. Meireles, V.; Rosado, T.; Barroso, M.; Soares, S.; Gonçalves, J.; Luís, Â.; Caramelo, D.; Simão, A.Y.; Fernández, N.; Duarte, A.P.; et al. *Mitragyna speciosa*: Clinical, toxicological aspects and analysis in biological and non-biological samples. *Medicines* **2019**, *6*, 35. [CrossRef] [PubMed]

27. Tavares, W.R.; Seca, A.M.L. The current status of the pharmaceutical potential of *Juniperus* L. metabolites. *Medicines* **2018**, *5*, 81. [CrossRef] [PubMed]

28. Pinto, D.C.G.A.; Rahmouni, N.; Beghidja, N.; Silva, M.A.S. *Scabiosa* genus: A rich source of bioactive metabolites. *Medicines* **2018**, *5*, 110. [CrossRef]

29. Mossa, A.-T.H. Green pesticides: Essential oils as biopesticides in insect-pest management. *J. Environ. Sci. Technol.* **2016**, *9*, 354–378. [CrossRef]

30. Echeverría, J.; Albuquerque, R.D.D.G. Nanoemulsions of essential oils: New tool for control of vector-Borne diseases and in vitro effects on some parasitic agents. *Medicines* **2019**, *6*, 42. [CrossRef] [PubMed]

31. Chen, R.; Wong, H.L.; Burns, B.P. New approaches to detect biosynthetic gene clusters in the environment. *Medicines* **2019**, *6*, 32. [CrossRef] [PubMed]

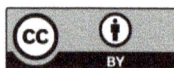

medicines

MDPI

Article

Antiproliferative Activity of (-)-Rabdosiin Isolated from *Ocimum sanctum* L.

Alexandros Flegkas [1], Tanja Milosević Ifantis [1], Christina Barda [1], Pinelopi Samara [2], Ourania Tsitsilonis [2] and Helen Skaltsa [1,*]

[1] Department of Pharmacognosy and Chemistry of Natural Products, Faculty of Pharmacy, National and Kapodistrian University of Athens, Panepistimiopolis, Zografou, 15771 Athens, Greece; alexflegas@yahoo.com (A.F.); kgtanja@yahoo.com (T.M.I.); cbarda@pharm.uoa.gr (C.B.)
[2] Department of Biology, National and Kapodistrian University of Athens, Panepistimiopolis Zografou, 15784 Athens, Greece; psamara@biol.uoa.gr (P.S.); rtsitsil@biol.uoa.gr (O.T.)
* Correspondence: skaltsa@pharm.uoa.gr

Received: 31 January 2019; Accepted: 7 March 2019; Published: 12 March 2019

Abstract: Background: *Ocimum sanctum* L. (holy basil; Tulsi in Hindi) is an important medicinal plant, traditionally used in India. **Methods:** The phytochemical study of the nonpolar (dichloromethane 100%) and polar (methanol:water; 7:3) extracts yielded fourteen compounds. Compounds **6**, **7**, **9**, **11**, **12**, and **13**, along with the methanol:water extract were evaluated for their cytotoxicity against the human cancer cell lines MCF-7, SKBR3, and HCT-116, and normal peripheral blood mononuclear cells (PBMCs). **Results:** Five terpenoids, namely, ursolic acid (**1**), oleanolic acid (**2**), betulinic acid (**3**), stigmasterol (**4**), and β-caryophyllene oxide (**5**); two lignans, i.e., (-)-rabdosiin (**6**) and shimobashiric acid C (**7**); three flavonoids, luteolin (**8**), its 7-*O*-β-D-glucuronide (**9**), apigenin 7-*O*-β-D-glucuronide (**10**); and four phenolics, (*E*)-p-coumaroyl 4-*O*-β-D-glucoside (**11**), 3-(3,4-dihydroxyphenyl) lactic acid (**12**), protocatechuic acid (**13**), and vanillic acid (**14**) were isolated. Compound **6** was the most cytotoxic against the human cancer lines assessed and showed very low cytotoxicity against PBMCs. **Conclusions:** Based on these results, the structure of compound **6** shows some promise as a selective anticancer drug scaffold.

Keywords: *Ocimum sanctum*; Lamiaceae; (-)-rabdosiin; cytotoxic activity; triterpenoids; phenolic derivatives

1. Introduction

Indigenous to India and parts of North and Eastern Africa, China, Hainan Island, and Taiwan, Tulsi (*Ocimum sanctum* L.; syn. *Ocimum tenuiflorum* L.) is referred to as "the elixir of life" or "the queen of herbs" and is believed to promote longevity [1,2]. Various parts of the plant are used in Ayurveda and Siddha traditional medicine to treat coughs, bronchitis, fever, bile disturbances, and has been also used as an anthelminthic, antiemetic, anticancer, antiseptic, antioxidant, antidiabetic anti-inflammatory, antiulcer, hepatoprotective, cardioprotective, anticoagulant, anticataract, and analgesic agent. Additionally, it has been reported that extracts of the plant can serve as vitalizers and rejuvenators, and are thought to increase life-expectancy and promote disease-free living [3–17].

Despite its wide therapeutic range, special care should be taken in case of the use of Tulsi in conjunction with other prescribed medicines since it exhibits various drug interactions. For example, its concomitant use with anticoagulants, such as heparin, warfarin, aspirin, clopidogrel, etc., is contraindicated due to allergic reactions that may occur. In addition, Tulsi increases the activity of phenobarbital and consequently may stimulate uterine contractions; thus, its use during pregnancy and lactation is not recommended [18,19].

The genus *Ocimum* L. is abundant in methylated flavones of the apigenin and luteolin types: cirsimartin, cirsilineol, isothymusin, and isothymonin. Terpenes such as triterpenic acids, ursolic, oleanolic acids, the oxygenated monoterpene carvacrol, the sesquiterpene hydrocarbon caryophyllene, the phenylpropenes eugenol and its methyl ether, as well as caffeic and rosmarinic acid are also present in significant amounts s. According to literature data, *O. sanctum* contains flavonoids, phenolics, neolignans, tannins, triterpenoids, sterols, cerebrosides, alkaloids, and saponin; most of them are well known for their in vitro and in vivo biological activities, such as antioxidant or prooxidant, cytotoxic, antitumor, anticarcinogenic, hepatoprotective, anti-inflammatory, as well as antiviral [3–6,19–23]. Moreover, the essential oil of *O. sanctum* contains high amount of eugenol (70%), also known for its antioxidant, anti-inflammatory, antimicrobial, and cytotoxic activities [24,25].

Based on the above, the plant is of high pharmacological importance, although it is still not fully chemically investigated. In this study, we analyzed both nonpolar and polar extracts of *O. sanctum* and studied the cytotoxic activity of its secondary metabolites.

2. Materials and Methods

2.1. Plant Material

Aerial parts of *O. sanctum* L. were collected in flowering stage at Suriname, as previously described [21]. A voucher specimen (ATHS 093) has been deposited in the Herbarium of the Laboratory of Pharmacognosy, National and Kapodistrian University of Athens.

2.2. General Experimental Procedures

^{1}H, ^{13}C, and 2D NMR spectra were recorded in CDCl$_3$ and CD$_3$OD on Bruker DRX 400 and Bruker AC 200 (50.3 MHz for ^{13}C NMR) instruments at 295 K. Chemical shifts are given in ppm (δ) and were referenced to the solvent signals at 7.24/3.31 and 77.0/49.0 ppm for ^{1}H-/^{13}C-NMR, respectively. COSY, HSQC, HMBC, HSQC-TOCSY (Heteronuclear Single Quantum Coherence-Total Correlation Spectroscopy), NOESY, and ROESY (Rotating-frame nuclear Overhauser Effect correlation SpectroscopY; mixing time 950 ms) were performed using standard Bruker microprograms. The solvents used were of spectroscopic grade (Merck). The $[\alpha]_D^{20}$ values were obtained in CHCl$_3$ or MeOH on a Perkin-Elmer 341 Polarimeter. FT-IR spectra were recorded on a Perkin Elmer PARAGON 500 spectrophotometer. UV spectra were recorded on a Shimadzu UV-160 A spectrophotometer according to Mabry et al. (1970) [26]. GC–MS analyses were performed on a Hewlett-Packard 5973–6890 system operating in EI mode (70 eV) equipped with a split/splitless injector (220 °C), a split ratio 1/10, using a fused silica HP-5 MS capillary column (30 m x 0.25 mm (i.d.), film thickness: 0.25 μm) with a temperature program for HP-5 MS column from 60 °C (5 min) to 280 °C at a rate of 4 °C/min and helium as a carrier gas at a flow rate of 1.0 mL/min. Vacuum liquid chromatography (VLC): silica gel 60H (Merck, Art. 7736) [27]. Column chromatography (CC): silica gel (Merck, Darmstadt, Germany, Art. 9385), gradient elution with the solvent mixtures indicated in each case. Preparative thin layer chromatography (pTLC) was performed on silica gel (Merck, Art. 5721) and cellulose (Merck, Art. 5716). MPLC (Medium Pressure Liquid Chromatography) support: reversed-phase column (Merck, 10167): 36 × 3.6 cm (Büchi Borosilikat 3.3, Code 19674), 24 × 1.5 cm (Büchi Borosilikat 3.3, Code 2813) on a system (Büchi Pump C-615). HPLC (High Performance Liquid Chromatography) support: preparative HPLC was performed using (a) Kromasil 100 si Semi-prep 25 cm × 10 mm and (b) Kromasil C$_{18}$ 25 cm × 10 mm columns on a HPLC system (Jasco PU-2080) equipped with a RI detector (Shimadzu 10 A). Fractionation was always monitored by TLC silica gel 60 F-254, (Merck, Art. 5554) with visualization under UV (254 and 365 nm) and spraying with vanillin–sulfuric acid reagent (vanillin Merck, Art. No. S26047 841) and with Neu's reagent for phenolics [28].

2.3. Extraction and Isolation

The initial extraction was previously described [21]. In brief, the aerial parts of *O. sanctum* L. (0.40 kg) were air-dried and finely ground, and then extracted at room temperature using dichloromethane and methanol, successively.

Part of the dichloromethane residue (11.9 g) was re-extracted at room temperature with ethyl acetate (EtOAc) and *n*-BuOH, yielding two fractions (A and B). Fraction A (7.8 g) was fractionated by VLC on silica gel using mixtures of cyclohexane and EtOAc of increasing polarity (100:0; 90:10; 80:20; 70:30; 60:40; 50:50; 40:60; 30:70) and yielded 8 subfractions (A_1–A_8). Subfractions A_3 (eluted with cyclohexane:EtOAc 80:20) and A_4 (eluted with cyclohexane:EtOAc 70:30) were combined to group AA (401.7 mg), subjected to CC over silica gel using mixtures of cyclohexane and EtOAc and yielded 81 fractions combined to 11 groups (AA_1–AA_{11}). Purification on preparative TLC of fraction AA_3 (51.8 mg; eluted with cyclohexane:EtOAc 95:5) yielded compound **5** (1.3 mg). Fractions AA_6 (34.7 mg; eluted with cyclohexane:EtOAc 97:3) and AA_8 (34.4 mg; eluted with cyclohexane:EtOAc 85:15) were further fractionated by normal-phase HPLC (isocratic elution cyclohexane:EtOAc 75:25) and yielded compounds **4** (t_R 21.84 min; 3.2 mg), **2** (t_R 16.01 min; 1.7 mg), and **3** (t_R 14.84 min; 5.5 mg). Fraction B purified by CC on silica gel using mixtures of cyclohexane and EtOAc yielded 131 fractions combined to 18 groups (B_1–B_{18}). Fraction B_5 (eluted with cyclohexane:EtOAc 80:20) was identified as compound **1** (1.8 mg), while fraction B_8 (eluted with cyclohexane:EtOAc 70:30) as compound **14** (2.3 mg).

Part of the methanol residue (3.6 g) was subjected to RP_{18}-MPLC using a H_2O:MeOH gradient system (100:0; 90:10; 85:15; 80:20; 75:25; 50:50; 0:100; 0:100; 50 min each) and yielded 8 fractions (M_1–M_8). Group M_2 (eluted with H_2O:MeOH 90:10) was applied to CC on silica gel with mixtures of dichloromethane:methanol:water of increasing polarity to give 151 fractions (combined to 14 groups; M_{2-1}–M_{2-14}) and afforded compounds **13** (M_{2-5} eluted with DM:MeOH: H_2O 95:5:0.3; 40.5 mg), **11** (M_{2-11} eluted with DM:MeOH:H_2O 70:30:3; 1.6 mg), and **12** (M_{2-12}; 4.3 mg; eluted with DM:MeOH:H_2O 40:60:6). M_3 (290.0 mg) was further purified on Sephadex LH-20 eluted with MeOH (100%) and yielded 30 fractions combined in 10 subfractions (M_{3-1}–M_{3-10}). M_{3-6} (57.0 mg) was subjected to reversed-phase HPLC (isocratic elution; methanol:AcOH 5% 7:3) to give compounds **6** (t_R 23.90 min; 7.5 mg), **9** (t_R 29.30 min; 1.9 mg), and **7** (t_R 35.20 min; 3.7 mg). M_6 (674.2 mg) was similarly fractionated by CC over silica gel with mixtures of CH_2Cl_2:MeOH:H_2O of increasing polarity and yielded 135 fractions combined in 25 subgroups (M_{6-1}–M_{6-25}). Subgroup M_{6-24} (eluted with CH_2Cl_2:MeOH:H_2O 70:30:3; 69.4 mg) was subjected to CC on silica gel as previously described to give 75 fractions; fraction 8 (1.3 mg) was identified as compound **10**. Another part of the methanol extract (7.7 g) was redissolved in water and extracted at room temperature with EtOAc and *n*-BuOH, affording three fractions (MA-MC). MB (eluted with *n*-BuOH; 5.3 g) was subjected to RP_{18}-MPLC using a H_2O:MeOH gradient system (100% H_2O→100% MeOH; steps of 10% MeOH) and yielded 11 fractions (MB_1-MB_{10}). Fraction MB_3 (eluted with H_2O:MeOH 80:20) was identified as compound **8** (13.6 mg).

It is notable that during the fractionation and isolation procedures, all extracts and subfractions were continuously monitored by analytical TLC and ^{1}H-NMR. All obtained fractions were concentrated to dryness under vacuum (30 °C) and placed in activated desiccators with P_2O_5 until their weights were stabilized.

2.4. Cytotoxic Effects against Cancer Cell Lines

The cytotoxic activity of the compounds, as well as of the initial methanol extract, were tested against three human cancer cell lines: MCF-7 (breast; estrogen receptor positive (ER+), progesterone receptor (PR)+, and HER2 negative (-)), SKBR3 (breast; ER-, PR-, and HER2+), and HCT-116 (colon). All cell lines were maintained in RPMI-1640, supplemented with 10% heat-inactivated fetal bovine serum (FBS), 10 mM Hepes, 10 U/mL penicillin, 10 U/mL streptomycin, and 5 mg/mL gentamycin (all from Lonza, Cologne, Germany) (thereafter referred to as complete medium) at 37 °C in a humidified 5% CO_2 incubator.

Compounds were prepared at a stock solution of 10.0 mg/mL in DMSO and the extract at 20.0 mg/mL in DMSO. Prior to their use, they were diluted in plain RPMI-1640. Cytotoxicity was evaluated by the MTT reduction assay [29], which determines the effect of treatment with an exogenously added agent on the viability of the cell population. Briefly, cells were plated in 96-well plates (Greiner Bio-One GmbH, Frickenhausen, Germany; 5×10^3 cells/well) and incubated at 5% CO_2 and 95% air at 37 °C for 24 h, in order to adhere. Further, cells were incubated with the compounds for 72 h at 37 °C in a 5% CO_2 incubator. The MTT reagent (Sigma-Aldrich, Darmstadt, Germany; 1 mg/mL in phosphate buffered saline (PBS); 100 µL/well) was added during the last 4 h of incubation. The formazan crystals formed were dissolved by adding 0.1 M HCl in 2-propanol (100 µL/well) and absorption was measured using an ELISA reader (Denley WeScan, Finland) at 545 nm with reference filter set at 690 nm. All cultures were set in triplicate, whereas cells incubated in complete medium or in medium containing the equivalent amount of DMSO, as well as cells incubated in the presence of doxorubicin (Sigma-Aldrich) were used as negative and positive controls, respectively. The half maximal inhibitory concentration (IC_{50}) was calculated according to the formula: $100(A_0 - A)/A_0 = 50$, where A and A_0 are optical densities of wells exposed to the compounds and control wells, respectively.

The compounds were tested at a concentration range of 200.0 to 6.25 µg/mL and the extract at 750.0 to 1.25 µg/mL. Doxorubicin was used as a standard cytotoxic agent and showed IC_{50} values $\leq$ 0.2 µM in all cell lines tested. All experiments were performed at least three times.

2.5. Flow Cytometry Analysis

MCF-7, SKBR3 and HCT-116 cells were incubated with compound **6** and analyzed with flow cytometry following staining with annexin V and propidium iodide (PI). Cells were plated into 24-well plates (Greiner Bio-One; 3×10^5/mL; 2 mL/well), let adhere overnight, and incubated with the mean IC_{50} value (80 µg/mL) and 40 µg/mL of compound **6** for 72 h. Cells were detached with 2 mM EDTA in Dulbecco's PBS (DPBS), harvested, centrifuged in cold PBS (1500 rpm; 5 min), and stained with the Annexin V-FITC Apoptosis Detection Kit (BioLegend, Fell, Germany; cat# 640914), according to the manufacturers' instructions. In brief, cells were resuspended in binding buffer, then annexin V-FITC (5 µL) and PI (10 µL; 0.03 µg/sample) were added, mixed, and incubated with the cells for 15 min in the dark at room temperature. The volume was adjusted to 500 µL with binding buffer and the cell suspension was immediately analyzed in a FACSCanto II (BD Biosciences, San Diego, CA, USA) using FACSDiva software (V7, BD Biosciences).

2.6. Cytotoxic Effect against Human Peripheral Blood Mononuclear Cells

Compound **6** was additionally assessed for its cytotoxicity against human peripheral blood mononuclear cells (PBMCs) isolated from healthy blood donors' peripheral blood as previously described [30]. Prior to blood draw, individuals gave their informed consent according to the regulations approved by the 2nd Peripheral Blood Transfusion Unit and Hemophiliac Centre, "Laikon" General Hospital Institutional Review Board, Athens, Greece. PBMCs were seeded in 24-well plates (5×10^5/mL; 2 mL/well) and exposed to 2 concentrations of compound **6**: 80 µg/mL and 40 µg/mL. PBMCs were collected, stained as described in 2.5 and analyzed by flow cytometry.

3. Results and Discussion

3.1. Secondary Metabolites Isolated from O. sanctum

The phytochemical study of both nonpolar and polar extracts from *O. sanctum* aerial parts led to the isolation of 14 compounds identified on the basis of their spectra. More specifically, five terpenoids, i.e., ursolic acid (**1**) [31], oleanolic acid (**2**) [32], betulinic acid (**3**) [32,33], stigmasterol (**4**) [33], and β-caryophyllene oxide (**5**) [34]; two lignans, (-)-rabdosiin (**6**) [35,36] and shimobashiric acid C (**7**) [37]; three flavonoids, luteolin (**8**) [38], its 7-*O*-β-D-glucuronide (**9**) [39–41], and apigenin 7-*O*-β-D-glucuronide (**10**) [42,43]; and phenolic compounds, (E)-*p*-coumaroyl 4-*O*-β-D-glucoside

(11) [44], 3-(3,4-dihydroxyphenyl) lactic acid (12) [45], protocatechuic acid (13) [46], and vanillic acid (14) [46] were isolated. This is the first time that compounds 6, 7, 11, and 12 were isolated from this plant.

According to the literature, the taxonomic description of the genus *Ocimum* L. is still debatable. It is composed of three subgenera, namely subgenus Ocimum (comprising three sections: Ocimum, Gratissima and Hiantia), subgenus Nautochilus, and subgenus Gymnocimum. The species (*O. sanctum* L.) under investigation has been located in the subgenus Gymnocimum. This subgenus can be distinguished because of the existence of flavonoid glucuronides, which are found in plants of the subgenera Nautochilus and Ocimum [38]. Consequently, our work is in agreement with previous studies regarding the chemical profile of the subgenus Gymnocimum. Moreover, it was previously shown that 3-(3,4-dihydroxyphenyl) lactic acid is a precursor of the nonenzymatic synthesis of (*S*)-(-)-rosmarinic acid and (+)-rabdosiin [47], therefore its identification (compound 12) could be related to the biosynthesis of (-)-rabdosiin (6) [48].

Compound (-)-rabdosiin (6) (Figure 1) is a caffeic acid tetramer connected to a lignan skeleton. Originally, it has been isolated and identified from the stem of *Rabdosia japonica*, Labiatae [35], while both enantiomers (-)-rabdosiin and (+)-rabdosiin were later isolated from *Macrotomia euchroma*, Boraginaceae [49] and also from other plants of this family such as *Lithospermum erythrorhizon* [50] and *Eritrichium sericeum* [36]. Based on the fact that the entire fractionation and isolation procedures were continuously monitored by ^{1}H-NMR, the active compound 6 was not detected in other fractions (NMR data of 6 are provided as Supplementary Materials, Tables S1 and S2, Figures S1–S6). Consequently, being a minor compound of the plant, its activity could derive in synergy with other constituents.

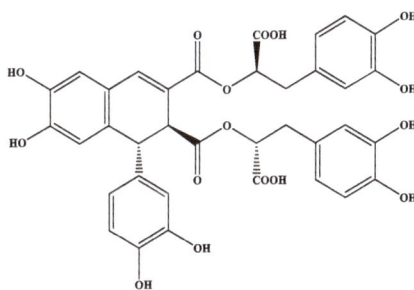

Figure 1. Chemical structures of (-)-rabdosiin (6) isolated from *O. sanctum*.

According to published data, rabdosiin and the similar caffeic acid derivatives have been suggested as potential anti-HIV and antiallergic agents. Moreover, studies showed that rabdosiin is an antioxidant factor (acting as an effective scavenger of reactive oxygen species), as well as a possible inhibitor of hyaluronidase and β-hexosaminidase release [51,52]. Nevertheless, to the best of our knowledge, the antiproliferative activity of rabdosiin is reported for the first time.

3.2. Antiproliferative Activityod of Secondary Metabolites of O. sanctum

Using the MTT dye reduction assay, the methanol:water extract (7:3) and 6 purified secondary metabolites (compounds 6, 7, 9, 11, 12, and 13) were screened for their cytotoxic/cytostatic activity against human breast and colon cell lines. Our results showed that the extract was cytotoxic against all cell lines, with an IC$_{50}$ range of 45 ± 2.12 to 57 ± 14.14 μg/mL (Table 1). Based on these data, we further proceeded to the screening of the isolated natural products 6, 7, 9, 11, 12, and 13 against MCF-7 cells which was the mostly affected cell line exposed to the methanol extract of *O. sanctum* L. The IC$_{50}$ values calculated are presented in Table 1. Among the purified compounds, the most prominent was 6, which was further tested against SKBR3 and HCT-116 cells. Overall, compound 6 demonstrated a considerable cytotoxic activity, with IC_{50} values 75 ± 2.12, 83 ± 3.54 and 84 ± 7.78 µg/mL against MCF-7, SKBR3, and HCT-116, respectively.

Table 1. In vitro cytotoxicity of the methanol extract and isolated compounds from Tulsi on human cancer cell lines.

	$IC_{50} \pm SD$ (in µg/mL) [a]							$IC_{50} \pm SD$ (in µM)
Compounds	6	7	9	11	12	13	Extract *	Doxorubicin
MCF-7	75 ± 2.12 [a]	142 ± 3.54	141 ± 1.41	139 ± 7.78	140 ± 12.02	140 ± 4.95	45 ± 2.12	0.092 ± 0.007
SKBR3	83 ± 3.54	NT	NT	NT	NT	NT	46 ± 5.66	0.095 ± 0.008
HCT-116	84 ± 7.78	NT	NT	NT	NT	NT	57 ± 14.14	0.192 ± 0.029

* Methanol:water 70:30 [a] IC_{50} values were determined after 72 h of exposure to each compound and represent means $\pm$ standard deviation (SD) of three independent experiments performed; Doxorubicin was used as positive control and showed $IC_{50} \leq 0.20$ µM for all cell lines assayed.

To analyze the type of cell death (apoptosis or necrosis) induced by compound **6** on MCF-7, SKBR3, and HCT-116 cells, cells were stained with annexin V which binds phosphatidylserine exposed on the surface of apoptotic cells and PI which intracellulary stains the DNA of necrotic cells. As shown in Figure 2, 80 µg/mL of compound **6** drove ca. 50% of all cells to apoptosis. Specifically, 44.9% of MCF-7 were annexin V+ and 12.3% annexin V+/PI+, suggesting that cells exposed to compound **6** underwent early apoptosis and a small percentage thereof late apoptosis/necrosis. Analogous percentages were obtained for SKBR3 (40.1% early apoptotic; 9.1% late apoptotic/necrotic) and HCT-116 (43.1% early apoptotic; 10.2% late apoptotic/necrotic) cells. When the same cell lines were exposed to 40 µg/mL of compound **6**, the percentages of early apoptotic and late apoptotic/necrotic cells were reduced ca. by 50% (13.5–20.1% and 3.9–6.5%, respectively), suggesting that induction of apoptosis by compound **6** is concentration-dependent.

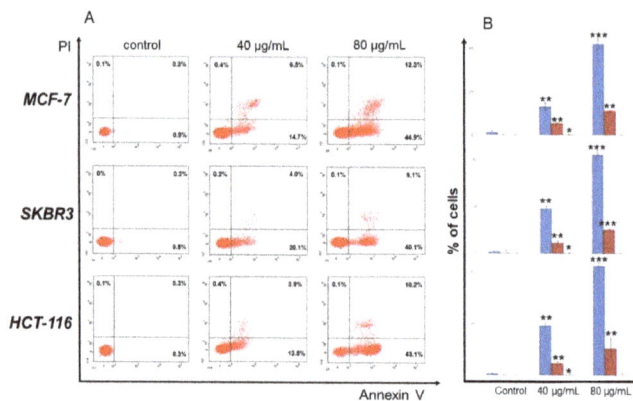

Figure 2. Compound **6** induced apoptosis to human cancer cells. MCF-7, SKBR3, and HCT-116 cells were exposed to 40 and 80 µg/mL of compound **6** for 72 h, stained with annexin V and PI, and analyzed by flow cytometry. Control cells were incubated in complete medium supplemented with 0.5% DMSO. Flow cytometry analysis was performed using FACS Diva software. (**A**). Representative dot plots from cells treated with compound **6**. Percentages of early apoptotic (lower right), late apoptotic/necrotic (upper right), and necrotic (upper left) are shown in each quadrat. (**B**). Histograms of apoptotic and necrotic cells after exposure to compound **6**. Blue columns show percentages of early apoptotic, red columns of late apoptotic and green columns of necrotic cells. Mean values $\pm$ SD from 3 experiments are shown. *, $p < 0.05$; **, $p < 0.01$; ***, $p < 0.001$, in all cases compared to control after Student's unpaired *t*-tests.

Based on the significant cytotoxic activity of compound **6** against cancer cell lines we further tested whether it may also be toxic against normal cells, i.e., PBMCs isolated from two different healthy blood donors. PBMCs were incubated for 24 h with the IC_{50} and the 1/2 concentration of **6**, stained and analyzed by flow cytometry. Interestingly, the IC_{50} of compound **6** (80 μg/mL) induced early and late apoptosis/necrosis in a small percentage of PBMCs (2.8% and 3.0% for donor 1; 4.3% and 3.1% for donor 2, respectively). At half concentration, the percentages were highly reduced and much less early apoptotic and late apoptotic/necrotic cells were detected (1.8% and 1.7% for donor 1; 2.1% and 1.9% for donor 2, respectively) (Figure 3).

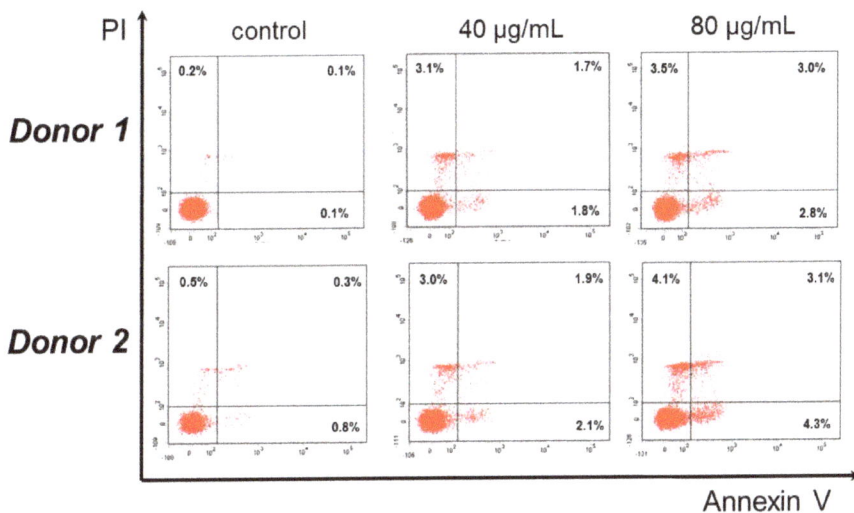

Figure 3. Compound **6** does not induce apoptosis or necrosis to peripheral blood mononuclear cells (PBMCs). PBMCs were isolated from 2 different donors (1 and 2) and incubated with 40 and 80 μg/mL of compound **6** for 24 h. Other details as in Legend of Figure 2. Representative dot plots from both donors are shown from one experiment performed in duplicate.

The good antitumor activity of compound **6** against human cancer cells and the simultaneous marginal cytotoxicity of the same compound when tested against normal human cells (PBMCs), suggest that (-)-rabdosiin may display less toxic side effects when administered in vivo. In support of our results, the few studies carried out in the last decade on the potential anticancer activity of *O. sanctum* extracts and its essential oil with different human cancer cell lines, clearly suggest that Tulsi may be used as a supplement to enhance anticancer chemotherapy without causing severe damage to normal epithelial cells [25,53,54]. Botanical drugs are currently approved in therapy with specific indications and in the last decades, research has focused on the anticancer effect of plant extracts.

Taken altogether, (-)-rabdosiin displays an interesting proapoptotic activity against cancer cell lines and in parallel shows a noticeable selectivity to malignant cells. It is noteworthy that the cytotoxic response of the extract is better compared to the other isolated compounds, including compound **6**. As (-)-rabdosiin is a minor compound of the plant, we assume that it contributes to the improved antiproliferative activity of the methanol extract, and that it is probably synergistically with other active metabolites. The good activity of the polar extract, as well as of compound **6** against a series of human cancer cell lines and its marginal cytotoxicity against PBMCs, give evidence toward the effective use of this plant for the prevention of human cancer. Moreover, the core structure of (-)-rabdosiin could be considered as drug lead in anticancer drug design.

Supplementary Materials: The following are available online at http://www.mdpi.com/2305-6320/6/1/37/s1, Table S1: ^{1}H-NMR of **6** (CD$_3$OD, 400 MHz); Table S2: ^{13}C-NMR of **6** (CD$_3$OD, 400 MHz); Figure S1: ^{1}H-NMR spectrum of **6** (CD$_3$OD, 400 Hz); Figure S2: COSY spectrum of **6** (CD$_3$OD, 400 Hz); Figure S3: ^{13}C NMR spectrum of **6** (CD$_3$OD, 400 Hz); Figure S4: HSQC spectrum of **6** (CD$_3$OD, 400 Hz); Figure S5: HMBC spectrum of **6** (CD$_3$OD, 400 Hz); Figure S6: Most important HMBC signals of compound **6**.

Author Contributions: Investigation, A.F., T.M.I., and P.S.; Supervision, O.T. and H.S.; Writing—Original Draft, C.B.

Funding: This research received no external funding.

Conflicts of Interest: The authors declare no conflicts of interest.

References

1. Prajapati, N.D.; Purohit, S.S.; Sharma, A.K.; Kumar, T.A. *Hand Book of Medicinal Plant*, 1st ed.; Agrobios: Jodhpur, India, 2003; p. 367.
2. Cohen, M.M. Tulsi-*Ocimum sanctum*: A herb for all reasons. *J. Ayurveda Integr. Med.* **2014**, *5*, 251–259. [CrossRef] [PubMed]
3. Pandey, B. Anita. In *Economic Botany*; Chand and Company Ltd.: New Delhi, India, 1990; p. 294.
4. Rajeshwari, S. *Ocimum sanctum*: The Indian home remedy. In *Current Medical Scene*; Cipla Ltd.: Bombay, India, 1992.
5. Gupta, S.K.; Prakash, J.; Srivastava, S. Validation of traditional claim of Tulsi, *Ocimum sanctum* Linn. as a medicinal plant. *Indian J. Exp. Biol.* **2002**, *40*, 765–773.
6. Das, S.K.; Vasudevan, D.M. Tulsi: The Indian holy power plant. *Nat. Prod. Radiance* **2006**, *5*, 279–283.
7. Mondal, S.; Mirdha, B.R.; Mahapatra, S.C. The Science behind sacredness of Tulsi (*Ocimum sanctum* L.). *Indian J. Physiol. Pharmacol.* **2009**, *53*, 291–306. [PubMed]
8. Pandey, G.; Madhuri, S. Pharmacological activities of *Ocimum sanctum* (Tulsi): A review. *JPSR* **2010**, *5*, 61–66.
9. Mohan, L.; Amberkar, M.V.; Kumari, M. *Ocimum sanctum* linn (TULSI)—An overview. *JPSR* **2011**, *7*, 51–53.
10. Pattanayak, P.; Pritishova, B.; Debajyoti, D.; Panda, S.K. *Ocimum sanctum* Linn. A reservoir plant for therapeutic applications: An overview. *Pharmacogn. Rev.* **2010**, *4*, 95–105. [CrossRef] [PubMed]
11. Khanna, N.; Bhatia, J. Antinociceptive action of *Ocimum sanctum* (Tulsi) in mice: Possible mechanisms involved. *J. Ethnopharmacol.* **2003**, *88*, 293–296. [CrossRef]
12. Babu, K.; Uma Maheswari, K.C. In vivo studies on the effect of *Ocimum sanctum* L. leaf extract in mordifying the genotoxicity induced by chromium and mercury in *Allium* root meristems. *J. Environ. Biol.* **2006**, *27*, 93–95.
13. Narendhirakannan, R.T.; Subramanian, S.; Kandaswamy, M. Biochemical evaluation of antidiabetogenic properties of some commonly used Indian plants on streptozotocin-induced diabetes in experimental rats. *Clin. Exp. Pharmacol. Physiol.* **2006**, *33*, 1150–1157. [CrossRef]
14. Hannan, J.M.; Marenah, L.; Ali, L.; Rokeya, B.; Flatt, P.R.; Abdel-Wahab, Y.H. *Ocimum sanctum* leaf extracts stimulate insulin secretion from perfusd pancreas, isolated islets and clonal pancreatic beta-cells. *J. Endocrinol.* **2006**, *189*, 127–136. [CrossRef] [PubMed]
15. Grovel, J.K.; Vats, V.; Yadav, S.S. Pterocarpus marsupium extract (Vijayasar) prevented the alteration in metabolic patterns induced in the normal rat by feeding an adequate diet containing fructose as sole carbohydrate. *Diabetes Obes. Metab.* **2005**, *7*, 414–420. [CrossRef] [PubMed]
16. Suzuki, A.; Shirota, O.; Mori, K.; Sekita, S.; Fuchino, H.; Takano, A.; Kuroyanagi, M. Leishmanicidal active constituents from Nepalese medicinal plant Tulsi (*Ocimum sanctum* L.). *Chem. Pharm. Bull.* **2009**, *57*, 245–251. [CrossRef] [PubMed]
17. Jamshidi, J.; Cohen, M.M. The Clinical Efficacy and Safety of Tulsi in Humans: A Systematic Review of the Literature. *Evid. Based Complement. Altern. Med.* **2017**. [CrossRef] [PubMed]
18. Available online: http://www.himalayawellness.com/herbfinder/ocimum-tenuiflorum.htm (accessed on 31 January 2019).
19. Skaltsa, H.; Tzakou, O.; Singh, M. Polyphenols of *Ocimum sanctum* L. from Suriname. *Pharm. Biol.* **1999**, *37*, 92–94. [CrossRef]
20. Skaltsa, H.; Couladi, M.; Philianos, S.; Singh, M. Phytochemical Study of the leaves of *Ocimum sanctum* L. *Fitoterapia* **1987**, *4*, 286.

21. Skaltsa, H.; Tzakou, O.; Loukis, A.; Argyriadou, N. Analyse de l'huile essentielle d'*Ocimum sanctum* L. *Plant. Méd. Phytoth.* **1990**, *2*, 79–81.

22. Kumar, S.; Pandey, A.K. Chemistry and Biological Activities of Flavonoids: An Overview. *Sci. World J.* **2013**. [CrossRef]

23. Desai, S.; Desai, D.G.; Kaur, H. Saponins and their biological activities. *Pharma Times* **2009**, *41*, 13–16.

24. Bezerra, D.P.; Militão, G.C.G.; Castro de Morais, M.; Pergentino de Sousa, D. The Dual Antioxidant/Prooxidant Effect of Eugenol and Its Action in Cancer Development and Treatment. *Nutrients* **2017**, *9*, 1367. [CrossRef]

25. Manaharan, T.; Thirugnanasampandan, R.; Jayakumar, R.; Kanthimathi, M.S.; Ramya, G.; Gogul Ramnath, M. Purified essential oil from *Ocimum sanctum* Linn. triggers the apoptotic mechanism in human breast cancer cells. *Pharmacogn. Mag.* **2016**, *12*, S327–S331.

26. Mabry, T.G.; Markham, K.R.; Thomas, M.B. *The Systematic Identification of Flavonoids*; Springer Science & Business Media: Berlin/Heidelberg, Germany; New York, NY, USA, 1970.

27. Coll, J.C.; Bowden, B.F. The application of Vacuum Liquid Chromatography to the separation of terpene mixtures. *J. Nat. Prod.* **1986**, *49*, 934–936. [CrossRef]

28. Neu, R. Chelate von Diarylborsäuren mit aliphatischen oxyalkylaminen als reagenzien für den nachweis von oxyphenyl-benzo-γ-pyronen. *Die Naturwissenschaften* **1957**, *44*, 181. [CrossRef]

29. Mosman, T. Rapid colorimetric assay for cellular growth and survival: Application to proliferation and cytotoxicity assays. *J. Immunol. Methods* **1983**, *65*, 55–63. [CrossRef]

30. Ioannou, K.; Derhovanessian, E.; Tsakiri, E.; Samara, P.; Kalbacher, H.; Voelter, W.; Trougakos, I.P.; Pawelec, G.; Tsitsilonis, O.E. Prothymosin α and a prothymosin α-derived peptide enhance TH1-type immune responses against defined HER-2/neu epitopes. *BMC Immunol.* **2013**, *14*, 43–55. [CrossRef]

31. Liu, J. Pharmacology of oleanolic acid and ursolic acid. *J. Ethnopharmacol.* **1995**, *49*, 57–58.

32. Moghaddam, G.M.; Ahmad, F.; Samzadeh-Kermani, A. Biological Activity of Betulinic Acid: A Review. *Pharmacol. Pharm.* **2012**, *3*, 119–123. [CrossRef]

33. Batta, A.K.; Xu, G.; Honda, A.; Miyazaki, T.; Salen, G. Stigmasterol reduces plasma cholesterol levels and inhibits hepatic synthesis and intestinal absorption in the rat. *Metabolism* **2006**, *55*, 292–299. [CrossRef] [PubMed]

34. Ghelardini, C.; Galeotti, N.; Di Cesare, L.; Mazzanti, G.; Bartolini, A. Local anaesthetic activity of β-caryophyllene. *Farmaco* **2001**, *56*, 5–7. [CrossRef]

35. Agata, I.; Hatanp, T.; Okudaq, T.A. Tetrameric derivative of caffeic acid from *Rabdosia japonica*. *Phytochemistry* **1989**, *28*, 2447–2450. [CrossRef]

36. Inyushkina, V.Y.; Bulgakov, P.V.; Veselova, V.M.; Bryukhanov, M.V.; Zverev, F.Y.; Lampatov, V.V.; Azarova, V.O.; Tchernoded, K.G.; Fedoreyev, A.S.; Zhuravlev, N.Y. High Rabdosiin and Rosmarinic acid production in *Eritrichium sericeum* callus cultures and the effect of the calli on *Masugi-Nephritis* in rats. *Biosci. Biotechnol. Biochem.* **2007**, *71*, 1286–1293. [CrossRef]

37. Murata, T.; Miyase, T.; Yoshizaki, F. Hyalurodinase inhibitors from *Keiskea japonica*. *Chem. Pharm. Bull.* **2008**, *60*, 121–128. [CrossRef]

38. López-Lázaro, M. Distribution and biological activities of the flavonoid luteolin. *Mini Rev. Med. Chem.* **2009**, *9*, 31–59. [CrossRef] [PubMed]

39. Grayer, R.J.; Kite, G.C.; Veitch, N.C.; Eckert, M.; Marin, P.D.; Senanayake, P.; Paton, A.J. Leaf flavonoid glycosides as chemosystematic characters in *Ocimum*. *Biochem. Syst. Ecol.* **2002**, *30*, 327–342. [CrossRef]

40. Markham, R.K.; Porter, J.L.; Mues, R.; Zinsmeister, D.H.; Brehmm, G.B. Flavonoid variation in the liverwort *Conocephalum conicum*: Evidence for geographic races. *Phytochemistry* **1976**, *15*, 147–150. [CrossRef]

41. Lu, Y.; Foo, L.Y. Flavonoid and phenolic glycosides from *Salvia officinalis*. *Phytochemistry* **2000**, *55*, 263–267. [CrossRef]

42. Agrawal, P.K.; Bansal, M.C. Flavonoid glycosides. In *Carbon-13 NMR of Flavonoids*; Agrawal, P.K., Ed.; Elsevier: Amsterdam, The Netherlands, 1989; pp. 283–364.

43. Markham, K.R.; Geiger, H. [^1]H NMR spectroscopy of flavonoids and their glycosides in DMSO-d6. In *The Flavonoids, Advances in Research Since 1986*; Harborne, J.B., Ed.; Chapman and Hall: London, UK, 1994; pp. 441–497.

44. Foo, L.Y.; Molan, A.L.; Woodfield, D.R.; McNabb, W.C. The phenols and prodelphinidins of white cover flowers. *Phytochemistry* **2000**, *54*, 539–548. [CrossRef]

45. Yahara, S.; Satoshiro, M.; Nishioka, I.; Nagasawa, T.; Oura, H. Isolation and Characterization of Phenolic Compounds from *Coptidis Rhizoma*. *Chem. Pharm. Bull.* **1985**, *33*, 527. [CrossRef]
46. Norr, H.; Wagner, H. New constituents from *Ocimum sanctum*. *Planta Med.* **1992**, *58*, 574. [CrossRef]
47. Bogucki, D.; Charlton, J. A non-enzymatic synthesis of (S)-(-)-rosmarinic acid and a study of a biomimetic route to (+)-rabdosiin. *Can. J. Chem.* **1997**, *75*, 1783–1794. [CrossRef]
48. Agata, I.; Hatano, T.; Nishibe, S.; Okuda, T. Rabdosiin, a new rosmarinic acid dimer with a lignan skeleton, from *Rabdosia japonica*. *Chem. Pharm. Bull.* **1988**, *36*, 3223–3225. [CrossRef]
49. Nishizawa, M.; Tsuda, M.; Hayashi, K. Two caffeic acid tetramers having enantiomeric phenyldihydronaphthalene moieties from *Macrotomia euchroma*. *Phytochemistry* **1990**, *29*, 2645–2649. [CrossRef]
50. Yamamoto, H.; Inoue, K.; Yazaki, K. Cafeic acid oligomers in Lithospermum erythrorhizon cell suspension cultures. *Phytochemistry* **2000**, *53*, 651–657. [CrossRef]
51. Ito, H.; Miyazaki, T.; Ono, M.; Sakurai, H. Antiallergic activities of rabdosiin and its related compounds: Chemical and biochemical evaluations. *Bioorg. Med. Chem.* **1988**, *6*, 1051–1056. [CrossRef]
52. Kashiwada, Y.; Nishizawa, M.; Yamagishi, T.; Tanaka, T.; Nonaka, G.; Cosentino, L.M.; Snoder, J.V.; Lee, K. Anti-AIDS agents, 18. Sodium and potassium salts of caffeic acid tetramers from *Arnebia euchromaas* anti-HIV agents. *J. Nat. Prod.* **1995**, *58*, 392–400. [CrossRef] [PubMed]
53. Dhandayuthapani, S.; Azad, H.; Rathinavelu, A. Apoptosis Induction by *Ocimum sanctum* extract in LNCaP prostate cancer cells. *J. Med. Food* **2015**, *18*, 776–785. [CrossRef] [PubMed]
54. Bhattacharyya, P.; Bishayee, A. *Ocimum sanctum* Linn. (Tulsi): An ethnomedicinal plant for the prevention and treatment of cancer. *Anticancer Drugs* **2013**, *24*, 659–666. [CrossRef] [PubMed]

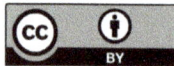

medicines

MDPI

Article

Semi-Synthesis and Evaluation of Sargahydroquinoic Acid Derivatives as Potential Antimalarial Agents

Tatenda C. Munedzimwe [1], Robyn L. van Zyl [2], Donovan C. Heslop [2], Adrienne L. Edkins [3] and Denzil R. Beukes [4],*

[1] Faculty of Pharmacy, Rhodes University, Grahamstown 6139, South Africa; tatendamunedzimwe@gmail.com
[2] Pharmacology Division, Department of Pharmacy and Pharmacology, WITS Research Institute for Malaria (WRIM), MRC Collaborating Centre for Multidisciplinary Research on Malaria, Faculty of Health Sciences, University of the Witwatersrand, Johannesburg 2000, South Africa; robyn.vanzyl@wits.ac.za (R.L.v.Z.); donoheslop@gmail.com (D.C.H.)
[3] Biomedical Biotechnology Research Unit (BioBRU), Department of Biochemistry and Microbiology, Rhodes University, Grahamstown 6139, South Africa; a.edkins@ru.ac.za
[4] School of Pharmacy, University of the Western Cape, Bellville 7535, South Africa
* Correspondence: dbeukes@uwc.ac.za; Tel.: +27-021-959-2352

Received: 25 February 2019; Accepted: 28 March 2019; Published: 1 April 2019

Abstract: Background: Malaria continues to present a major health problem, especially in developing countries. The development of new antimalarial drugs to counter drug resistance and ensure a steady supply of new treatment options is therefore an important area of research. Meroditerpenes have previously been shown to exhibit antiplasmodial activity against a chloroquinone sensitive strain of *Plasmodium falciparum* (D10). In this study we explored the antiplasmodial activity of several semi-synthetic analogs of sargahydroquinoic acid. **Methods:** Sargahydroquinoic acid was isolated from the marine brown alga, *Sargassum incisifolium* and converted, semi-synthetically, to several analogs. The natural products, together with their synthetic derivatives were evaluated for their activity against the FCR-3 strain of *Plasmodium falciparum* as well as MDA-MB-231 breast cancer cells. **Results:** Sarganaphthoquinoic acid and sargaquinoic acid showed the most promising antiplasmodial activity and low cytotoxicity. **Conclusions:** Synthetic modification of the natural product, sargahydroquinoic acid, resulted in the discovery of a highly selective antiplasmodial compound, sarganaphthoquinoic acid.

Keywords: sargaquinoic acid; sarganaphthoquinoic acid; antiplasmodial; malaria

1. Introduction

Despite the impressive breakthroughs in the treatment of malaria [1], it remains a life-threatening disease. Southeast Asia and sub-Saharan Africa account for the vast majority of the estimated 219 million malaria cases reported worldwide, leading to 435,000 deaths [2]. More than 90% of malaria cases and deaths occur in Africa, of which more than 70% are children under five years of age [2]. The prospect of resistance to current drugs appears inevitable and paints a bleak picture indeed [3]. Although the reasons for this dire situation are complex, there is undoubtedly a need for the continued search for and development of new antimalarial drugs. Natural products have historically offered some of the most effective antimalarial drugs [4]. In a previous study, we reported on the antiplasmodial activity of natural products isolated from the South African brown seaweed, *Sargassum incisifolium*, against a chloroquine sensitive strain of *Plasmodium falciparum* (D10) [5]. *S. incisifolium* is relatively abundant along the South African coastline and produces sargahydroquinoic acid (**1**) as the major metabolite. The accessibility of **1** thus provided an opportunity to explore the structure activity relationships of analogs of this natural product. Herein we report on the antiplasmodial activity of semi-synthetic analogs of sargahydroquinoic acid (**1**) (Figure 1).

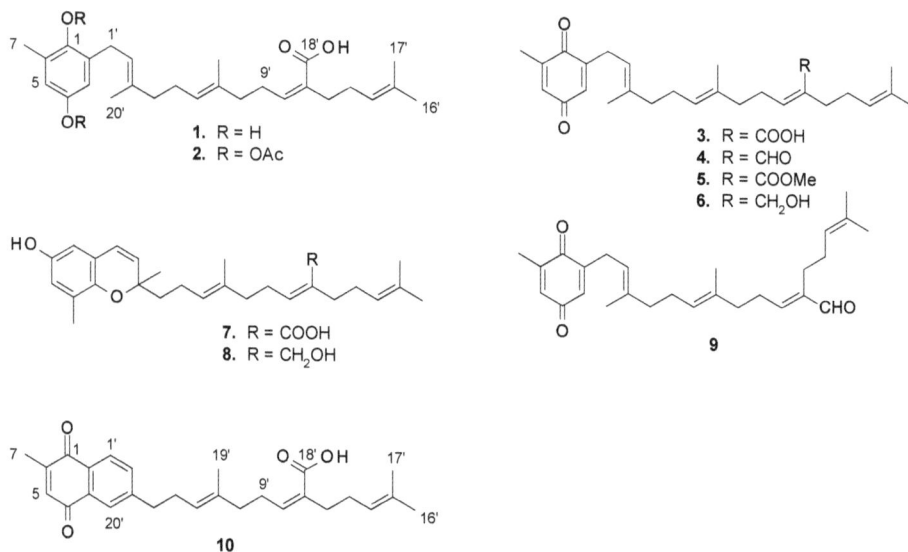

Figure 1. Natural and semi-synthetic derivatives of sargahydroquinoic acid (**1**).

2. Materials and Methods

2.1. General Experimental

All solvents were of chromatographic grade (Merck, Darmstadt, Germany) and used without further purification. Column chromatography was performed on silica gel (40–63 μm particle size) from Merck, Darmstadt, Germany. Normal Phase HPLC was carried out using a Whatman Partisil 10 semi-preparative column (Sigma-Aldrich, Schnelldorf, Germany) (10 mm × 500 mm, 10 μm), while a Phenomenex Luna C_{18} column (Sigma-Aldrich, Schnelldorf, Germany, 10 mm × 250 mm, 10 μm) was used for reversed phase HPLC. NMR spectra were recorded on Bruker Avance 400 and 600 MHz spectrometers (Bruker Biospin, Rheinstetten, Germany) and referenced to residual undeuterated $CDCl_3$ solvent signals (δ_H 7.26 ppm and δ_C 77.0 ppm). UV spectra were measured on a Perkin Elmer Lambda 25 UV/Vis spectrometer (Perkin-Elmer, Norwalk, CT, USA) while FT-IR data was obtained using a Perkin Elmer Spectrum 100 FT-IR spectrometer (Perkin-Elmer, Norwalk, CT, USA). High resolution electrospray ionization mass spectroscopy (HR-ESIMS) spectra were obtained on a Waters Synapt G2 mass spectrometer (Waters Corporation, Milford, MA, USA) at 20 V.

2.2. Extraction and Isolation of Natural Products

Specimens of *Sargassum incisifolium* were collected from Port Alfred (collection code PA071b) on the south east coast of South Africa on 21 September 2007 and stored at −20 °C. The samples were authenticated by comparison with voucher specimens from previous studies [5]. Voucher specimens are stored at the School of Pharmacy, University of the Western Cape.

The following isolation protocol is representative and was repeated several times in order to generate sufficient quantities of **1** for synthetic modification. The frozen alga (38.77 g, extracted dry weight) was allowed to thaw at room temperature after which it was soaked in methanol for one hour. The methanol was removed and the alga extracted three times with MeOH-CH_2Cl_2 (1:2) at 40 °C for 30 min. Extracts were pooled and separated into aqueous and organic phases by the addition of distilled water. Concentration of the organic phase under reduced pressure gave a dark green residue (3.87 g). A portion of the organic fraction (1.09 g) was fractionated by step-gradient elution on a silica gel column (10 g) using solvents of increasing polarity (*n*-hexane-EtOAc) to give seven fractions as follows: Fr A (H-E, 10:0, 8.6 mg), Fr B (H-E, 9:1, 27 mg), Fr C (H-E, 8:2, 132 mg), Fr D (H-E, 6:4, 218 mg), Fr E (H-E, 4:6, 65 mg), Fr F (H-E, 2:8, 9.7 mg) and Fr G (H-E, 0:10, 50 mg) followed by MeOH-EtOAc (1:1), Fr 7H (238 mg). Fraction B (19 mg) was further purified by silica gel column chromatography using a mobile phase of *n*-hexane-EtOAc (9:1) to give 1.7 mg of sargaquinal (**9**). Fraction C (40 mg) was purified by normal phase HPLC using *n*-hexane-EtOAc as mobile phase (8:2) to give 15 mg of sargaquinoic acid (**3**). Fraction D (20 mg) was purified by reversed phase HPLC using MeOH-H$_2$O phase (90:10) as the mobile phase to give sargahydroquinoic acid (**1**) (6.8 mg) and sargachromenol (**7**) (2.4 mg), respectively. The isolation of compounds **1**, **3**, **7** and **9** is summarised in Scheme S1 and their structures were confirmed by spectroscopic methods, which were in agreement with literature data (Table S1) [5]. The NMR spectra for compounds **1** (Figures S1 and S2), **3** (Figures S3 and S4), **7** (Figures S5 and S6) and **9** (Figures S7 and S8) are presented in the Supplementary Materials.

2.3. Sargaquinoic Acid (3) and Sarganaphthoquinoic Acid (10)

To a solution of **1** (154.0 mg, 0.36 mmol) in a mixture of CHCl$_3$ (8 mL) and MeOH (7 mL) was added Ag$_2$O (100 mg, 0.43 mmol). The reaction mixture was stirred at room temperature for 24 h, after which the resulting suspension was filtered through diatomaceous earth and concentrated under reduced pressure. The crude product was filtered through a plug of charcoal (*n*-hexane-EtOAc, 4:6) to give a yellow mixture of compounds which was separated by silica gel column chromatography (*n*-hexane-EtOAc, 7:3) to give sargaquinoic acid (**3**) (80 mg, 70%) and compound **10** (9.8 mg, 6%) as light yellow oils. NMR spectra for compound **10** (Figures S9–S14) can be found in the Supplementary Materials.

Sarganaphthoquinonoic acid (**10**): IR (film) ν$_{max}$ (cm^{-1}): 1600, 1663, 2850, 2924; ^{1}H and ^{13}C NMR data see Table 1; HRESIMS *m/z* 419.2222 [M-H] (calcd. for C$_{27}$H$_{35}$O$_3$, 419.2221)

Table 1. NMR spectroscopic data for sarganaphthoquinoic aicd (**10**) (600 and 125 MHz, CDCl$_3$).

Carbon Number	δ$_C$	Type	δ$_H$, mult, *J* (Hz)	COSY	HMBC
1	185.4	C	-		
2	130.2	C	-		
3	132.2	C	-		
4	185.4	C	-		
5	136.0	CH	6.81, s	H-7	
6	149.0	C	-		
7	16.4	CH$_3$	2.18, s,	H-5	C-6, C-5
1'	126.7	CH	8.00, d, 7.9	H-2'	C-2, C-1
2'	133.8	CH	7.51, d, 7.9	H-4', H-20'	C-1, C-20'
3'	148.2	C	-		
4'	36.2	CH$_2$	2.77, t, 7.6	H-5'	C-5', C-3'
5'	29.1	CH$_2$	2.36, m	H-4', H-6'	C-4', C-6', C-7'
6'	123.2	CH	5.17, m		
7'	136.0	C	-		
8'	39.0	CH$_2$	2.08, m	H-9'	C-6'
9'	28.2	CH$_2$	2.57, m	H-10'	C-8', C-10'
10'	145.0	CH	5.96, t, 7.3	H-9'	C-8'
11'	130.6	C	-		
12'	27.8	CH$_2$	2.26, m	H-13', H-14' (lr)	C-13', C-14'
13'	28.2	CH$_2$	2.11, m	H-14'	C-15', C-11'
14'	123.4	CH	5.17, t, 7.0	H-13', H-14' (lr)	
15'	132.3	C	-		
16'	25.6	CH$_3$	1.68, s	H-14' (lr)	C-15', C-14'
17'	17.7	CH$_3$	1.59, s	H-14' (lr)	C-16'
18'	171.9	C	-		
19'	15.9	CH$_3$	1.58, s	H-6'	C-6'
20'	125.9	CH	7.86, s	H-4'	C-4', C-4

COSY: ^{1}H-^{1}H Correlation spectroscopy; HMBC: ^{1}H-^{13}C Heteronuclear multiple-bond correlation spectroscopy.

2.4. Sargaquinoic Acid Methyl ester (5)

To a solution of **1** (122.4 mg, 0.29 mmol) dissolved in 2 mL acetone, was added K_2CO_3 (207.4 mg, 1.50 mmol) in 5 mL acetone and dimethylsulphate (250 µL, 2.63 mmol). The mixture was heated at 40 °C for 8 h followed by stirring at room temperature for 16 h. The reaction mixture was filtered, concentrated under reduced pressure and separated by silica gel column chromatography (*n*-hexane-EtOAc, 8:2) to give the methyl ester of **1**, which, upon exposure to air was completely oxidized to **5**. NMR spectra for compound **5** (Figures S15–S16) can be found in the Supplementary Materials.

Yellow oil, ^{1}H NMR (400 MHz, CDCl$_3$) δ 6.52 (1H, s, H-3), 6.44 (1H, s, H-5), 5.83 (1H, t, *J* = 7.0 Hz, H-10'), 5.10 (3H, m, H-2', H-6', H-14'), 3.71 (3H, s, OMe), 3.11 (2H, d, *J* = 6.8 Hz, H-1'), 2.49 (2H, m, H-9'), 2.22 (2H, m, H-12'), 2.05 (2H, m, H-4') 2.03-2.05 (6H, m, H-5', H-8', H-13'), 1.65 (6H, s, H-7, H-19'), 1.61 (3H, s, H-20'), 1.58 (3H, s, H-16'), 1.55 (3H, s, H-17'); 188.0 (C-1, C-4), 168.4 (C-18'), 148.4 (C-6), 145.8 (C-2), 142.1 (C-10'), 140.0 (C-3') 134.8 (C-7') 133.1 (C-3, C-15'), 132.1 (C-5), 131.4 (C-11'), 124.4 (C-6'), 123.5 (C-14'), 118.0 (C-2'), 51.0 (OMe), 39.8 (C-4'), 39.1 (C-8'), 34.7 (C-12'), 28.0 (C-9'), 27.8 (C13'), 27.5 (C-1'), 26.4 (C-5'), 25.6 (C-16'), 17.6 (C-17'), 16.1 (C-7), 15.9 (C-19'); HRESIMS *m/z* 437.2710 [M-H] (calcd. for $C_{28}H_{37}O_4$, 437.2692).

2.5. Diacetyl Sargahydroquinoic Acid (2)

To sargahydroquinoic acid (**1**) (110.0 mg, 0.26 mmol) was added acetic anhydride (3 mL, 31.8 mmol) and pyridine (2 mL, 24.8 mmol). The reaction mixture was stirred at room temperature for 30 h. The crude product was acidified with 1 M HCl (10 mL) and extracted with EtOAc (5 mL × 3). The organic layer was collected and concentrated under reduced pressure to give a crude product which was further purified by silica gel column chromatography (*n*-hexane:EtOAc, 7:3) to give compound **2** (12.8 mg, 12%) as a yellow oil. The structure of compound **2** was confirmed by spectroscopic methods, which were in agreement with literature data [6,7]. NMR spectra for compound **2** (Figures S17 and S18) can be found in the Supplementary Materials.

2.6. Sargaquinol (6) and Sargachromendiol (8)

To a solution of sargahydroquinoic acid (**1**) (140.7 mg, 0.33 mmol) dissolved in anhydrous THF (5 mL), was added LiAlH$_4$ (0.104 g, 2.74 mmol). The reaction mixture was stirred at room temperature, under a nitrogen atmosphere for 1.25 h. The reaction was quenched with a few drops of EtOAc, concentrated and partitioned between EtOAc (10 mL^{-2}) and H$_2$O (5 mL). The organic layer was concentrated under reduced pressure to give a crude product which was purified by silica gel chromatography (*n*-hexane:EtOAc, 8:2) to give sargaquinol (**6**) (12.2 mg, 30%) and the alcohol derivative of sargachromenol (**8**) (2.8 mg, 3.5%). The structure of compound **6** was confirmed by spectroscopic methods, which were in agreement with literature data (Table S1) [7]. NMR spectra for compounds **6** (Figures S19 and S20) and **8** (Figures S21 and S22) can be found in the Supplementary Materials.

Sargaquinol (**6**) yellow oil; ^{1}H NMR (400 MHz, CDCl$_3$) δ 6.54 (s, 1H) (H-3), 6.46 (s, 1H) (H-5), 5.15 (dd, *J* = 21.0, 13.2 Hz) (H- 2', 6', 14'), 4.11 (s) (H-18'), 3.63 (t, *J* = 6.5 Hz) (H-10'), 3.12 (d, *J* = 7.1 Hz) (H-1'), 2.12 (s) (H-5', 9', 13'), 2.05 (s) (H-4', 8'), 1.67 (s) (H- 7, 16'), 1.60 (s) (H-19', 20'), 1.57 (s) (H-17'). ^{13}C NMR (100 MHz, CDCl$_3$) δ 188.0 (C-1), 187.97 (C-4), 148.5 (C-6), 145.9 (C-2), 139.7 (C-3'), 135.0 (C-7'), 133.1 (C-3), 131,2 (C-11'), 132.24 (C-5), 133.7 (C-15'), 124.7 (C-6'), 124.2 (C-14'), 118.1 (C-2'), 71.8 (C-18'), 62.8 (C-10'), 39.8 (C-4'), 39.5 (C-8'), 35.2 (C-12'), 27.1 (C-13'),27.5 (C-1'), 26.2 (C-5'), 26.3 (C-9'), 25.6 (C-16'), 17.7 (C-7), 16.11 (C-17'), 16.07 (C-19'), 16.0 (C-20').

Sargachromendiol (**8**) yellow oil; ^{1}H NMR (400 MHz, CDCl$_3$) δ 6.47 (d, *J* = 2.4 Hz) (H-5), 6.32 (d, *J* = 2.5 Hz) (H-2), 6.26 (s) (H-2'), 5.98 (t, *J* = 7.2 Hz) (H-9'), 5.57 (d, *J* = 9.8 Hz) (H-3'), 5.12 (dt, *J* = 19.0, 6.4 Hz) (H-5', 14'), 2.59 (q, *J* = 7.3 Hz (H-8'), 2.27 (t, *J* = 7.4 Hz), 2.13 (s) (H-12'), 2.09–2.04 (m) (H-4', 7'), 1.68 (s) (H-8), 1.58 (d, *J* = 3.5 Hz) (H-17', 19'), 1.36 (s) (20'); ^{13}C NMR (100 MHz, CDCl$_3$) δ 148.6 (C-5), 145.0 (C-10'), 144.8 (C-8), 134.7 (C-7'), 131.8 (C-15'), 130.6 (C-11'), 126.3 (C-3), 124.7 (C-6'), 124.1 (C-1'), 122.9 (C-14'), 121.3 (C-2), 117.0 (C-4), 110.3 (C-6), 77.8 (C-3'), 60.3 (C-18'), 40.7 (C-4'), 39.8 (C-8'), 35.1

(C-12′), 35.3 (C-12′), 27.0 (C-9′), 26.1 (C-13′), 25.9 (C-20′), 25.7 (C-16′), 22.6 (C-5′), 17.7 (17′), 15.9 (C-7), 15.5 (C-19′).

2.7. Z-sargaquinal (4)

To a solution of sargaquinol (6) (37.2 mg, 0.09 mmol) dissolved in anhydrous CH_2Cl_2 (8 mL), Dess-Martin Periodinane (107 mg, 0.26 mmol) was added. The reaction mixture was stirred at room temperature for 2 h after which it was quenched with CH_2Cl_2 (10 mL) and de-ionized water (10 mL). The organic phase was separated and washed with saturated solutions of $NaHCO_3$ (10 mL × 3) and $Na_2S_2O_3$ (10 mL × 3), dried over anhydrous Na_2SO_4 and concentrated under reduced pressure. The crude product was purified by silica gel column chromatography (*n*-hexane:EtOAc, 8:2) to give compound 4 (42%, 14.9 mg), as a yellow oil. The structure of compound 4 was confirmed by spectroscopic methods, which were in agreement with literature data (Table S1) [7]. NMR spectra for compound 4 (Figures S23 and S24) can be found in the Supplementary Materials.

2.8. Antiplasmodial Assays

All compounds were tested in triplicate against the chloroquine-resistant Gambian FCR-3 strain of *P. falciparum*. The in vitro erythrocytic stage of the parasite was maintained using the method outlined by Trager and Jensen [8]. The antimalarial activity of the compounds was determined using the tritiated hypoxanthine incorporation assay using a 0.5% parasitaemia and 1% haematocrit [9]. All assays were carried out using untreated parasites and uninfected red blood cells as controls. The concentration that inhibited 50% parasite growth (IC_{50} value) was determined from the log sigmoid dose response curve using GraphPad Prism. Quinine was used as the reference antiplasmodial agent. The selectivity index for the compounds was determined from the ratio of cytotoxicity IC_{50} to antimalarial IC_{50}.

2.9. Cytotoxicity Assay

All compounds were tested in triplicate against MDA-MB-231 breast carcinoma cells, which were purchased from the ATCC (Catalogue number HTB-26, Manassas, VA, USA). The cytotoxicity of the compounds was determined using the WST-1 assay method (Roche). The cells were treated with a range of concentrations of the test compounds or vehicle control (DMSO). Cells treated with DMSO were considered to represent 100% viability and the viability of cells at each dose was represented relative to this value. The concentration resulting in a decrease of cell viability to 50% was calculated from the linear portion of the dose response curve.

3. Results and Discussion

3.1. Isolation and Synthetic Modification of Sargahydroquinoic Acid Derivatives

Sargahydroquinoic acid (1) is the major component of the CH_2Cl_2-MeOH extract of *Sargassum incisifolium* and has also been reported from several other *Sargassum* spp. [5–7]. This compound slowly converts to sargaquinoic acid (3) and sargachromenol (7) on storage of the seaweed, the extract and during purification. Specimens of *S. incisifolium* (PA071b) were collected from Port Alfred on the south eastern coast of South Africa and extracted with CH_2Cl_2-MeOH. The crude extract was first fractionated by silica gel column chromatography, followed by normal or reversed phase HPLC to give compounds 1, 3, 7 and 9. The identities of all isolated compounds were confirmed by comparison of their NMR spectroscopic data (Table S1) to literature values [5]. The above protocol yielded sufficient quantities of 1 to perform structural modifications and biological assays.

Sargaquinoic acid (3) is normally isolated from fresh seaweed in relatively small quantities; however, it can be produced more efficiently by the oxidation of 1 [7,10]. Thus, treatment of 1 with Ag_2O gave 3 in moderate to good yields. Interestingly, although this conversion is facile, we consistently observed a series of unusual peaks between δ_H 7 and 8 in the ^1H NMR spectrum of the crude reaction product. The compound (**10**) responsible for these peaks was isolated and its structure was elucidated by NMR spectroscopy and mass spectrometry.

The HRESIMS spectrum of compound **10** showed a molecular ion peak at *m/z* 419.2222 [M-H] which corresponds to a molecular formula of $C_{27}H_{31}O_4$. Characteristic deshielded methine resonances at δ_H 8.00 (d, *J* = 7.9), δ 7.98 (s) and δ 7.51 (d, *J* = 7.9) were evident in its ^{1}H NMR spectrum. In addition, one of the aromatic singlets had shifted downfield from δ_H 6.46 in **3** to δ_H 6.81 in **10**. Data from the ^{13}C NMR spectrum of compound **10** revealed no change in the number of carbon atoms when compared to the starting material (**1**). It revealed the presence of two quinone carbonyls signals at (δ_C 185.4 and δ 185.4) and a carboxylic acid moiety (δ_C 171.9). In addition, the DEPT-135 NMR spectrum indicated the loss of one methyl signal (δ_C 16.1, C-20′) and a methylene signal (δ_C 27.5, C-1′) when compared to **3**, together with the appearance of two additional olefinic methine signals at δ_C 126.7 (C-1′) and 125.9 (C-20′). HMBC correlations (Figure 2) from the doublet at δ_H 8.00 (H-1′) to carbon signals at δ_C 126.7 (C-1′) and δ_C 133.8 (C-2′); the methine signal at δ_H 7.51 (H-2′) to the carbon signal at δ_C 125.9 (C-20′) and from δ_H 7.86 (H-20′) to carbon signals at δ_C 36.2 (C-4′) and δ_C 185.4 (C-4), allowed for the assignment of the naphthoquinone moiety. All other spectroscopic data are consistent with a polyprenyl side chain with a 6′*E*,10′*Z*-double bond geometry (as in **3**). We assigned the name sarganaphthoquinoic acid to this new compound. A related compound, chabrolonaphthoquinone, had previously been reported from the Taiwanese soft coral, *Nephthea chabrolii* [11]. The main differences between the two compounds are the methyl substituent at C-6 and the 10-double bond geometry in compound **10**.

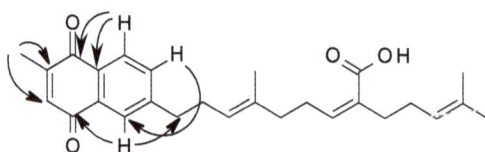

Figure 2. Key HMBC correlations for **10**.

The direct conversion of prenylated hydroquinones to naphthoquinones is uncommon and presents a novel approach to the synthesis of this important group of compounds. To the best of our knowledge there is only a single report describing the formation of a naphthoquinone as a side-product in the synthesis of chromenes from prenylated quinones [12]. Naphthoquinones are typically synthesized by Diels-Alder reactions between *p*-benzoquinones and dienes or by the prenylation of halogenated naphthoquinone moieties [13–15]. Compound **10** is proposed to form via tautomerism and oxidation of the intermediate quinone (**3**) followed by 6πelectrocyclization and further oxidation (Scheme 1).

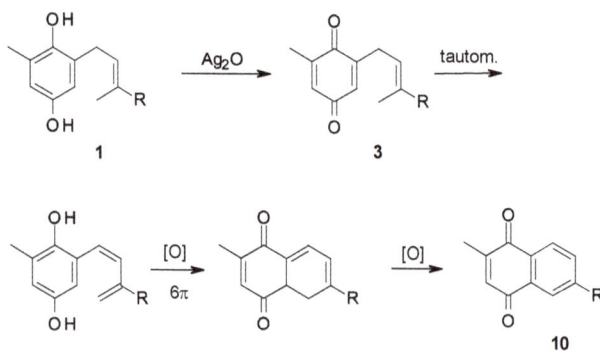

Scheme 1. Proposed mechanism for the synthesis of sarganaphthoquinoic acid (**10**).

In order to establish preliminary structure-antiplasmodial activity relationships for this series of sargahydroquinoic acid derivatives, we focused our attention on modification of the carboxylic acid and quinone moieties. Acetylation of **1** with acetic anhydride/pyridine gave the diacetate (**2**), while its reduction with lithium aluminium hydride gave a mixture of sargaquinol (**6**) and sargachromendiol (**8**). The facile conversion of the hydroquinone to a mixture of the quinone and chromene on exposure to air is often seen in this series of compounds [6,7]. Spectroscopic evidence for the identity of alcohols **6** and **8** were provided by the disappearance of the ^{13}C NMR signal due to the carboxylic acid group at δ_C 172 ppm and the appearance of an oxymethylene carbon signal at δ_C 60.3 ppm in both compounds.

Mild oxidation of **6** with Dess-Martin periodinane, gave 10Z-sargaquinal (**4**). The structures of aldehydes **4** and **9** were confirmed by comparison of their spectroscopic data with literature values [5,7]. A comparison of the ^{1}H NMR spectra of the natural and semi-synthetic aldehydes revealed differences in chemical shifts of both proton and carbon atoms associated with the aldehyde group. The ^{1}H and ^{13}C NMR spectra of the semi-synthetic aldehyde (**4**) showed signals at δ_H 10.1 and δ_C 190.9 ppm compared to δ_H 9.55 and δ_C 205.4 ppm in the natural aldehyde (**9**). ^{1}H-^{1}H NOESY correlations in both compounds confirmed the difference in the geometry of the Δ^{10} double bond with the semi-synthetic aldehyde (**4**) bearing a 10Z-geometry and the natural aldehyde (**9**) a 10E-geometry. The formation of 2'E,6'E,10'Z-sargaquinal (**4**) from 2'E,6'E,10'Z-sargahydroquinoic acid (**1**) has been reported in the literature [7]. However, this is the first report of its ^{13}C and 2D NMR data.

Interestingly, methylation of **1** with dimethylsulphate/potassium carbonate did not produce the dimethyl ether, but instead produced sargaquinoic acid methyl ester (**5**). This was confirmed by the appearance of an additional methyl signal at δ_C 51.0 and an upfield shift of the C-18' carbonyl signal from δ_C 172 to δ 168.4 ppm in the ^{13}C NMR spectrum of **5** (Table S1).

3.2. Biological Assays

The ten sargahydroquinoic acid derivatives were assessed for both antiplasmodial and cytotoxic activity against the chloroquine-resistant Gambian FCR-3 strain of *P. falciparum* and MDA-MB-231 breast cells, respectively (Table 2). All compounds showed moderate to good antiplasmodial activity. However, the most promising compound in this series is the naphthoquinone **10** which not only revealed good antiplasmodial activity (IC$_{50}$ 5.4 µM), but also very low cytotoxicity (IC$_{50}$ 2410 µM), resulting in a high selectivity index of 443. Sargaquinoic acid (**3**) also shows promising antiplasmodial activity (IC$_{50}$ 10.8 µM), but is slightly more toxic (IC$_{50}$ 658 µM) than **10**. It appears that the carboxylic acid in the prenyl side chain is important for activity since both aldehydes (**4**) and (**9**) and the alcohol (**6**) showed decreased antiplasmodial activity. The quinone/naphthoquinone scaffold is present in several antimalarial natural products and drugs [16]. It is therefore likely that the mode of action of the compounds reported here is related to this important pharmacophore [16–20].

Table 2. Bioassay results for compounds **1**–**10**.

Compound	IC$_{50}$ (µM)			Selectivity Index
	D10 [1]	FCR-3	MDA-MB-231	
Sargahydroquinoic acid (**1**)	15.2	38.6	70	1.8
Sargahydroquinoic acid di-acetate (**2**)	-	84.3	286	3.4
Sargaquinoic acid (**3**)	12.0	10.8	658	60.9
10Z-sargaquinal (**4**)	-	72.6	211	2.9
Sargaquinoic acid methyl ester (**5**)	-	8.2	70	8.6
Sargaquinol (**6**)	-	93.1	99	1.1
Sargachromenol (**7**)	-	114.8	56	0.5
Sargachromendiol (**8**)	-	34.2	187	5.5
10E-sargaquinal (**9**)	2.0	104.4	69	0.7
Sarganaphthoquinone (**10**)	-	5.4	2410	443
Quinine		0.17	-	-

[1] From reference [5].

4. Conclusions

In this study we isolated the relatively abundant antiplasmodial natural product, sargahydroquinoic acid (**1**) and converted it to several analogs which were evaluated for antiplasmodial and cytotoxic activity. The serendipitous formation of sarganaphthoquinoic acid (**10**) gave a compound with good antiplasmodial activity while being almost non-toxic. Due to the small number of compounds no clear structure activity relationships can be established, however it appears that the presence of a quinone and carboxylic acid are important for selective activity against *P. falciparum*. Further studies are warranted to explore the mode of action of these compounds and to further improve on its antiplasmodial activity.

Supplementary Materials: The following are available online at http://www.mdpi.com/2305-6320/6/2/47/s1, Scheme S1: Isolation of compounds **1**, **3**, **7** and **9**, Table S1: Comparison of ^{13}C NMR data for compounds **1**, **3–9**, Figure S1: ^{1}H NMR spectrum of sargahydroquinoic acid (**1**) (400 MHz, CDCl$_3$), Figure S2: ^{13}C NMR spectrum of sargahydroquinoic acid (**1**) (100 MHz, CDCl$_3$), Figure S3: ^{1}H NMR spectrum of sargaquinoic acid (**3**) (400 MHz, CDCl$_3$), Figure S4: ^{13}C NMR spectrum of compound **3** (400 MHz, CDCl$_3$), Figure S5: ^{1}H NMR spectrum of sargachromenol (**7**) (400 MHz, CDCl$_3$), Figure S6: ^{13}C NMR spectrum of sargachromenol (**7**) (100 MHz, CDCl$_3$), Figure S7: ^{1}H NMR spectrum of 10′E-sargaquinal (**9**) (400 MHz, CDCl$_3$), Figure S8: ^{13}C NMR spectrum of 10′E-sargaquinal (**9**) (100 MHz, CDCl$_3$), Figure S9: ^{1}H NMR spectrum of sarganaphthoquinoic acid (**10**) (400 MHz, CDCl$_3$), Figure S10: ^{13}C NMR spectrum of sarganaphthoquinoic acid (**10**) (100 MHz, CDCl$_3$), Figure S11: DEPT-135 NMR spectrum of sarganaphthoquinoic acid (**10**) (100 MHz, CDCl$_3$), Figure S12: HSQC NMR spectrum of sarganaphthoquinoic acid (**10**) (CDCl$_3$), Figure S13: COSY NMR spectrum of sarganaphthoquinoic acid (**10**) (CDCl$_3$), Figure S14: HMBC NMR spectrum of sarganaphthoquinoic acid (**10**) (CDCl$_3$). Figure S15: ^{1}H NMR spectrum of sargaquinoic acid methyl ester (**5**) (400 MHz, CDCl$_3$), Figure S16: ^{13}C NMR spectrum of sargaquinoic acid methyl ester (**5**) (100 MHz), Figure S17: ^{1}H NMR spectrum of sargahydroquinoic acid diacetate (**2**) (400 MHz, CDCl$_3$), Figure S18: ^{13}C NMR spectrum of sargahydroquinoic acid diacetate (**2**) (100 MHz, CDCl$_3$), Figure S19: ^{1}H NMR spectrum of sargaquinol (**6**) (400 MHz, CDCl$_3$), Figure S20: ^{13}C NMR spectrum of sargaquinol (**6**) (100 MHz, CDCl$_3$), Figure S21: ^{1}H NMR spectrum of sargachromendiol (**8**) (400 MHz, CDCl$_3$), Figure S22: ^{13}C NMR spectrum of sargachromendiol (**8**) (100 MHz, CDCl$_3$), Figure S23: ^{1}H NMR spectrum of 10′Z-sargaquinal (**4**) (600 MHz, CDCl$_3$), Figure S24: ^{13}C NMR spectrum of 10′Z-sargaquinal (**4**) (100 MHz, CDCl$_3$).

Author Contributions: D.R.B. conceived and designed the work. T.C.M. isolated the natural products and synthesized the analogs, R.L.v.Z. and D.C.H conducted the antiplasmodial assays. Cytotoxicity studies were done by A.L.E. D.R.B. and T.C.M. drafted the manuscript. All authors read and approved the final version of manuscript.

Funding: This research was funded by Rhodes University, University of the Witwatersrand and the University of the Western Cape. A.L.E is funded by the South African Research Chairs Initiative of the Department of Science and Technology (DST) and National Research Foundation of South Africa (NRF) (Grant No 98566), and National Research Foundation CPRR (Grant No 105829).

Acknowledgments: T.C.M. acknowledges Rhodes University and the Andrew W. Mellon Foundation for a Masters scholarship.

Conflicts of Interest: The authors declare no conflict of interest.

References

1. Okombo, J.; Chibale, K. Recent updates in the discovery and development of novel antimalarial drug candidates. *Med. Chem. Commun.* **2018**, *9*, 437–453. [CrossRef] [PubMed]
2. World Health Organization. *World Malaria Report*; World Health Organization: Geneva, Switzerland, 2018.
3. Amato, R.; Pearson, R.D.; Almagro-Garcia, J.; Amaratunga, C.; Lim, P.; Suon, S.; Sreng, S.; Drury, E.; Stalker, J.; Miotto, O.; et al. Origins of the current outbreak of multidrug-resistant malaria in southeast Asia: A retrospective genetic study. *Lancet Infect. Dis.* **2018**, *18*, 337–345. [CrossRef]
4. Fernández-Álvaro, E.; Hong, W.D.; Nixon, G.L.; O'Neill, P.M.; Calderón, F. Antimalarial chemotherapy: Natural product inspired development of preclinical and clinical candidates with diverse mechanisms of action. *J. Med. Chem.* **2016**, *59*, 5587–5603. [CrossRef] [PubMed]
5. Afolayan, A.F.; Bolton, J.J.; Lategan, C.A.; Smith, P.J.; Beukes, D.R. Fucoxanthin, tetraprenylated toluquinone and toluhydroquinone metabolites from *Sargassum heterophyllum* inhibit the in vitro growth of the malaria parasite *Plasmodium falciparum*. *Z. Naturforsch.* **2008**, *63c*, 848–852. [CrossRef]

6. Segawa, M.; Shirahama, H. New plastoquinones from the brown alga *Sargassum sagamianum* var. *yezoense*. *Chem. Lett.* **1987**, 1365–1366. [CrossRef]

7. Kusumi, T.; Ishitsuka, M.; Kinoshita, T.; Kakisawa, H.; Shibata, Y. Structures of new plastoquinones from the brown alga *Sargassum serratifolium*. *Chem. Lett.* **1979**, *8*, 277–278. [CrossRef]

8. Trager, W.; Jensen, J.B. Human malaria parasites in continuous culture. *Science* **1976**, *193*, 673–675. [CrossRef] [PubMed]

9. Desjardins, R.E.; Canfield, C.J.; Haynes, J.D.; Chulay, J.D. Quantitative assessment of antimalarial activity in vitro by a semiautomated microdilution technique. *Antimicrob. Agents Chemother.* **1979**, *16*, 710–718. [CrossRef] [PubMed]

10. Perez-Castorena, A.; Arciniegas, A.; Apan, M.T.R.; Villasenor, J.L.; de Vivar, A. Evaluation of the anti-inflammatory and antioxidant activities of the plastoquinones derivatives isolated from *Roldana barba-johanis*. *Planta Med.* **2002**, *68*, 645–647. [CrossRef] [PubMed]

11. Sheu, J.-H.; Su, J.-H.; Sung, P.-J.; Wang, G.-H.; Dai, H. Novel meroditerpenoid-related metabolites from the formosan soft coral *Nephthea chabrolii*. *J. Nat. Prod.* **2004**, *67*, 2048–2052. [CrossRef] [PubMed]

12. Chan, S.T.S.; Pullar, M.A.; Khalil, I.M.; Allouche, E.; Barker, D.; Copp, B.R. Bio-inspired dimerisation of prenylated quinones directed towards the synthesis of the meroterpenoid natural products, the scabellones. *Tetrahedron Lett.* **2015**, *56*, 1486–1488. [CrossRef]

13. Alonso, M.A.; Lopez-Alvarado, P.; Avendano, C.; Menendez, J.C. Regioselective Diels-Alder reactions of 3-vinylindoles with quinones. *Lett. Org. Chem.* **2004**, *1*, 20–22. [CrossRef]

14. de Koning, C.B.; Rousseau, A.L.; van Otterlo, W.A.L. Modern methods for the synthesis of substituted naphthalenes. *Tetrahedron* **2003**, *59*, 7–36. [CrossRef]

15. Couladouros, E.A.; Plyta, Z.F.; Papageorgiou, V.P. A general procedure for the efficient synthesis of (alkylamino)naphthoquinones. *J. Org. Chem.* **1996**, *61*, 3031–3033. [CrossRef] [PubMed]

16. Nixon, G.L.; Moss, D.M.; Shone, A.E.; Lalloo, D.G.; Fisher, N.; O'Neill, P.M.; Ward, S.A.; Biagini, G.A. Antimalarial pharmacology and therapeutics of atovaquone. *J. Antimicrob. Chemother.* **2013**, *68*, 977–985. [CrossRef] [PubMed]

17. Olliaro, P. Mode of action and mechanisms of resistance for antimalarial drugs. *Pharmacol. Ther.* **2001**, *89*, 207–219. [CrossRef]

18. Vennerstrom, J.L.; Eaton, J.W. Oxidants, oxidant drugs, and malaria. *J. Med. Chem.* **1988**, *31*, 1269–1277. [CrossRef] [PubMed]

19. Brandão, G.C.; Rocha Missias, F.C.; Arantes, L.M.; Soares, L.F.; Roy, K.K.; Doerksen, R.J.; Braga de Oliveira, A.; Pereira, G.R. Antimalarial naphthoquinones. Synthesis via click chemistry, in vitro activity, docking to PfDHOD and SAR of lapachol-based compounds. *Eur. J. Med. Chem.* **2018**, *145*, 191–205. [CrossRef] [PubMed]

20. Imperatore, C.; Persico, M.; Senese, M.; Aiello, A.; Casertano, M.; Luciano, P.; Basilico, N.; Parapini, S.; Paladino, A.; Fattorusso, C.; et al. Exploring the antimalarial potential of the methoxy-thiazinoquinone scaffold: Identification of a new lead candidate. *Bioorg. Chem.* **2019**, *85*, 240–252. [CrossRef] [PubMed]

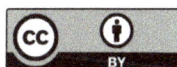

medicines

MDPI

Article

In Vitro Evaluation of the Phytopharmacological Potential of *Sargassum incisifolium* for the Treatment of Inflammatory Bowel Diseases

Mutenta N. Nyambe [1], Trevor C. Koekemoer [1], Maryna van de Venter [1,*], Eleonora D. Goosen [2] and Denzil R. Beukes [3]

[1] Department of Biochemistry and Microbiology, P.O. Box 7700, Nelson Mandela University, Port Elizabeth 6031, South Africa; mutentanyambe@gmail.com (M.N.N.); trevor.koekemoer@mandela.ac.za (T.C.K.)

[2] Faculty of Pharmacy, Division of Pharmaceutical Chemistry, P.O. Box 94, Rhodes University, Grahamstown 6140, South Africa; l.goosen@ru.ac.za

[3] School of Pharmacy, Private Bag X17, University of the Western Cape, Bellville 7535, South Africa; dbeukes@uwc.ac.za

* Correspondence: maryna.vandeventer@mandela.ac.za; Tel.: +27-041-504-2813

Received: 28 February 2019; Accepted: 28 March 2019; Published: 6 April 2019

Abstract: Background: Comprised of Crohn's disease and ulcerative colitis, inflammatory bowel diseases (IBD) are characterized by chronic inflammation of the gastro-intestinal tract, which often results in severe damage to the intestinal mucosa. This study investigated metabolites from the South African endemic alga, *Sargassum incisifolium*, as potential treatments for IBD. Phytochemical evaluation of *S. incisifolium* yielded prenylated toluhydroquinones and toluquinones, from which semi-synthetic analogs were derived, and a carotenoid metabolite. The bioactivities of *S. incisifolium* fractions, natural products, and semi-synthetic derivatives were evaluated using various in vitro assays. **Methods:** Sargahydroquinoic acid isolated from *S. incisifolium* was converted to several structural derivatives by semi-synthetic modification. Potential modulation of IBD by *S. incisifolium* crude fractions, natural compounds, and sargahydroquinoic acid analogs was evaluated through in vitro anti-inflammatory activity, anti-oxidant activity, cytotoxicity against HT-29 and Caco-2 colorectal cancer cells, and PPAR-γ activation. **Results:** Sargahydroquinoic acid acts on various therapeutic targets relevant to IBD treatment. **Conclusions:** Conversion of sargahydroquinoic acid to sarganaphthoquinoic acid increases peroxisome proliferator activated receptor gamma (PPAR-γ) activity, compromises anti-oxidant activity, and has no effect on cytotoxicity against the tested cell lines.

Keywords: PPAR-γ; sargahydroquinoic acid; sarganaphthoquinoic acid; sargachromenoic acid; inflammation; bowel diseases

1. Introduction

The incidence of the two major types of inflammatory bowel diseases (IBDs), Crohn's disease (CD) and ulcerative colitis (UC), has become a global health challenge. A systematic review of studies reporting the prevalence and incidence of IBDs, performed by Ng et al., revealed that while the incidence has stabilised in the westernised world, it has steadily been increasing in developing countries over the past decade or two [1]. CD and UC are characterised by chronic inflammation of the intestine with many associated symptoms, complications, and an increased risk for colorectal cancer [2]. Conventional treatment is aimed at reducing intestinal inflammation and modulating the immune system. The most commonly used treatments are aminosalicylate anti-inflammatories (5-ASA, sulfasalazine, mesalamine and derivatives), corticosteroids (prednisone, prednisolone, budesonide,

budesonide MMX), immunosuppressives (thiopurines, methotrexate) and TNF antagonists (infliximab, adalimumab, certolizumab pegol, golimumab). More recent developments include integrin antagonists to inhibit T cell adhesion and antagonists of the pro-inflammatory interleukins IL-12 and -23 [2]. None of these medications come without problems such as safety, efficacy, or cost implications and the search for new alternatives continues [2,3].

Oxidative stress signalling has been implicated in the pathogenesis and progression of IBD [4]. Although its exact role and mechanism is not fully understood, it is accepted that oxidative stress plays a role in the initiation and development of the disease and is not merely a result of chronic inflammation in the gut. Antioxidants may therefore have potential therapeutic effects especially if administered in combination with conventional therapies [4].

The nuclear receptor PPAR-γ, well known for its role in adipocyte differentiation, has also been identified as a potential therapeutic target for IBD [5,6]. It plays a role in regulation of inflammation in the intestine, where it is expressed at high levels in epithelial cells and at lower levels in macrophages and lymphocytes [7]. Peroxisome proliferator-activated receptor gamma (PPAR-γ) agonists inhibit the inflammatory response in intestinal epithelial cells [4,5] and macrophages [8]. Activation of PPAR-γ also slows down the proliferation of colon cancer cells [9] and protects against the development of colorectal cancer [10].

Secondary metabolites from natural products have been an important source of lead compounds for drug development. Advances in chemical techniques and functional, as well as phenotypic, bioassays have led to a revived interest in this field [11,12]. The multi-target nature of pleiotropic natural products holds many advantages in the treatment of complex diseases [13].

The brown seaweed *Sargassum incisifolium* is found in South Africa (from the Western Cape through the Eastern Cape and KwaZulu-Natal), southern Mozambique, and south-east Madagascar [14]. An aqueous extract of this species was shown to exhibit no antimicrobial activity on its own but surprisingly enhanced the antimicrobial potential of silver nanoparticles [15]. The same authors have reported a high polyphenol content of 150 μg/mg for the aqueous extract and high antioxidant activity, with a total reducing power of 75 ascorbic acid equivalents (AAE), measured in μg/mg of dried extract. Partitioning of the aqueous extract with organic solvent increased the polyphenol content to 235 μg/mg and the reducing power to 95 μg/mL. Although IC_{50} values were not reported by the authors, the extract and organic partition were non-toxic to MCF-7 cells at 100 μg/mL, while reducing HT-29 and MCF-12a cell viability to between 45% and 70% [15].

This study investigated the potential of metabolites from the South African endemic alga *Sargassum incisifolium* (Figure S1) in the treatment of inflammatory bowel diseases (IBD). Phytochemical evaluation of *Sargassum incisifolium* yielded known compounds consisting of prenylated metabolites and a carotenoid. The isolated natural compounds were sargahydroquinoic acid (SHQA, **1**), sargaquinoic acid (SQA, **2**), fucoxanthin (**3**), and sargaquinal (**4**). Since SQA (**2**) was isolated in minute quantities, it was further semi-synthesized from SHQA (**1**) (65.1% yield). Sarganaphthoquinoic acid (SNQA, **5**) and sargachromenoic acid (SCA, **6**) were semi-synthesized from sargaquinoic acid (**2**) and sargahydroquinoic acid (SHQA, **1**), respectively (Figure 1). The bioactivities of *S. incisifolium* fractions, compounds, and semi-synthetic derivatives were evaluated as potential modulators of inflammatory bowel diseases using various in vitro assays.

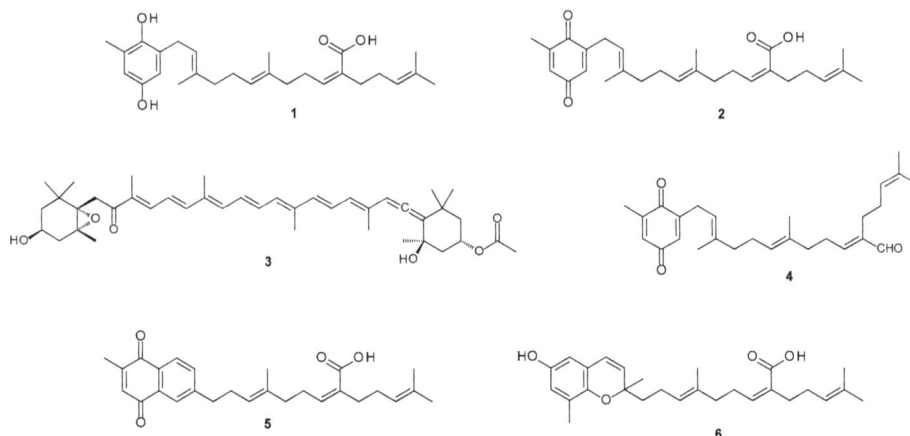

Figure 1. *Sargassum incisifolium* metabolites sargahydroquinoic acid (**1**), sargaquinoic acid (**2**), fucoxanthin (**3**) and sargaquinal (**4**), and semi-synthetic derivatives sarganaphthoquinoic acid (**5**) and sargachromenoic acid (**6**).

2. Materials and Methods

2.1. Reagents

Culture mediums were sourced from Sigma Aldrich® (Johannesburg, South Africa) and Hyclone® (Thermo Fisher, Logan, UT, USA) while Fetal Bovine Serum (FBS) was obtained from LONZA® (Basel, Switzerland). Chang Liver cells (HeLa derivative) were purchased from Highveld Biologicals, Johannesburg, South Africa and HT29 and Caco2 colorectal carcinoma cell lines from the American Type Culture Collection (Manassas, VA, USA). The EC_{50} values of the test compounds were calculated from a minimum 5-point dose-response curve using a GraphPad Prism 4 software package (GraphPad, San Diego, CA, USA). Liquid chromatography utilised HPLC grade solvents supplied by Lichrosolv® (Merck, Germany). NMR experiments were obtained on a Bruker Avance 400 MHz NMR spectrometer (Bruker Corporation, Billerica, MA, USA) using standard pulse sequences. All HPLC solvents were filtered through a 0.45 μm filter before use. Normal phase HPLC was performed using a Spectra-Physics IsoChrom pump (Spectra-Physics, Santa Clara, CA, USA), a Whatman® Partisil 10 (9.5 mm × 500 mm) semi-preparative column (GE healthcare, Chicago, IL, USA) and a Waters 410 differential refractometer (Waters Corporation, Milford, MA, USA) attached to a 100 mV full scale Rikadenki chart recorder (Rikadenki Electronics GmbH, Freiburg im Breisgau, Germany).

2.2. Algal Material

The algal specimen of *S. incisifolium* (collection voucher NDK101124) was collected from Noordhoek, near Port Elizabeth, on the southeast coast of South Africa on 24 November 2010. A specimen (Figure S1) is kept in the seaweed collection at the School of Pharmacy, University of the Western Cape. The algal specimen was transported to the laboratory on ice where it was immediately frozen and stored until the time of extraction. For purposes of identification and authentication, the algal material was morphologically compared with previous voucher specimens of *S. incisifolium*. A voucher specimen (NDK06-5) is kept at the Division of Pharmaceutical Chemistry, Rhodes University, Makhanda, South Africa.

2.3. Extraction and Isolation of Bioactive Metabolites

The algal extraction procedure was consistent with previously reported methods [16]. The frozen alga (NDK101124) was allowed to defrost under running distilled water. The defrosted alga was then soaked in MeOH for 1 h, after which the MeOH was decanted and the retained algae heated at 40 °C for 30 min in CH_2Cl_2/MeOH (2:1, 150 mL × 3). MeOH and CH_2Cl_2/MeOH (2:1) mixtures were pooled and sufficient water added to allow for the separation of the CH_2Cl_2 and the MeOH/H_2O phases. The CH_2Cl_2 phase was then collected and dried in vacuo to yield the desired crude extract (12.4 g). A portion of the crude extract (0.95 g) was applied to a silica gel column (10 g) and the column eluted using a series of solvents (50 mL each) of increasing polarity. This yielded the following fractions: **Fr A** (*n*-hexane-EtOAc, 10:0, 17.2 mg), **Fr B** (*n*-hexane-EtOAc, 9:1, 20.7 mg), **Fr C** (*n*-hexane-EtOAc, 8:2, 143.1 mg), **Fr D** (*n*-hexane-EtOAc, 7:3, 284.5 mg), **Fr E** (*n*-hexane-EtOAc, 6:4, 32.6 mg), **Fr F** (*n*-hexane-EtOAc, 4:6, 35.5 mg), **Fr G** (*n*-hexane-EtOAc, 2:8, 6.6 mg), **Fr H** (EtOAc, 2.5 mg), and **Fr I** (MeOH-EtOAc, 1:1, 207.7 mg). **Fr D** contained pure sargahydroquinoic acid (SHQA, **1**, 284.5 mg, 30% extracted yield). Normal phase HPLC of **Fr B** (20.7 mg) using *n*-hexane/EtOAc (9:1) yielded sargaquinal (**4**, 3.0 mg, 15.4% dry weight). **Fr F** contained pure fucoxanthin (**3**, 35.5 mg, 3.74% extracted yield). The structures for compounds **1**, **3**, and **4** were confirmed by spectroscopic methods consistent with previously reported data [17,18]. A summary of the isolation process (Scheme S1) as well as the NMR spectra for compounds **1** (Figures S2 and S3), **4** (Figures S4 and S5) and **3** (Figures S6 and S7) are provided in the Supplementary Materials.

2.4. Semi-Synthetic Derivatization of Sargahydroquinoic Acid (1) Analogs

2.4.1. Oxidation of Sargahydroquinonic Acid (**1**) to Sargaquinoic Acid (**2**)

As previously reported [19].

2.4.2. Conversion of Sargahydroquinoic Acid (**1**) to Sarganaphthoquinoic Acid (**5**)

As previously reported [19].

2.4.3. Conversion of Sargaquinoic Acid (**2**) to Sargachromenoic Acid (**6**)

As previously reported [19]. The ^1H NMR spectra for compounds **2**, **5** and **6** (Figure S2) and a summary of their derivatization (Scheme S2) are provided in the Supplementary Materials.

2.5. Anti-Inflammatory Assay

The murine peritoneal macrophage cells (RAW267.4) were cultured in DMEM containing 10 % FCS. Cells were seeded into 96 well plates at a density of 8×10^4 cells/well and allowed to attach overnight. The cells were then treated with 1 μg/mL of bacterial lipopolysaccharide (LPS) (SIGMA®) and two concentrations of the test sample (12.5 and 25 μg/mL) for 18 h. To measure nitrate levels, 50 μL of the spent culture medium was removed and added to an equal volume of Griess reagent (SIGMA®). The absorbance was measured at 540 nm using a microplate reader and the nitrate concentrations were calculated by comparison with the absorbance to sodium nitrate standard solutions. Aminogaunidine (Sigma®) was used as positive control to demonstrate the inhibition of nitrate production. Cell viability was simultaneously measured using the standard MTT assay.

2.6. 2,2-diphenyl-1-picrylhydrazyl (DPPH) Radical Scavenging Assay

Test samples were diluted in EtOH/H_2O (1:1) from 10 mg/100 μL stocks prepared in DMSO. A total of 5 μL of each sample was placed into each well of a 96-well plate, followed by the addition of 120 μL of Tris-HCl buffer (50 mM, pH7.4) and 120 μL of freshly prepared DPPH solution (0.1 mM in EtOH). The plate was incubated for 20 min at room temperature, with the absorbance read at 513 nm. The percentage of DPPH radical scavenging was calculated as $((A - B/A) \times 100)$ where A represents the absorbance in the absence of test samples and B represents the absorbance in the presence of test samples. Ascorbic acid was used as a positive control (EC_{50} = 24.07 μg/mL).

2.7. 3-(4,5-dimethylthiazol-2-yl)-2,5-diphenyltetrazolium Bromide (MTT) Cytotoxicity Assay

HT-29 and Caco-2 cells were seeded into 96-well culture plates (TTP) at 5 000 cells/well in DMEM supplemented with 10% fetal bovine serum (FBS) and left for 24 h. Algal extracts were added and the cells incubated for a further 48 h, after which the medium was replaced with 200 μL MTT (Sigma®) (0.5 mg/mL in DMEM). After 3 h of incubation at 37 °C, the MTT was removed and the purple formazan product dissolved in 200 μL DMSO.

HeLa derivative cells were seeded into 96-well culture plates (TTP) at 10,000 cells/well in EMEM supplemented with 10% fetal bovine serum (FBS) and left for 24 h. Algal extracts and compounds were added and the cells incubated for a further 48 h after which the medium was replaced with 200 μL of MTT (Sigma®) (0.5 mg/mL in EMEM). After a further 2 h of incubation at 37 °C, the MTT was removed and the purple formazan product dissolved in 200 μL of DMSO.

Absorbance was measured at 560 nm using a multiwell scanning spectrophotometer (Multiscan MS, Labsystems). All incubation steps were carried out in a 37 °C humidified incubator with 5% CO_2. IC_{50} and EC_{50} values were calculated from a minimum 5-point dose-response curves using the GraphPad Prism 4 software package.

2.8. 3T3-L1 Preadipocyte Differentiation Assay

Prior to the induction of differentiation, 3T3-L1 cells were routinely maintained in DMEM containing newborn calf serum. Cells were seeded at a density of 3000 cells/well into 96-well plates and allowed to reach 100% confluence. Two days post-confluence, the cells were treated for a further two days with DMEM medium, now supplemented with FBS (to induce mitotic clonal expansion) and the indicated concentrations of test compounds or the control substances rosiglitazone and troglitazone (1 μM, final concentration). Cells were then cultured for an additional 7 days in normal culture medium (DMEM, 10% FBS with inducers) and the medium replaced every two to three days. Triglyceride accumulation, a marker for adipocyte differentiation, was measured by Oil red-O staining. The Oil Red-O stained lipids were extracted in isopropanol and measured at 510 nm. The sample results were then compared to controls using a two-tailed Student's t-test assuming equal variances.

3. Results

3.1. Anti-Inflammatory Potential of S. incisifolium

S. incisifolium fractions were evaluated for anti-inflammatory activity. Fractions **Fr C**, **Fr D** (SHQA, **1**), and **Fr F** (fucoxanthin, **3**) produced a significant decrease in LPS-stimulated nitrate production at both test concentrations, with **Fr C** being relatively less potent by only having a significant effect at the highest test concentration (Figure 2). SHQA (**1**) significantly attenuated nitrate production, indicating that this compound may also be considered to possess anti-inflammatory properties. Under the conditions of the anti-inflammatory assay there was no evidence for cytotoxicity toward the RAW 267.4 cells and, thus, it can be assumed that the inhibition of nitrate production was not due to differences in the relative cytotoxicity. In naïve cells, i.e., in the absence of LPS, no response was induced by any of the samples.

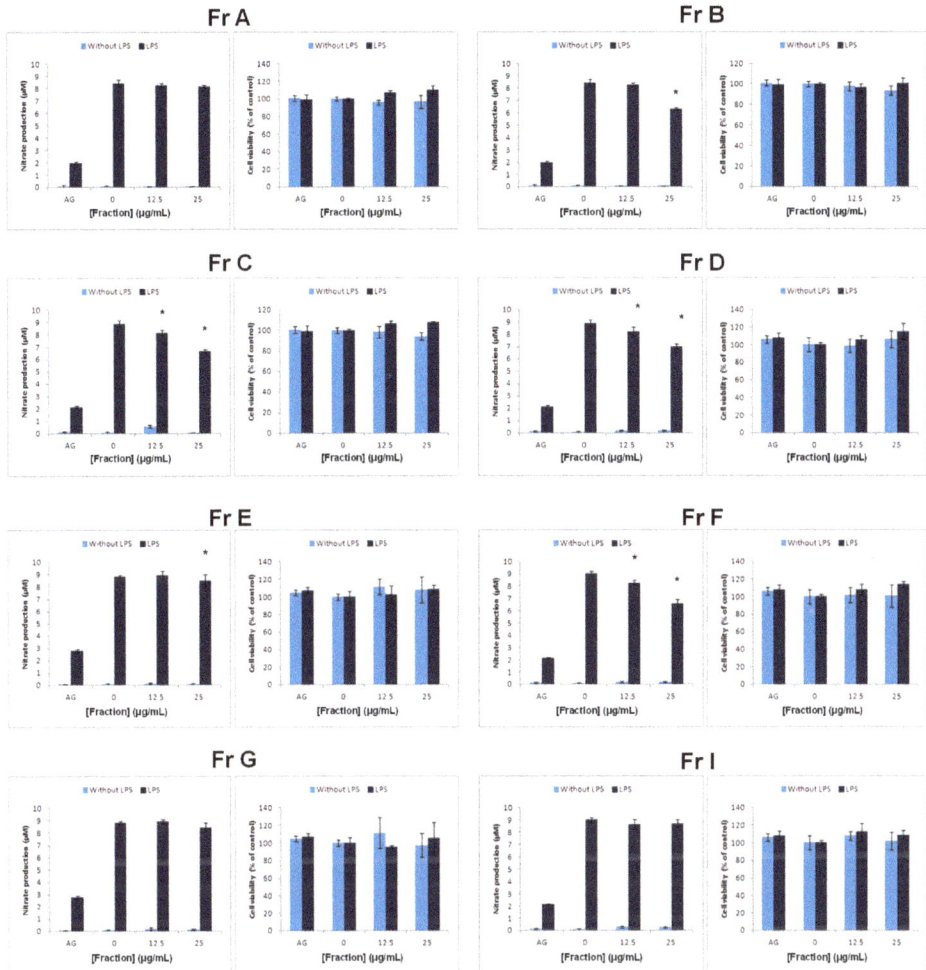

Figure 2. Nitrate production in LPS activated and naïve RAW 264.7 macrophages treated with *S. incisifolium* fractions **Fr A–I**. Aminogaunidine (AG) was used as positive control. Data represents the mean $\pm$ SD (n = 4). Significant ($p < 0.05$) reductions in the levels of nitrate are indicated as (*).

3.2. Antioxidant Activity of S. incisifolium Fractions, Metabolites, and Derivatives

S. incisifolium crude fractions were evaluated for DPPH radical scavenging activity using ascorbic acid as the standard. **Fr C** (EC_{50} = 19.48 µg/mL), **Fr D** (SHQA, **1**) (EC_{50} = 4.01 µg/mL), and **Fr E** (EC_{50} = 3.32 µg/mL) exhibited strong DPPH radical scavenging activity more potent than ascorbic acid (EC_{50} = 24.07 µg/mL) (Table 1). There should be background fucoxanthin absorbance in **Fr F**, which would interfere with the DPPH quantification and, as such, it was not possible to reliably determine its antioxidant activity under these experimental conditions. However, extensive research has already been undertaken to show, among many others, the anti-oxidant, anti-inflammatory and anticancer activity of fucoxanthin (**3**) [20]. SCA (**6**, EC_{50} = 6.99 µg/mL) and SHQA (**1**, EC_{50} = 4.01 µg/mL) exhibited stronger DPPH radical scavenging activity than ascorbic acid. SNQA (**5**, EC_{50} = 226.5 µg/mL) showed the least DPPH radical scavenging activity. The DPPH titration curves for fractions **FrA-G** (Figure S8) and compounds **1** and **6** (Figure S9) are provided in the Supplementary Materials.

Table 1. DPPH radical scavenging activity of *S. incisifolium* fractions, compounds and analogs.

Fraction/Compound	EC$_{50}$ (µg/mL)
Ascorbic Acid	24.7
Fr A	>500
Fr B	113.9
Fr C	19.48
Fr D (SHQA, **1**)	4.01
Fr E	3.32
Fr F (fucoxanthin, **3**)	N.D [1]
Fr G	43.14
Sargaquinal (**4**)	N.D [1]
SQA (**2**)	95.76
SNQA (**5**)	226.5
SCA (**6**)	6.99

[1] N.D = Not determined.

3.3. Cytotoxicity of S. incisifolium Fractions Against HT-29 and Caco-2 Cancer Cells

Cytotoxicity towards HT-29 and Caco-2 colorectal cancer cell lines was evaluated for *S. incisifolium* extracts. The most cytotoxic *S. incisifolium* fractions yielded IC$_{50}$ values < 50 µg/mL on HT-29 and Caco-2 cells (Table 2). This is consistent with studies that have been done to show the selectivity of *Sargassum* extracts towards HT-29 and Caco-2 cell apoptosis [21]. **Fr F** (fucoxanthin, **3**) was the most potent sample tested. **Fr D**, (SHQA, **1**) was found to be more selective towards Caco-2 than HT-29 cells (SI = 1.97). Taken together these results indicate the presence of multiple cytotoxic compounds in the *S. incisifolium* extract. Dose-response curves showing the inhibition of HeLa (Figure S10), HT-29 (Figure S11) and Caco-2 (Figure S12) cell proliferation by **FrA-I** are provided in the Supplementary Materials.

Table 2. Cytotoxicity of *S. incisifolium* fractions against proliferating HT-29 and Caco-2 cells. IC$_{50}$ values as determined using MTT viability assay after 48 h of treatment.

Fraction/Compound	IC$_{50}$ (µg/mL)		Selectivity Index *
	HT-29	**Caco-2**	
Fr A	150.2	126.8	1.2
Fr B	25.9	14.06	1.8
Fr C	35.06	23.12	1.5
Fr D (SHQA, **1**)	114.8	58.25	1.97
Fr E	369.5	114.1	3.2
Fr F (fucoxanthin, **3**)	19.83	14.82	1.3
Fr G	116.5	117.6	1.0
Fr I	Non-toxic	Non-toxic	-

* Selectivity index: IC$_{50}$ (HT-29)/IC$_{50}$ (Caco-2).

3.4. PPAR-γ Agonist Activity of SHQA (1) and Derivatives

Adipocyte differentiation can be used as a convenient indicator of PPAR-γ activation, due to its essential role in adipogenesis [22]. The most significant PPAR-γ response was observed with SNQA (**5**). At test concentrations of 1 µg/mL (0.24 µM) and 5 µg/mL (1.19 µM), SNQA (**5**) produced a response similar to that of rosiglitazone at 1 µM (Figures 3 and 4). SCA (**6**) also induced a strong PPAR-γ response, but it was only significant at 5 µg/mL (1.14 µM). The PPAR-γ activity of SHQA (**1**) was weakly positive at 5 µg/mL (1.17 µM) while SQA (**2**) did not reveal any PPAR-γ activity at all test concentrations. To our knowledge, this is the first report on the PPAR-γ activity of SNQA (**5**).

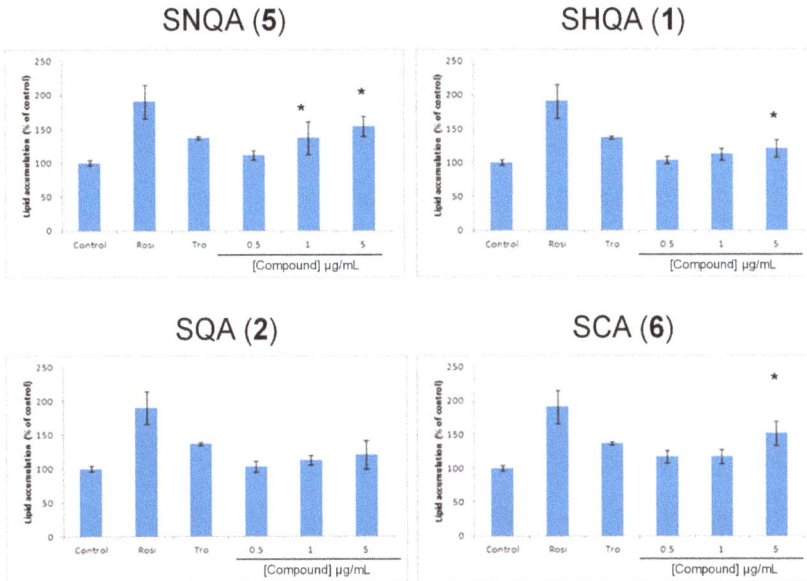

Figure 3. Dose-dependent lipid accumulation in differentiating 3T3-L1 cells after treatment with sargahydroquinoic acid (**1**), sargaquinoic acid (**2**), sarganaphthoquinoic acid (**5**), and sargachromenoic acid (**6**). A total of 1 µM each of rosiglitazone (Rosi) and troglitazone (Tro) was used as positive control. Each data point represents the mean ± SD (n = 3) while the asterisks (*) indicate a significant increase in lipid accumulation.

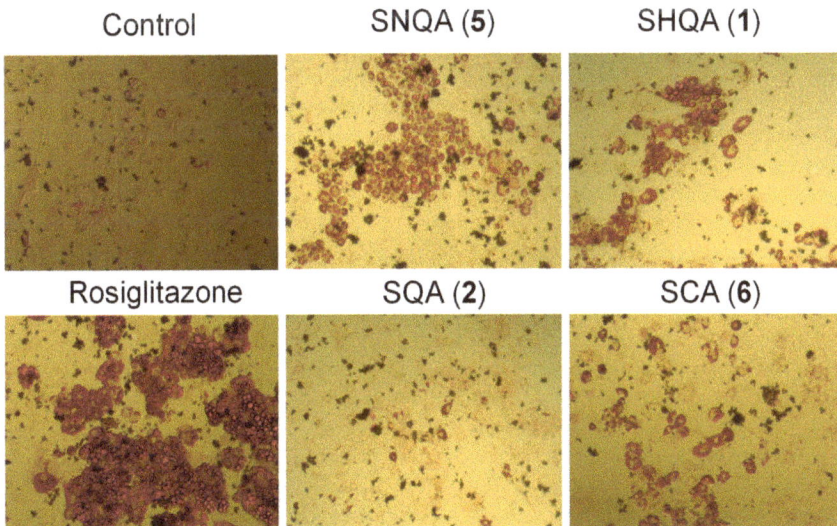

Figure 4. Representative images of oil red O stained 3T3-L1 cells after treatment with sargahydroquinoic acid (**1**), sargaquinoic acid (**2**), sarganaphthoquinoic acid (**5**), sargachromenoic acid (**6**) and rosiglitazone. Original magnification 200×.

Fucoxanthin (**3**) and sargaquinal (**4**) showed the strongest cytotoxic activity against HeLa cells with IC_{50} values of 12.11 and 13.59 µg/mL respectively (Table 3). SHQA (**1**) (IC_{50} = 43.16 µg/mL) showed similar activity compared to SNQA (**5**) (IC_{50} = 43.50 µg/mL) and SCA (**6**) (IC_{50} = 53.56 µg/mL), but stronger than its quinone congener, SQA (**2**) (IC_{50} = 92.85 µg/mL). Dose-response curves for the inhibition of HeLa derivative cells (Figure S13) are provided in the Supplementary Materials.

Table 3. Cytotoxicity assay results for compounds **1–6** against HeLa derivative cells.

Compound	HeLa IC_{50} (µg/mL)
SHQA (**1**)	43.16
SQA (**2**)	92.85
Fucoxanthin (**3**)	12.11
Sargaquinal (**4**)	13.59
SNQA (**5**)	43.50
SCA (**6**)	53.56

4. Discussion

Phytochemical analysis of the major fractions obtained from *S. incisifolium* dichloromethane extract identified SHQA (**1**), SQA (**2**), fucoxanthin (**3**), and sargaquinal (**4**) as the most prominent metabolites present. These represent common constituents often reported to occur in *Sargassum* species. While the biological properties of fucoxanthin (**3**) are plentifully described in the literature, SHQA (**1**), SQA (**2**), and sargaquinal (**4**) remain poorly explored.

Considering that inflammation represents the predominant therapeutic target against IBD [3], the anti-inflammatory potential of the fractions was investigated using LPS activated RAW 264.7 macrophages as a model. Both SHQA (**1**) and fucoxanthin (**3**) revealed a concentration-dependent inhibition in nitrate production, indicating potential anti-inflammatory activity. Concurrent cell viability measurements confirmed that these effects were not due to cytotoxicity. The anti-inflammatory activity of fucoxanthin (**3**) is in accord with previous studies [20]. Similarly, research on the anti-inflammatory activity of plastoquinone derivatives isolated from natural sources also reported that SHQA (**1**) significantly reduced TPA-induced mouse ear oedema [23]. The precise mechanism through which SHQA (**1**) exerts this anti-inflammatory response however awaits further studies. Our results suggest that SHQA (**1**) may, at least in part, directly target macrophage function. In contrast to the anti-inflammatory activity, treatment of naïve RAW 264.7 cells did not reveal any potential risk to induce a pro-inflammatory effect, which could exacerbate inflammation.

Oxidative stress is currently considered as a contributory factor in the initiation, progression, and severity of IBD and is regarded as more than just a simple consequence of chronic inflammation associated with the disease. Although the underlying mechanisms are yet to be thoroughly elucidated, strategies to reduce oxidative stress are anticipated to improve therapeutic outcome. Antioxidants, especially those derived from natural products, have attracted attention as acceptable ingredients to target oxidative stress in IBD [4]. Compounds with dual anti-inflammatory and antioxidant activity may be particularly relevant to the treatment of IBD. The DPPH radical scavenging activity of SHQA (**1**) and SCA (**6**) has been previously documented [23]. Reduced forms of vitamin E and coenzyme Q groups, such as hydroquinones, chromanols, and chromenols normally function as protective anti-oxidants. However, the ability of such compounds to function in these capacities of electron transfer and antioxidant activity directly depend upon the oxidation potential of the compound, which is also partly dependent upon the nuclear substituents [24]. Not surprisingly, SHQA (**1**) showed more potent DPPH radical scavenging activity than SQA (**2**, EC_{50} = 95.76 µg/mL), as it is generally known that hydroquinones are more potent radical scavengers than their quinone congeners. We, therefore, identify SHQA (**1**) as an anti-inflammatory compound with potent radical scavenging activity. In the DPPH assay, SHQA (**1**) was greater than 5-fold more active relative to the standard antioxidant, ascorbic acid.

It is well recognised that patients with IBD show a higher incidence of developing colon cancer [4], primarily believed to be the result of chronic intestinal inflammation. Subsequently, many IBD patients also develop the requirement for cancer therapy, which is accompanied by unique challenges associated with this comorbidity. Often chemotherapeutic drugs damage the intestine, resulting in the remission of IBD. It thus follows that although cytotoxicity towards cancer cells may have an advantage in cancer treatment, it is also at risk of aggravating intestinal inflammation and thus, IBD. Evaluation of the fractions obtained from *S. incisifolium* revealed significant toxicity towards colon cancer cell lines Caco-2 and HT-29 with fucoxanthin (**3**) being the most potent. This is consistent with previous studies which report fucoxanthin (**3**) to inhibit the proliferation of HT-29 and Caco-2 cells through inducing cell cycle arrest in the Go/G1 phase at low concentrations (25 μM) and apoptosis at higher concentrations [25]. SHQA (**1**) was also significantly cytotoxic towards these colon cancer cells.

The adipocyte has been described as "a dynamic cell that plays a fundamental role in energy balance and overall body homeostasis" [26]. The formation of adipocytes (adipogenesis) is a differentiation process governed by transcriptional cascades involving a regulated set of gene expression events [22]. The peroxisome proliferator-activated receptor gamma (PPAR-γ) has been termed as the 'master regulator' of adipogenesis sufficient to differentiate fibroblasts into mature adipocytes [27]. The PPAR-γ is therefore not only crucial for adipogenesis but is also a requirement for the maintenance of the differentiated state. Hence, a compound or extract that stimulates the differentiation of preadipocytes into mature adipocytes is considered as a PPAR-γ agonist. The PPAR-γ is predominantly expressed in adipose tissue with lower levels of expression in other tissues, such as cardiac, renal, and hepatic tissues [28]. The association of PPAR-γ activation and consequent adipogenesis with an increase in tissue insulin sensitivity provided the basis for the development of thiazolidinediones as a class of anti-diabetic drugs. Other known PPAR isoforms include α and β/δ, for which dual and pan agonists have been identified.

The high relative expression of PPAR-γ in the colon has stimulated many studies on the role of PPAR-γ in gut health. While early studies focused heavily on the involvement of PPAR-γ in the process of colonic tumor suppression, more recently, research has expanded to include intestinal inflammation and fibrosis, major factors in the pathogenesis of IBD. Identification of the direct involvement of PPAR-γ in the mechanism of action of mesalazine, a clinically effective drug often used to treat ulcerative colitis, has highlighted the anti-inflammatory role of PPAR-γ and renewed the search for novel PPAR-γ agonists to treat IBD [9]. Fibrosis, excessive deposition of extracellular matrix components including collagen, is a common complication of IBD, leading to obstruction and loss of function of the intestine. PPAR-γ agonists can diminish fibrogenesis through the antagonist effects on TGF signalling. Given that the anti-inflammatory drugs currently used to treat IBD are unable to attenuate intestinal fibrosis, new therapeutic approaches are sought with PPAR-γ agonists holding considerable promise. Taken together, it is clear that PPAR-γ has again emerged as an important therapeutic target for the development of new drugs to treat IBD.

Previously Kim et al. demonstrated that SHQA (**1**) and SQA (**2**) could activate PPAR-γ [29]. However, under our experimental conditions, only SHQA (**1**) revealed a statistically significant enhancement in 3T3-L1 differentiation, a marker for PPAR-γ agonist activity. Considering that Kim et al. [29] used 10 μM each of SHQA (**1**) and SQA (**2**) for the induction of differentiation while we used a maximum of 1.17 μM of SHQA (**1**) and 1.18 μM of SQA (**2**), it is highly possible that increasing the test concentrations would also result in an increased PPAR-γ activity of these compounds. To further explore SHQA (**1**) as a potential chemical scaffold in the development of new PPAR-γ agonists, we synthesized derivatives of SHQA (**1**), namely sargaquinoic acid (SQA, **2**), sarganaphthoquinoic acid (SNQA, **5**), and sargachromenoic acid (SCA, **6**). The most significant response was obtained from SNQA (**5**), which at test concentrations of 1 μg/mL (0.24 μM) and 5 μg/mL (1.19 μM), produced a response similar to that of rosiglitazone at 1 μM. SCA (**6**) also induced a PPAR-γ response, but it was only significant at 5 μg/mL (1.14 μM).

The structural derivatives were also evaluated for antioxidant activity and cytotoxicity against HeLa derivative cells. SNQA (**5**) showed a dramatic decrease in radical scavenging activity while SCA (**6**) antioxidant activity remained essentially unchanged. Cytotoxicity towards HeLa derivative cells, a cell line previously shown to be devoid of PPAR-γ protein [30], was unchanged relative to SHQA (**1**).

To our knowledge, this is the first report on the PPAR-γ-mediated activity of SNQA (**5**). In an attempt to improve the side effect profiles of current PPAR-γ agonists, research has explored the replacement of the thiazolidine ring with other 'acidic head groups', which have lesser side effects. Such examples include a study performed by Sundriyal et al. in which, after replacement of the thiazolidine ring with a 1,4-naphthoquinone moiety, the newly synthesized compounds still retained PPAR-γ activity comparable to pioglitazone [31]. This shows that the 1,4-naphthoquinone, SNQA (**5**), is a potential PPAR-γ agonist similar to the well-known thiazolidinediones and supports our findings and potential for the treatment of IBD. Additionally, 1,4-naphthoquinones are commercially available, less costly, and easily derivatized.

5. Conclusions

SHQA (**1**) is identified as a promising lead compound due to its effects on multiple therapeutic targets relevant to IBD. Derivatization to SNQA (**5**) significantly improved the PPAR-activity. However, this dramatically reduced its antioxidant activity and had minimal effect on cytotoxicity.

Supplementary Materials: The following are available online at http://www.mdpi.com/2305-6320/6/2/49/s1, Figure S1: Photograph of *S. incisifolium* specimen used in this study, Figure S2: ^{1}H NMR spectra (CDCl$_3$, 400 MHz) for sargahydroquinoic acid (**1**), sargaquinoic acid (**2**), sargachromenoic acid (**6**) and sarganaphthoquinoic acid (**5**), Figure S3: ^{13}C NMR spectrum (CDCl$_3$, 100 MHz) of sargahydroquinoic acid (**1**), Figure S4: ^{1}H NMR spectrum (CDCl$_3$, 400 MHz) of 10′*E*-sargaquinal (**4**), Figure S5: ^{13}C NMR spectrum (CDCl$_3$, 100 MHz) of 10′*E*-sargaquinal (**4**), Figure S6: ^{1}H NMR spectrum (CDCl$_3$, 400 MHz) of fucoxanthin (**3**), Figure S7: ^{13}C NMR spectrum (CDCl$_3$, 100 MHz) of fucoxanthin (**3**), Figure S8: Titration curves for the DPPH radical scavenging activity of *Sargassum incisifolium* crude fractions **Fr A**, **Fr B**, **Fr C**, **Fr D**, **Fr E** and **Fr G**, Figure S9: Titration curves for the DPPH radical scavenging activity of SHQA (**1**) and SCA (**6**), Figure S10: Dose-dependent inhibition of HeLa cell viability by *S. incisifolium* fractions **Fr A–I**, Figure S11: Dose-dependent inhibition of HT-29 cell viability by *S. incisifolium* fractions, Figure S12: Dose-dependent inhibition of Caco-2 cell viability by *S. incisifolium* fractions, Figure S13: Dose-dependent inhibition of HeLa cell viability by sarganaphthoquinoic acid (**5**), sargahydroquinoic acid (**1**), sargaquinoic acid (**2**) and sargachromenoic acid (**6**), Scheme S1: Isolation of compounds **1**, **3**, and **4** from *S. incisifolium*, Scheme S2: Semi-synthetic derivatization of sargahydroquinoic acid (**1**) analogs; **2**, **5**, and **6**.

Author Contributions: Conceptualization, T.C.K. and D.R.B.; Data curation, M.N.N.; Formal analysis, M.N.N., T.C.K., E.D.G., and D.R.B.; Funding acquisition, M.v.d.V. and D.R.B.; Investigation, M.N.N. and T.C.K.; Methodology, M.N.N., T.C.K., E.D.G., and D.R.B.; Project administration, M.v.d.V. and D.R.B.; Resources, M.v.d.V., E.D.G., and D.R.B.; Supervision, M.v.d.V., E.D.G., and D.R.B.; Writing—original draft, M.N.N., T.C.K., and M.v.d.V.; Writing—review & editing, M.v.d.V. and D.R.B..

Funding: This research was funded by the Beit Trust Scholarship, Rhodes University, and Nelson Mandela University.

Conflicts of Interest: The authors declare no conflict of interest.

References

1. Ng, S.C.; Shi, H.Y.; Hamidi, N.; Underwood, F.E.; Tang, W.; Benchimol, E.I.; Panaccione, R.; Ghosh, S.; Wu, J.C.Y.; Chan, F.K.L.; et al. Worldwide incidence and prevalence of inflammatory bowel disease in the 21st century: A systematic review of population-based studies. *Lancet* **2017**, *390*, 2769–2778. [CrossRef]

2. Duijvestein, M.; Battat, R.; Vande Casteele, N.; D'Haens, G.R.; Sandborn, W.J.; Khanna, R.; Jairath, V.; Feagan, B.G. Novel Therapies and Treatment Strategies for Patients with Inflammatory Bowel Disease. *Curr. Treat. Opt. Gastroenterol.* **2018**, *16*, 129–146. [CrossRef]

3. Verstockt, B.; Ferrante, M.; Vermeire, S.; Van Assche, G. New treatment options for inflammatory bowel disease. *J. Gasteroenterol.* **2018**, *53*, 585–590. [CrossRef] [PubMed]

4. Tian, T.; Wang, Z.; Zhang, J. Pathomechanisms of oxidative stress in inflammatory bowel disease and potential antioxidant therapies. *Oxid. Med. Cell. Longev.* **2017**, *2017*, 1–18. [CrossRef] [PubMed]

5. Su, C.G.; Wen, X.; Bailey, S.T.; Jiang, W.; Rangwala, S.M.; Keilbaugh, S.A.; Flanigan, A.; Murthy, S.; Lazar, M.A.; Wu, G.D. A novel therapy for colitis utilizing PPAR-γ ligands to inhibit the epithelial inflammatory response. *J. Clin. Investig.* **1999**, *104*, 383–389. [CrossRef] [PubMed]

6. Dubuquoy, L.; Rousseaux, C.; Thuru, X.; Peyrin-Biroulet, L.; Romano, O.; Chavatte, P.; Chamaillard, M.; Desreumaux, P. PPARγ as a new therapeutic target in inflammatory bowel diseases. *Gut* **2006**, *55*, 1341–1349. [CrossRef]

7. Annese, V.; Rogai, F.; Settesoldi, A.; Bagnoli, S. PPARγ in inflammatory bowel disease. *PPAR Res.* **2012**, *2012*, 1–9. [CrossRef]

8. Wang, X.; Sun, Y.; Zhao, Y.; Ding, Y.; Zhang, X.; Kong, L.; Li, Z.; Guo, Q.; Zhao, L. Oroxyloside prevents dextran sulfate sodium-induced experimental colitis in mice by inhibiting NF-ḳB pathway through PPARγ activation. *Biochem. Pharmacol.* **2016**, *106*, 70–81. [CrossRef]

9. Schwab, M.; Reynders, V.; Loitsch, S.; Shastri, Y.M.; Steinhilber, D.; Schröder, O.; Stein, J. PPARγ is involved in mesalazine-mediated induction of apoptosis and inhibition of cell growth in colon cancer cells. *Carcinogenesis* **2008**, *29*, 1407–1414. [CrossRef] [PubMed]

10. Stolfi, C.; Pallone, F.; Monteleone, G. Colorectal cancer chemoprevention by mesalazine and its derivatives. *J. Biomed. Biotech.* **2012**, *2012*, 1–6. [CrossRef] [PubMed]

11. Harvey, A.; Edrada-Ebel, R.; Quinn, R.J. The re-emergence of natural products for drug discovery in the genomics era. *Nat. Rev. Drug Discov.* **2015**, *14*, 111–129. [CrossRef] [PubMed]

12. Dias, D.A.; Urban, S.; Roessner, U. A historical overview of natural products in drug discovery. *Metabolites* **2012**, *2*, 303–336. [CrossRef]

13. Poornima, P.; Kumar, J.D.; Zhao, Q.; Blunder, M.; Efferth, T. Network pharmacology of cancer: From understanding of complex interactomes to the design of multi-target specific therapeutics from nature. *Pharmacol. Res.* **2016**, *111*, 290–302. [CrossRef] [PubMed]

14. Mattio, L.; Anderson, R.J.; Bolton, J.J. A revision of the genus Sargassum (Fucales, Phaeophyceae) in South Africa. *S. Afr. J. Bot.* **2015**, *98*, 95–107. [CrossRef]

15. Mmola, M.; Le Roes-Hill, M.; Durrell, K.; Bolton, J.J.; Sibuyi, N.; Meyer, M.E.; Beukes, D.R.; Antunes, E. Enhanced antimicrobial and anticancer activity of silver and gold nanoparticles synthesised using *Sargassum incisifolium* aqueous extracts. *Molecules* **2016**, *21*, 1633. [CrossRef]

16. Afolayan, F.; Bolton, J.; Lategan, A.; Smith, P.; Beukes, D. Fucoxanthin, Tetraprenylated Toluquinone and Toluhydroquinone Metabolites from Sargassum heterophyllum Inhibit the in vitro Growth of the Malaria Parasite Plasmodium falciparum. *Z. Naturforsch.* **2008**, *63*, 848–852. [CrossRef]

17. Kusumi, T.; Shibata, Y.; Ishitsuka, M.; Kinoshita, T.; Kakisawa, H. Structures of new plastoquinones from the brown alga Sargassum serratifolium. *Chem. Lett.* **1979**, *8*, 277–278. [CrossRef]

18. Mori, K.; Ooi, T.; Hiraoka, M.; Oka, N.; Hamada, H.; Tamura, M.; Kusumi, T. Fucoxanthin and Its Metabolites in Edible Brown Algae Cultivated in Deep Seawater. *Mar. Drugs* **2004**, *2*, 63–72. [CrossRef]

19. Munedzimwe, T.C.; van Zyl, R.L.; Heslop, D.C.; Edkins, A.L.; Beukes, D.R. Semi-synthesis and evaluation of sargahydroquinoic acid derivatives as potential antimalarial agents. *Medicines* **2019**, *6*, 47. [CrossRef]

20. Peng, J.; Yuan, J.; Wu, C.; Wang, J. Fucoxanthin, a marine carotenoid present in brown seaweeds and diatoms: Metabolism and bioactivities relevant to human health. *Mar. Drugs* **2011**, *9*, 1806–1828. [CrossRef]

21. Khanavi, M.; Nabavi, M.; Sadati, N.; Ardekani, M.S.; Sohrabipour, J.; Nabavi, S.M.; Ghaeli, P.; Ostad, S.N. Cytotoxic activity of some marine brown algae against cancer cell lines. *Biol. Res.* **2010**, *43*, 31–37. [CrossRef] [PubMed]

22. Moseti, D.; Regassa, A.; Kim, W.K. Molecular regulation of adipogenesis and potential anti-adipogenic bioactive molecules. *Int. J. Mol. Sci.* **2016**, *17*, 124. [CrossRef] [PubMed]

23. Pérez-Castorena, A.L.; Arciniegas, A.; Apan, M.T.; Villaseñor, J.L.; de Vivar, A.R. Evaluation of the anti-inflammatory and antioxidant activities of the plastoquinone derivatives isolated from *Roldana barba-johannis*. *Planta Medica* **2002**, *68*, 645–647. [CrossRef]

24. Moore, H.W.; Schwab, D.E.; Folkers, K. Coenzyme, Q. LVII. Synthesis of new analogs of coenzyme Q4 for biochemical mechanism studies. *Biochemistry* **1964**, *3*, 1586–1588. [CrossRef]

25. Das, S.K.; Hashimoto, T.; Shimizu, K.; Yoshida, T.; Sakai, T.; Sowa, Y.; Komoto, A.; Kanazawa, K. Fucoxanthin induces cell cycle arrest at G0/G1 phase in human colon carcinoma cells through up-regulation of p21WAF1/Cip1. *Biochim. Biophys. Acta (BBA)—Gen. Subj.* **2005**, *1726*, 328–335. [CrossRef]

26. Bernlohr, D.A.; Jenkins, A.E.; Benaars, A.A. Adipose tissue and lipid metabolism. In *Biochemistry of Lipids, Lipoproteins and Membranes*, 4th ed.; Vance, D.E., Vance, J.E., Eds.; Elsevier Science B. V.: Amsterdam, The Netherlands, 2002; pp. 263–289.
27. Ma, X.; Wang, D.; Zhao, W.; Xu, L. Deciphering the Roles of PPARγ in Adipocytes via Dynamic Change of Transcription Complex. *Front. Endocrinol.* **2018**, *9*, 473. [CrossRef] [PubMed]
28. Janani, C.; Ranjitha, K.B.D. PPAR gamma gene: A review. *Diabetes Metab. Syndr. Clin. Res. Rev.* **2015**, *9*, 46–50. [CrossRef] [PubMed]
29. Kim, S.N.; Choi, H.Y.; Lee, W.; Park, G.M.; Shin, W.S.; Kim, Y.K. Sargaquinoic acid and sargahydroquinoic acid from *Sargassum yezoense* stimulate adipocyte differentiation through PPARα/γ activation in 3T3-L1 cells. *FEBS Lett.* **2008**, *582*, 3465–3472. [CrossRef]
30. Lin, Y.; Wang, F.; Yang, L.; Chun, Z.; Bao, J.; Zhang, G. Anti-inflammatory phenanthrene derivatives from stems of *Dendrobium denneanum*. *Phytochemistry* **2013**, *95*, 242–251. [CrossRef]
31. Sundriyal, S.; Viswanad, B.; Bharathy, E.; Ramarao, P.; Chakraborti, A.K.; Bharatam, P.V. New PPARγ ligands based on 2-hydroxy-1,4-naphthoquinone: Computer-aided design, synthesis, and receptor-binding studies. *Bioorgan. Med. Chem. Lett.* **2008**, *18*, 3192–3195. [CrossRef]

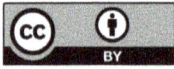

medicines

MDPI

Article

Assessment of Artemisinin Contents in Selected *Artemisia* Species from Tajikistan (Central Asia)

Sodik Numonov [1,2,3], **Farukh Sharopov** [1,2,4], **Aminjon Salimov** [5], **Parviz Sukhrobov** [2], **Sunbula Atolikshoeva** [2], **Ramazon Safarzoda** [4], **Maidina Habasi** [1,2,*] and **Haji Akber Aisa** [2,*]

[1] Research Institution "Chinese-Tajik Innovation Center for Natural Products" of the Tajikistan Academy of Sciences, Ayni str. 299/2, Dushanbe 734063, Tajikistan; sodikjon82@gmail.com (S.N.); shfarukh@mail.ru (F.S.)

[2] Key Laboratory of Plant Resources and Chemistry in Arid Regions, Xinjiang Technical Institute of Physics and Chemistry, Chinese Academy of Sciences, Urumqi 830011, China; parviz@gmail.com (P.S.); sunbula87@mail.ru (S.A.)

[3] Center for Research in Innovative Technologies, Academy of Sciences of the Republic of Tajikistan, Dushanbe 734062, Tajikistan

[4] Department of Pharmaceutical Technology, Avicenna Tajik State Medical University, Rudaki 139, Dushanbe 734003, Tajikistan; safarzoda90@yandex.ru

[5] V.I. Nikitin Institute of Chemistry of the Tajikistan Academy of Sciences, Ayni str. 299/2, Dushanbe 734063, Tajikistan; amin-jon-86@mail.ru

* Correspondence: maidn@ms.xjb.ac.cn (M.H.); haji@ms.xjb.ac.cn (H.A.A.);
  Tel.: +86-991-3835679 (M.H. & H.A.A.); Fax: +86-991-3838957 (M.H. & H.A.A.)

Received: 15 January 2019; Accepted: 31 January 2019; Published: 31 January 2019

Abstract: Background: Central Asia is the center of origin and diversification of the *Artemisia* genus. The genus *Artemisia* is known to possess a rich phytochemical diversity. Artemisinin is the shining example of a phytochemical isolated from *Artemisia annua*, which is widely used in the treatment of malaria. There is great interest in the discovery of alternative sources of artemisinin in other *Artemisia* species. **Methods:** The hexane extracts of *Artemisia* plants were prepared with ultrasound-assisted extraction procedures. Silica gel was used as an adsorbent for the purification of *Artemisia annua* extract. High-performance liquid chromatography with ultraviolet detection was performed for the quantification of underivatized artemisinin from hexane extracts of plants. **Results:** Artemisinin was found in seven *Artemisia* species collected from Tajikistan. Content of artemisinin ranged between 0.07% and 0.45% based on dry mass of *Artemisia* species samples. **Conclusions:** The artemisinin contents were observed in seven *Artemisia* species. *A. vachanica* was found to be a novel plant source of artemisinin. Purification of *A. annua* hexane extract using silica gel as adsorbent resulted in enrichment of artemisinin.

Keywords: *Artemisia* species; *Artemisia vachanica*; artemisinin; HPLC-PAD; Tajikistan

---

1. Introduction

As reported by the World Health Organization (WHO), in the last four years (2015–2018), nearly half of the population of the world (3.2 billion people) was at risk of malaria. In 2017, there were 435,000 deaths from malaria globally, 61% (266,000) of which were of children younger than five years [1].

At present, artemisinin-based combination treatments are effective and accepted as being among the best malaria treatments [2]. Artemisinin is the bioactive compound produced by the plant *Artemisia annua* L. Artemisinin has saved the lives of millions of malarial patients worldwide and served as the standard regimen for treating *Plasmodium falciparum* infection [3].

With 500 species, the genus *Artemisia* L. is the largest and the most widely distributed genus of the Asteraceae, and Central Asia is the center of origin and diversification of the genus [4]. Many

Artemisia species grow in Tajikistan [5]. The genus *Artemisia* is known to possess rich phytochemical diversity [6–9]. Almost 600 secondary metabolites have been characterized from *A. annua* alone [10].

Artemisinin is the shining example of a phytochemical isolated from *A. annua*, and is widely used in the treatment of malaria. Artemisinin is a natural sesquiterpene lactone with an unusual 1,2,4-trioxane substructure (Figure 1). It is soluble in most aprotic solvents and is poorly soluble in water. It decomposes in protic solvents, probably by the opening of the lactone ring [11]. The artemisinin biosynthesis proceeds via the tertiary allylic hydroperoxide, which is derived from the oxidation of dihydroartemisinic acid [10].

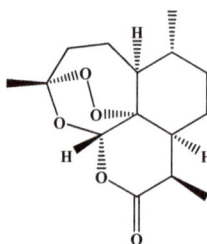

Figure 1. Artemisinin structure.

The mechanism of artemisinin action is controversial [12,13]. It is related to the presence of an endoperoxide bridge, which by breaking creates a powerful free radical form of the artemisinin, which attacks the parasite proteins without harming the host [14].

The presence of artemisinin has been reported in many *Artemisia* species, including *A. absinthium*, *A. anethifolia*, *A. anethoides*, *A. austriaca*, *A. aff. tangutica*, *A. annua*, *A. apiacea*, *A. bushriences*, *A. campestris*, *A. cina*, *A. ciniformis*, *A. deserti*, *A. diffusa*, *A. dracunculus*, *A. dubia*, *A. incana*, *A. indica*, *A. fragrans*, *A. frigida*, *A. gmelinii*, *A. japonica*, *A. khorassanica*, *A. kopetdaghensis*, *A. integrifolia*, *A. lancea*, *A. macrocephala*, *A. marschalliana*, *A. messerschmidtiana*, *A. moorcroftiana*, *A. parviflora*, *A. pallens*, *A. roxburghiana*, *A. scoparia*, *A. sieberi*, *A. sieversiana*, *A. spicigeria*, *A. thuscula*, *A. tridentata*, *A. vestita*, and *A. vulgaris* [9,15–32].

The chemical structure of artemisinin provided a foundation for several synthetic antimalarial drugs including pyronaridine, lumefantrine (benflumetol), naphthoquine, and so on [33]. Recently, research interest in biotechnological approaches for enhanced artemisinin production in *Artemisia* have increased due to the global needs and low amounts of artemisinin and its derivatives in *Artemisia* plants [34]. Various biotechnological approaches such as the transformation of genes for production of artemisinin to cells of eukaryotic and prokaryotic organisms and to genetically engineered yeast were developed to enhance the production of artemisinin and its derivatives [35–38].

In addition, artemisinin and its bioactive derivatives have a second career as antitumor agents [39]. They demonstrated high efficiency against a variety of cancer cells, with minor side effects to normal cells in cancer patients [40,41]. The investigation of the biological activity of *Artemisia* species and their constituents is required to explore the full potential of diverse *Artemisia* species and their chemical ingredients against cancer, malaria, and infections [42]. Artemisinin can also exert beneficial effects in treatment of the wide-spectrum diseases such as obesity, diabetes, and aging-related disorders [43].

Natural conditions influence the biotransformation and accumulation of artemisinin in plants. For example, Ferreira et al. reported that that biosynthesis of artemisinin is affected by light intensity [44]. The relatively large number of sunny days per year in Tajikistan is essential for artemisinin accumulation in *Artemisia* species.

Accordingly, there is great interest in the discovery of artemisinin in *Artemisia* species growing wild in Tajikistan. The purpose of the current investigation was to evaluate the presence of artemisinin in eight *Artemisia* species.

2. Materials and Methods

2.1. Plant Materials

The aerial parts of eight *Artemisia* species including *A. annua*, *A. vachanica*, *A. vulgaris*, *A. makrocephala*, *A. leucotricha*, *A. dracunculus*, *A. absinthium*, and *A. scoparia* were collected during their vegetative and flowering period from three regions of Tajikistan. The voucher specimen numbers, local names, collection time, and location of plants are summarized in Table 1. These species were identified with regards to specimens in the herbarium of the Institute of Botany, Plant Physiology and Genetics of Tajikistan Academy of Sciences. The voucher specimens of the plant material were deposited at the Chinese-Tajik Innovation Center for Natural Products research institution of the Tajikistan Academy of Sciences.

Table 1. *Artemisia* species collected from Tajikistan.

Species	Local Name	Collection Site	Time	Voucher Number
A. annua	говчорӯб (govjorub), бургун (burghun)	Ziddeh, Varzob Region	15.07.2018	CTICNPG 2018 - 5
A. vachanica	пуши оддӣ (pushi oddi)	Khaskhorugh, Ishkoshim Region	25.08.2018	CTICNPG 2018 - 6
A. vulgaris	сафедчорӯб (safedjorub), явшон (yavshon)	Khaskhorugh, Ishkoshim Region	22.08.2018	CTICNPG 2018 - 7
A. mackrocephala	пуши калонгул (pushi kalongul)	Khaskhorugh, Ishkoshim Region	21.08.2018	CTICNPG 2018 - 8
A. leucotricha	пуши сафед (pushi safed)	Khaskhorugh, Ishkoshim Region	22.08.2018	CTICNPG 2018 - 9
A. dracunculus	тархун (tarkhun), гӯда (ghuda)	Ziddeh, Varzob Region	15.07.2018	CTICNPG 2018 - 10
A. absinthium	тахач (takhach)	Guli Bodom, Yovon Region	20.07.2018	CTICNPG 2018 - 11
A. scoparia	туғак (tughak), маҳинчорӯб (mahinjorub)	Guli Bodom, Yovon Region	20.07.2018	CTICNPG 2018 - 12

2.2. Preparation of Hexane Extracts

The extraction process of dried aerial parts of *Artemisia* plants were prepared by the following procedure: 10 g of plant materials were crushed into smaller pieces and weighed in a 250-mL flask, into which 150 mL of hexane were added at room temperature. The prepared plant mixtures were sonicated in an ultrasonic bath at a frequency of 35 kHz for 15 min at room temperature. Then, plant mixtures were allowed to stand for 12 h at room temperature. After 12 h, they were filtered through Whatman filter paper and used for the designed chemical analysis.

The yield of hexane extracts were calculated using following Equation (1):

$$\omega(\%) = \frac{a * 100\%}{b},\tag{1}$$

where ω is the yield of hexane extract (%), a is the weight of hexane extract; and b is the weight of plant sample.

2.3. Quantitative Analysis of Artemisinin Using HPLC

A number of studies have been addressed for the development of HPLC methodology for quantification of artemisinin in plant material and extracts [44,45]. The best separation of artemisinin was achieved on columns Luna 5 μm C18 250 × 4.6 mm (Phenomenex, Torrance, CA, USA) and Betasil C18 5 μm 250 × 4.6 mm (Thermo Fisher Scientific, Waltham, MA, USA), using acetonitrile:water (65:35, v/v) as the mobile phase [44,45].

In addition, artemisinin analysis by HPLC-PAD at 192 nm, compared to HPLC with evaporative light scattering detection (HPLC-ELSD), was very accurate, precise, and reproducible [44].

Artemisia extracts were analyzed by HPLC UltiMate 3000 system with DAD detector (Thermo Fisher Scientific, Waltham, MA, USA). Extracts of *Artemisia* plants (10 mg/mL) were prepared in methanol and the solution was filtered using a 0.45-μm syringe filter for HPLC analysis. Analysis was performed on a Waters Bridge C18 5 μm (250 × 4.6 mm, Waters, Milford, MA, USA) and XSelect CSH™ C18 5 μm (250 × 4.6 mm, Waters, Milford, MA, USA) columns. The mobile phase consisted of water (A) and acetonitrile (B). The gradient elution program was as follows: 0–7 min, hold 60% of B; 17–30 min, 60–100% of B; 30–35 min, 100% of B. The detection wavelengths were 192, 210, 254, and 320 nm, the flow rate was 1 mL/min, the injection volume was 5 μL, and the oven temperature was set to 30 °C.

Quantification of the artemisinin was performed using a linear calibration graph with increasing amounts of artemisinin and their peak area response with UV detection (192 nm) (Figure 2). Standard solutions with seven different concentrations (between 0.05 and 5 mg/mL) were prepared by solving the standard artemisinin in methanol.

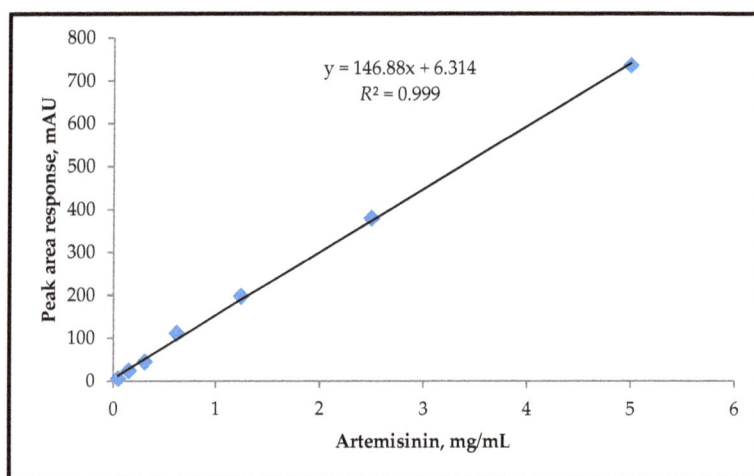

Figure 2. Linear calibration graph for the standard artemisinin.

2.4. Purification of Artemisia annua Extract

Silica gel as adsorbent (10.0 g dry weight) was added to 100 mL of *A. annua* extract (10 mg/mL in hexane) in a 250-mL flask while agitating on a shaker at room temperature until the adsorption reached equilibrium. After reaching the adsorption equilibrium, the silica gel was filtered from the mixture and then washed with hexane 3–4 times until decolorization of the filtrate. The filtrate was evaporated using a rotary evaporator.

3. Results

The yields of hexane extract, number of components detected at 192 nm, and content of artemisinin per dry weight plant are summarized in Table 2. The hexane percentage yield of *Artemisia* species ranged from 2.3% to 8.1%. The hexane extract of *A. vachanica* had the highest yield (8.1%), followed by *A. annua* (5.8%) and *A. absinthium* (5.4%), while *A. vulgaris* had the lowest yield (2.3%). A total of 83, 90, 95, 94, 75, 100, 98, and 90 components (peaks on the chromatograms) were detected in *A. annua*; *A. vachanica*; *A. vulgaris*; *A. makrocephala*; *A. leucotricha*; *A. dracunculus*; *A. absinthium*, and *A. scoparia*, respectively.

Table 2. Extraction yield, componential composition, and artemisinin content in *Artemisia* species.

Species	Yield of Hexane Extract, %	Number of Components	Content of Artemisinin in Dry Weight Plant, %
Artemisia annua	5.80 ± 0.05	83	0.45 ± 0.03
Artemisia vachanica	8.09 ± 0.1	90	0.34 ± 0.02
Artemisia vulgaris	2.32 ± 0.02	95	0.18 ± 0.01
Artemisia makrocephala	3.01 ± 0.02	94	0.20 ± 0.01
Artemisia leucotricha	3.19 ± 0.03	75	Not detected
Artemisia dracunculus	3.78 ± 0.04	100	0.07 ± 0.01
Artemisia absinthium	5.41 ± 0.05	98	0.09 ± 0.01
Artemisia scoparia	3.39 ± 0.02	90	0.11 ± 0.02

The content of artemisinin per dry weight of *Artemisia* species ranged from 0.07% to 0.45%. The highest content of artemisinin was observed in *A. annua* (0.45%), followed by *A. vachanica* (0.34%), while *A. dracunculus* had the lowest artemisinin content (0.07%). The HPLC chromatograms of *Artemisia* species with standard of artemisinin are showed in Figures S1–S5.

After treatment of *A. annua* extract with silica gel as an adsorbent, the total peaks in the chromatograms decreased from 83 to 47, while the content of artemisinin in *A. annua* extract increased from 4.5 mg/g to 10.2 mg/g. The results of *A. annua* extract treatment are given in Figure 3.

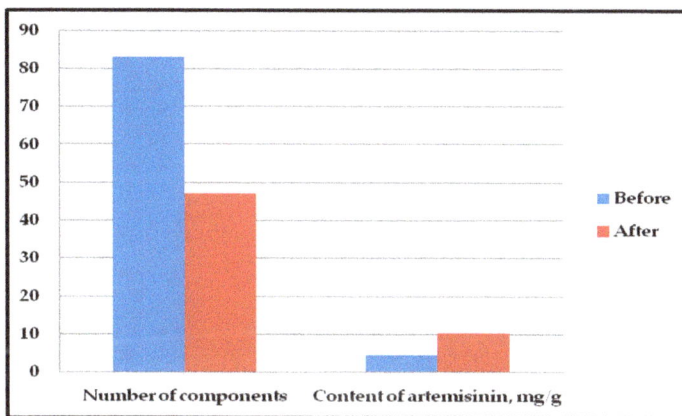

Figure 3. Total components number and artemisinin content in *A. annua* extract before and after purification.

4. Discussion

There are many factors such as environmental, genetic, etc. that can influence the variation in artemisinin concentration [17]. Ranjbar and co-authors have reported that there is a relationship between the increased expression of some genes and the enhancement of artemisinin content in *Artemisia* species at the vegetative, budding, and flowering stages [22]. Recently, Salehi et al. investigated the expression of artemisinin biosynthesis and trichome formation genes in five *Artemisia* species and concluded that there is a relationship between the enhancement of artemisinin content and increased expression of some genes [23].

Previous works have reported that artemisinin concentration varied due to differences in methods of artemisinin extraction as well as the solvents used [40,41]. Literature reports indicated that extraction of artemisinin has been carried out by different extraction methods: traditional solvent extraction, microwave-assisted extraction, ultrasound-aided extraction, and supercritical fluid extraction method using CO_2 as a solvent [20,46]. *n*-hexane [38], toluene [40], chloroform [41], petroleum ether [44], acetone, and ethanol [47] were the solvents most widely used for artemisinin extraction from *Artemisia* species.

According to our results, ultrasound-aided extraction and *n*-hexane as a solvent for artemisinin extraction were suitable for the extraction of artemisinin from *Artemisia* species. Our experiments are in agreement with previous reports that the yield of artemisinin extraction is enhanced by ultrasound-aided extraction when compared to comparable conventional extraction processes [46].

Various methods such as thin-layer chromatography (TLC), high-performance liquid chromatography (HPLC) with evaporative light scattering detection (ELSD), ultraviolet detection (PAD), diode array detection (DAD), gas chromatography (GC) combined with flame ionization detector (FID), and mass spectrometry (MS) have been proposed and assessed to detect and quantify artemisinin [48,49]. Recently, a fully electrochemical molecularly imprinted polymer sensor was developed for the sensitive detection of artemisinin with a detection limit of 0.02 μM in plant matrix [50].

In the present work, HPLC-PAD was used to analyze artemisinin in *Artemisia* species. Researchers have reported that HPLC-PAD is readily applicable for quality control of herbals and artemisinin-related pharmaceutical compounds and it was validated for the quantification of underivatized artemisinin, dihydroartemisinic acid, and artemisinic acid from crude plant samples [44].

The literature reports with respect to artemisinin content in *Artemisia* species up to now are summarized in Table 3. Artemisinin was found at least in 40 *Artemisia* species [9,15–32]. The artemisinin content ranged from 0.0005% to 1.38% on dried parts of *Artemisia* species.

Table 3. Summary of literature reports showing presence of artemisinin in *Artemisia* species.

Artemisia Species	Part Used	Artemisinin, %	Ref.
A. absinthium	Flowers, leaves, stem, and roots	0.02–0.35	[17,22,24]
A. austriaca	Leaves	0.05	[23]
A. aff. tangutica	Flowers, leaves, stem, and roots	0.02–0.11	[17]
A. anethifolia	Leaves	0.05	[30]
A. anethoides	Leaves	0.006	[30]
A. annua	Flowers, leaves, stem, and roots	0.02–1.4	[17,25–28,51,52]
A. arborescens	Leaves	0.001	[30]
A. apiacea	Leaves	Not shown	[21]
A. bushriences	Flowers, leaves, stem, and roots	0.01–0.34	[17]
A. campestris	Leaves, buds, and flowers	0.05–0.1	[22]
A. cina	Shoots	0.0006	[16]
A. ciniformis	Leaves	0.22	[23]
A. deserti	Leaves	0.4–0.6	[23]
A. diffusa	Leaves, buds, and flowers	0.05–0.15	[22]
A. dracunculus	Flowers, leaves, stem, and roots	0.01–0.27	[17]
A. dubia	Flowers, leaves, stem, and roots	0.01–0.07	[17,19]
A. incana	Leaves	0.25	[23]
A. indica	Flowers, leaves, stem, and roots	0.01–0.10	[17,19]
A. fragrans	Leaves	0.2	[23]
A. frigida	Leaves	0.007	[30]
A. gmelinii	Leaves	0.038	[30]
A. japonica	Flowers, leaves, stem, and roots	0.01–0.08	[17]
A. kopetdaghensis	Leaves	0.18	[23]
A. integrifolia	Leaves	0.036	[30]
A. lancea	Leaves	Not shown	[21]
A. macrocephala	Leaves	0.011	[30]
A. marschalliana	Leaves	0.38	[23]
A. messerschmidtiana	Leaves	0.032	[30]
A. moorcroftiana	Flowers, leaves, stem, and roots	0.01–0.16	[17]
A. parviflora	Flowers, leaves, stem, and roots	0.03–0.15	[17]
A. pallens	Leaves and flowers	0.1	[31]

Table 3. *Cont.*

Artemisia Species	Part Used	Artemisinin, %	Ref.
A. roxburghiana	Flowers, leaves, stem, and roots	0.02–0.22	[17]
A. scoparia	Leaves, buds, and flowers	0.1–0.18	[22,32]
A. sieberi	Aerial parts	0.1–0.2	[22,23]
A. sieversiana	Flowers, leaves, stem, and roots	0.05–0.20	[17]
A. spicigeria	Leaves, buds, and flowers	0.05–0.14	[22]
A. thuscula (syn. *A. canariensis*)	Leaves	0.045	[30]
A. tridentata Nutt. subsp. *vaseyana*	Leaves	0.0005	[30]
A. vestita	Flowers, leaves, stem, and roots	0.04–0.20	[17]
A. vulgaris	Flowers, leaves, stem, and roots	0.02–0.18	[17,22]

The highest content of artemisinin was found in *A. annua* (up to 1.4%) [51], followed by *A. deserti* (0.4–0.6%), *A. marschalliana* (up to 0.38%) [23] and *A. absinthium* (up to 0.35%) [17,22,24].

The current study observed the presence of artemisinin in eight of the various *Artemisia* species growing wild in Tajikistan. *A. vachanica* was found to be a novel plant source of artemisinin. The content of artemisinin in *A. macrocephala* was found almost 20-fold higher than a previous study [30]. Hence, no significant difference was detectable between the artemisinin content of *A. annua*, *A. absinthium*, *A. dracunculus*, and *A. vulgaris* growing in Tajikistan. Generally, previous studies reported that the artemisinin content in *A. annua* was higher than in other *Artemisia* species [15,17,21,22,24]. Artemisinin was not detected in *A. leucotricha*.

The extracts obtained from plant material using organic solvent extractions are very complex, and have several unwanted components such as chlorophylls and other colored organic molecules from the feed material. Removal of the contaminants from the extracts has been performed with charcoal and clays [53,54].

In this work, purification of *A. annua* hexane extract by using silica gel as adsorbent resulted in the enrichment of artemisinin. The concentration of artemisinin increased 2.3 times and 35 unwanted components were purified out by silica gel.

A selective sorption method has resulted in the increase of artemisinin to a final purity up to 90% using a polymeric adsorbent loaded with specific ligands [53]. Using silica gel compared to an adsorbent with specific ligands was less effective. However, silica gel is a cheap alternative that can be used for primary treatment of crude artemisinin extracts from the feed material.

5. Conclusions

The study demonstrated the presence of artemisinin, a biologically important natural sesquiterpene lactone in several *Artemisia* species growing wild in Tajikistan. The content of artemisinin ranged between 0.07% and 0.45% on a dry weight basis of *Artemisia* species. *A. vachanica* was found to be a novel plant source of artemisinin. Treatment of *A. annua* hexane extract with silica gel as adsorbent resulted in enrichment of artemisinin.

Supplementary Materials: The following are available online at http://www.mdpi.com/2305-6320/6/1/23/s1, Figure S1: HPLC chromatogram of the pure artemisinin (Rt 4.257 min) (A) and hexane extract of *Artemisia annua* (B), Figure S2: HPLC chromatogram of hexane extract of *Artemisia vachanica* (A) and *Artemisia vulgaris* (B), Figure S3: HPLC chromatogram of hexane extract of *Artemisia makrocephala* (A) and *Artemisia leucotricha* (B), Figure S4: HPLC chromatogram of hexane extract of *Artemisia dracunculus* (A) and *Artemisia absinthium* (B), Figure S5: HPLC chromatogram of hexane extract of *Artemisia scoparia* (A) and mixture *Artemisia annua* and pure artemisinin (B).

Author Contributions: F.S., S.N., and S.A. performed the phytochemical investigation, designed the study, and wrote the manuscript; F.S., P.S., and A.S. analyzed the data; R.S., M.H., and H.A.A. made revisions to the manuscript.

Acknowledgments: The authors are grateful for financial support from the Central Asian Drug Discovery & Development Centre of Chinese Academy of Sciences (Grant No. CAM201808) and PIFI PostDoctoral scholarship for Sodik Numonov (No. 2019PB0043).

Conflicts of Interest: The authors declare no conflict of interest.

References

1. WHO. *World Malaria Report 2018*; WHO: Geneva, Switzerland, 2018; p. 165.
2. Nosten, F.; White, N.J. Artemisinin-Based Combination Treatment of Falciparum Malaria. *Am. J. Trop. Med. Hyg.* **2007**, *77*, 181–192. [CrossRef] [PubMed]
3. Guon, Z. Artemisinin anti-malarial drugs in china. *Acta Pharm. Sin. B* **2016**, *6*, 115–124.
4. Sanz, M.; Vilatersana, R.; Hidalgo, O.; Garcia-Jacas, N.; Susanna, A.; Schneeweiss, G.M.; Valls, J. Molecular phylogeny and evolution of floral characters of *Artemisia* and Allies (Anthemideae, Asteracea): Evidence from nrdna ets and its sequences. *Taxon* **2008**, *57*, 66–78.
5. Sharopov, F.; Setzer, W.N. Medicinal plants of Tajikistan. In *Vegetation of Central Asia and Environs*; Egamberdieva, D., Öztürk, M., Eds.; Springer Nature: Cham, Switzerland, 2018; pp. 163–210.
6. Sharopov, F.S.; Sulaimonova, V.A.; Setzer, W.N. Composition of the essential oil of *Artemisia absinthium* from Tajikistan. *Rec. Nat. Prod.* **2012**, *6*, 127–134.
7. Sharopov, F.S.; Setzer, W.N. Thujone-rich essential oils of *Artemisia rutifolia* stephan ex spreng. Growing wild in Tajikistan. *J. Essent. Oil-Bear. Plants* **2011**, *14*, 136–139. [CrossRef]
8. Sharopov, F.S.; Setzer, W.N. The essential oil of *Artemisia scoparia* from Tajikistan is dominated by phenyldiacetylenes. *Nat. Prod. Commun.* **2011**, *6*, 119–122. [PubMed]
9. Tan, R.X.; Zheng, W.F.; Tang, H.Q. Biologically active substances from the genus *Artemisia*. *Planta Med.* **1998**, *64*, 295–302. [CrossRef]
10. Brown, G.D. The biosynthesis of artemisinin (qinghaosu) and the phytochemistry of *Artemisia annua* L. (qinghao). *Molecules* **2010**, *15*, 7603–7698. [CrossRef]
11. Rydén, A.M.; Kayser, O. Chemistry, biosynthesis and biological activity of artemisinin and related natural peroxides. In *Bioactive Heterocycles III*; Springer: Berlin/Heidelberg, Germany, 2007; Volume 9, pp. 1–32.
12. Yarnell, E. *Artemisia annua* (sweet annie), other *Artemisia* species, artemisinin, artemisinin derivatives, and malaria. *J. Restor. Med.* **2014**, *3*, 69–85. [CrossRef]
13. Krishna, S.; Uhlemann, A.C.; Haynes, R.K. Artemisinins: Mechanisms of action and potential for resistance. *Drug Resist. Updat.* **2004**, *7*, 233–244. [CrossRef]
14. Meshnick, S.R. Artemisinin: Mechanisms of action, resistance and toxicity. *Int. J. Parasitol.* **2002**, *32*, 1655–1660. [CrossRef]
15. Arab, H.A.; Rahbari, S.; Rassouli, A.; Moslemi, M.H.; Khosravirad, F.D.A. Determination of artemisinin in *Artemisia sieberi* and anticoccidial effects of the plant extract in broiler chickens. *Trop. Anim. Health Prod.* **2006**, *38*, 497–503. [CrossRef] [PubMed]
16. Aryanti; Bintang, M.; Ermayanti, T.M.; Mariska, I. Production of antileukemic agent in untransformed and transformed root cultures of *Artemisia cina*. *Ann. Bogor.* **2001**, *8*, 11–16.
17. Mannan, A.; Ahmed, I.; Arshad, W.; Asim, M.F.; Qureshi, R.A.; Hussain, I.; Mirza, B. Survey of artemisinin production by diverse *Artemisia* species in northern Pakistan. *Malar. J.* **2010**, *9*, 310. [CrossRef] [PubMed]
18. Mannan, A.; Ahmed, I.; Arshad, W.; Hussain, I.; Mirza, B. Effects of vegetative and flowering stages on the biosynthesis of artemisinin in *Artemisia* species. *Arch. Pharm. Res.* **2011**, *34*, 1657–1661. [CrossRef] [PubMed]
19. Mannan, A.; Shaheen, N.; Arshad, W.; Qureshi, R.A.; Zia, M.; Mirza, B. Hairy roots induction and artemisinin analysis in *Artemisia dubia* and *Artemisia indica*. *Afr. J. Biotechnol.* **2008**, *7*, 3288–3292.
20. Bayarmaa, J.; Zorzi, G.D. Determination of artemisinin content in *Artemisia annua* L. *Mong. J. Boil. Sci.* **2011**, *9*, 47–51.
21. Hsu, E. The history of qing hao in the Chinese materia medica. *Trans. R. Soc. Trop. Med. Hyg.* **2006**, *100*, 505–508. [CrossRef] [PubMed]
22. Ranjbar, M.; Naghavi, M.R.; Alizadeh, H.; Soltanloo, H. Expression of artemisinin biosynthesis genes in eight *Artemisia* species at three developmental stages. *Ind. Crop. Prod.* **2015**, *76*, 836–843. [CrossRef]
23. Salehi, M.; Karimzadeh, G.; Naghavi, M.R.; Badi, H.N.; Monfared, S.R. Expression of artemisinin biosynthesis and trichome formation genes in five *Artemisia* species. *Ind. Crop. Prod.* **2018**, *112*, 130–140. [CrossRef]
24. Zia, M.; Abdul, M.; Chaudhary, M.F. Effect of growth regulators and amino acids on artemisinin production in the callus of *Artemisia absinthium*. *Pak. J. Bot.* **2007**, *39*, 799–805.
25. Charles, D.J.; Simon, J.E.; Wood, K.V.; Heinstein, P. Germplasm variation in artemisinin content of *Artemisa annua* using an alternative method of artemisinin analysis from crude plant extracts. *J. Nat. Prod.* **1990**, *53*, 157–160. [CrossRef]

26. Dayrit, F.M. *From Artemisia annua L. to Artemisinins: The Discovery and Development of Artemisinins and Antimalarial Agents*; Academic Press: Cambridge, MA, USA, 2017.

27. Singh, A.; Vishwakarma, R.A.; Husain, A. Evaluation of *Artemisia annua* strains for higher artemisinin production. *Planta Med.* **1988**, *54*, 475–477. [CrossRef]

28. Woerdenbag, H.J.; Pras, N.; Chan, N.G. Artemisinin, related sesquiterpenes, and essential oil in *Artemisia annua* during a vegetation period in Vietnam. *Planta Med.* **1994**, *60*, 272–275. [CrossRef] [PubMed]

29. Hamidi, F.; Karimzadeh, G.; Monfared, S.R.; Salehi, M. Assessment of Iranian endemic *Artemisia khorassanica*: Karyological, genome size, and gene expressions involved in artemisinin production. *Turk. J. Boil.* **2018**, *42*, 322–333. [CrossRef]

30. Pellicera, J.; Saslis-Lagoudakis, C.H.; Carrió, E.; Ernst, M.; Garnatje, T.; Grace, O.M.; Gras, A.; Mumbrú, M.; Vallès, J.; Vitales, D.; et al. A phylogenetic road map to antimalarial *Artemisia* Species. *J. Ethnopharmacol.* **2018**, *225*, 1–9. [CrossRef] [PubMed]

31. Suresh, J.; Singh, A.; Vasavi, A.; Ihsanullah, M.; Mary, S. Phytochemical and pharmacological properties of *Artemisia pallens*. *Int. J. Pharm. Sci. Res.* **2011**, *5*, 3090–3091.

32. Singh, A.; Sarin, R. *Artemisia scoparia*: A new source of artemisinin. *Bangladesh J. Pharmacol.* **2010**, *5*, 17–20. [CrossRef]

33. Liu, C.X. Discovery and development of artemisinin and related compounds. *Chin. Herb. Med.* **2017**, *9*, 101–114. [CrossRef]

34. Kayani, W.K.; Kiani, B.H.; Dilshad, E.; Mirza, B. Biotechnological approaches for artemisinin production in *Artemisia. World J. Microbiol. Biotechnol.* **2018**, *34*, 54. [CrossRef]

35. Zeng, Q.P.; Qiu, F.; Yuan, L. Production of artemisinin by genetically-modified microbes. *Biotechnol. Lett.* **2008**, *30*, 581–592. [CrossRef] [PubMed]

36. Arsenault, P.R.; Wobbe, K.K.; Weathers, P.J. Recent advances in artemisinin production through heterologous expression. *Curr. Med. Chem.* **2008**, *15*, 2886. [CrossRef] [PubMed]

37. Hommel, M. The future of artemisinins: Natural, synthetic or recombinant? *J. Boil.* **2008**, *7*, 38. [CrossRef] [PubMed]

38. Badshah, S.L.; Ullah, A.; Ahmad, N.; Almarhoon, Z.M.; Mabkhot, Y. Increasing the strength and production of artemisinin and its derivatives. *Molecules* **2018**, *23*, 100. [CrossRef] [PubMed]

39. Efferth, T. Artemisinin–second career as anticancer drug? *World J. Tradit. Chin. Med.* **2015**, *1*, 2–25. [CrossRef]

40. Zhang, Y.; Xu, G.; Zhang, S.; Wang, D.; Prabha, P.S.; Zuo, Z. Antitumor research on artemisinin and its bioactive derivatives. *Nat. Prod. Bioprospect.* **2018**. [CrossRef] [PubMed]

41. Efferth, T. From ancient herb to modern drug: *Artemisia annua* and artemisinin for cancer therapy. *Semin. Cancer Boil.* **2017**, *46*, 65–83. [CrossRef]

42. Naß, J.; Efferth, T. The activity of *Artemisia* spp. and their constituents against *Trypanosomiasis*. *Phytomedicine* **2018**, *47*, 184–191. [CrossRef]

43. Yuan, D.S.; Chen, Y.P.; Tan, L.L.; Huang, S.Q.; Li, C.Q.; Wang, Q.; Zeng, Q.P. Artemisinin: A panacea eligible for unrestrictive use? *Front. Pharmacol.* **2017**, *8*, 737. [CrossRef]

44. Ferreira, J.F.S.; Gonzalez, J.M. Analysis of underivatized artemisinin and related sesquiterpene lactones by high-performance liquid chromatography with ultraviolet detection. *Phytochem. Anal.* **2009**, *20*, 91–97. [CrossRef]

45. Lapkin, A.A.; Walker, A.; Sullivan, N.; Khambay, B.; Mlambo, B.; Chemat, S. Development of HPLC Analytical Protocol for Artemisinin Quantification in Plant Materials and Extracts. *J. Pharm. Biomed. Anal.* **2009**, *49*, 908–915. [CrossRef] [PubMed]

46. Paniwnyk, L.; Briars, R. Examining the extraction of artemisinin from *Artemisia annua* using ultrasound. In *International Congress on Ultrasonics*; Linde, B.B.J., Pączkowski, J., Ponikwicki, N., Eds.; American Institute of Physics: Gdańsk, Poland, 2011; pp. 581–585.

47. Huter, M.J.; Schmidt, A.; Mestmäcker, F.; Sixt, M.; Strube, J. Systematic and model-assisted process design for the extraction and purification of frtemisinin from *Artemisia annua* L.—Part iv: Crystallization. *Processes* **2018**, *6*, 181. [CrossRef]

48. Liu, C.Z.; Zhou, H.Y.; Zhao, Y. An effective method for fast determination of artemisinin in *Artemisia annua* L. by high performance liquid chromatography with evaporative light scattering detection. *Anal. Chim. Acta* **2007**, *581*, 298–302. [CrossRef] [PubMed]

49. Peng, C.A.; Ferreira, J.F.S.; Wood, A.J. Direct analysis of artemisinin from *Artemisia annua* L. using high-performance liquid chromatography with evaporative light scattering detector, and gas chromatography with flame ionization detector. *J. Chromatogr. A* **2006**, *1133*, 254–258. [CrossRef] [PubMed]

50. Waffo, A.F.T.; Yesildag, C.; Caserta, G.; Katz, S.; Zebger, I.; Lensen, M.C.; Wollenberger, U.; Scheller, F.W.; Altintas, Z. Fully electrochemical mip sensor for artemisinin. *Sens. Actuators B. Chem.* **2018**, *275*, 163–173. [CrossRef]

51. Czechowski, T.; Larson, T.R.; Catania, T.M.; Harvey, D.; Wei, C.; Essome, M.; Brown, G.D.; Graham, I.A. Detailed phytochemical analysis of high- and low artemisinin-producing chemotypes of *Artemisia annua*. *Front. Plant Sci* **2018**, *9*, 641. [CrossRef]

52. Liersch, R.; Soicke, H.; Stehr, C.; Tüllner, H.U. Formation of artemisinin in *Artemisia annua* during one vegetation period. *Planta Med.* **1986**, *52*, 387–390. [CrossRef] [PubMed]

53. Patil, A.R.; Arora, J.S.; Gaikar, V.G. Purification of artemisinin from *Artemisia annua* extract by sorption on different ligand loaded polymeric adsorbents designed by molecular simulation. *Sep. Sci. Technol.* **2012**, *47*, 1156–1166. [CrossRef]

54. Chemat-Djenni, Z.; Sakhri, A. Purification of artemisinin excerpt from *Artemisia annua* L. In *MATEC*; EDP Sciences: Les Ulis, France, 2013.

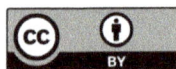

medicines

MDPI

Article

Development and Validation of an HPLC-PDA Method for Biologically Active Quinonemethide Triterpenoids Isolated from *Maytenus chiapensis*

Vito Alessandro Taddeo [1,2], **Ulises Guardado Castillo** [3], **Morena Lizette Martínez** [3],
Jenny Menjivar [4], **Ignacio Antonio Jiménez** [1], **Marvin José Núñez** [3] and **Isabel López Bazzocchi** [1,*]

[1]   Instituto Universitario de Bio-Orgánica Antonio González, Departamento de Química Orgánica,
     Universidad de La Laguna, Avenida Astrofísico Francisco Sánchez 2, 38206 La Laguna, Tenerife, Spain;
     taddeovitoalessandro@gmail.com (V.A.T.); ignadiaz@ull.edu.es (I.A.J.)
[2]   Dipartimento di Farmacia, Università degli Studi "G. d'Annunzio" Chieti-Pescara, Via dei Vestini 31,
     66100 Chieti, Italy
[3]   Laboratorio de Investigación en Productos Naturales, Facultad de Química y Farmacia,
     Universidad de El Salvador, Final Av. de Mártires y Héroes del 30 de Julio, San Salvador 1101, El Salvador;
     ulises.guardado@ues.edu.sv (U.G.C.); morena.martinez@ues.edu.sv (M.L.M.);
     marvin.nunez@ues.edu.sv (M.J.N.)
[4]   Museo de Historia Natural de El Salvador, Ministerio de Cultura, San Salvador 1101, El Salvador;
     jmenjivar@cultura.gob.sv
*   Correspondence: ilopez@ull.edu.es

Received: 24 January 2019; Accepted: 4 March 2019; Published: 7 March 2019

Abstract: Background: Quinonemethide triterpenoids, known as celastroloids, constitute a relatively small group of biologically active compounds restricted to the Celastraceae family and, therefore, they are chemotaxonomic markers for this family. Among this particular type of metabolite, pristimerin and tingenone are considered traditional medicines in Latin America. The aim of this study was the isolation of the most abundant celastroloids from the root bark of *Maytenus chiapensis*, and thereafter, to develop an analytical method to identify pristimerin and tingenone in the Celastraceae species. **Methods**: Pristimerin and tingenone were isolated from the *n*-hexane-Et$_2$O extract of the root bark of *M. chiapensis* through chromatographic techniques, and were used as internal standards. Application of a validated RP HPLC-PDA method was developed for the simultaneous quantification of these two metabolites in three different extracts, *n*-hexane-Et$_2$O, methanol, and water, to determine the best extractor solvent. **Results**: Concentration values showed great variation between the solvents used for extraction, with the *n*-hexane–Et$_2$O extract being the richest in pristimerin and tingenone. **Conclusions**: *M. chiapensis* is a source of two biologically active quinonemethide triterpenoids. An analytical method was developed for the qualification and quantification of these two celastroloids in the root bark extracts of *M. chiapensis*. The validated method reported herein could be extended and be useful in analyzing Celastraceae species and real commercial samples.

Keywords: *Maytenus chiapensis*; Celastraceae; quinonemethide triterpenoids; pristimerin; tingenone; HPLC-PDA

---

1. Introduction

Species of the Celastraceae family have had a long history in traditional medicine and agriculture in North Africa, South and Central America, and Central and East Asia [1]. The therapeutic potential of Celastraceae species has been mainly attributed to the presence of quinonemethide triterpenoids (QMTs), a group of triterpenoids with unique structural features [2]. QMTs contain a *D:A*-friedo-nor-oleanane skeleton characterized by a particular oxygenation pattern with an unsaturated system involving rings A and B, and the majority of them bear a highly oxidized ring E [2]. QMTs constitute a relatively small group of biologically active compounds restricted to the Celastraceae family, commonly referred to as the bittersweet family [3] and, therefore, they are considered to be chemotaxonomic markers for this family. For this reason, QMTs and their structurally related congeners, phenolic triterpenoids, and triterpene dimers and trimers, were given the general name celastroloids by Brüning and Wagner [4]. QMTs have been reported mainly in the *Maytenus* [5], *Celastrus* [6], and *Tripterygium* [7] genera. This particular class of naturally occurring products, which are exclusively accumulated in the root barks of the plants that contain them, show a wide range of bioactivities, including cytotoxic [8,9], anti-inflammatory [10], antioxidant [11], antimicrobial [12], antiparasitic [13], and insecticidal [14] properties.

Since 1936, when celastrol, the most extensively studied quinonemethide, was isolated from *Tripterygium wilfordii* [15], a variety of QMTs have been reported from Celastraceae species. In particular, pristimerin and tingenone, isolated for the first time from *Pristimera indica* [16] and *Euonymus tingens* [17], respectively, are the most frequently reported celastroloids. These two naturally occurring quinonemethide triterpenoid orange pigments are traditional medicines derived from the Celastraceae family and have long been used for the treatment of a variety of ailments [3,7]. Pristimerin has been reported to have promising clinical potential as both a therapeutic and chemopreventive agent for various types of cancer, including breast [18], glioma [19], prostate [20], pancreatic [21], ovarian [22], colon [23], esophageal squamous [24], osteosarcoma [25], and uveal [26] cancer, via a number of mechanisms [27]. Moreover, tingenone displays antinociceptive [28] and antiprotozoal [29] activities. Since there is pharmacological interest in this type of metabolite and their synthesis is not commercially viable, some research groups have investigated in vitro plant systems to increase their production [30].

In the course of the search for bioactive metabolites from species of the Celastraceae family, phytochemical studies on *Maytenus chiapensis*—a Celastraceae species collected in El Salvador and commonly named "Escobo blanco"—have reported the isolation of sesquiterpenoids [31–33] and tetracyclic and pentacyclic triterpenoids [34–36] from the areal parts of the plant.

Taking into consideration the relevance of QMTs from a chemotaxonomic and therapeutic point of view, the aim of our study is to develop a validated analytical method to identify pristimerin and tingenone in the root barks of Celastraceae species. To perform this task and to investigate the previously unreported pristimerin and tingenone content in *M. chiapensis* root bark, the two known QMTs were isolated, characterized, and subsequently used as pure standard samples in HPLC analysis. Moreover, the successful application of a validated RP HPLC-PDA method is developed for the qualification and quantification of these two pharmacologically relevant QMTs in *M. chiapensis* extracts. Three different solvents were used to optimize the extraction procedure of the QMTs under study. The validated method reported herein could be extended and be useful in analyzing commercial samples.

2. Materials and Methods

2.1. Chemical

The solvents, methanol (HPLC-grade), water (HPLC-grade), *n*-hexane, diethyl ether, dichloromethane, and chloroform, and formic acid were purchased from Sigma-Aldrich (St. Louis, MO, USA) and used without further purification. Pristimerin and tingenone were isolated from the root bark of *Maytenus chiapensis* and used as pure standards (purity ≥99%) after their NMR characterization (see Figures S1 and S2 in the Supplementary Material).

2.2. Plant Material

The root bark of *Maytenus chiapensis* Lundell (Celastraceae) was collected at Montecristo National Park (latitude: 14°23′39″ N, longitude: 89°23′10″ W, elevation: 1617 msnm) in the municipality of Metapán, Santa Ana, El Salvador, in March 2018, and was identified by Jenny Elizabeth Menjívar Cruz, curator of the

Herbarium at the Museo de Historia Natural de El Salvador. A voucher specimen (J. Menjívar et al. 4255) was deposited in the Herbarium at the Museo de Historia Natural de El Salvador, El Salvador.

2.3. Extraction and Isolation of Pristimerin and Tingenone

The root bark (650 g) of *M. chiapensis* was extracted with *n*-hexane–Et$_2$O in a Soxhlet apparatus as previously reported [37]. The extract (27.2 g) was chromatographed on Sephadex LH-20 (*n*-hexane–CHCl$_3$–MeOH, 2:1:1) to afford 15 final fractions after combination on the basis of their TLC profile. Fractions 7 and 8, after successive chromatographies on Sephadex LH-20 (*n*-hexane–CHCl$_3$–MeOH, 2:1:1), silica gel (CH$_2$Cl$_2$–Et$_2$O of increasing polarity), and preparative HPTLC developed with *n*-hexane–Et$_2$O (4:6), gave rise to pristimerin (680 mg, R$_f$ 0.35) and tingenone (210 mg, R$_f$ 0.56). Their structures were identified by comparison of their ^{1}H and ^{13}C NMR (Bruker Avance 500 spectrometer, Bruker, Billerica, MA, USA) and MS (Micromass Autospec spectrometer, Micromass, Manchester, UK) data with those previously reported [38].

2.4. Preparation of Plant Extracts for HPLC Analysis

The methanolic and *n*-hexane–Et$_2$O (1:1) extracts were prepared by dissolving 2.5 g of dried powdered root bark into 100 mL of organic solvents, and afterwards macerated for 72 hours at 25 °C. Both extracts were concentrated under reduced pressure at 40 °C to obtain 700 mg and 350 mg of crude residues, respectively.

The water extraction was carried out by dissolving 2.5 g of powdered root bark with 100 mL of water by magnetic stirrer ultrasonic (VWR, model 97043-988, operating frequency at 35 kHz) for 90 min at 25 °C. The aqueous extract was further filtered in Whatman No. 91 paper. The filtrate was frozen at −20 °C in an ultra-low temperature freezer (Fischer Scientific, Waltham, MA, USA) and lyophilized in a lyophilizator under 0.1 mmHg pressure at −50 °C (Labconco, Freezone, Kansas City, MO, USA) for 72 h. The resulting powder (130 mg) was stored at −20 °C until used.

2.5. HPLC-PDA Apparatus and Conditions

The chromatographic system consisted of an Alliance W2690 separation module equipped with an online degasser, an automatic injector, and a W2487 photodiode array detector set at 420 nm for the detection of pristimerin and tingenone. Data were collected and processed using Empower v.2 software for HPLC system (Waters, Milford, MA, USA). Separation was performed with a column Supelco Ascentis RP C18 (150 mm × 4.6 mm; particle size 5 μm, Sigma-Aldrich, St. Louis, MO, USA) column equipped with a Sentry Guard Cartridge (3.9 mm x 20 mm; Waters, Sigma-Aldrich, St. Louis, MO, USA) guard column. Both columns were maintained at 25 ± 1 °C. The mobile phase consisted of water with 0.4% of formic acid (v/v) (solvent A) and methanol (solvent B), using a gradient elution program for 10 min with a flow rate of 1.2 mL/min as follows: linear gradient ratio A/B 90:10 from the beginning of the chromatographic run to 6.0 min, A/B 90:10 to A/B 70:30 gradient from 6.01 min to 10.0 min, and finally, linear gradient ratio A/B 90:10 from 10.01 min to 15.0 min.

2.6. Preparation of Samples

A total of 10.0 mg of each extract was dissolved in 10 mL of methanol, using an ultrasonic bath (VWR, model 97043-988, operating frequency at 35 kHz) at room temperature. The sample solutions were filtrated through a 0.22 μm membrane filter before being subjected to HPLC analysis.

2.7. Method Validation

2.7.1. Calibration, Linearity and Quality Control Samples

Standard solutions of pristimerin and tingenone (quality control samples, QC samples) were prepared in methanol at a concentration of 1000 μg/mL. Combined working solutions of mixed standards (QC samples) at concentrations of 10, 15, 30, 50, 80, and 100 μg/mL were obtained by the dilution of mixed stock solutions at 1000 µg/mL in a volumetric flask containing methanol. Calibration curves obtained at 420 nm were plotted using a weighted linear least-squares regression analysis. Concentrations of the QMTs (QC samples) were calculated by interpolating their peak areas on the calibration curve. The linearity of the investigated compounds was obtained by using the plant extract samples spiked at different concentrations. However, the slopes obtained from samples were different from those of the standard solution.

2.7.2. Limit of Detection (LOD) and Limit of Quantification (LOQ)

The quality control samples (QC) were prepared to determine the limit of quantification (LOQ), the intra- and inter-assay precision and accuracy of the method, and defined according to International Guidelines, International Conference on Harmonisation (ICH) Q2 (R1). QC samples at three different concentration levels (QC low = 15.0, QC medium = 50.0, and QC high = 80.0 µg/mL) were used to validate the analytical method. The limit of detection (LOD) was calculated from the calibration graphic and was defined as 3 times the standard deviation of blank samples divided by the analytical sensitivity. The LOQ was defined as the lowest concentration on the calibration curve, which could be measured ($n = 5$) with a precision (RSD%) not exceeding 20% and with an accuracy between 80% and 120%. The method's efficiency was measured by comparing the peak areas obtained from several samples obtained using pretreatment extraction processes and different extraction solvent systems. Analysis of these results allowed for an evaluation of the best extraction procedures, leading to the maximum recovery for the cited metabolites, minimizing solvent consumption and time.

3. Results and Discussion

3.1. Isolation of Pristimerin and Tingenone from Maytenus chiapensis

Following the methodology previously established in our laboratory [37], multiple chromatographic steps of the root bark extract (*n*-hexane–Et$_2$O, 1:1, 27.2 g) of the plant were carried out to yield pristimerin (680 mg) and tingenone (210 mg). The structures of these two known quinonemethide triterpenoids (Figure 1) were identified by comparison of their spectroscopic and spectrometric data with values reported in the literature [38] (see Figures S1 and S2 in the Supplementary Material). Following this, these compounds were used as internal standards in the HPLC analysis.

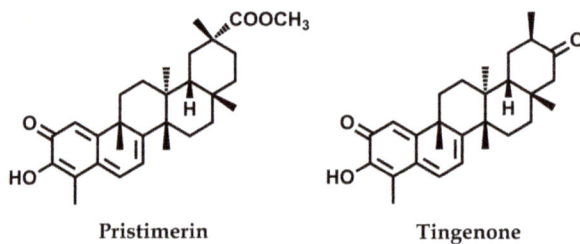

Figure 1. Structure of the main quinonemethide triterpenoids isolated from the root bark of *Maytenus chiapensis*.

3.2. HPLC Analysis

The relevance of QMTs from a chemotaxonomic and therapeutic point of view has led several research groups to study their content in Celastraceae species, and some HPLC analyses have been reported. Thus, an HPLC method for the quantification of quinonemethide derivatives of five Brazilian morphological types of *Maytenus ilicifolia* has been reported [39]. Some years later, analysis by HPLC-DAD of *M. ilicifolia* extracts from root barks of adult plants and roots of seedlings indicated that pristimerin is the major component of both extracts [11]. Nossack and co-workers quantified pristimerin and tingenone (maitenin) in hydroalcoholic and aqueous extracts from the leaves and root bark of *Maytenus aquifolium* ("espinheira santa") by HPLC-UV coupled with mass spectrometry (LC-MS) as a procedure for assessing the quality of this phytomedicine [40]. Moreover, a simple HPLC method was developed for the identification and comparison of quinonemethide triterpenes in wild *Hippocratea excelsa* and "cancerina", a method useful for the control of this herb used in Mexican traditional medicine as an alternative cancer treatment [41]. In addition, Roca-Mézquita and co-workers performed quantitative analysis of pristimerin and tingenone in a dichloromethane extract of *Elaeodendron trichotomum*, revealing that this species contains both celastroloids, although, unexpectedly, pristimerin was present in very low concentration [29].

In the current study, the successful application of a validated RP HPLC-PDA method was performed for the qualification and quantification of pristimerin and tingenone in three different extracts of *Maytenus chiapensis*, using different solvents to optimize the extraction procedure. To carry out this task, a gradient mobile phase had been tested in order to obtain separation of both QMTs. The Supelco Ascentis C18 column was chosen owing to the good separation with respect to peak symmetry, resolution, and total analysis time. A mobile phase system consisting of water with 0.4% of formic acid (v/v) (solvent A) and methanol (solvent B) was used. Under these conditions, the peak retention times of pristimerin and tingenone were 6.04 ($\pm$ 0.4) min and 2.25 ($\pm$ 0.3) min, respectively (see Figure S3 in the Supplementary Material).

Calibration curves, obtained at 420 nm, were plotted using weighted ($1/x^2$) linear least-squares regression analysis. The calibration curves were linear over the concentration range tested, with the coefficient of determination $r^2 \geq 0.9981$ as reported in Table 1. The within-assay precision (repeatability) of the method was determined by performing three consecutive assays in the same day on QMTs samples spiked at three different standard concentration levels, i.e., 15 (low level), 50 (medium level), and 80 µg/mL (high level), which are within the range of the calibration curve. The results obtained are shown in Table 2.

Table 1. Mean linear calibration curve parameters obtained by weighted linear least-squares regression analysis of three independent six non-zero concentration points.

Compound	Linearity Range (µg/mL)	Slope	Intercept	Determination Coefficient (r^2)
Pristimerin	1–100	74653–79342	−19550 to −4325	0.9981
Tingenone	1–100	45234–49342	−2345 to 13456	0.9990

Table 2. Assay precision (RSD%) and trueness (bias%) of the analytical method obtained from the analysis of quinonemethide triterpenoids (QMTs) samples.

Parameters	Pristimerin	Tingenone
Theoretical [a]	15.0	
Mean back-calculated [a]	14.90	15.02
RSD%	4.45	2.34
Bias%	1.45	2.65
Theoretical [a]	50.0	
Mean back-calculated [a]	50.10	49.80
RSD%	4.60	2.80
Bias%	1.80	2.10
Theoretical [a]	80.0	
Mean back-calculated [a]	89.87	88.99
RSD%	5.76	6.42
Bias%	4.56	4.1

[a] Concentration expressed as µg/mL

3.3. Simultaneous Quantification of Pristimerin and Tingenone

HPLC analysis was used for the simultaneous determination of pristimerin and tingenone from *M. chiapensis* root bark in different solvents. Triplicate measurements were performed to determine the mean amount of both metabolites. The results indicate the influence of the solvent used in the extraction process (Table 3). A mixture of *n*-hexane–Et$_2$O (1:1) was the best extractor solvent since it extracted the highest quantity of pristimerin and tingenone, whereas water was the worst extractor solvent as neither of the two compounds could be detected.

Table 3. Pristimerin and tingenone content in *M. chiapensis* root bark.

Solvent	Extraction Method	Content in Pristimerin			Content in Tingenone		
		µg/mL [a]	mg/g Extract	mg/g dry Material	µg/mL	mg/g Extract	mg/g Dry Material
n-hexane–Et$_2$O (1:1)	Maceration	46.41 ± 0.10	46.41 mg	6.50 mg	31.66 ± 0.15	31.66 mg	4.43 mg
Methanol	Maceration	18.01 ± 0.20	18.01 mg	5.04 mg	10.15 ± 0.18	10.15 mg	2.84 mg
H$_2$O	UAE [b]	ND [c]	ND [c]	ND [c]	ND [c]	ND [c]	ND [c]

[a] Data are expressed as µg/mL of dry plant; [b] UAE: ultrasound-assisted extraction; [c] ND: not detected.

This study revealed that *Maytenus chiapensis* is a source of pristimerin and tingenone, two components with great potential in drug development. Moreover, an RP HPLC-PDA method was developed and validated for their quantification in root bark extracts of this species. The results indicate that a mixture of *n*-hexane–Et$_2$O (1:1) is the optimal extractor solvent for these two promising bioactive naturally occurring compounds. The methodology described herein could be extended to other Celastraceae species, and be useful in the analysis of commercial samples.

Supplementary Materials: The following are available online at http://www.mdpi.com/2305-6320/6/1/36/s1, Figure S1: ^{1}H and ^{13}C NMR spectra of pristimerin in CDCl$_3$ (500 and 125 MHz, respectively), Figure S2: ^{1}H and ^{13}C NMR spectra of tingenone in CDCl$_3$ (500 and 125 MHz, respectively), Figure S3: HPLC chromatograms with UV detection at 420 nm of (A) standard compounds, tingenone and pristimerin, and (B) *n*-hexane–Et$_2$O (1:1) extract (for chromatographic protocol, see Experimental section).

Author Contributions: V.A.T. and M.J.N. conceived and planned the experiments; U.G.C. and M.L.M. carried out the experiments; J.M. identified the plant material; V.A.T., M.J.N. and I.A.J. contributed to the interpretation of the results; I.L.B. was involved in planning and supervising the work; U.G.C., V.A.T. and M.J.N. writing—original draft preparation; I.L.B. writing—review and editing.

Funding: This study was supported by the SAF2015-65113-C2-1-R Spanish MINECO co-funded by the European Regional Development Fund (FEDER).

Acknowledgments: M.J.N. thanks the Dirección General de Ecosistemas y Vida Silvestre, Ministerio de Medio Ambiente Recursos Naturales, for supplying the species *Maytenus chiapensis*. V.A.T. thanks the "G. d'Annunzio" Chieti-Pescara University for a doctoral grant.

Conflicts of Interest: The authors declare no conflicts of interest.

References

1. González, A.G.; Bazzocchi, I.L.; Moujir, L.M.; Jiménez, I.A. Ethnobotanical uses of Celastraceae: Bioactive metabolites. In *Studies in Natural Products Chemistry Bioactive Natural Product (Part D)*; Atta-ur-Rahman, Ed.; Elsevier: Amsterdam, The Netherlands, 2000; Volume 23, pp. 649–738.
2. Gunatilaka, A.A.L. Triterpenoid quinonemethides and related compounds (Celastroloids). In *Progress in the Chemistry of Organic Natural Products*; Springer-Verlag/Wien: New York, NY, USA, 1996; Volume 67, pp. 1–123.
3. Alvarenga, N.; Ferro, E.A. Bioactive triterpenes and related compounds from Celastraceae. In *Studies in Natural Products Chemistry (Part K)*; Atta-ur-Rahman, Ed.; Elsevier: Amsterdam, The Netherlands, 2006; Volume 33, pp. 239–307.

4. Brüning, R.; Wagner, H. Übersicht über die celastraceen-inhaltsstoffe: Chemie, chemotaxonomie, biosynthese, pharmakologie. *Phytochemistry* **1978**, *17*, 1821–1858. [CrossRef]

5. Muñoz, O.; Gonzalez, A.; Ravelo, A.; Estevez, A. Triterpenoid and phenolic compounds from two Chilean Celastraceae. *Z. Naturforsch* **1999**, *54c*, 144–145. [CrossRef]

6. Chen, M.X.; Wang, D.Y.; Guo, J. 3-Oxo-11β-hydroxyfriedelane from the roots of *Celastrus monospermus*. *J. Chem. Res.* **2010**, *34*, 114–117. [CrossRef]

7. Brinker, A.M.; Ma, J.; Lipsky, P.E.; Raskin, I. Medicinal chemistry and pharmacology of genus *Tripterygium* (Celastraceae). *Phytochemistry* **2007**, *68*, 732–766. [CrossRef] [PubMed]

8. Li, P.P.; He, W.; Yuan, P.F.; Song, S.S.; Lu, J.T.; Wei, W. Celastrol induces mitochondria-mediated apoptosis in hepatocellular carcinoma Bel-7402 cells. *Am. J. Chin. Med.* **2015**, *43*, 137–148. [CrossRef] [PubMed]

9. Rodrigues, A.C.B.C.; Oliveira, F.P.; Dias, R.B.; Sales, C.B.S.; Rocha, C.A.G.; Soares, M.B.P.; Costa, E.V.; Silva, F.M.A.; Rocha, W.C.; Koolen, H.H.F.; et al. In vitro and in vivo anti-leukemia activity of the stem bark of *Salacia impressifolia* (Miers) A. C. Smith (Celastraceae). *J. Ethnopharmacol.* **2019**, *231*, 516–524. [CrossRef] [PubMed]

10. Dai, W.; Wang, X.; Teng, H.; Li, C.; Wang, B.; Wang, J. Celastrol inhibits microglial pyroptosis and attenuates inflammatory reaction in acute spinal cord injury rats. *Int. Immunopharmacol.* **2019**, *66*, 215–223. [CrossRef] [PubMed]

11. Santos, V.A.F.F.M.; Santos, D.P.; Castro-Gamboa, I.; Zanoni, M.V.B.; Furlan, M. Evaluation of antioxidant capacity and synergistic associations of quinonemethide triterpenes and phenolic substances from *Maytenus ilicifolia* (Celastraceae). *Molecules* **2010**, *15*, 6956–6973. [PubMed]

12. de León, L.; López, M.R.; Moujir, L. Antibacterial properties of zeylasterone, a triterpenoid isolated from *Maytenus blepharodes*, against *Staphylococcus aureus*. *Microbiol. Res.* **2010**, *165*, 617–626. [CrossRef] [PubMed]

13. Liao, L.M.; Silva, G.A.; Monteiro, M.R.; Albuquerque, S. Trypanocidal activity of quinonemethide triterpenoids from *Cheiloclinium cognatum* (Hippocrateaceae). *Z. Naturforsch. C* **2008**, *63*, 207–210. [CrossRef] [PubMed]

14. Avilla, J.; Teixidó, A.; Velázquez, C.; Alvarenga, N.; Ferro, E.; Canela, R. Insecticidal activity of *Maytenus* species (Celastraceae) nortriterpene quinone methides against Codling Moth, *Cydia pomonella* (L.) (Lepidoptera: Tortricidae). *J. Agric. Food Chem.* **2000**, *48*, 88–92. [CrossRef] [PubMed]

15. Chou, T.Q.; Mei, P.F. The principle of Chinese drug Lei-Kung-Teng, *Tripterygium wilfordii* Hook. The coloring substance and the sugars. *Chin. J. Physiol.* **1936**, *10*, 259–534.

16. Bhatnagar, S.S.; Divekar, P.V. Pristimerin, the antibacterial principle of *Pristimera indica*. I. Isolation, toxicity, and antibacterial action. *J. Sci. Ind. Res.* **1951**, *10B*, 56–61.

17. Brown, P.M.; Moir, M.; Thomson, R.H.; King, T.J.; Krishnamoorthy, V.; Seshadri, T.R. Tingenone and hydroxytingenone, triterpenoid quinone methides from *Euonymus tingens*. *J. Chem. Soc. Perkin Trans. 1* **1973**, *22*, 2721–2725. [CrossRef]

18. Cevatemre, B.; Erkısa, M.; Aztopal, N.; Karakas, D.; Alper, P.; Tsimplouli, C.; Sereti, E.; Dimas, K.; Armutak, E.I.I.; Gurevin, E.G.; et al. A promising natural product, pristimerin, results in cytotoxicity against breast cancer stem cells in vitro and xenografts in vivo through apoptosis and an incomplete autopaghy in breast cancer. *Pharmacol. Res.* **2018**, *129*, 500–514. [CrossRef] [PubMed]

19. Yan, Y.Y.; Bai, J.P.; Xie, Y.; Yu, J.Z.; Ma, C.G. The triterpenoid pristimerin induces U87 glioma cell apoptosis through reactive oxygen species-mediated mitochondrial dysfunction. *Oncol. Lett.* **2013**, *5*, 242–248. [CrossRef] [PubMed]

20. Lee, S.-O.; Kim, J.-S.; Lee, M.-S.; Lee, H.-J. Anti-cancer effect of pristimerin by inhibition of HIF-1a involves the SPHK-1 pathway in hypoxic prostate cancer cells. *BMC Cancer* **2016**, *16*, 701–710. [CrossRef] [PubMed]

21. Deeb, D.; Gao, X.; Liu, Y.B.; Pindolia, K.; Gautam, S.C. Pristimerin, a quinonemethide triterpenoid, induces apoptosis in pancreatic cancer cells through the inhibition of pro-survival Akt/NF-κB/ mTOR signaling proteins and anti-apoptotic Bcl-2. *Int. J. Oncol.* **2014**, *44*, 1707–1715. [CrossRef] [PubMed]

22. Gao, X.; Liu, Y.; Deeb, D.; Arbab, A.S.; Gautam, S.C. Anticancer activity of pristimerin in ovarian carcinoma cells is mediated through the inhibition of prosurvival Akt/NF-κB/mTOR signaling. *J. Exp. Ther. Oncol.* **2014**, *10*, 275–283. [PubMed]

23. Park, J.-H.; Kim, J.-K. Pristimerin, a naturally occurring triterpenoid, attenuates tumorigenesis in experimental colitis-associated colon cancer. *Phytomedicine* **2018**, *42*, 164–171. [CrossRef] [PubMed]

24. Tu, Y.; Tan, F.; Zhou, J.; Pan, J. Pristimerin targeting NF-κB pathway inhibits proliferation, migration, and invasion in esophageal squamous cell carcinoma cells. *Cell Biochem. Funct.* **2018**, *36*, 228–240. [CrossRef] [PubMed]

25. Mori, Y.; Shirai, T.; Terauchi, R.; Tsuchida, S.; Mizoshiri, N.; Hayashi, D.; Arai, Y.; Kishida, T.; Mazda, O.; Kubo, T. Antitumor effects of pristimerin on human osteosarcoma cells in vitro and in vivo. *OncoTargets Ther.* **2017**, *10*, 5703. [CrossRef] [PubMed]

26. Zhang, B.; Zhang, J.; Pan, J. Pristimerin effectively inhibits the malignant phenotypes of uveal melanoma cells by targeting NF-kB pathway. *Int. J. Oncol.* **2017**, *51*, 887–898. [CrossRef] [PubMed]

27. Yousef, B.A.; Hassan, H.M.; Zhang, L.-Y.; Jiang, Z.-Z. Anticancer potential and molecular targets of pristimerin: A Mini-Review. *Curr. Cancer Drug Targets* **2017**, *17*, 100–108. [CrossRef] [PubMed]

28. Veloso, C.C.; Ferreira, R.C.M.; Rodrigues, V.G.; Duarte, L.P.; Klein, A.; Duarte, I.D.; Romero, T.R.L.; Perez, A.C. Tingenone, a pentacyclic triterpene, induces peripheral antinociception due to cannabinoid receptors activation in mice. *Inflammopharmacol.* **2018**, *26*, 227–233. [CrossRef] [PubMed]

29. Roca-Mézquita, C.; Graniel-Sabido, M.; Moo-Puc, R.E.; Leon-Déniz, L.V.; Gamboa-Leon, R.; Arjona-Ruiz, C.; Tun-Garrido, J.; Miron-Lopez, G.; Mena-Rejón, G.J. Antiprotozoal activity of extracts of *Elaeodendron trichotomum* (Celastraceae). *Afr. J. Tradit. Complement. Altern. Med.* **2016**, *13*, 162–165. [CrossRef] [PubMed]

30. Inácio, M.C.; Paz, T.A.; Pereira, A.M.S.; Furlan, M. Endophytic *Bacillus megaterium* and exogenous stimuli affect the quinonemethide triterpenes production in adventitious roots of *Peritassa campestris* (Celastraceae). *Plant Cell Tissue Organ Cult. PCTOC* **2017**, *131*, 15–26. [CrossRef]

31. Núñez, M.J.; Cortés-Selva, F.; Bazzocchi, I.L.; Jiménez, I.A.; González, A.G.; Ravelo, A.G.; Gavin, J.A. Absolute configuration and complete assignment of ^{13}C NMR data for new sesquiterpenes from *Maytenus chiapensis*. *J. Nat. Prod.* **2003**, *16*, 572–574. [CrossRef] [PubMed]

32. Núñez, M.J.; Guadaño, A.; Jiménez, I.A.; Ravelo, A.G.; González-Coloma, A.; Bazzocchi, I.L. Insecticidal sesquiterpene pyridine alkaloids from *Maytenus chiapensis*. *J. Nat. Prod.* **2004**, *67*, 14–18. [CrossRef] [PubMed]

33. Núñez, M.J.; Jiménez, I.A.; Mendoza, C.R.; Chavez-Sifontes, M.; Martínez, M.L.; Ichiishi, E.; Tokuda, R.; Tokuda, H.; Bazzocchi, I.L. Dihydro-β-agarofuran sesquiterpenes from Celastraceae species as anti-tumour-promoting agents: Structure-activity relationship. *Eur. J. Med. Chem.* **2016**, *111*, 95–102. [CrossRef] [PubMed]

34. Núñez, M.J.; López, M.R.; Jiménez, I.A.; Moujir, L.M.; Ravelo, A.G.; Bazzocchi, I.L. First examples of tetracyclic triterpenoids with a D:B-friedobaccharane skeleton. A tentative biosynthetic route. *Tetrahedron Lett.* **2004**, *45*, 7367–7370. [CrossRef]

35. Núñez, M.J.; Reyes, C.P.; Jiménez, I.A.; Moujir, L.; Bazzocchi, I.L. Lupane triterpenoids from *Maytenus* species. *J. Nat. Prod.* **2005**, *68*, 1018–1021. [CrossRef] [PubMed]

36. Reyes, C.P.; Núñez, M.J.; Jiménez, I.A.; Busserolles, J.; Alcaraz, M.J.; Bazzocchi, I.L. Activity of lupane triterpenoids from *Maytenus* species as inhibitors of nitric oxide and prostaglandin E2. *Bioorg. Med. Chem.* **2006**, *14*, 1573–1579. [CrossRef] [PubMed]

37. González, A.G.; Alvarenga, N.L.; Rodríguez, F.; Ravelo, A.G.; Jiménez, I.A.; Bazzocchi, I.L.; Gupta, M.P. New phenolic and quinone-methide triterpenes from *Maytenus* species (Celastraceae). *Nat. Prod. Lett.* **1995**, *7*, 209–218. [CrossRef]

38. Gunatilaka, A.A.L.; Fernando, H.C. ^{1}H and ^{13}C NMR analysis of three quinone-methide triterpenoids. *Magn. Reson. Chem.* **1989**, *27*, 803–811. [CrossRef]

39. Filho, W.B.; Corsino, J.; Bolzani, V.S.; Furlan, M.; Pereira, A.M.S.; França, S.C. Quantitative determination of cytotoxic friedo-nor-oleanane derivatives from five morphological types of *Maytenus ilicifolia* (Celastraceae) by reverse-phase highperformance liquid chromatography. *Phytochem. Anal.* **2002**, *13*, 75–78. [CrossRef] [PubMed]

40. Nossack, A.C.; Celeghini, R.M.S.; Lanças, F.M.; Yariwake, J.H. HPLC-UV and LC-MS Analysis of quinonemethides triterpenes in hydroalcoholic extracts of "espinheira santa" (*Maytenus aquifolium* Martius, Celastraceae) leaves. *J. Braz. Chem. Soc.* **2004**, *15*, 582–586. [CrossRef]

41. Leon, J.-A.A.; Ciau, D.-V.R.; Martinez, T.-I.C.; Ciau, Z.-O.C. Comparative fingerprint analyses of extracts from the root bark of wild *Hippocratea excelsa* and "cancerina" by high-performance liquid chromatography. *J. Sep. Sci.* **2015**, *38*, 3870–3875. [CrossRef] [PubMed]

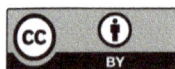

medicines
MDPI

Article

Protein Targets of Frankincense: A Reverse Docking Analysis of Terpenoids from *Boswellia* Oleo-Gum Resins

Kendall G. Byler [1] and William N. Setzer [1,2,*]

[1] Department of Chemistry, University of Alabama in Huntsville, Huntsville, AL 35899, USA;
    kendall.byler@uah.edu
[2] Aromatic Plant Research Center, 230 N 1200 E, Suite 102, Lehi, UT 84043, USA
*   Correspondence: wsetzer@chemistry.uah.edu; Tel.: +1-256-824-6519

Received: 19 July 2018; Accepted: 28 August 2018; Published: 31 August 2018

Abstract: Background: Frankincense, the oleo-gum resin of *Boswellia* trees, has been used in traditional medicine since ancient times. Frankincense has been used to treat wounds and skin infections, inflammatory diseases, dementia, and various other conditions. However, in many cases, the biomolecular targets for frankincense components are not well established. **Methods:** In this work, we have carried out a reverse docking study of *Boswellia* diterpenoids and triterpenoids with a library of 16034 potential druggable target proteins. **Results:** *Boswellia* diterpenoids showed selective docking to acetylcholinesterase, several bacterial target proteins, and HIV-1 reverse transcriptase. *Boswellia* triterpenoids targeted the cancer-relevant proteins (poly(ADP-ribose) polymerase-1, tankyrase, and folate receptor β), inflammation-relevant proteins (phospholipase A2, epoxide hydrolase, and fibroblast collagenase), and the diabetes target 11β-hydroxysteroid dehydrogenase. **Conclusions:** The preferential docking of *Boswellia* terpenoids is consistent with the traditional uses and the established biological activities of frankincense.

Keywords: frankincense; *Boswellia*; cembranoids; cneorubenoids; boswellic acids; molecular docking

---

1. Introduction

The genus *Boswellia* (Burseraceae) is made up of resiniferous trees and shrubs that are distributed across India, the Arabian peninsula, and Africa [1,2]. The genus is known for its aromatic terpenoid oleo-gum resin, frankincense. Frankincense has been a part of human religious ceremonies and ethnobotany for thousands of years [3]. Important frankincense-producing species include *B. carteri*, which grows in Somaliland and Puntland [1], *B. sacra*, found in Yemen, southern Oman, Somalia, and Somaliland [2], *B. frereana*, which is endemic to Somalia [2], *B. papyrifera*, primarily found in Sudan, Eritrea, and Ethiopia [4], and *B. serrata*, which grows primarily in India [5].

Frankincense oleo-gum resin has been used traditionally to treat wounds [6], to treat inflammatory diseases [7], for oral hygiene [8], as well as for its psychoactive effects [9,10]. The biological activities of frankincense have been attributed to its essential oils [11] and its non-volatile diterpenoids and triterpenoids [6]. Although frankincense has been used for various maladies and conditions, and numerous biological activities have been attributed to frankincense, the particular biological targets are not well established. In this work, we have carried out a reverse molecular docking study of *Boswellia* cembranoid diterpenoids (Figure 1), cneorubenoid diterpenoids (Figure 2), and triterpenoids (Figure 3) against a library of 16,034 potential druggable target proteins.

The cembranoids incensole and incensole acetate were detected in the oleo-gum resin of *B. papyrifera*, while serratol was found in *B. carteri*, *B. sacra*, and *B. serrata* [12]. The boscartins have been isolated from the oleo-gum resin of *B. carteri* [13]. Incensole oxide has been isolated from *B. carteri* and the X-ray crystal structure determined [13,14]; both incensole oxide and incensole oxide acetate have been detected in small concentrations in the essential oil from the resin of *B. papyrifera* [15]. Isoincensole oxide [16,17] and isoincensolol [17] were isolated from *B. carteri* resin. Verticilla-4(20),7,11-triene and serratol and were isolated from *B. carteri* [18] and *B. serrata* [19], respectively.

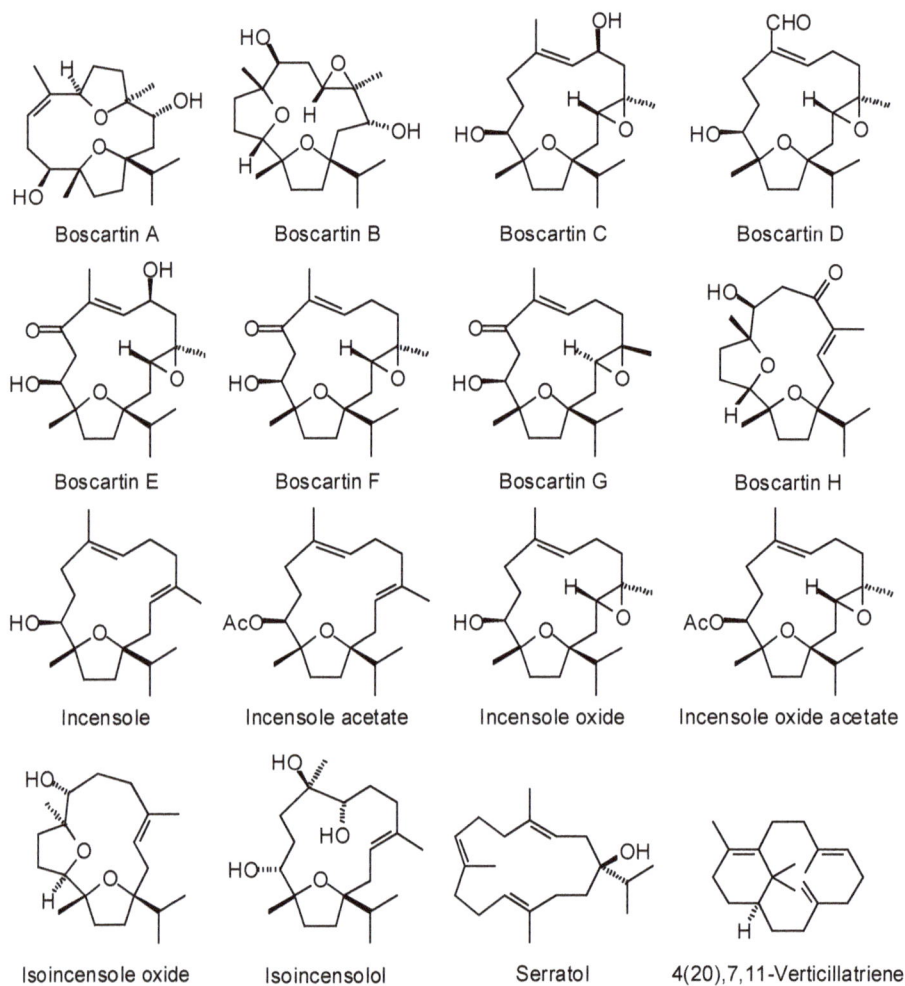

Figure 1. Macrocyclic diterpenoids found in *Boswellia* species.

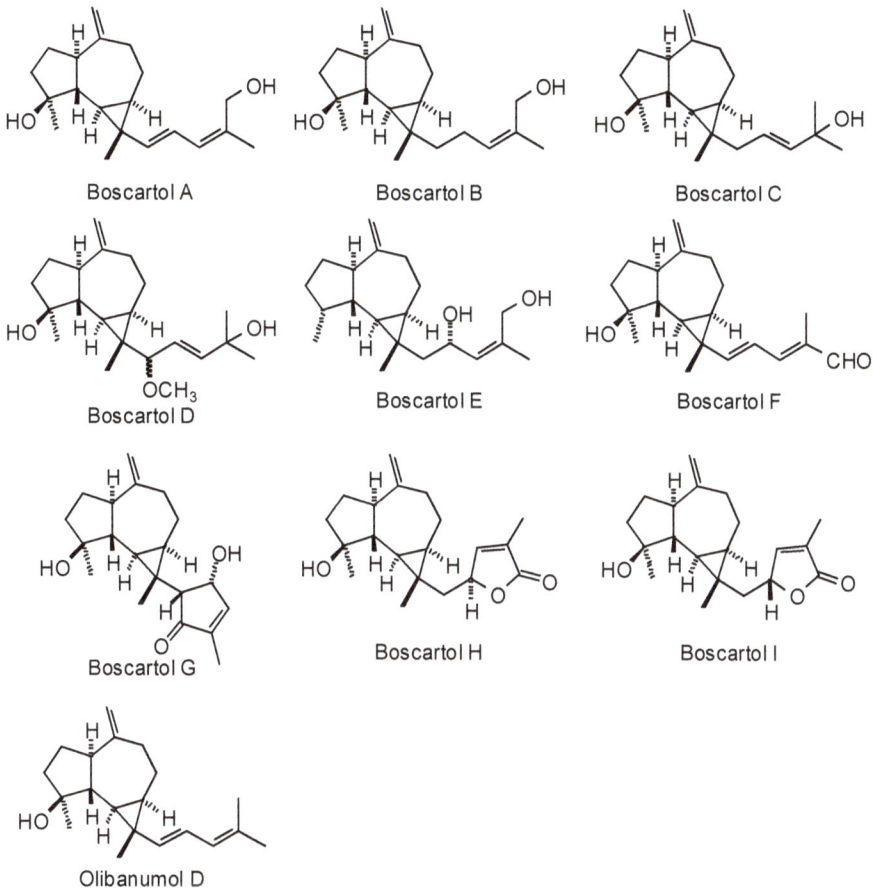

Figure 2. Cneorubenoid diterpenoids isolated from *Boswellia carteri*.

Boswellia carteri oleo-gum resin is the source of several prenylated aromadendrane (cneorubenoid) diterpenoids (Figure 2) [20,21].

Numerous ursane, oleanane, lupane, dammarane, and tirucallane triterpenoids have been isolated and characterized from *Boswellia* species (Figure 3) [22]. *Boswellia serrata* has yielded α-boswellic acid, β-boswellic acid, 3-acetyl-α-boswellic acid, 3-acetyl-β-boswellic acid, 11-keto-β-boswellic acid, and 3-acetyl-11-keto-β-boswellic acid [23]. *Boswellia carteri* has yielded the oleanane triterpenoids α-boswellic acid, and 3-acetyl-α-boswellic acid; the ursane triterpenoids β-boswellic acid, 3-acetyl-β-boswellic acid, 11-keto-β-boswellic acid, 3-acetyl-11-keto-β-boswellic acid, 3-acetyl-11α-methoxy-β-boswellic acid, 9,11-dehydro-β-boswellic acid, and 3-acetyl-9,11-dehydro-β-boswellic acid; the lupane triterpenoids lupeolic acid and 3-acetyl lupeolic acid; and the tirucallane triterpenoids α-elemolic acid, β-elemonic acid, 3α-hydroxytirucalla-7,24-dien-21-oic acid, 3α-acetoxytirucalla-7,24-dien-21-oic acid, and 3β-hydroxytirucalla-7, 24-dien-21-oic acid [24]. Olibanumols A, B, C, H, I, J′ [25], E, F, G [20], K, L′, M, and N [26] have been isolated from the oleo-gum resin of *B. carteri*. *B. carteri* resin has also yielded boscartenes L, M, and N, as well as trametenolic acid B, 3-oxotirucalla-7,9(11),24-trien-21-oic acid, and (20S)-3,7-dioxo-tirucalla-8,24,-dien-21-oic acid [27].

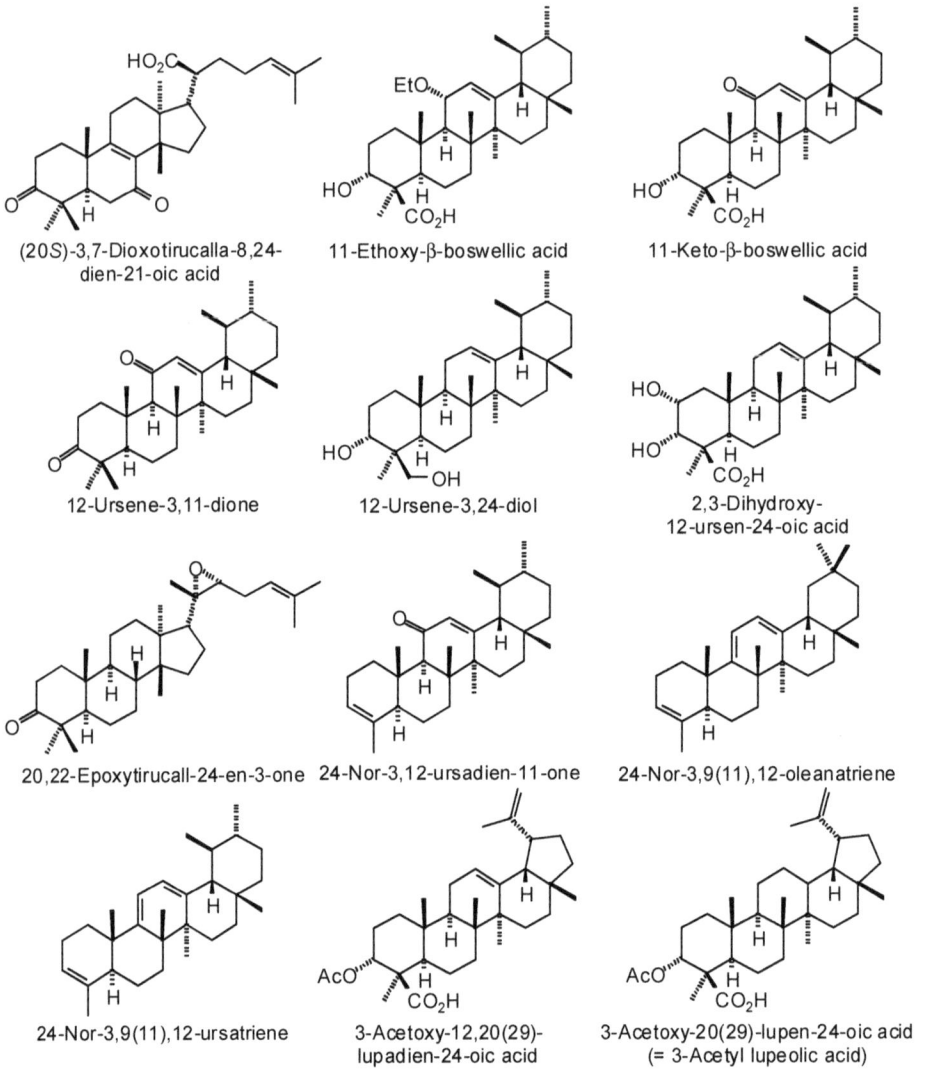

(20*S*)-3,7-Dioxotirucalla-8,24-
dien-21-oic acid

11-Ethoxy-β-boswellic acid

11-Keto-β-boswellic acid

12-Ursene-3,11-dione

12-Ursene-3,24-diol

2,3-Dihydroxy-
12-ursen-24-oic acid

20,22-Epoxytirucall-24-en-3-one

24-Nor-3,12-ursadien-11-one

24-Nor-3,9(11),12-oleanatriene

24-Nor-3,9(11),12-ursatriene

3-Acetoxy-12,20(29)-
lupadien-24-oic acid

3-Acetoxy-20(29)-lupen-24-oic acid
(= 3-Acetyl lupeolic acid)

Figure 3. *Cont.*

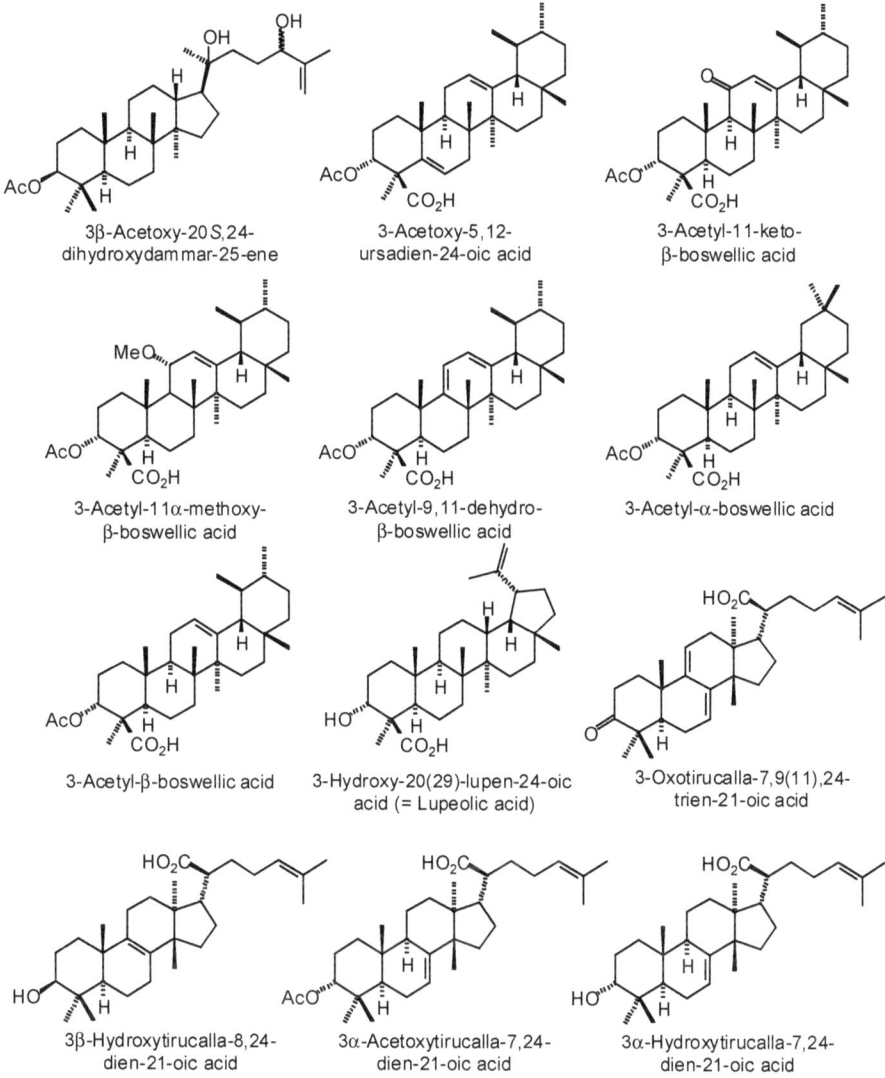

3β-Acetoxy-20S,24-
dihydroxydammar-25-ene

3-Acetoxy-5,12-
ursadien-24-oic acid

3-Acetyl-11-keto-
β-boswellic acid

3-Acetyl-11α-methoxy-
β-boswellic acid

3-Acetyl-9,11-dehydro-
β-boswellic acid

3-Acetyl-α-boswellic acid

3-Acetyl-β-boswellic acid

3-Hydroxy-20(29)-lupen-24-oic
acid (= Lupeolic acid)

3-Oxotirucalla-7,9(11),24-
trien-21-oic acid

3β-Hydroxytirucalla-8,24-
dien-21-oic acid

3α-Acetoxytirucalla-7,24-
dien-21-oic acid

3α-Hydroxytirucalla-7,24-
dien-21-oic acid

Figure 3. *Cont.*

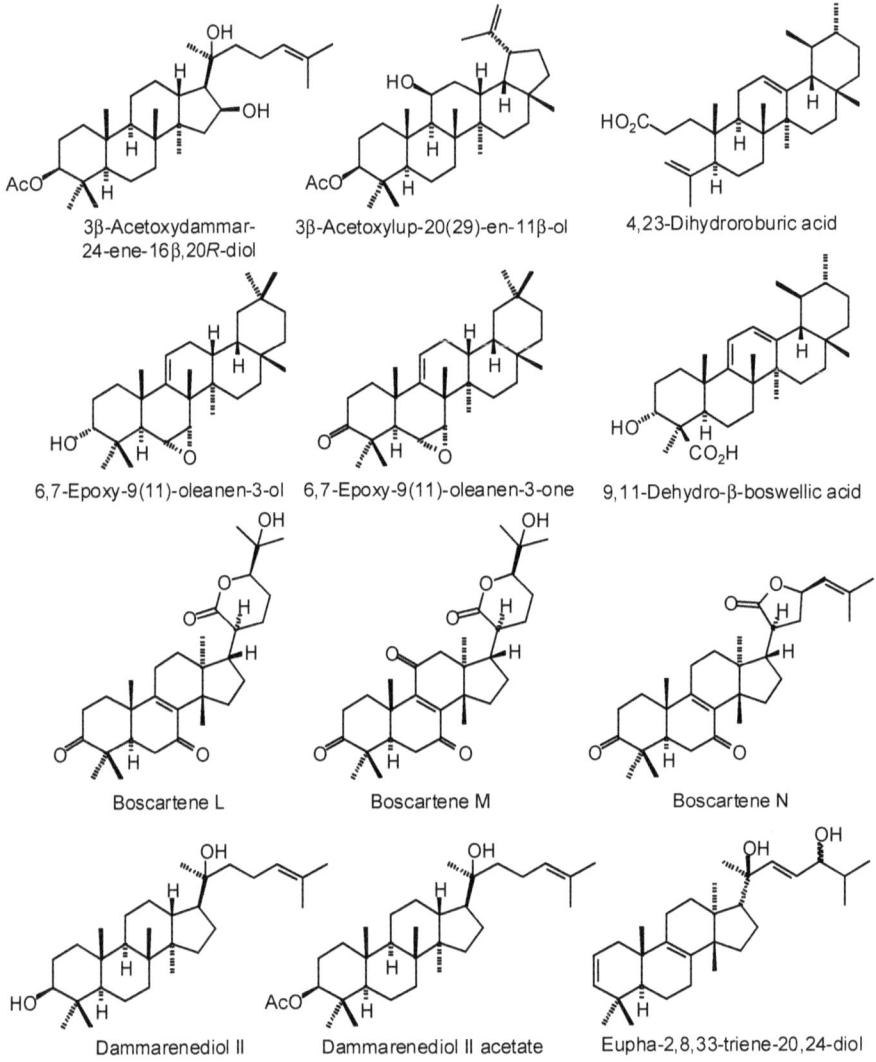

3β-Acetoxydammar-24-ene-16β,20R-diol

3β-Acetoxylup-20(29)-en-11β-ol

4,23-Dihydroroburic acid

6,7-Epoxy-9(11)-oleanen-3-ol

6,7-Epoxy-9(11)-oleanen-3-one

9,11-Dehydro-β-boswellic acid

Boscartene L

Boscartene M

Boscartene N

Dammarenediol II

Dammarenediol II acetate

Eupha-2,8,33-triene-20,24-diol

Figure 3. *Cont.*

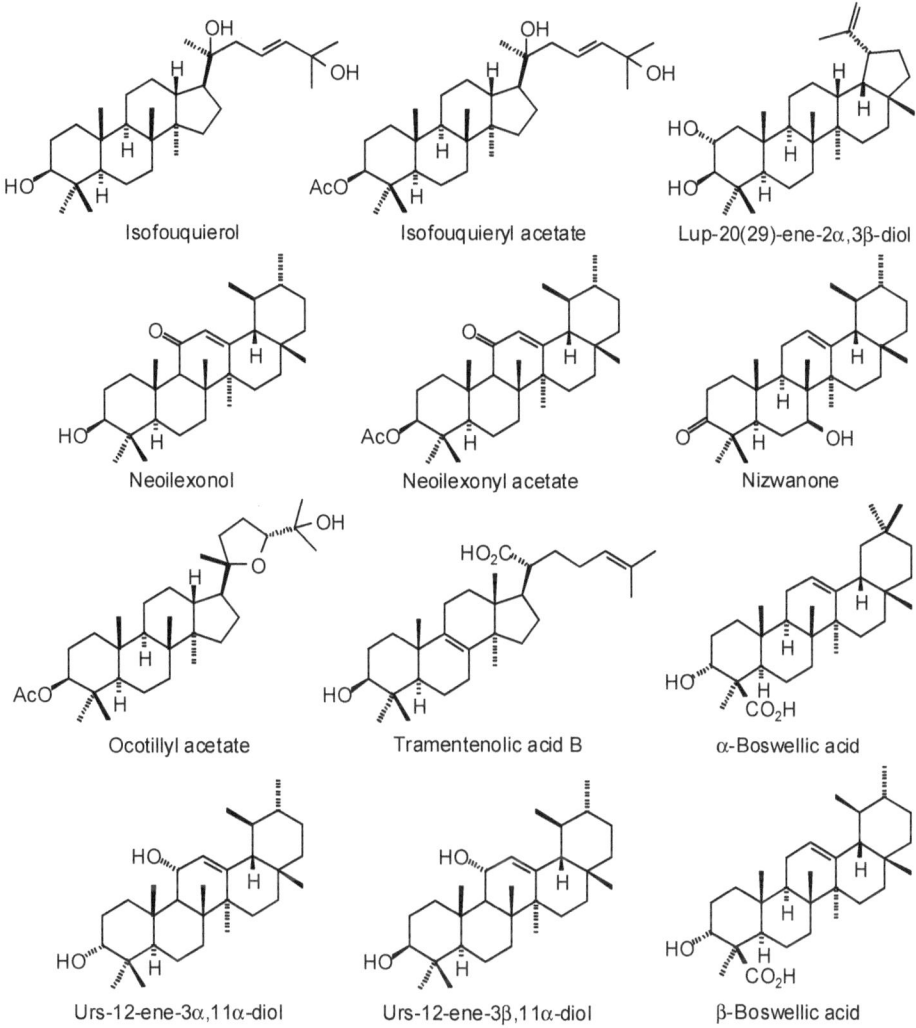

Isofouquierol

Isofouquieryl acetate

Lup-20(29)-ene-2α,3β-diol

Neoilexonol

Neoilexonyl acetate

Nizwanone

Ocotillyl acetate

Tramentenolic acid B

α-Boswellic acid

Urs-12-ene-3α,11α-diol

Urs-12-ene-3β,11α-diol

β-Boswellic acid

Figure 3. *Cont.*

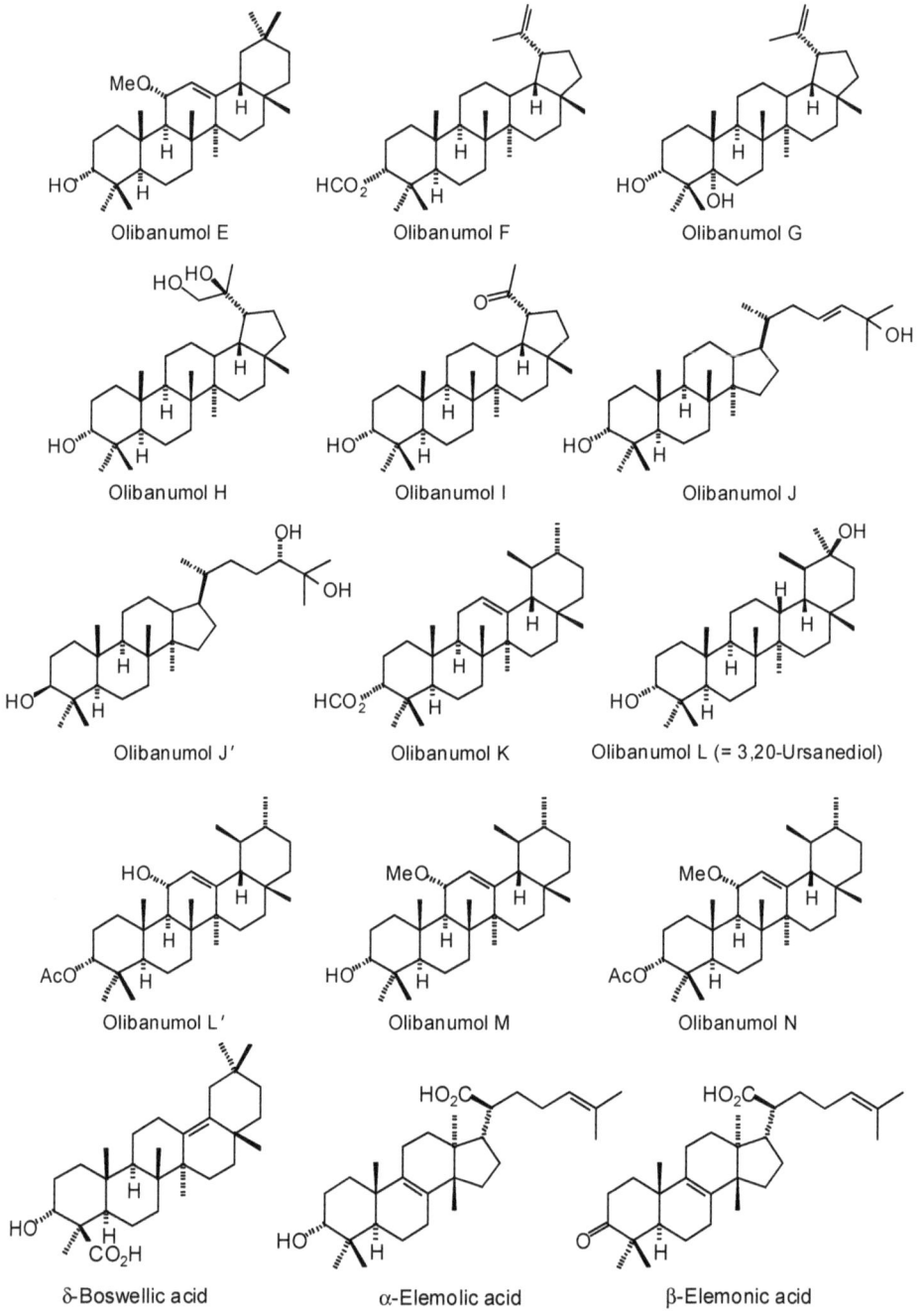

Figure 3. Triterpenoids isolated from *Boswellia* species.

2. Materials and Methods

2.1. Ligand Preparation

Each ligand structure was prepared using Spartan'16 v. 2.0.7 (Wavefunction, Inc., Irvine, CA, USA). The lowest-energy conformations of the ligands were determined using the Merck Molecular Force Field (MMFF) [28]. In the case of the cembranoid macrocyclic ligands, further conformational analysis was carried out using density functional theory at the M06-2X/6-31G* level [29] with SM8 [30] aqueous solvent model [31].

2.2. Reverse Molelcular Docking

A reverse molecular docking study was carried out on each of the *Bosellia* terpenoids with the sc-PDB database of druggable binding sites [32]. Each compound was examined against the 16034 protein targets contained in the sc-PDB database. Prior to docking, all solvent molecules were removed from the protein structures. Co-crystallized enzyme cofactors were retained as cofactors and co-crystallized substrates or inhibitors were retained as ligands. Molecular docking was carried out using Molegro Virtual Docker v. 6.0.1 (Molegro ApS, Aarhus, Denmark) [33] as previously reported [34]. A python script was written to generate the Molegro input files; the jobs were run as a batch from the mvd.exe command line executable. The script took the co-crystallized ligands in each protein and wrote an input file that defined the search space for that docking as a sphere centered on the ligand's center of mass. A 15-Å radius sphere was centered on the binding sites of each protein structure in order to permit each ligand to search. Standard protonation states of each protein, based on neutral pH, were used and charges were assigned based on standard templates as part of the Molegro Virtual Docker program. Each protein was used as a rigid model without protein relaxation. Flexible-ligand models were used in the docking optimizations. Different orientations of the ligands were search and ranked based on their "rerank" energy scores. A total of 100 runs for each ligand were carried out.

2.3. Conformational Analysis of Boscartol D

All calculations were carried out using Spartan'16 for Windows (Wavefunction, Inc., Irvine, CA, USA). Conformational profiles were carried out using molecular mechanics with the MMFF force field. Conformations with relative energies <20 kJ/mol were re-evaluated, with geometry optimization, using density functional theory (DFT, M06-2X/6-31G*) with a nonpolar solvent ($CHCl_3$) model.

3. Results and Discussion

3.1. Cembranoid Diterpenoids

The macrocyclic cembranoid diterpenoids examined in this study are shown in Figure 1. The top-binding protein targets for each of the *Boswellia* cembranoids are summarized in Table 1. Included in Table 1 are the median docking energies for comparison. The top binding proteins for boscartin A were acetylcholinesterase (AChE) enzymes, *Torpedo californica* (TcAChE) and human (HsAChE). Boscartin B docked preferentially with human *N*-acetylgalactosaminyltransferase (HsGTA) as well as with the bacterial targets *Serratia marcescens* chitinase B (SmChiB), *Helicobacter pylori* peptide deformylase (HpPDF), and *Mycobacterium tuberculosis* 7,8-diaminopelargonic acid synthase (MtBioA). The proteins with the most exothermic docking for boscartin C were *Escherichia coli* aspartate transaminase (EcAspTA), murine acetylcholinesterase (MmAChE), and *Daboia russelii* (Russell's viper) phospholipase A$_2$ (DrPLA2). Boscartin D showed excellent docking with TcAChE (PDB 2cek, E_{dock} = −115.3 kJ/mol) and EcAspTA. The best protein targets for boscartin E were TcAChE, HpPDF, and MtBioA. Boscartin F showed preferential docking energies with human pyruvate kinase M2 (HsPKM2), TcAChE, and HpPDF. Boscartin G showed excellent docking properties with acetylcholinesterases TcAChE and HsAChE. The proteins with the most exothermic docking energies with boscartin H were human N-acetylgalactosaminyltransferase (HsGTA), DrPLA2, SmChiB, and MmAChE.

Table 1. Protein targets with the most exothermic docking energies (E_{dock}, kJ/mol) for *Boswellia* cembranoid ligands.

Ligand	PDB [a]	E_{dock}	Target Protein
Boscartin A	1e66	−119.7	*Torpedo californica* acetylcholinesterase (TcAChE)
	2cek	−123.7	*Torpedo californica* acetylcholinesterase (TcAChE)
	4bdt	−113.5	human acetylcholinesterase (HsAChE)
		−79.2	Median docking energy
Boscartin B	1h0g	−107.8	*Serratia marcescens* chitinase B (SmChiB)
	2ew5	−104.6	*Helicobacter pylori* peptide deformylase (HpPDF)
	3tfu	−107.5	*Mycobacterium tuberculosis* 7,8-diaminopelargonic acid synthase (MtBioA)
	3v0o	−110.4	human fucosylgalactoslde α N acetylgalactosaminyltransferase (HsGTA)
		−80.5	Median docking energy
Boscartin C	1ahg	−112.5	*Escherichia coli* aspartate aminotransferase (EcAspTA)
	1fv0	−108.2	*Daboia russelii* (Russell's viper) phospholipase A_2 (DrPLA2)
	1q83	−110.4	murine acetylcholinesterase (MmAChE)
	4g1n	−106.5	human pyruvate kinase isozyme M2 (HsPKM2)
		−91.2	Median docking energy
Boscartin D	1ahg	−114.4	*Escherichia coli* aspartate aminotransferase (EcAspTA)
	1xzq	−106.3	*Thermotoga maritima* GTP-binding protein TrmE (TmTrmE)
	2cek	−115.3	*Torpedo californica* acetylcholinesterase (TcAChE)
		−82.0	Median docking energy
Boscartin E	1ahg	−110.4	*Escherichia coli* aspartate aminotransferase (EcAspTA)
	1e66	−111.7	*Torpedo californica* acetylcholinesterase (TcAChE)
	2ew5	−107.5	*Helicobacter pylori* peptide deformylase (HpPDF)
		−68.4	Median docking energy
Boscartin F	2ew5	−109.5	*Helicobacter pylori* peptide deformylase (HpPDF)
	3i6m	−107.3	*Torpedo californica* acetylcholinesterase (TcAChE)
	4g1n	−108.5	human pyruvate kinase isozyme M2 (HsPKM2)
		−82.9	Median docking energy
Boscartin G	1e66	−126.4	*Torpedo californica* acetylcholinesterase (TcAChE)
	2cek	−116.8	*Torpedo californica* acetylcholinesterase (TcAChE)
	4bdt	−118.7	human acetylcholinesterase (HsAChE)
		−89.9	Median docking energy
Boscartin H	1fv0	−106.9	*Daboia russelii* (Russell's viper) phospholipase A_2 (DrPLA2)
	1w1t	−106.0	*Serratia marcescens* chitinase B (SmChiB)
	2gyw	−105.9	murine acetylcholinesterase (MmAChE)
	3v0o	−109.3	human fucosylgalactoside α N-acetylgalactosaminyltransferase (HsGTA)
		−88.4	Median docking energy
Incensole	2cek	−111.9	*Torpedo californica* acetylcholinesterase (TcAChE)
	3ugr	−109.7	human aldo-keto reductase 1C3 (HsAKR1C3)
	1h0g	−102.4	*Serratia marcescens* chitinase B (SmChiB)
		−78.1	Median docking energy
Incensole acetate	1ahg	−106.9	*Escherichia coli* aspartate aminotransferase (EcAspTA)
	3jun	−103.7	*Burkholderia cepacia* phenazine biosynthesis protein A/B (BcPhzA/B)
		−69.5	Median docking energy
Incensole oxide	1ahg	−108.6	*Escherichia coli* aspartate aminotransferase (EcAspTA)
	2cek	−103.1	*Torpedo californica* acetylcholinesterase (TcAChE)
	3jup	−103.5	*Burkholderia cepacia* phenazine biosynthesis protein A/B (BcPhzA/B)
	3mee	−106.7	HIV-1 reverse transcriptase (HIV-1 RT)
		−74.6	Median docking energy
Incensole oxide acetate	1ahg	−119.0	*Escherichia coli* aspartate aminotransferase (EcAspTA)
	1q83	−109.6	murine acetylcholinesterase (MmAChE)
	2cek	−110.4	*Torpedo californica* acetylcholinesterase (TcAChE)
	3i6m	−114.3	*Torpedo californica* acetylcholinesterase (TcAChE)
	3mee	−113.5	HIV-1 reverse transcriptase (HIV-1 RT)
		−91.9	Median docking energy
Isoincensole oxide	3jup	−103.3	*Burkholderia cepacia* phenazine biosynthesis protein A/B (BcPhzA/B)
		−80.5	Median docking energy

Table 1. *Cont.*

Ligand	PDB [a]	E_{dock}	Target Protein
Isoincensolol	1fv0	−108.2	*Daboia russelii* (Russell's viper) phospholipase A_2 (DrPLA2)
	1jus	−107.9	*Staphylococcus aureus* multidrug binding protein (SaQacR)
	2qp4	−102.2	human dehydroepiandrosterone sulfotransferase (HsSULT2A1)
		−74.0	Median docking energy
Serratol	1e66	−104.1	*Torpedo californica* acetylcholinesterase (TcAChE)
	2cek	−106.1	*Torpedo californica* acetylcholinesterase (TcAChE)
	2ew5	−103.2	*Helicobacter pylori* peptide deformylase (HpPDF)
	4bdt	−103.0	human acetylcholinesterase (HsAChE)
		−78.1	Median docking energy
Verticillatriene	1w4l	−104.3	*Torpedo californica* acetylcholinesterase (TcAChE)
	3i6m	−100.8	*Torpedo californica* acetylcholinesterase (TcAChE)
	3i6z	−103.2	*Torpedo californica* acetylcholinesterase (TcAChE)
		−63.6	Median docking energy

[a] PDB: Protein Data Bank code.

Incensole docked well with TcAChE, human aldo-keto reductase 1C3 (HsAKR1C3), and SmChiB. Incensole acetate preferentially targeted bacterial proteins EcAspTA, HpPDF, and *Burkholderia cepacia* phenazine biosynthesis protein A/B (BcPhzA/B). The preferred protein targets for incensole oxide were EcAspTA, human immunodeficiency virus type 1 reverse transcriptase (HIV-1-RT), TcAChE, BcPhzA/B, and MtBioA. Incensole oxide acetate gave excellent docking energies to EcAspTA, TcAChE, MmAChE, and HIV-1-RT. Isoincensole oxide docked well to BcPzhA/B and TcAChE. The protein targets that showed the best docking energies with isoincensolol were DrPLA2, *Staphylococcus aureus* multidrug binding protein QacR (SaQacR), and human dehydroepiandrosterone sulfotransferase (HsSULT2A1).

Every cembranoid ligand showed excellent docking properties to acetylcholinesterases (Table 2). Acetylcholinesterase has been identified as a target for treatment of Alzheimer's disease [35]. This is notable because frankincense (*Boswellia* spp.) resins have been used in Persian traditional medicine as an anti-Alzheimer's agent [36,37]. Animal models (rat) of Alzheimer's disease [38–40] and human clinical trials [41,42] showed beneficial effects on memory with frankincense.

Table 2. MolDock molecular docking energies (kJ/mol) of *Boswellia* cembranoids with acetylcholinesterase protein targets. [a]

Ligand	TcAChE 1e66	TcAChE 1h22	TcAChE 1w4l	TcAChE 2cek	TcAChE 3i6m	TcAChE 3i6z	MmAChE 1q83	MmAChE 2gyw	HsAChE 4bdt
Boscartin A	−119.7	−98.4	−99.5	−123.7	−98.2	−100.6	−95.9	−101.4	−113.5
Boscartin B	−95.1	−98.8	−92.5	−106.3	−99.2	−94.5	−94.3	−85.8	−106.3
Boscartin C	−87.7	−90.8	−94.7	−96.9	−104.1	−94.2	−110.4	−94.0	−86.6
Boscartin D	−99.7	−102.8	−93.1	−115.3	−103.7	−93.9	−92.5	−93.6	−90.2
Boscartin E	−111.7	−96.5	−94.5	−108.7	−95.5	−92.9	−86.0	−94.8	−90.6
Boscartin F	−93.2	−97.0	−98.5	−104.8	−107.3	−95.8	−101.1	−82.4	−77.3
Boscartin G	−126.4	−99.4	−94.5	−116.8	−101.5	−95.6	−111.1	−94.1	−118.7
Boscartin H	−100.1	−106.3	−103.6	−105.6	−103.0	−104.2	−98.8	−105.9	−97.8
Incensole	−89.7	−92.1	−89.5	−111.9	−94.1	−89.6	−90.3	−87.7	−53.4
Incensole acetate	−88.6	−97.2	−102.8	−102.5	−102.3	−101.7	−87.5	−85.0	−42.3
Incensole oxide	−89.6	−93.2	−92.7	−103.1	−96.9	−89.3	−119.9	−95.5	−93.5
Incensole oxide acetate	−109.8	−98.7	−96.8	−110.4	−114.3	−95.8	−109.6	−97.7	−102.6
Isoincensole oxide	−92.9	−98.9	−96.4	−103.6	−98.1	−89.9	−89.9	−90.3	−94.1
Isoincensolol	−88.5	−99.5	−92.4	−101.5	−98.3	−91.2	−77.0	−80.4	−73.6
Serratol	−104.1	−95.7	−92.2	−106.1	−94.5	−88.1	−96.4	−89.3	−104.0
Verticillatriene	−82.5	−91.2	−104.3	−85.3	−100.8	−103.2	−73.9	−98.1	−61.2

[a] TcAChE = *Torpedo californica* acetylcholinesterase. MmAChE = *Mus musculus* (murine) acetylcholinesterase. HsAChE = human acetylcholinesterase.

The lowest-energy docked pose of boscartin G with TcAChE (PDB 1e66, Figure 4A) shows the ligand to adopt the lowest-energy conformation as calculated by density functional theory at the

M06-2X/6-31G*/SM8 level [31]. Key interactions between boscartin G and TcAChE are hydrophobic interactions between the ligand and aromatic amino acid side chains of Trp84, Phe330, and His440 (Figure 4B). In addition, there are hydrogen-bonding interactions between the oxirane ring of the ligand and the phenolic -OH of Tyr121 and the C(11)-OH of the ligand and the peptide C=O of His440 (Figure 4B).

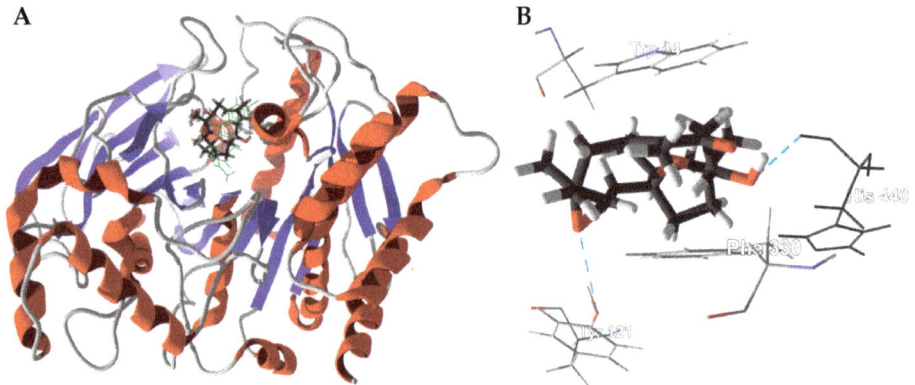

Figure 4. Lowest-energy docked pose of boscartin G with *Torpedo californica* acetylcholinesterase (TcAChE, PDB 1e66). (**A**): Ribbon structure of TcAChE with boscartin G in the active site; the co-crystallized ligand (huprene X) is shown as a green wire figure. (**B**): Key interactions of boscartin G with amino acids in the active site of TcAChE; hydrogen bonds are shown as blue dashed lines.

Boscartin A occupies the active site of TcAChE (Figure 5A, PDB 2cek). As observed for boscartin G with TcAChE, key interactions between the docked ligand and the protein are hydrophobic interactions with Trp84, Phe330, and His440, and a hydrogen-bond between the C(11)-OH of the ligand and the His440 peptide C=O. The conformation of the lowest energy docked pose of boscartin A (Figure 5A) is the same as the lowest-energy calculated (M06-2X/6-31G*/SM8, Figure 5B) [31] and not that found in the X-ray crystal structure [13].

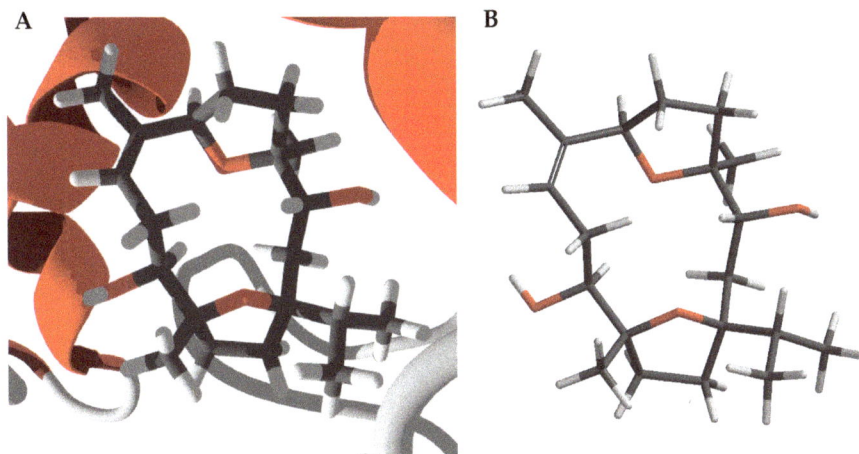

Figure 5. Boscartin A. (**A**): Lowest-energy docked pose of boscartin A with *Torpedo californica* acetylcholinesterase (PDB 2cek). (**B**): Calculated lowest-energy conformation of boscartin A at the M06-2X/6-31G*/SM8 level of theory [31].

A number of bacterial proteins were targeted by *Boswellia* cembranoids (Table 3). *Helicobacter pylori* peptide deformylase (HpPDF) and *Escherichia coli* aspartate transaminase (EcAspTA) were particularly well targeted, while boscartin C and E and incensole oxide acetate showed remarkably exothermic docking energies. *Boswellia* resin extracts have shown in-vitro antibacterial activity [43–45], and frankincense resins have been used traditionally to treat wounds [6,46] and for oral hygiene [8]. Furthermore, *B. papyrifera* resin has shown activity against methicillin-resistant *Staphylococcus aureus* (MRSA) [47] and *B. serrata* resin showed activity in a clinical trial against plaque-induced gingivitis [48]. The selective targeting of bacterial proteins by *Boswellia* cembranoids corroborates the traditional medicinal uses and the demonstrated antibacterial activities of frankincense.

The potent docking properties of *Boswellia* cembranoids with HpPDF are particularly noteworthy. There is a strong association between colonization of the human stomach by *Helicobacter pylori* and gastrointestinal illnesses such as chronic gastritis and peptic ulcers [49]. Frankincense has been used traditionally to treat stomach disturbances [4] and ulcers [46]. In addition, *Boswellia* extracts have been shown in clinical studies to be helpful in treating ulcerative colitis [50].

Boscartin G is the strongest binding *Boswellia* cembranoid ligand with HpPDF (PDB 2ew5). The lowest-energy docked pose is shown in Figure 6. Boscartin G occupies the active site of HpPDF at the same location as the co-crystallized ligand, 4-{(1*E*)-3-oxo-3-[(2-phenylethyl)amino]-prop-1-en-1-yl}-1,2-phenylene diacetate, a cavity surrounded by Ile45, Gly95, Glu94, His138, Cys96, and Gly46 (Figure 6B). The ligand forms two hydrogen-bonds with the peptide N-H groups of Ile45 and Gly46. The docked structure of boscartin G with HpPDF shows the same conformation (Figure 6C) as that predicted from DFT calculations (Figure 6D) [31].

Table 3. MolDock molecular docking energies (kJ/mol) of *Boswellia* cembranoids with bacterial target proteins. [a]

Ligand	EcAspTA	SmChiB	SmChiB	SmChiB	SaQacR	SaQacR	SaQacR	SaQacR	HpPDF	BcPhzA/B	BcPhzA/B	MtBioA
	1ahg	1h0g	1w1t	3wd2	1jus	1rpw	3br2	3bti	2ew5	3jun	3jup	3tfu
Boscartin A	−116.9	−93.6	−99.4	−96.3	−99.4	−104.1	−94.9	−95.7	−101.8	−100.3	−107.8	−104.9
Boscartin B	−98.2	−107.8	−103.7	−91.5	−98.1	−106.5	−94.7	−96.5	−104.6	−98.4	−93.9	−107.5
Boscartin C	−112.5	−96.3	−97.3	−90.6	−100.0	−98.5	−98.4	−102.3	−106.2	−99.3	−106.4	−100.4
Boscartin D	−114.4	−99.7	−105.3	−91.5	−95.2	−106.2	−100.1	−96.3	−104.9	−98.0	−95.8	−99.3
Boscartin E	−110.4	−101.0	−105.9	−105.4	−99.2	−101.3	−95.3	−95.3	−107.5	−84.7	−96.7	−107.7
Boscartin F	−99.7	−97.3	−103.7	−89.9	−101.0	−95.7	−94.4	−85.2	−109.5	−87.7	−98.0	−95.1
Boscartin G	−105.5	−90.8	−93.0	−93.8	−95.1	−98.2	−92.2	−88.7	−112.7	−95.4	−92.6	−108.5
Boscartin H	−104.1	−103.6	−106.0	−104.4	−97.2	−98.8	−97.4	−94.5	−100.9	−93.4	−101.5	−99.5
Incensole	−104.3	−102.4	−101.1	−96.2	−85.0	−96.3	−90.7	−95.0	−94.0	−92.9	−93.0	−95.7
Incensole acetate	−109.9	−102.3	−96.2	−98.1	−96.6	−104.5	−96.1	−98.8	−96.2	−103.7	−91.5	−96.2
Incensole oxide	−108.6	−92.0	−93.5	−90.3	−97.4	−99.8	−94.2	−95.6	−101.4	−97.1	−103.5	−103.5
Incensole oxide acetate	−119.0	−101.1	−98.9	−96.4	−96.7	−98.7	−99.2	−100.0	−106.9	−105.5	−99.4	−100.0
Isoincensole oxide	−96.2	−87.6	−93.5	−89.9	−98.5	−97.5	−98.5	−92.7	−88.9	−87.5	−103.3	−91.2
Isoincensolol	−87.3	−91.2	−88.9	−87.9	−107.9	−90.0	−99.6	−87.8	−99.7	−91.5	−100.0	−95.2
Serratol	−90.2	−90.1	−89.9	−82.2	−90.1	−91.4	−97.6	−89.1	−103.2	−87.4	−92.7	−93.4
Verticillatriene	−74.0	−69.5	−69.0	−69.5	−81.2	−87.2	−85.5	−78.5	−77.3	−76.5	−89.9	−84.4

[a] EcAspTA = *Escherichia coli* aspartate transaminase. SmChiB = *Serratia marcescens* chitinase. SaQacR = *Staphylococcus aureus* multidrug binding protein. HpPDF = *Helicobacter pylori* peptide deformylase. BcPhzA/B = *Burkholderia cepacia* phenazine biosynthesis protein A/B. MtBioA = *Mycobacterium tuberculosis* 7,8-diaminopelargonic acid synthase.

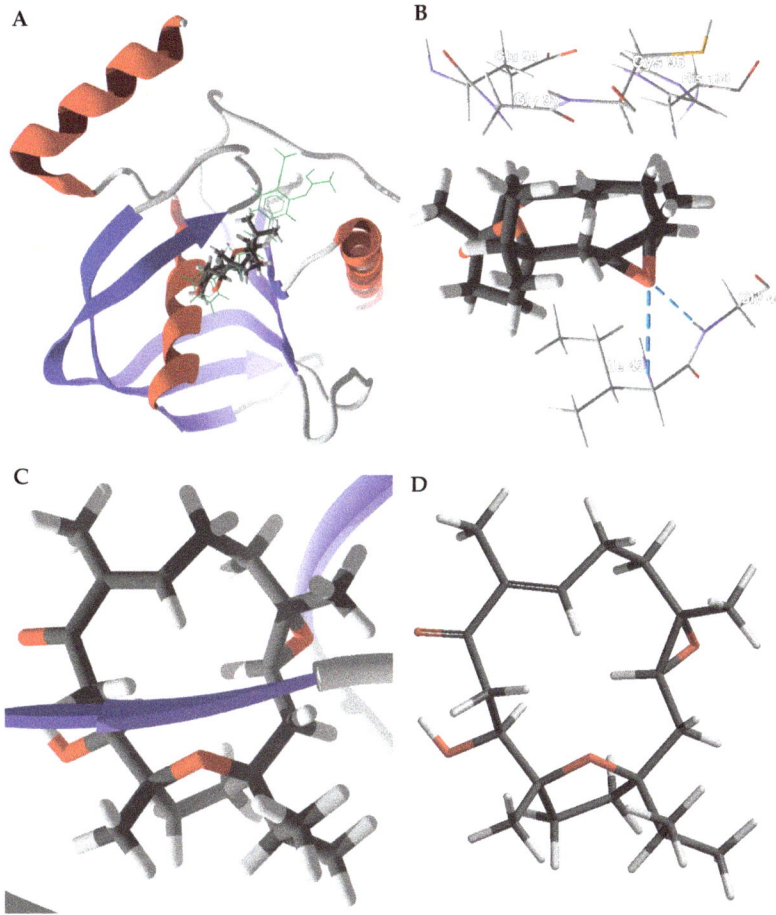

Figure 6. Docking of boscartin G with *Helicobacter pylori* peptide deformylase (HpPDF, PDB 2cek). (**A**): Ribbon structure of HpPDF showing boscartin G in the active site; the co-crystallized ligand, 4-{(1*E*)-3-oxo-3-[(2-phenylethyl)amino]prop-1-en-1-yl}-1,2-phenylene diacetate, is shown as a green stick figure. (**B**): Key interactions of boscartin G in the active site of HpPDF; hydrogen-bonds are shown as blue dashed lines. (**C**): Conformation of boscartin G docked to HpPDF. (**D**): Lowest-energy conformation of boscartin G determined by density functional calculations (M06-2X/6-31G*/SM8) [31].

Several *Boswellia* cembranoids showed selective docking to HIV-1 reverse transcriptase (HIV1-RT) (Table 4). In particular, incensole oxide acetate showed excellent docking ($E_{dock} < -100$ kJ/mol) to four of the seven HIV1-RT protein crystal structures. The lowest-energy docked pose of incensole oxide acetate with HIV-1 reverse transcriptase (PDB 3mee) is shown in Figure 7. Key interactions between the ligand and the protein are Tyr181, Tyr188, Leu100, Trp229, and Lys103 (Figure 7B). Interestingly, the docking energies for the cembranoids to PDB 3lal and 3t19 are, on average, lower than for the other protein structures. The differences in docking energies can be attributed to the arrangements of the amino acid residues at the binding sites, resulting in different orientations of the docked ligands. Thus, for example, the key amino acids interacting with incensole oxide acetate in PDB 3lal are Tyr188, Leu100, Tyr181, Phe227, and Tyr318 (Figure 7C), while PDB 3t19 had Leu100, Tyr188, Val106, Tyr318, and Tyr181 (Figure 7D). That is, binding sites of the protein crystal structures are heavily influenced by the co-crystallized ligands. Both methanol and aqueous extracts of *Boswellia carteri* have demonstrated HIV-1 reverse transcriptase activity [51].

Table 4. MolDock molecular docking energies (kJ/mol) of *Boswellia* cembranoids with human immunodeficiency virus type 1 reverse transcriptase (HIV1-RT).

Ligand	1eet	2hnz	3irx	3is9	3mee	3lal	3t19
Boscartin A	−99.1	−101.7	−96.8	−93.8	−96.0	−69.4	−75.4
Boscartin B	−94.1	−98.5	−100.2	−94.7	−95.6	−72.2	−97.8
Boscartin C	−104.2	−91.5	−97.0	−101.3	−100.5	−87.8	−84.0
Boscartin D	−89.2	−100.5	−97.1	−97.1	−96.4	−78.7	−83.2
Boscartin E	−97.2	−100.6	−91.7	−97.0	−89.4	−60.8	−72.0
Boscartin F	−88.9	−93.8	−98.1	−98.1	95.1	−88.1	−69.4
Boscartin G	−92.8	−88.7	−97.6	−95.4	−113.8	+9.3	−82.3
Boscartin H	−98.2	−90.4	−96.9	−97.1	−98.2	−86.9	−56.2
Incensole	−83.8	−101.5	−88.8	−88.3	−86.8	−84.0	−94.7
Incensole acetate	−95.6	−92.6	−97.9	−97.0	−84.6	−95.9	−91.6
Incensole oxide	−105.1	−93.2	−94.9	−98.7	−106.7	−81.7	−79.0
Incensole oxide acetate	−107.2	−84.5	−106.8	−106.2	−113.5	−87.8	−87.1
Isoincensole oxide	−97.8	−86.5	−89.4	−90.2	−98.7	−77.5	−57.7
Isoincensolol	−95.2	−85.6	−98.2	−85.4	−85.9	−70.6	−72.5
Serratol	−90.4	−87.9	−86.8	−89.3	−90.1	−56.0	−48.9
Verticillatriene	−81.6	−67.1	−78.4	−81.0	−82.5	−76.9	−25.5

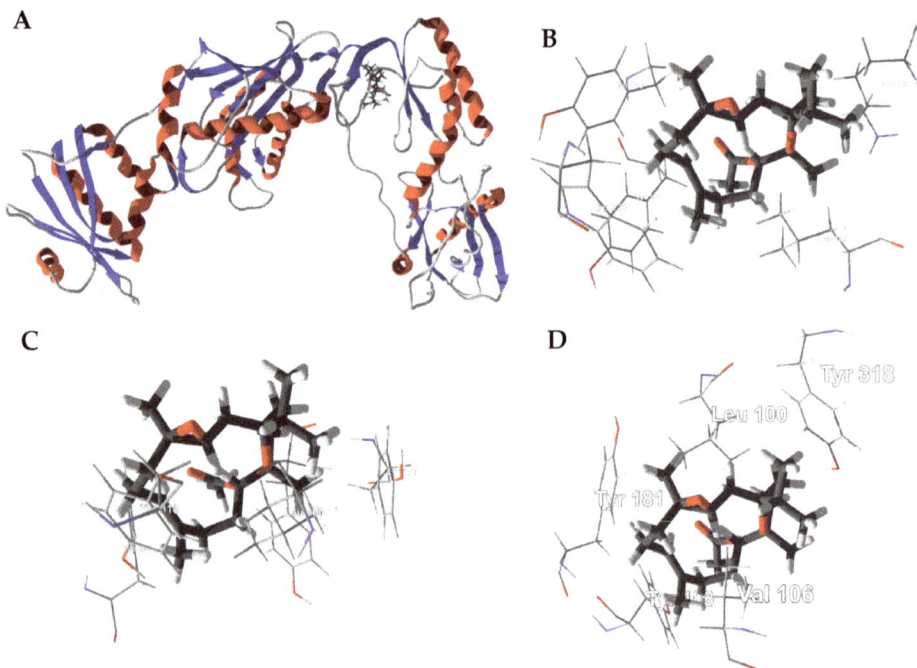

Figure 7. Molecular docking of incensole oxide acetate with HIV-1 reverse transcriptase. (**A**): Ribbon structure of HIV1-RT (PDB 3mee) showing incensole oxide acetate in the active site. (**B**): Key interactions of incensole oxide acetate in the active site of HIV1-RT (PDB 3mee). (**C**): Key interactions of incensole oxide acetate in the active site of HIV1-RT (PDB 3lal). (**D**): Key interactions of incensole oxide acetate in the active site of HIV1-RT (PDB 3t19).

3.2. Cneorubenoid Diterpenoids

The cneorubenoid diterpenoids, boscartols A–I and olibanumol D, can be considered to be prenylated aromadendranes (Figure 2), and have been isolated from the oleo-gum resin of *Boswellia carteri* [21]. The absolute configuration of the C(15) of boscartol D was not experimentally determined [21]. Nevertheless, both diastereomers, (15*R*)-boscartol D and (15*S*)-boscartol D were used in the reverse docking. In addition, the stereochemistry of C(15) was determined theoretically using density functional theory (DFT) conformational analysis carried out at the M06-2X/6-31G* level of theory, including a non-polar ($CHCl_3$) solvent model. A complete conformational analysis of (15*R*)-boscartol D was carried out giving 20 low-energy conformations (E_{rel} < 14.0 kJ/mol, accounting for 100% of the Boltzmann distribution of conformers). Similarly, conformational analysis of (15*S*)-boscartol D returned 13 low-energy (E_{rel} < 13.0 kJ/mol). For each of the conformations, the H-C(15)-C(16)-H dihedral angle was determined and the corresponding vicinal coupling constants ($^3J_{HH}$) calculated using both the original Karplus equation [52] and the Haasnoot/Altona generalized Karplus equation that includes correction terms for the electronegativity of substituents [53]. Accounting for the Boltzmann distribution, (15*R*)-boscartin D is predicted to have $^3J_{HH}$ of 4.3 and 5.1 Hz, respectively. The (15*S*)-diastereomer, on the other hand, is calculated to have $^3J_{HH}$ of 6.3 and 6.5 Hz, respectively. The reported $^3J_{HH}$ coupling constant was 7.6 Hz [21]. Based on the calculated $^3J_{HH}$ coupling constants, the stereochemistry of boscartol D is predicted to be (15*S*).

The protein targets that showed the best docking properties with *Boswellia* cneorubenoids are listed in Table 5, along with median docking energies. The protein that was best targeted by *Boswellia* cneorubenoids was *Bacillus anthracis* nucleotide adenylyltransferase (BaNadD, PDB 3hfj) with seven of the 11 ligands showing docking energies <−120 kJ/mol. Human folate receptor β (HsFRβ, PDB 4kn0 and 4kn1) was also well targeted with 7/11 cneorubenoids with E_{dock} < −120 kJ/mol. The strongest docking ligands were boscartol E and boscartol I, and both of these ligands targeted BaNadD (PDB 3 hfj) and HsFRβ (PDB 4kn0) very well.

Table 5. Protein targets with the most exothermic docking energies (E_{dock}, kJ/mol) for *Boswellia* cneorubenoid ligands.

Ligand	PDB [a]	E_{dock}	Target Protein
Boscartol A	3hfj	−124.2	*Bacillus anthracis* nucleotide adenyltransferase (BaNadD)
	4kn0	−125.6	human folate receptor β (HsFRβ)
	4kn1	−127.5	human folate receptor β (HsFRβ)
		−89.7	Median docking energy
Boscartol B	3hfj	−124.2	*Bacillus anthracis* nucleotide adenyltransferase (BaNadD)
	4kn0	−127.8	human folate receptor β (HsFRβ)
	4kn1	−126.8	human folate receptor β (HsFRβ)
		−91.6	Median docking energy
Boscartol C	3bt9	−120.2	*Staphylococcus aureus* multidrug binding protein (SaQacR)
		−85.8	Median docking energy
(15*R*)-Boscartol D	2cek	−120.9	*Torpedo californica* acetylcholine esterase (TcAChE)
	3bt9	−122.7	*Staphylococcus aureus* multidrug binding protein (SaQacR)
	3lal	−125.5	HIV-1 reverse transcriptase
	3t19	−123.1	HIV-1 reverse transcriptase
		−87.6	Median docking energy
(15*S*)-Boscartol D	3lal	−120.6	HIV-1 reverse transcriptase
		−81.8	Median docking energy
Boscartol E	1s9d	−125.9	bovine guanine nucleotide exchange factor (BtGEF)
	3hjf	−135.1	*Bacillus anthracis* nucleotide adenyltransferase (BaNadD)
	4b80	−124.1	murine acetylcholinesterase (MmAChE)
	4kn0	−124.2	human folate receptor β (HsFRβ)
		−85.0	Median docking energy

Table 5. *Cont.*

Ligand	PDB [a]	E_{dock}	Target Protein
Boscartol F	1s9d	−124.5	bovine guanine nucleotide exchange factor (BtGEF)
	3hfj	−123.1	*Bacillus anthracis* nucleotide adenylyltransferase (BaNadD)
	4kn1	−122.3	human folate receptor β (HsFRβ)
		−84.6	Median docking energy
Boscartol G	3hfj	−125.8	*Bacillus anthracis* nucleotide adenylyltransferase (BaNadD)
		−80.3	Median docking energy
Boscartol H	1dx4	−123.6	*Drosophila melanogaster* acetylcholine esterase (DmAChE)
	3bt9	−122.0	*Staphylococcus aureus* multidrug binding protein (SaQacR)
	3hfj	−127.9	*Bacillus anthracis* nucleotide adenyltransferase (BaNadD)
	4kn0	−124.6	human folate receptor β (HsFRβ)
		−85.9	Median docking energy
Boscartol I	3hfj	−133.8	*Bacillus anthracis* nucleotide adenylyltransferase (BaNadD)
	3p2v	−121.1	human aldose reductase (HsAR)
	4kn0	−127.3	human folate receptor β (HsFRβ)
		−91.4	Median docking energy
Olibanumol D	4kn1	−120.6	human folate receptor β (HsFRβ)
		−78.4	Median docking energy

[a] PDB: Protein Data Bank code.

Nicotinate mononucleotide adenylyltransferase (NadD) has been identified as a target for development of antibacterial agents. The excellent docking of cneorubenoids with BaNadD, along with the known antibacterial activity of frankincense [43–45], corroborates the traditional uses of frankincense to treat wounds [6,46].

Bacillus anthracis NadD (PDB 3hfj) is a dimeric structure with the active site at the interface of the two protein monomers (Figure 8). The active site is a hydrophobic pocket formed by Trp116A, Trp116B, Tyr112A, Tyr112B, Lys115A, and Lys115B (Figure 8B).

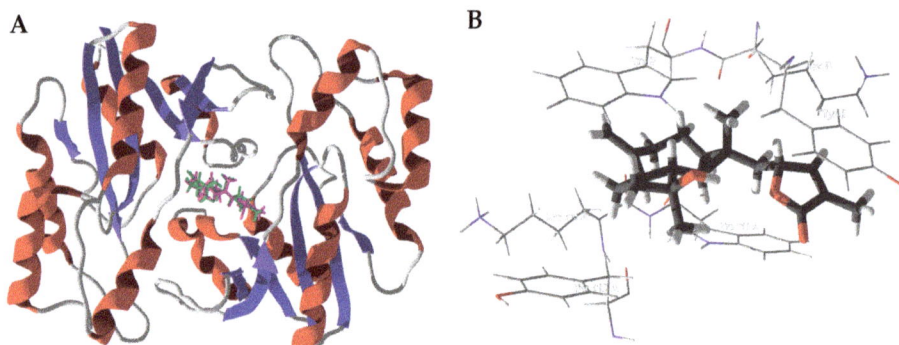

Figure 8. *Bacillus anthracis* nucleotide adenylyltransferase (BaNadD, PDB 3hfj). (**A**): Lowest-energy docked poses of boscartol E (magenta) and boscartol I (green) in the active site of the dimeric enzyme. (**B**): Boscartol I in the hydrophobic pocket formed at the interface of the two protein monomers.

Human folate receptor β (HsFRβ) is overexpressed in activated macrophages associated with pathogenesis of inflammatory and autoimmune diseases [54] as well as neoplastic tissues [55]. Thus, antifolates that target folate receptors could be useful for the treatment of cancer and inflammatory diseases [56]. Clinical trials have demonstrated the encouraging results of frankincense treatment for inflammatory and autoimmune diseases such as rheumatoid arthritis, osteoarthritis, Crohn's disease, and collagenous colitis [57]. *Boswellia* cneorubenoids may be playing a role in the anti-inflammatory activity of frankincense.

The boscartols docked with HsFRβ in the folate binding site (Figure 9). The cyclopropazulane ring is surrounded by aromatic amino acids Trp187, Tyr101, Tyr76, and Phe78 (Figure 9B). In the case of boscartol A and boscartol B, the terminal –OH group is held in place by hydrogen bonds to Ser73 and Phe78 (Figure 9B).

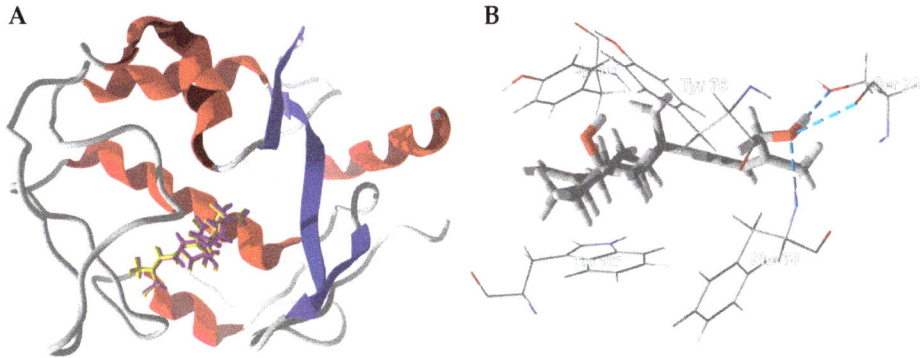

Figure 9. Human folate receptor β (HsFRβ, PDB 4kn1). (**A**): Ribbon structure of protein showed the docked poses of boscartin A (yellow) and boscartin B (purple). (**B**): Lowest-energy docked pose of boscartin A in the binding site of HsFRβ. Hydrogen-bonds are shown as blue dashed lines.

3.3. Boswellia Triterpenoids

The *Boswellia* triterpenoids examined in this reverse docking study are shown in Figure 3 and the target proteins with the best docking energies for each triterpenoid ligand are summarized in Table 6. The most receptive protein targets for *Boswellia* triterpenoids were *Staphylococcus aureus* multidrug binding protein (SaQacR, PDB 3bt9) with an average docking energy (E_{dock}) of −111.9 kJ/mol and human fibroblast collagenase (PDB 1cgl) with an average docking energy (E_{dock}) of −110.5 kJ/mol.

Table 6. Protein targets with the most exothermic docking energies (E_{dock}, kJ/mol) for *Boswellia* triterpenoid ligands.

Ligand	PDB [a]	E_{dock}	Target
(20*S*)-3,7-Dioxotirucalla-8,24-dien-21-oic acid	3l3m	−141.8	Human poly(ADP-ribose) polymerase-1 (HsPARP-1) (anticancer target)
	3ua9	−140.3	Human tankyrase-2 (HsTANK2) = human poly(ADP-ribose) polymerase-5b (HsPARP-5b) (antitumor target)
	3g49	−132.4	*Cavia porcellus* 11β-hydroxysteroid dehydrogenase type 1 (Cp11βHSD1) (diabetes target)
	2b03	−127.4	Porcine pancreatic phospholipase A2 (SsPLA2) (anti-inflammatory target)
		−91.3	Median docking energy
11-Ethoxy-β-boswellic acid	3i6m	−124.6	*Torpedo californica* acetylcholinesterase (TcAChE) (Alzheimer's target)
		−63.0	Median docking energy
11-Keto-β-boswellic acid	4b84	−125.3	Murine acetylcholinesterase (MmAChE) (Alzheimer's target)
	3i6m	−120.8	*Torpedo californica* acetylcholinesterase (TcAChE) (Alzheimer's target)
		−59.9	Median docking energy
12-Ursen-3,11-dione	1h22	−118.8	*Torpedo californica* acetylcholinesterase (TcAChE) (Alzheimer's target)
		−64.2	Median docking energy
12-Ursen-3,24-diol	1h22	−123.8	*Torpedo californica* acetylcholinesterase (TcAChE) (Alzheimer's target)
		+17.4	Median docking energy
2,3-Dihydroxy-12-ursen-24-oic acid	4b84	−128.0	Murine acetylcholinesterase (MmAChE) (Alzheimer's target)
		+16.2	Median docking energy
20,22-Epoxytirucall-24-en-3-one	3l3m	−133.5	Human poly(ADP-ribose) polymerase-1 (HsPARP-1) (anticancer target)
	3g49	−125.0	*Cavia porcellus* 11β-hydroxysteroid dehydrogenase type 1 (Cp11βHSD1) (diabetes target)
		−88.9	Median docking energy
24-Nor-3,12-ursadien-11-one	1h22	−121.0	*Torpedo californica* acetylcholinesterase (TcAChE) (Alzheimer's target)
	4b84	−120.9	Murine acetylcholinesterase (MmAChE) (Alzheimer's target)
		+30.9	Median docking energy
24-Nor-3,9(11),12-oleanatriene	3lz6	−112.6	*Cavia porcellus* 11β-hydroxysteroid dehydrogenase type 1 (Cp11βHSD1) (diabetes target)
		−31.2	Median docking energy
24-Nor-3,9(11),12-ursatriene	1h22	−118.4	*Torpedo californica* acetylcholinesterase (TcAChE) (Alzheimer's target)
		+15.1	Median docking energy

Table 6. *Cont.*

Ligand	PDB [a]	E_{dock}	Target
3-Acetoxy-12,20(29)-lupadien-24-oic acid	1uk1	−118.4	Human poly(ADP-ribose) polymerase-1 (HsPARP-1) (anticancer target)
	3bti	−117.9	*Staphylococcus aureus* multidrug binding protein (SaQacR)
		+16.4	Median docking energy
3-Acetoxy-20(29)-lupen-24-oic acid (= 3-Acetyl lupeolic acid)	1cgl	−117.5	Human fibroblast collagenase (HsMMP-1) (arthritis target)
		+8.0	Median docking energy
3β-Acetoxy-20S,24R-hydroxydammar-25-ene [b]	2aba	−144.7	*Enterobacter cloacae* pentaerythritol tetranitrate reductase (EcPETNR) (antibacterial target)
	3lz6	−141.8	*Cavia porcellus* 11β-hydroxysteroid dehydrogenase type 1 (Cp11βHSD1) (diabetes target)
	1h36	−136.4	*Alicyclobacillus acidocardarius* oxidosqualene cyclase (Aa OSC) (cholesterol-lowering)
		−64.6	Median docking energy
3β-Acetoxy-20S,24S-dihydroxydammar-25-ene [b]	2aba	−149.9	*Enterobacter cloacae* pentaerythritol tetranitrate reductase (EcPETNR) (antibacterial target)
	3g49	−139.7	*Cavia porcellus* 11β-hydroxysteroid dehydrogenase type 1 (Cp11βHSD1) (diabetes target)
	3lz6	−136.2	*Cavia porcellus* 11β-hydroxysteroid dehydrogenase type 1 (Cp11βHSD1) (diabetes target)
	3tfu	−134.5	*Mycobacterium tuberculosis* 7,8-diaminopelargonic acid synthase (MtBioA)
		−73.7	Median docking energy
3-Acetoxy-5,12-ursadien-24-oic acid	3i6m	−131.7	*Torpedo californica* acetylcholinesterase (TcAChE) (Alzheimer's target)
		−66.7	Median docking energy
3-Acetyl-11-keto-β-boswellic acid	3i6m	−129.7	*Torpedo californica* acetylcholinesterase (TcAChE) (Alzheimer's target)
		−70.7	Median docking energy
3-Acetyl-11α-methoxy-β-boswellic_acid	3i6m	−129.0	*Torpedo californica* acetylcholinesterase (TcAChE) (Alzheimer's target)
		−72.2	Median docking energy
3-Acetyl-9,11-dehydro-β-boswellic_acid	3i6m	−124.0	*Torpedo californica* acetylcholinesterase (TcAChE) (Alzheimer's target)
		−64.4	Median docking energy
3-Acetyl-α-boswellic acid	2b03	−112.7	Porcine pancreatic phospholipase A2 (SsPLA2) (anti-inflammatory target)
		−64.8	Median docking energy
3-Acetyl-β-boswellic acid	3i6m	−128.3	*Torpedo californica* acetylcholinesterase (TcAChE) (Alzheimer's target)
		−71.5	Median docking energy
3-Hydroxy-20(29)-lupen-24-oic acid (= Lupeolic acid)	3bt9	−119.3	*Staphylococcus aureus* multidrug binding protein (SaQacR)
		−55.8	Median docking energy
3-Oxotirucalla-7,9(11),24-trien-21-oic acid	3ua9	−151.0	Human tankyrase-2 (HsTANK2) = human poly(ADP-ribose) polymerase-5b (HsPARP-5b) (antitumor target)
	3l3m	−137.6	Human poly(ADP-ribose) polymerase-1 (HsPARP-1) (anticancer target)
	3h6k	−130.9	Human 11β-hydroxysteroid dehydrogenase type 1 (11βHSD1) (diabetes target)
	1w6j	−127.5	Human oxidosqualene cyclase (HsOSC) (hypercholesterolemia target)
	3bt9	−127.1	*Staphylococcus aureus* multidrug binding protein (SaQacR)
		−96.8	Median docking energy
3β-Hydroxytirucalla-8,24-dien-21-oic acid	3ua9	−144.5	Human tankyrase-2 (HsTANK2) = human poly(ADP-ribose) polymerase-5b (HsPARP-5b) (antitumor target)
	3l3m	−133.0	Human poly(ADP-ribose) polymerase-1 (HsPARP-1) (anticancer target)
	3g49	−132.3	*Cavia porcellus* 11β-hydroxysteroid dehydrogenase type 1 (Cp11βHSD1) (diabetes target)
	2ilt	−129.1	Human 11β-hydroxysteroid-dehydrogenase (Hs11β-HSDH) (diabetes target)
	4krs	−127.7	Human tankyrase-1 (HsTANK1) (anticancer target)
	4l0i	−127.3	Human tankyrase-2 (HsTANK2) (anticancer target)
		−85.6	Median docking energy
3α-Acetoxytirucalla-7,24-dien-21-oic acid	3ua9	−147.1	Human tankyrase-2 (HsTANK2) = human poly(ADP-ribose) polymerase-5b (HsPARP-5b) (antitumor target)
	4krs	−134.1	Human tankyrase-1 (HsTANK1) (anticancer target)
	1cgl	−129.9	Human fibroblast collagenase (HsMMP-1) (arthritis target)
	4gv0	−128.4	Human poly(ADP-ribose) polymerase-1 (HsPARP-1) (anticancer target)
	4l0i	−128.4	Human tankyrase-2 (HsTANK2) (anticancer target)
	3lep	−126.8	Human aldose reductase (HsAR) (diabetes target)
		−102.1	Median docking energy
3α-Hydroxytirucalla-7,24-dien-21-oic acid	3ua9	−154.3	Human tankyrase-2 (HsTANK2) = human poly(ADP-ribose) polymerase-5b (HsPARP-5b) (antitumor target)
	3g49	−128.9	*Cavia porcellus* 11β-hydroxysteroid dehydrogenase type 1 (Cp11βHSD1) (diabetes target)
	3l3m	−126.7	Human poly(ADP-ribose) polymerase-1 (HsPARP-1) (anticancer target)
	3tfu	−126.4	*Mycobacterium tuberculosis* 7,8-diaminopelargonic acid synthase (MtBioA)
		−88.7	Median docking energy
3β-Acetoxydammar-24-ene-16β,20R-diol	3lz6	−149.6	*Cavia porcellus* 11β-hydroxysteroid dehydrogenase type 1 (Cp11βHSD1) (diabetes target)
	2aba	−141.1	*Enterobacter cloacae* pentaerythritol tetranitrate reductase (EcPETNR) (antibacterial target)
	1h36	−139.2	*Alicyclobacillus acidocardarius* oxidosqualene cyclase (AaOSC) (cholesterol-lowering)
	1s0x	−131.2	Human retinoic acid-related orphan receptor α (HsRORα) (may regulate lipid metabolism)
		−54.0	Median docking energy
3β-Acetoxylup-20(29)-en-11β-ol	1ukl	−121.9	Human poly(ADP-ribose) polymerase-1 (HsPARP-1) (anticancer target)
		−50.4	Median docking energy
4,23-Dihydroburic acid	1h22	−135.8	*Torpedo californica* acetylcholinesterase (TcAChE) (Alzheimer's target)
	4b84	−127.8	Murine acetylcholinesterase (MmAChE) (Alzheimer's target)
	1jtx	−125.1	*Staphylococcus aureus* multidrug binding protein (SaQacR)
		+11.7	Median docking energy
6,7-Epoxy-9(11)-oleanen-3-ol	4hai	−111.6	Human soluble epoxide hydrolase (HsEPHX2) (anti-inflammatory target)
		−60.7	Median docking energy
6,7-Epoxy-9(11)-oleanen-3-one	1ry0	−113.7	Human prostaglandin F synthase (HsPGFS) (hypertension target)
		−49.1	Median docking energy
9,11-Dehydro-β-boswellic acid	1qvu	−114.3	*Staphylococcus aureus* multidrug binding protein (SaQacR)
		−60.8	Median docking energy
Boscartene L	3l3m	−131.0	Human poly(ADP-ribose) polymerase-1 (HsPARP-1) (anticancer target)
		−87.6	Median docking energy
Boscartene M	3l3m	−133.7	Human poly(ADP-ribose) polymerase-1 (HsPARP-1) (anticancer target)
		−89.4	Median docking energy
Boscartene N	3ua9	−157.2	Human tankyrase-2 (HsTANK2) = human poly(ADP-ribose) polymerase-5b (HsPARP-5b) (antitumor target)
	3bt9	−136.7	*Staphylococcus aureus* multidrug binding protein (SaQacR)
	3l3m	−133.3	Human poly(ADP-ribose) polymerase-1 (HsPARP-1) (anticancer target)
	1xl5	−125.2	HIV-1 protease
		−95.1	Median docking energy
Dammarenediol II	1w6k	−135.1	Human oxidosqualene cyclase (HsOSC) (hypercholesterolemia target)
	3lz6	−134.6	*Cavia porcellus* 11β-hydroxysteroid dehydrogenase type 1 (Cp11βHSD1) (diabetes target)
	1h36	−129.2	*Alicyclobacillus acidocardarius* oxidosqualene cyclase (AaOSC) (cholesterol-lowering)
		−72.1	Median docking energy

Table 6. *Cont.*

Ligand	PDB [a]	E_{dock}	Target
Dammarenediol II acetate	3lz6	−142.8	*Cavia porcellus* 11β-hydroxysteroid dehydrogenase type 1 (Cp11βHSD1) (diabetes target)
	1h36	−138.9	*Alicyclobacillus acidocardarius* oxidosqualene cyclase (AaOSC) (cholesterol-lowering)
	2aba	−136.4	*Enterobacter cloacae* pentaerythritol tetranitrate reductase (EcNETNR) (antibacterial target)
	4kn0	−132.3	Human folate receptor β (HsFRβ) (anticancer target)
		−77.7	Median docking energy
Eupha-2,8,22-triene-20,24R-diol [b]	3l3m	−139.8	Human poly(ADP-ribose) polymerase-1 (HsPARP-1) (anticancer target)
	3ua9	−135.3	Human tankyrase-2 (HsTANK2) = human poly(ADP-ribose) polymerase-5b (HsPARP-5b) (antitumor target)
	4dbs	−124.0	Human estrogenic 17β-hydroxysteroid dehydrogenase (17β-HSD1)
		−94.9	Median docking energy
Eupha-2,8,22-triene-20,24S-diol [b]	1uk1	−137.6	Human poly(ADP-ribose) polymerase-1 (HsPARP-1) (anticancer target)
	3ua9	−135.8	Human tankyrase-2 (HsTANK2) = human poly(ADP-ribose) polymerase-5b (HsPARP-5b) (antitumor target)
	4dbs	−127.4	Human estrogenic 17β-hydroxysteroid dehydrogenase (17β-HSD1)
		−85.1	Median docking energy
Isofouquierol	3lz6	−134.1	*Cavia porcellus* 11β-hydroxysteroid dehydrogenase type 1 (Cp11βHSD1) (diabetes target)
	2aba	−131.3	*Enterobacter cloacae* pentaerythritol tetranitrate reductase (EcPETNR) (antibacterial target)
	4kn0	−130.4	Human folate receptor β (HsFRβ) (anticancer target)
		−83.2	Median docking energy
Isofouquieryl acetate	3lz6	−150.1	*Cavia porcellus* 11β-hydroxysteroid dehydrogenase type 1 (Cp11βHSD1) (diabetes target)
	2aba	−137.9	*Enterobacter cloacae* pentaerythritol tetranitrate reductase (EcPETNR) (antibacterial target)
	4kn0	−137.0	Human folate receptor β (HsFRβ) (anticancer target)
	1s0x	−135.7	Human retinoic acid-related orphan receptor α (HsRORα) (may regulate lipid metabolism)
	1h35	−135.5	*Alicyclobacillus acidocardarius* oxidosqualene cyclase (AaOSC) (cholesterol-lowering)
	2w4q	−132.7	Human zinc-binding alcohol dehydrogenase 1 (HsZADH1)
	3g49	−132.4	*Cavia porcellus* 11β-hydroxysteroid dehydrogenase type 1 (Cp11βHSD1) (diabetes target)
	2zxm	−131.0	Rat vitamin D receptor (RnVDR) (target for psoriasis)
		−79.3	Median docking energy
Lup-20(29)-ene-2α,3β-diol	1xu9	−112.5	Human 11β-hydroxysteroid dehydrogenase type 1 (11βHSD1) (diabetes target)
	3wd2	−112.4	*Serratia marcescens* chitinase B (SmChiB)
	1xl5	−112.2	HIV-1 protease
		−62.2	Median docking energy
Neoilexonol	1h22	−118.2	*Torpedo californica* acetylcholinesterase (TcAChE) (Alzheimer's target)
		−66.7	Median docking energy
Neoilexonyl acetate	2ilt	−118.8	Human 11β-hydroxysteroid-dehydrogenase (Hs11β-HSDH) (diabetes target)
	4b84	−118.5	Murine acetylcholinesterase (MmAChE) (Alzheimer's target)
		−74.8	Median docking energy
Nizwanone	4b84	−123.2	Murine acetylcholinesterase (MmAChE) (Alzheimer's target)
		−63.3	Median docking energy
Ocotillyl acetate	1gsz	−144.6	*Alicyclobacillus acidocardarius* oxidosqualene cyclase (AaOSC) (cholesterol-lowering)
	2aba	−130.1	*Enterobacter cloacae* pentaerythritol tetranitrate reductase (EcPETNR) (antibacterial target)
	4jbs	−127.7	Human endoplasmic reticulum aminopeptidase 2 (HsERAP2) (immune response target)
		−70.7	Median docking energy
Olibanumol E	2ilt	−109.5	Human 11β-hydroxysteroid-dehydrogenase (Hs11β-HSDH) (diabetes target)
		−63.5	Median docking energy
Olibanumol F	1cgl	−110.1	Human fibroblast collagenase (HsMMP-1) (arthritis target)
	3bt9	−108.8	*Staphylococcus aureus* multidrug binding protein (SaQacR)
		−36.7	Median docking energy
Olibanumol G	3bt9	−117.4	*Staphylococcus aureus* multidrug binding protein (SaQacR)
		−53.0	Median docking energy
Olibanumol H	3bt9	−121.6	*Staphylococcus aureus* multidrug binding protein (SaQacR)
		−60.9	Median docking energy
Olibanumol I	3bt9	−115.7	*Staphylococcus aureus* multidrug binding protein (SaQacR)
		−63.2	Median docking energy
Olibanumol J	1rpw	−135.5	*Staphylococcus aureus* multidrug binding protein (SaQacR)
	1cr6	−133.3	Murine soluble epoxide hydrolase (MmEPHX2) (anti-inflammatory target)
	3bti	−132.6	*Staphylococcus aureus* multidrug binding protein (SaQacR)
	3gyt	−132.1	*Strongyloides stercoralis* nuclear receptor DAF-12 (SsDAF12) (antiparasitic target)
		−55.5	Median docking energy
Olibanumol J′	3l3m	−132.2	Human poly(ADP-ribose) polymerase-1 (HsPARP-1) (anticancer target)
	3g49	−129.0	*Cavia porcellus* 11β-hydroxysteroid dehydrogenase type 1 (Cp11βHSD1) (diabetes target)
	3w5e	−128.8	Human phosphodiesterase 4B (HsPDE4B) (anti-inflammatory target)
	3bt9	−123.4	*Staphylococcus aureus* multidrug binding protein (SaQacR)
		−74.7	Median docking energy
Olibanumol K	4b84	−122.9	Murine acetylcholinesterase (MmAChE) (Alzheimer's target)
	3i6m	−122.1	*Torpedo californica* acetylcholinesterase (TcAChE) (Alzheimer's target)
		−64.8	Median docking energy
Olibanumol L	1ry0	−116.2	Human prostaglandin F synthase (HsPGFS) (hypertension target)
	3g49	−111.1	*Cavia porcellus* 11β-hydroxysteroid dehydrogenase type 1 (Cp11βHSD1) (diabetes target)
		−27.6	Median docking energy
Olibanumol L′	4b84	−130.1	Murine acetylcholinesterase (MmAChE) (Alzheimer's target)
		−70.7	Median docking energy
Olibanumol M	1h22	−128.4	*Torpedo californica* acetylcholinesterase (TcAChE) (Alzheimer's target)
		−62.7	Median docking energy
Olibanumol N	4b84	−133.0	Murine acetylcholinesterase (MmAChE) (Alzheimer's target)
		−70.9	Median docking energy
Trametenolic acid B	3ua9	−131.6	Human tankyrase-2 (HsTANK2) = human poly(ADP-ribose) polymerase-5b (HsPARP-5b) (antitumor target)
	3g49	−127.1	*Cavia porcellus* 11β-hydroxysteroid dehydrogenase type 1 (11βHSD1) (diabetes target)
	3hfb	−126.6	Human tryptophan hydroxylase type 1 (HsTPH1) (biosynthesis of serotonin)
	1eve	−126.5	*Torpedo californica* acetylcholinesterase (TcAChE) (Alzheimer's target)
		−74.2	Median docking energy
Urs-12-ene-3α,11α-diol	1h22	−120.9	*Torpedo californica* acetylcholinesterase (TcAChE) (Alzheimer's target)
		−61.1	Median docking energy
Urs-12-ene-3β,11α-diol	4b84	−123.7	Murine acetylcholinesterase (MmAChE) (Alzheimer's target)
		−59.8	Median docking energy

Table 6. *Cont.*

Ligand	PDB [a]	E_{dock}	Target
α-Boswellic acid	3g49	−110.0	*Cavia porcellus* 11β-hydroxysteroid dehydrogenase type 1 (11βHSD1) (diabetes target)
		−65.7	Median docking energy
α-Elemolic acid	3ua9	−152.7	Human tankyrase-2 (HsTANK2) = human poly(ADP-ribose) polymerase-5b (HsPARP-5b) (antitumor target)
	1c3s	−136.9	*Aquifex aeolicus* histone deacetylase (AaHDAC) (anticancer target)
	3g49	−128.9	*Cavia porcellus* 11β-hydroxysteroid dehydrogenase type 1 (11βHSD1) (diabetes target)
		−87.8	Median docking energy
β-Boswellic acid	3i6m	−118.1	*Torpedo californica* acetylcholinesterase (TcAChE) (Alzheimer's target)
		+20.7	Median docking energy
β-Elemonic acid	3ua9	−147.3	Human tankyrase-2 (HsTANK2) = human poly(ADP-ribose) polymerase-5b (HsPARP-5b) (antitumor target)
	3l3m	−133.7	Human poly(ADP-ribose) polymerase-1 (HsPARP-1) (anticancer target)
	3g49	−131.9	*Cavia porcellus* 11β-hydroxysteroid dehydrogenase type 1 (11βHSD1) (diabetes target)
		−89.0	Median docking energy
δ-Boswellic acid	3g49	−106.7	*Cavia porcellus* 11β-hydroxysteroid dehydrogenase type 1 (11βHSD1) (diabetes target)
		−60.7	Median docking energy

[a] PDB: Protein Data Bank code. [b] The stereochemistry at C(24) was not experimentally determined for 3β-acetoxy-20*S*,24-dihydroxydammar-25-ene or for eupha-2,8,22-triene-20,24-diol; both diastereomers for each of these compounds were examined in this reverse docking study.

The best overall triterpenoid ligand-protein target pairs were boscartene N with human tankyrase 2 (HsTANK2, PDB 3ua9), E_{dock} = −157.2 kJ/mol; 3α-hydroxytirucalla-7,24-dien-21-oic acid with HsTANK2, E_{dock} = −154.3 kJ/mol; α-elemolic acid with HsTANK2, E_{dock} = −152.7 kJ/mol; 3-oxotirucalla-7,9(11),24-trien-21-oic acid with HsTANK2, E_{dock} = −151.0 kJ/mol; 3α-acetoxytirucalla-7,24-dien-21-oic acid with human glucokinase (PDB 4ixc), E_{dock} = −150.4 kJ/mol; isofouquieryl acetate with Guinea pig (*Cavia porcellus*) 11β-hydroxysteroid dehydrogenase type 1 (11βHSD1, PDB 3lz6), E_{dock} = −150.1 kJ/mol; 3β-acetoxy-20*S*,24*S*-dihydroxydammar-25-ene with *Enterobacter cloacae* pentaerythritol tetranitrate reductase (EcPETNR, PDB 2aba), E_{dock} = −149.9 kJ/mol; and 3β-acetoxydammar-24-ene-16β,20*R*-diol with Guinea pig 11β-hydroxysteroid dehydrogenase type 1 (Cp11βHSD1, PDB 3lz6), E_{dock} = −149.6 kJ/mol.

Frankincense oleo-gum resins have been used in traditional medicine to treat a variety of inflammatory conditions, including arthritis, colitis, and asthma [58,59]. Boswellic acids, including β-boswellic acid, 11-keto-β-boswellic acid, and acetyl-11-keto-β-boswellic acid, have been implicated in the anti-inflammatory properties of *Boswellia* resins; these triterpenoid components are involved in inhibition of 5-lipoxygenase (5-LOX), inducible nitric oxide synthase (iNOS), cyclooxygenase-1 (COX-1) and cyclooxygenase-2 (COX-2) [60].

In-silico screening of the *Boswellia* triterpenoids was carried out against molecular targets of inflammation, including human pancreatic secretory phospholipase A2 (HsPLA2), porcine pancreatic phospholipase A2 (SsPLA2), human phosphoinositide 3-kinase (HsPI3K), human interkeukin-1 receptor associated kinase 4 (HsIRAK4), human glutathione transferase omega 1 (HsGSTO1), human 5-lipoxygenase (Hs5-LOX), mouse inducible nitric oxide synthase (MmiNOS), ovine COX-1 (OaCOX-1), murine COX-2 (MmCOX-2), human fibroblast collagenase (matrix metalloproteinase-1, HsMMP-1), murine soluble epoxide hydrolase 2 (MmEPHX2), human endoplasmic reticulum aminopeptidase 2 (HsERAP2), human soluble epoxide hydrolase 2 (HsEPHX2), and human phosphodiesterase 4B (HsPDE4B). The docking energies of the triterpenoid ligands with inflammatory target proteins are shown in Table 7.

The *Boswellia* triterpenoids showed relatively weak docking to 5-LOX, iNOS, PI3K, IRAK4, or GSTO1, and no docking at all to either COX-1 or COX-2 (positive docking energies). However, several *Boswellia* triterpenoids showed relatively strong docking (E_{dock} < −120 kJ/mol) to human endoplasmic reticulum aminopeptidase 2 (HsERAP2), including 3β-acetoxy-20*S*,24*S*-dihydroxydammar-25-ene, 3β-acetoxydammar-24-ene-16β,20*R*-diol, isofouquieryl acetate, ocotillyl acetate, olibanumol J, and olibanumol J′. There is a significant association of ERAP2 with psoriatic arthritis [61], and notably, *Boswellia* triterpenoids have shown promise for the treatment of psoriasis [62]. Similarly, inhibitors of phosphodiesterase 4B have shown promise in the treatment of psoriasis and atopic dermatitis [63], and isofouquierol and olibanumol J′ showed good docking properties with HsPDE4B with docking energies of −128.3 and −128.8 kJ/mol, respectively.

The only other strong docking observed was olibanumol J with murine soluble epoxide hydrolase 2 (MmEPHX2), 3α-acetoxytirucalla-7,24-dien-21-oic acid with human matrix metalloproteinase-1 (HsMMP-1), (20S)-3,7-dioxotirucalla-8,24-dien-21-oic acid with porcine pancreatic phospholipase A2 (SsPLA2), and 3β-acetoxy-20S,24-dihydroxydammar-25-ene with human pancreatic secretory phospholipase A2 (HsPLA2). The targeting of matrix metalloproteinase-1 (fibroblast collagenase) is noteworthy; *B. serrata* extract has shown clinical efficacy as a treatment for osteoarthritis of the knee [64].

Note that β-boswellic acid, 11-keto-β-boswellic acid, and 3-acetyl-11-keto-β-boswellic acid had relatively weak docking with inflammation-relevant protein targets. It may be that these *Boswellia* triterpenoids, rather than inhibiting particular enzyme targets, are inhibiting the secretion of pro-inflammatory cytokines such as tumor necrosis factor α (TNFα), interleukin 1 (IL-1), IL-6, IL-12, IL-18, or interferon γ (IFN-γ) [65].

Olibanumols G, H, I, and J all showed selective docking to *S. aureus* multidrug binding protein (SaQacR). The olibanumols occupy the binding site of SaQacR, same site as the co-crystallized ligand in PDB 3bti (Figure 10). The site is made up of aromatic amino acids Trp61, Tyr93, and Tyr123, forming a hydrophobic pocket. The triterpenoid ligand olibanumol J also has a hydrogen-bonding interaction between C(3)-OH of the ligand and the amide C=O of Ala153. Other key interacting amino acids in the binding site are Ser86, Glu90, and Asn157. In addition to the olibanumols, six additional triterpenoids also showed selective docking to SaQacR, 3-acetoxy-12,20(29)-lupadien-24-oic acid, lupeolic acid, 3-oxotirucalla-7,9(11),24-trien-21-oic acid, 4,23-dihydroburic acid, 9,11-dehydro-β-boswellic acid, and boscartene N.

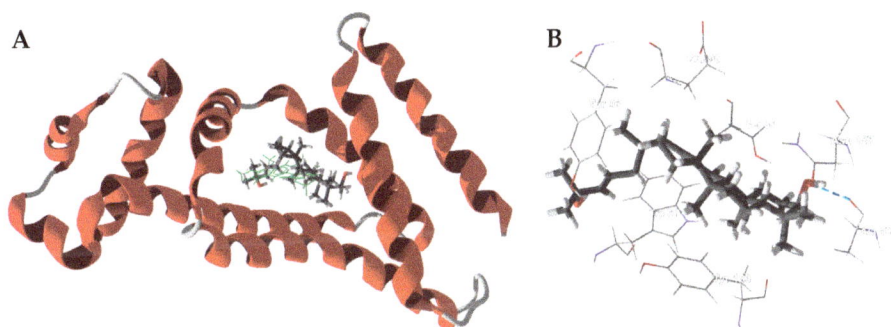

Figure 10. Lowest-energy docking pose of olibanumol J with *Staphylococcus aureus* multidrug binding protein (SaQacR, PDB 3bti). (**A**): Ribbon structure of SaQacR showing olibanumol J (E_{dock} = −132.6 kJ/mol) in the active site. The co-crystallized ligand, berberine (E_{dock} = −113.8 kJ/mol), is shown as a green wire structure. (**B**): Key interactions of olibanumol J in the active site of SaQacR. The hydrogen-bond is indicated by a blue dashed line.

Another antibacterial target protein that showed good docking properties was *Enterobacter cloacae* pentaerythritol tetranitrate reductase (EcPETNR) with seven *Boswellia* dammarane triterpenoids showing selective docking to this target, 3β-acetoxy-20S,24-dihydroxydammar-25-ene (both diastereomers), 3β-acetoxydammar-24-ene-16β,20R-diol, dammarenediol II acetate, isofouquierol, isofouquieryl acetate, and ocotillyl acetate. These dammarane triterpenoids occupy the active site of EcPETNR, near to the riboflavin monophosphate redox cofactor, with very similar docked poses (Figure 11). Key intermolecular contacts are hydrogen bonding of the C(3) acetoxygroup with Arg142, hydrogen-bonding of C(20)-OH with the riboflavin monophosphate cofactor and His184 (Figure 11B). In the case of 3β-acetoxy-20S,24S-dihydroxydammar-25-ene, there is also a hydrogen-bond between the C(24)-OH group and Asp274.

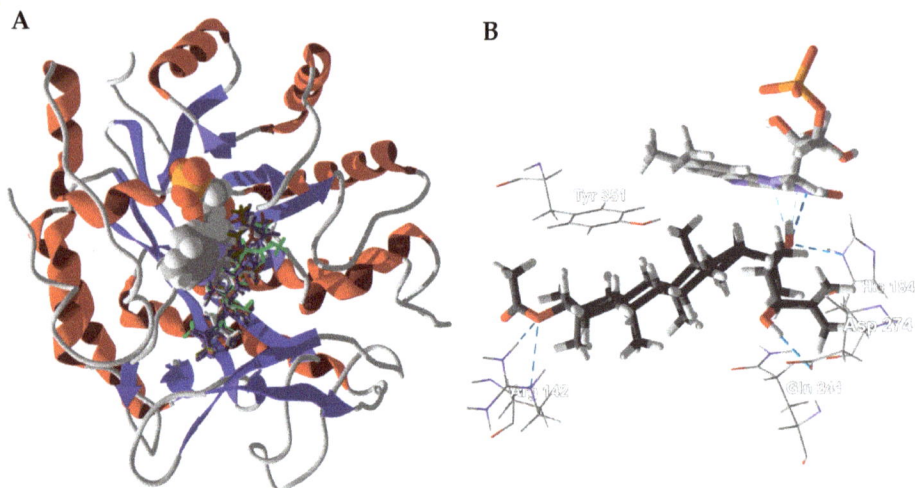

Figure 11. *Enterobacter cloacae* pentaerythritol tetranitrate reductase (EcPETNR, PDB 2aba). (**A**): Ribbon structure of EcPETNR with docked dammarane triterpenoids (stick figures). The riboflavin monophosphate cofactor is shown as a space-filling model. (**B**): Lowest-energy docked pose of 3β-acetoxy-20*S*,24*S*-dihydroxydammar-25-ene. Hydrogen-bonding interactions are indicated with blue dashed lines.

Drugs that reversibly inhibit acetylcholinesterase are currently being explored to treat Alzheimer's disease [66], and *Torpedo californica* and murine acetylcholinesterases have been used as model enzyme targets for anticholinesterase inhibition [67]. β-Boswellic acid and its derivatives (11-keto-β-boswellic acid, 11-ethoxy-β-boswellic acid, 3-acetyl-β-boswellic acid, and 3-acetyl-11-keto-β-boswellic acid) showed selective docking to *Torpedo californica* acetylcholinesterase (TcAChE, PDB 3i6m). Interestingly, increasing oxygenation resulted in more exothermic docking energies (−118.1, −120.8, −124.6, −128.3, and −129.7 kJ/mol, respectively). These β-boswellic acid derivatives all adopt the same lowest-energy poses in the active site of the enzyme (Figure 12). It is tempting to suggest that the ordering of docking energies is due to increasing hydrogen-bonding of the more oxygenated ligands. However, the only hydrogen bonding seen is with the C(3)-substituent of the ligand (either –OH or –OAc) with Tyr121 (see Figure 10B. Note that the active site of the acetylcholinesterase is surrounded by aromatic amino acids (Trp84, Tyr334, Tyr121, Phe330, Phe331, and Trp279). The more important interactions, therefore, are van der Waals hydrophobic interactions between the ligand and the aromatic amino acids. The trend in docking energies for these β-boswellic acid derivatives is likely due to the increased number of heavy atoms and increasing molecular weight. Olibanumols K, L', M, and N also showed selective docking to acetylcholinesterase proteins. The strongest-docking triterpenoid ligands to TcAChE were 4,23-dihydroburic acid (E_{dock} = −135.8 kJ/mol) and 3-acetoxy-5,12-ursadien-24-oic acid (E_{dock} = −131.7 kJ/mol); olibanumol N docked strongly with MmAChE (E_{dock} = −133.0 kJ/mol). The excellent docking properties of *Boswellia* triterpenoid ligands to acetylcholinesterase supports the clinical use of frankincense to treat Alzeimer's disease [41].

Table 7. MolDock docking energies (kJ/mol) of *Boswellia* triterpenoid ligands with inflammation-relevant protein targets.

Ligand	MmEPHX2 1cr6	HsEPHX2 4hai	HsMMP-1 1cgl	SsPLA2 2b03	HsPLA2 1j1a	Hs5-LOX 3v99	Mm iNOS 1m8d	HsPI3Kγ 2a5u	HsIRAK4 5tls	HsERAP2 4jbs	HsGSTO1 5v3q	HsPDE4B 3w5e
(20S)-3,7-Dioxotirucalla-8,24-dien-21-oic acid	−113.3	−114.1	−121.8	−127.4	−106.9	−103.1	−88.0	−87.7	−112.7	−107.3	−106.0	−114.0
11-Ethoxy-β-boswellic acid	−80.3	−96.3	−107.9	−100.9	−87.3	−85.8	−71.7	−82.5	−99.7	−104.5	−66.8	−101.5
11-Keto-β-boswellic acid	−75.7	−91.8	−100.7	−94.9	−85.3	−83.3	−64.2	−77.2	−89.7	−99.4	−70.7	2.8
12-Ursen-3,11-dione	−73.9	−88.8	−102.0	−102.4	−71.2	−75.8	−63.0	−74.9	−82.0	−98.6	−71.4	−99.9
12-Ursen-3,24-diol	−81.9	−84.5	−105.5	−88.7	−93.7	−77.4	−60.4	−76.9	−89.8	−96.4	−87.8	−101.1
2,3-Dihydroxy-12-ursen-24-oic acid	−78.8	−83.9	−98.9	−100.0	−91.1	−81.7	−30.0	−78.6	−91.7	−96.5	−74.8	−102.4
20,22-Epoxytirucall-24-en-3-one	−98.2	−102.5	−113.1	−111.0	−95.7	−90.2	−89.9	−82.5	−94.7	−105.1	−80.9	−99.3
24-Nor-3,12-ursadien-11-one	−84.1	−89.6	−99.9	−103.4	−95.6	−77.5	−71.8	−75.1	−64.1	−91.7	−50.1	−83.4
24-Nor-3,9(11),12-oleanatriene	−83.4	−94.7	−99.5	−99.9	−93.3	−70.8	−61.0	−75.2	−59.9	−95.3	−47.3	−90.8
24-Nor-3,9(11),12-ursatriene	−83.3	−89.4	−100.6	−99.3	−85.5	−81.4	−65.0	−75.3	−77.0	−86.3	−62.2	−91.2
3-Acetoxy-12,20(29)-lupadien-24-oic acid	−77.8	−85.2	−115.4	−87.5	−82.7	−83.7	−68.4	−93.6	−59.1	−105.0	−78.9	−97.8
3-Acetoxy-20(29)-lupen-24-oic acid (=3-Acetyl lupeolic acid)	−84.1	−83.5	−117.5	−86.7	−87.1	−82.7	−71.8	−92.9	−79.7	−104.5	−79.0	−92.8
3β-Acetoxy-20S,24R-dihydroxydammar-25-ene	−109.7	−109.3	−124.7	−118.5	−120.3	−100.8	−96.7	−94.4	−106.4	−119.1	−85.8	−116.3
3β-Acetoxy-20S,24S-dihydroxydammar-25-ene	−106.2	−109.2	−121.7	−115.6	−122.0	−100.3	−81.5	−93.9	−109.5	−126.1	−76.5	−111.0
3-Acetoxy-5,12-ursadien-24-oic acid	−92.6	−78.1	−121.1	−97.5	−81.7	−81.0	−73.3	−83.6	−70.4	−105.0	−70.2	−47.3
3-Acetyl-11-keto-β-boswellic acid	−87.3	−75.6	−107.6	−102.4	−74.0	−84.9	−67.7	−79.7	−71.9	−93.3	−71.6	−49.2
3-Acetyl-11α-methoxy-β-boswellic acid	−86.7	−91.1	−109.3	−91.0	−75.4	−87.3	−76.1	−79.5	−90.0	−101.9	−69.5	−52.0
3-Acetyl-9,11-dehydro-β-boswellic acid	−90.4	−80.3	−120.6	−98.5	−94.8	−82.7	−74.4	−82.7	−61.1	−103.7	−84.3	−50.3
3-Acetyl-α-boswellic acid	−79.0	−82.4	−109.7	−112.7	−97.2	−82.0	−70.5	−83.0	−83.8	−99.7	−72.7	−91.4
3-Acetyl-β-boswellic acid	−91.5	−83.1	−119.8	−99.4	−96.2	−85.1	−69.0	−79.4	−70.8	−90.2	−80.6	−91.8
3-Hydroxy-20(29)-lupen-24-oic acid (=Lupeolic acid)	−103.4	−105.0	−106.6	−82.6	−76.6	−79.2	−72.6	−81.8	−76.0	−103.4	−69.5	−87.3
3-Oxotirucalla-7,9(11),24-trien-21-oic acid	−113.1	−113.3	−123.3	−116.9	−113.5	−100.5	−86.3	−92.1	−103.6	−108.8	−99.8	−113.2
3β-Hydroxytirucalla-8,24-dien-21-oic acid	−110.8	−112.1	−118.6	−123.4	−106.5	−103.3	−97.3	−80.7	−107.8	−109.4	−94.6	−111.9
3α-Acetoxytirucalla-7,24-dien-21-oic acid	−115.5	−113.3	−129.9	−109.8	−116.2	−91.2	−95.4	−95.3	−109.7	−106.1	−91.4	−104.9
3α-Hydroxytirucalla-7,24-dien-21-oic acid	−110.8	−115.7	−115.4	−117.2	−110.1	−105.7	−84.1	−86.9	−102.8	−106.6	−82.9	−109.8
3β-Acetoxydammar-24-ene-16β,20R-diol	−102.8	−110.3	−125.7	−111.2	−109.3	−97.7	−97.0	−90.7	−107.9	−125.2	−79.8	−115.2
3β-Acetoxylup-20(29)-en-11β-ol	−94.6	−92.9	−109.8	−105.6	−90.8	−86.1	−87.1	−80.9	−93.2	−108.2	−74.5	−41.2
4,23-Dihydrobruric acid	−101.2	−101.6	−109.8	−120.9	−92.0	−88.3	−72.0	−84.3	−102.9	−110.2	−85.3	−107.7
6,7-Epoxy-9(11)-oleanen-3-ol	−53.0	−111.6	−100.2	−106.3	−89.8	−79.6	−64.5	−67.7	−66.2	−94.9	−68.6	−87.2
6,7-Epoxy-9(11)-oleanen-3-one	−66.0	−100.9	−105.0	−107.8	−93.3	−75.1	−68.5	−70.3	−40.3	−100.6	−66.1	−106.2
9,11-Dehydro-β-boswellic acid	−75.8	−85.7	−109.8	−96.8	−93.1	−79.8	−27.4	−73.6	−89.5	−91.2	−83.4	−62.6
Boscartene L	−83.2	−110.2	−104.4	−115.7	−77.4	−100.1	−81.6	−82.0	−100.0	−108.6	−62.6	−97.7
Boscartene M	−73.8	−110.8	−114.0	−107.0	−96.7	−102.9	−86.8	−83.4	−76.8	−110.4	−83.5	−91.5
Boscartene N	−110.2	−113.7	−116.6	−126.2	−106.6	−92.9	−85.8	−87.4	−109.6	−111.8	−100.1	−118.6
Dammarenediol II	−114.1	−112.3	−126.2	−103.7	−110.8	−95.8	−77.3	−87.2	−110.3	−108.4	−101.4	−120.5
Dammarenediol II acetate	−109.5	−109.5	−113.4	−101.8	−115.7	−105.2	−92.1	−97.4	−115.2	−107.2	−77.7	−104.9
Eupha-2,8,22-triene-20,24R-diol	−111.9	−106.1	−112.9	−121.3	−98.2	−97.9	−80.5	−85.9	−101.0	−106.4	−92.8	−104.5
Eupha-2,8,22-triene-20,24S-diol	−117.2	−104.4	−113.1	−115.5	−100.1	−97.8	−82.6	−87.3	−99.4	−103.0	−94.1	−105.8
Isofouquierol	−116.4	−103.7	−118.4	−113.5	−114.9	−104.0	−96.4	−93.2	−110.4	−114.1	−96.8	−128.3
Isofouquieryl acetate	−107.6	−119.6	−123.5	−122.4	−115.8	−96.8	−103.7	−86.4	−113.4	−124.4	−85.2	−106.6
Lup-20(29)-ene-2α,3β-diol	−101.4	−98.8	−106.0	−95.5	−83.0	−71.4	−87.9	−75.4	−89.8	−107.6	−73.2	−73.6
Neoilexonol	−73.0	−87.9	−101.1	−104.8	−71.4	−74.7	−62.8	−69.5	−52.3	−92.8	−73.9	−98.0
Neoilexonyl acetate	−86.0	−86.7	−108.2	−109.9	−83.8	−79.4	−68.2	−74.3	−87.5	−95.5	−69.4	−31.7
Nizwanone	−81.2	−89.7	−108.6	−89.5	−95.3	−78.5	−60.5	−70.1	−88.3	−98.1	−90.9	−106.3
Ocotillyl acetate	−94.4	−96.1	−121.5	−105.5	−107.2	−96.7	−72.8	−84.5	−108.2	−127.7	−77.5	−97.2

Table 7. *Cont.*

Ligand	MmEPHX2 1cr6	HsEPHX2 4hai	HsMMP-1 1cg1	SsPLA2 2b03	HsPLA2 1j1a	Hs5-LOX 3v99	Mm iNOS 1m8d	HsPI3Kγ 2a5u	HsIRAK4 5tls	HsERAP2 4jbs	HsGSTO1 5v3q	HsPDE4B 3w5e
Olibanumol E	−81.7	−82.4	−101.7	−98.7	−91.8	−82.2	−60.6	−79.4	−92.4	−97.9	−49.2	−99.2
Olibanumol F	−85.7	−108.9	−110.1	−86.1	−79.7	−87.6	−65.9	−86.4	−80.4	−95.0	−77.3	−46.1
Olibanumol G	−81.5	−95.3	−99.3	−82.4	−70.4	−80.0	−61.0	−77.9	−80.8	−93.2	−54.0	−72.7
Olibanumol H	−101.1	−113.9	−107.7	−102.3	−86.8	−82.6	−78.1	−88.4	−94.2	−103.8	−74.1	−55.0
Olibanumol I	−96.2	−97.4	−101.5	−93.4	−70.6	−81.9	−75.5	−78.2	−88.8	−96.9	−71.6	−79.2
Olibanumol J	−133.3	−119.3	−114.2	−112.5	−117.6	−106.1	−93.8	−88.4	−108.3	−123.8	−99.3	−112.3
Olibanumol J'	−108.2	−119.2	−112.7	−112.3	−118.8	−107.7	−84.4	−84.3	−109.2	−124.4	−84.6	−128.8
Olibanumol K	−88.8	−77.8	−110.3	−90.5	−94.9	−77.0	−64.9	−79.8	−76.2	−89.9	−78.8	−82.4
Olibanumol L	−78.1	−80.8	−109.6	−91.7	−98.1	−81.3	−67.6	−73.8	−82.4	−97.3	−64.1	−108.1
Olibanumol L'	−85.0	−74.1	−111.4	−97.1	−83.9	−84.7	−67.6	−77.4	−72.7	−92.4	−70.0	−37.9
Olibanumol M	−77.5	−89.2	−100.1	−95.5	−57.5	−83.9	−69.2	−77.1	−96.5	−93.1	−63.9	−100.0
Olibanumol N	−85.0	−76.5	−103.3	−84.5	−70.8	−86.3	−73.6	−79.7	−87.9	−96.8	−70.4	−50.1
Trametenolic acid B	−106.3	−107.3	−106.9	−107.3	−107.9	−99.7	−92.6	−84.0	−107.6	−115.0	−92.9	−111.6
Urs-12-ene-3α,11α-diol	−77.8	−78.6	−104.3	−94.2	−85.2	−84.4	−68.3	−77.7	−92.2	−90.9	−64.6	−100.1
Urs-12-ene-3β,11α-diol	−79.4	−74.8	−101.3	−108.0	−71.2	−76.9	−67.3	−69.9	−70.9	−93.8	−61.8	−114.1
α-Boswellic acid	−79.9	−87.8	−103.7	−100.2	−95.0	−80.7	−64.4	−79.4	−85.7	−94.8	−62.5	−62.0
α-Elemolic acid	−106.5	−110.5	−113.9	−124.4	−104.1	−99.7	−107.1	−84.0	−108.7	−111.1	−97.3	−110.3
β-Boswellic acid	−78.0	−87.8	−108.9	−94.2	−90.0	−82.5	−7.8	−76.7	−91.1	−94.4	−85.2	−95.5
β-Elemonic acid	−112.2	−113.8	−110.5	−123.3	−109.6	−100.4	−92.4	−86.3	−106.6	−107.1	−108.0	−112.6
δ-Elemonic acid	−110.0	−114.6	−120.2	−120.4	−106.3	−99.8	−98.8	−83.5	−109.2	−109.0	−103.6	−116.2
δ-Boswellic acid	−76.4	−90.4	−101.3	−89.6	−82.5	−74.7	−69.2	−80.7	−87.2	−96.4	−64.4	−76.4

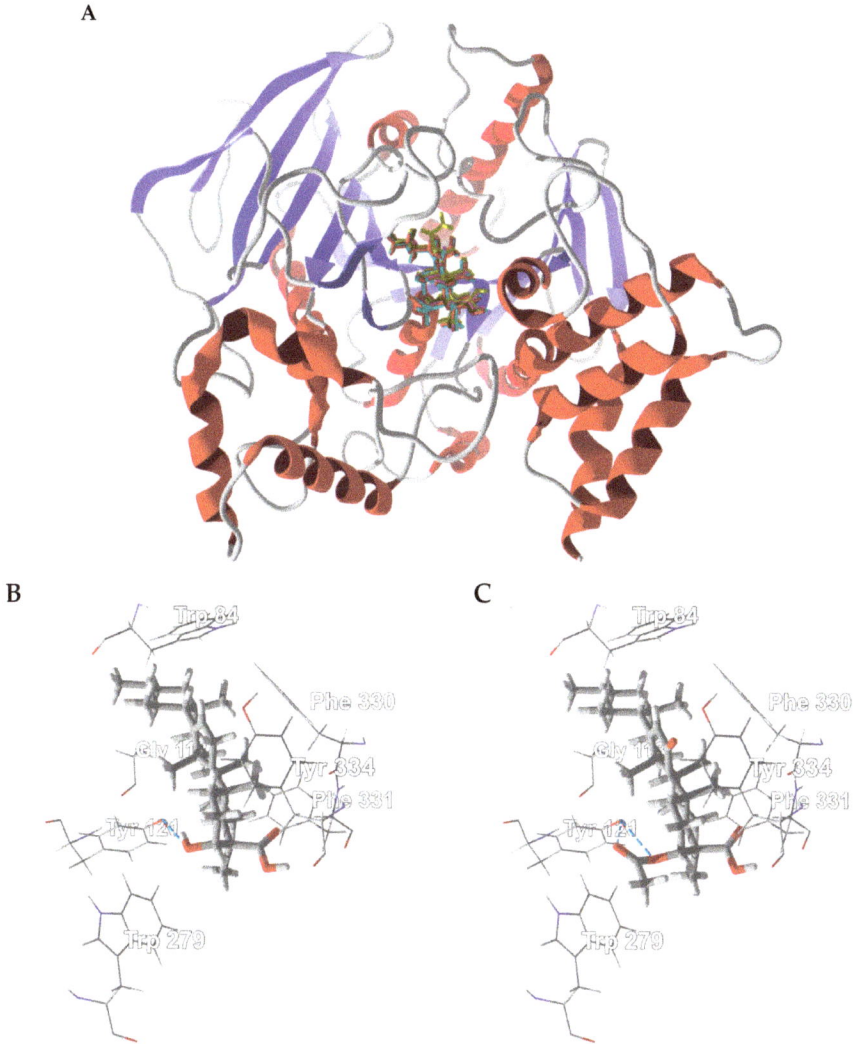

Figure 12. Lowest-energy docked poses of β-boswellic acid derivatives with *Torpedo californica* acetylcholinesterase (TcAChE, PDB 3i6m). (**A**): Ribbon structure with docked ligands, β-boswellic acid (brown), 11-keto-β-boswellic acid (magenta), 11-ethoxy-β-boswellic acid (yellow), 3-acetyl-β-boswellic acid (red), and 3-acetyl-11-keto-β-boswellic acid (aqua). (**B**): Molecular environment of docked β-boswellic acid in the active site of TcAChE. (**C**): Molecular environment of docked 3-acetyl-11-keto-β-boswellic acid in the active site of TcAChE.

Several protein targets related to cancer were targeted by *Boswellia* triterpenoids, including poly(ADP-ribose) polymerase-1 (PARP-1), tankyrase-1 (TANK1), tankyrase-2 (TANK2), folate receptor β (FRβ), and histone deacetylase (HDAC). Poly(ADP-ribose) polymerase-1 (PARP-1) is an important enzyme for the repair of single-strand DNA breaks, and inhibition of PARP-1 can cause multiple double strands DNA breaks to occur, leading to cell death [68]. Several types of cancers are more dependent on PARP-1 than normal cells, so PARP-1 has become an attractive target for cancer chemotherapy [69,70]. At least 15 *Boswellia* triterpenoids showed selective docking to PARP-1 (see Table 6). The strongest-docking ligands for human PARP-1 were (20*S*)-3,7-dioxotirucalla-8,24-dien-21-oic acid (E_{dock} = −141.8 kJ/mol) and eupha-2,8,22-triene-20,24*R*-diol (E_{dock} = −139.8 kJ/mol).

Folate receptors are overexpressed in cancer cells, presumably due to the increased requirement of cancer cells for folic acid needed in cell proliferation [71] and folate receptor-β is overexpressed in lung, liver, skin, and soft tissue tumors, as well as associated stromal cells. Folate receptors, therefore, show promise as chemotherapeutic targets for cancer and other human pathologies [72]. Three of the *Boswellia* triterpenoids in this study showed excellent docking properties to human folate receptor β (HsFRβ), namely dammarenediol II acetate, isofouquierol, and isofouquieryl acetate, with docking energies of −132.3, −130.4, and −137.0 kJ/mol, respectively.

Histone deacetylases (HDAC) are enzymes that remove acetyl groups from lysine residues of histones, which allow the histones to envelope DNA more tightly. Thus, HDACs can affect cell growth and differentiation and cell death [73,74]. Histone deacetylase has been recognized as a promising target for cancer chemotherapy [75,76]. Reverse docking of *Boswellia* triterpenoids has revealed α-elemolic acid to preferentially dock to *Aquifex aeolicus* histone deacetylase (AaHDAC).

Frankincense-containing formulations had been used in ancient Greece for treating various malignant tumors [77]. Frankincense has been used in the Indian traditional medicine (Ayurveda) and in Traditional Chinese Medicine (TCM) as a treatment for proliferative diseases [78]. In addition, extracts of frankincense oleo-gum resins have shown in-vitro cytotoxic activity on several human tumor-derived cell lines [58,79–81], and these activities have been attributed to boswellic acids [82]. Interestingly, although β-boswellic acid [83] and 3-acetyl-11-keto-β-boswellic acid [84] have shown antineoplastic activities, this reverse-docking study did not reveal particularly notable docking properties to cancer-relevant protein targets. It may be that the boswellic acids and derivatives are targeting inflammatory pathways [85,86] or multiple targets as their mechanisms of antineoplastic activities [82,84].

Several *Boswellia* triterpenoids showed good docking properties to 11β-hydroxysteroid dehydrogenase type 1 (11βHSD1). For example, the dammarane triterpenoids 3β-acetoxy-20*S*,24-dihydroxydammar-25-ene, 3β-acetoxydammar-24-ene-16β,20*R*-diol, dammarenediol II, dammarenediol II acetate, isofouquierol, and isofouquieryl acetate showed excellent docking energies with *Cavia porcellus* 11β-hydroxysteroid dehydrogenase type 1 (Cp11βHSD1, PDB 3lz6). These dammarane triterpenoids all occupy the same position in the active site of the enzyme, blocking access to the NADPH cofactor (Figure 13). The docked dammaranes are sandwiched between the NADPH cofactor and hydrophobic amino acids Tyr152, Tyr98, Tyr158, Leu192, and Tyr206 (Figure 13B). There are also close contacts, but no apparent hydrogen-bonds, with Thr197 and Asn99. 11β-Hydroxysteroid dehydrogenase type 1 mediates the interconversion of cortisone and cortisol and overexpression of 11βHSD1 can lead to metabolic disease, characterized by visceral obesity, hyperlipidemia, hypertension, glucose intolerance, insulin resistance, and type II diabetes [87,88]. Thus, inhibition of 11βHSD1 may serve as a treatment option for metabolic syndrome and type II diabetes [89,90].

Boswellia serrata is used traditionally by diabetic patients in Iran, and *B. serrata* supplementation has shown clinical benefit in blood lipid and glucose levels in type II diabetic patients [91,92]. Furthermore, *B. serrata* resin extract has been shown to prevent increase in blood glucose levels in streptozotocin-induced diabetic mice [93]. Similarly, *B. glabra* extracts have shown hypoglycemic effects in alloxan-induced diabetic rats [94]. The selective targeting of Guinea pig 11βHSD1 and human 11βHSD1 by *Boswellia* triterpenoids is consistent with the traditional use and anti-diabetic activities of *Boswellia* oleo-gum resin.

Oxidosqualene cyclases (OSCs) are enzymes that catalyze the cyclization of 2,3-epoxysqualene to form triterpenoids or steroids [95]. In mammals, cyclization of 2,3-epoxyaqualene leads to lanosterol, which can then be converted to cholesterol [96]. Inhibition of oxidosqualene cyclase, therefore, has emerged as a viable therapeutic option to treat hypercholesterolemia and atherosclerosis [97,98].

The oxidosqualene-hopene cyclase from the thermophilic bacterium *Alicyclobacillus acidocaldarius* is homologous to the human enzyme and has been crystallized with OSC inhibitors [99]. Several triterpenoid ligands, most notably ocotillyl acetate, 3β-acetoxydammar-24-ene-16β,20R-diol, and dammarenediol II acetate, docked well to AaOSC with docking energies of −144.6, −139.2, and −138.9 kJ/mol, respectively. These dammarane triterpenoids adopt the same positions in the active site of the enzyme (Figure 14). The active site of AaOSC is a hydrophobic pocket composed of Trp489, Trp169, Phe365, Ile261, Trp312, Phe601, and Tyr420. In addition, there is a hydrogen bond formed between the C(24)-OH of the ligand and the phenolic -OH of Tyr609. The structural similarities between triterpenoids and steroids are likely responsible for the docking properties of *Boswellia* triterpenoids to OSCs.

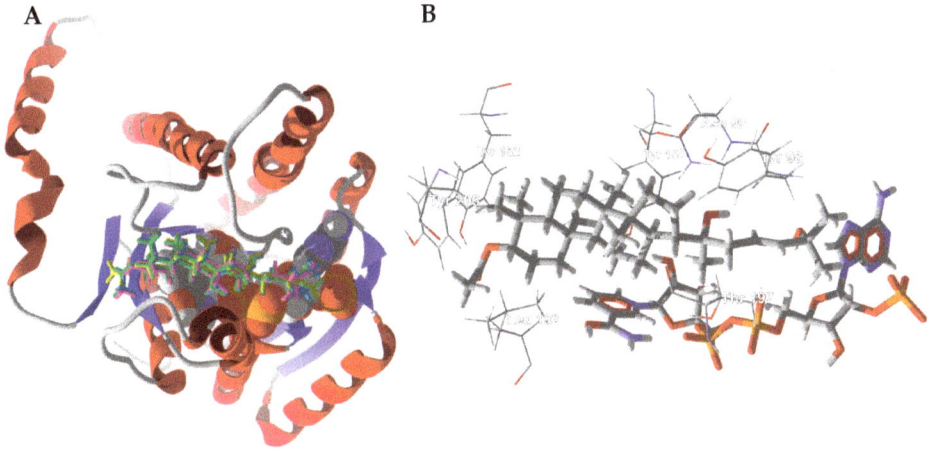

Figure 13. Guinea pig 11β-hydroxysteroid dehydrogenase type 1 (Cp11β-HSD, PDB 3lz6). (**A**): Lowest-energy docked poses of 3β-acetoxy-20S,24R-dihydroxydammar-25-ene (magenta), 3β-acetoxydammar-24-ene-16β,20R-diol (green), dammarenediol II acetate (yellow), and isofouquieryl acetate (blue) with Cp11β-HSD. The NADPH cofactor is shown as a space-filling model. (**B**): Isofouqueryl acetate in the active site of Cp11β-HSD showing the molecular environment.

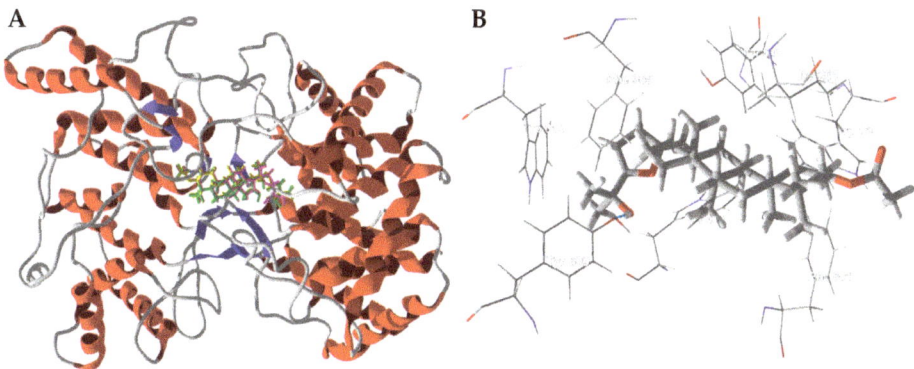

Figure 14. *Alicyclobacillus acidocaldarius* oxidosqualene cyclase (AaOSC, PDB 1h36). (**A**): Lowest energy docked poses of ocotillyl acetate (magenta), 3β-acetoxydammar-24-ene-16β,20R-diol (green), and dammarenediol II acetate (yellow) with AaOSC. (**B**): Molecular environment of docked ocotillyl acetate in the active site of AaOSC.

4. Conclusions

Numerous *Boswellia* terpenoid components have shown selective docking to bacterial protein targets, antineoplastic molecular targets, diabetes-relevant targets, protein targets involved in inflammatory disease conditions, and the Alzheimer's disease target acetylcholinesterase. The molecular docking properties of *Boswellia* terpenoid components corroborate the traditional uses of frankincense, the clinical efficacy of frankincense, and the biological activities of *Boswellia* oleo-gum resins and components. Furthermore, the biomolecular targets identified in this work should lead to further exploration of development and improvement of inhibitors to treat these various disease states.

Author Contributions: K.G.B. and W.N.S. contributed equally to the computational work and manuscript preparation.

Funding: This research was partially funded by dōTERRA International (Pleasant Grove, UT, USA).

Acknowledgments: This work was carried out as part of the activities of the Aromatic Plant Research Center (APRC, https://aromaticplant.org/). The authors are grateful to dōTERRA International (https://www.doterra.com/US/en) for financial support of the APRC.

Conflicts of Interest: The authors declare no conflicts of interest. The funding sponsor, dōTERRA International, played no role in the design of the study; in the collection, analysis, or interpretation of the data; conclusions of the study; or in the decision to publish the results.

References

1. Hepper, F.N. Arabian and African frankincense trees. *J. Egypt. Archaeol.* **1969**, *55*, 66–72. [CrossRef]
2. Thulin, M.; Warfa, A.M. The frankincense trees (*Boswellia* spp., *Burseraceae*) of northern Somalia and southern Arabia. *Kew Bull.* **1987**, *42*, 487–500. [CrossRef]
3. Langenheim, J.H. *Plant Resins: Chemistry, Evolution, Ecology, and Ethnobotany*; Timber Press, Inc.: Portland, OR, USA, 2003.
4. Gebrehiwot, K.; Muys, B.; Haile, M.; Mitloehner, R. Introducing *Boswellia papyrifera* (Del.) Hochst and its non-timber forest product, frankincense. *Int. For. Rev.* **2003**, *5*, 348–353. [CrossRef]
5. Murthy, T.K.; Shiva, M.P. Salai Guggul from *Boswellia serrata* Roxb.-its exploitation and utilisation. *Indian For.* **1977**, *103*, 466–473.
6. Moussaieff, A.; Mechoulam, R. *Boswellia* resin: From religious ceremonies to medical uses; a review of in-vitro, in-vivo and clinical trials. *J. Pharm. Pharmacol.* **2009**, *61*, 1281–1293. [CrossRef] [PubMed]
7. Frawley, D.; Lad, V. *The Yoga of Herbs: An Ayurvedic Guide to Herbal Medicine*, 2nd ed.; Lotus Press: Twin Lakes, WI, USA, 2001.
8. Mies, B.A.; Lavranos, J.J.; James, G.J. Frankincense on Soqotra island (*Boswellia*, Burseraceae; Yemen). *Cactus Succul. J.* **2000**, *72*, 265–278.
9. Getahon, A. *Some Common Medicinal and Poisonous Plants Used in Ethiopian Folkmedicine*; Addis Abeba University: Addis Abeba, Ethiopia, 1976.
10. Dannaway, F.R. Strange fires, weird smokes and psychoactive combustibles: Entheogens and incense in ancient traditions. *J. Psychoact. Drugs* **2010**, *42*, 485–497. [CrossRef] [PubMed]
11. Mertens, M.; Buettner, A.; Kirchhoff, E. The volatile constituents of frankincense—A review. *Flavour Fragr. J.* **2009**, *24*, 279–300. [CrossRef]
12. Paul, M.; Brüning, G.; Bergmann, J.; Jauch, J. A thin-layer chromatography method for the identification of three different olibanum resins (*Boswellia serrata*, *Boswellia papyrifera* and *Boswellia carterii*, respectively, *Boswellia sacra*). *Phytochem. Anal.* **2012**, *23*, 184–189. [CrossRef] [PubMed]
13. Ren, J.; Wang, Y.-G.; Wang, A.-G.; Wu, L.-Q.; Zhang, H.-J.; Wang, W.-J.; Su, Y.-L.; Qin, H.-L. Cembranoids from the gum resin of *Boswellia carterii* as potential antiulcerative colitis agents. *J. Nat. Prod.* **2015**, *78*, 2322–2331. [CrossRef] [PubMed]
14. Boscarelli, A.; Giglio, E.; Quagliata, C. Structure and conformation of incensole oxide. *Acta Crystallogr. Sect. B* **1981**, *37*, 744–746. [CrossRef]
15. Hamm, S.; Bleton, J.; Connan, J.; Tchapla, A. A chemical investigation by headspace SPME and GC–MS of volatile and semi-volatile terpenes in various olibanum samples. *Phytochemistry* **2005**, *66*, 1499–1514. [CrossRef] [PubMed]

16. Forcellese, M.L.; Nicoletti, R.; Petrossi, U. The structure of isoincensole-oxide. *Tetrahedron* **1972**, *28*, 325–331. [CrossRef]

17. Li, F.; Xu, K.; Yuan, S.; Yan, D.; Liu, R.; Tan, J.; Zeng, G.; Zhou, Y.; Tan, G. Macrocyclic diterpenes from *Boswellia carterii* Birdwood (frankincense). *Chin. J. Org. Chem.* **2010**, *30*, 107–111. (In Chinese)

18. Basar, S.; Koch, A.; König, W.A. A verticillane-type diterpene from *Boswellia carterii* essential oil. *Flavour Fragr. J.* **2001**, *16*, 315–318. [CrossRef]

19. Schmidt, T.J.; Kaiser, M.; Brun, R. Complete structural assignment of serratol, a cembrane-type diterpene from *Boswellia serrata*, and evaluation of its antiprotozoal activity. *Planta Med.* **2011**, *77*, 849–850. [CrossRef] [PubMed]

20. Morikawa, T.; Oominami, H.; Matsuda, H.; Yoshikawa, M. New terpenoids, olibanumols D–G, from traditional Egyptian medicine olibanum, the gum-resin of *Boswellia carterii*. *J. Nat. Med.* **2011**, *65*, 129–134. [CrossRef] [PubMed]

21. Wang, Y.; Ren, J.; Wang, A.; Yang, J.; Ji, T.; Ma, Q.-G.; Tian, J.; Su, Y. Hepatoprotective prenylaromadendrane-type diterpenes from the gum resin of *Boswellia carterii*. *J. Nat. Prod.* **2013**, *76*, 2074–2079. [CrossRef] [PubMed]

22. Zhang, Y.; Ning, Z.; Lu, C.; Zhao, S.; Wang, J.; Liu, B.; Xu, X.; Liu, Y. Triterpenoid resinous metabolites from the genus *Boswellia*: Pharmacological activities and potential species-identifying properties. *Chem. Cent. J.* **2013**, *7*, 153. [CrossRef] [PubMed]

23. Singh, S.; Khajuria, A.; Taneja, S.C.; Johri, R.K.; Singh, J.; Qazi, G.N. Boswellic acids: A leukotriene inhibitor also effective through topical application in inflammatory disorders. *Phytomedicine* **2008**, *15*, 400–407. [CrossRef] [PubMed]

24. Banno, N.; Akihisa, T.; Yasukawa, K.; Tokuda, H.; Tabata, K.; Nakamura, Y.; Nishimura, R.; Kimura, Y.; Suzuki, T. Anti-inflammatory activities of the triterpene acids from the resin of *Boswellia carteri*. *J. Ethnopharmacol.* **2006**, *107*, 249–253. [CrossRef] [PubMed]

25. Yoshikawa, M.; Morikawa, T.; Oominami, H.; Matsuda, H. Absolute stereostructures of olibanumols A, B, C, H, I, and J from olibanum, gum-resin of *Boswellia carterii*, and inhibitors of nitric xxide production in lipopolysaccharide-activated mouse peritoneal macrophages. *Chem. Pharm. Bull.* **2009**, *57*, 957–964. [CrossRef] [PubMed]

26. Morikawa, T.; Oominami, H.; Matsuda, H.; Yoshikawa, M. Four new ursane-type triterpenes, olibanumols K, L, M, and N, from traditional Egyptian medicine olibanum, the gum-resin of *Boswellia carterii*. *Chem. Pharm. Bull.* **2010**, *58*, 1541–1544. [CrossRef] [PubMed]

27. Yang, J.; Ren, J.; Wang, A. Isolation, characterization, and hepatoprotective activities of terpenes from the gum resin of *Boswellia carterii* Birdw. *Phytochem. Lett.* **2018**, *23*, 73–77. [CrossRef]

28. Halgren, T.A. Merck Molecular Force Field. I. Basis, form, scope, parameterization, and performance of MMFF94. *J. Comput. Chem.* **1996**, *17*, 490–519. [CrossRef]

29. Zhao, Y.; Truhlar, D.G. The M06 suite of density functionals for main group thermochemistry, thermochemical kinetics, noncovalent interactions, excited states, and transition elements: Two new functionals and systematic testing of four M06-class functionals and 12 other function. *Theor. Chem. Acc.* **2008**, *120*, 215–241. [CrossRef]

30. Marenich, A.V.; Olson, R.M.; Kelly, C.P.; Cramer, C.J.; Truhlar, D.G. Self-consistent reaction field model for aqueous and nonaqueous solutions based on accurate polarized partial charges. *J. Chem. Theory Comput.* **2007**, *3*, 2011–2033. [CrossRef] [PubMed]

31. Setzer, W.N. Conformational analysis of macrocyclic frankincense (*Boswellia*) diterpenoids. *J. Mol. Model.* **2018**, *24*, 74. [CrossRef] [PubMed]

32. Desaphy, J.; Bret, G.; Rognan, D.; Kellenberger, E. sc-PDB: A 3D-database of ligandable binding sites. Available online: http://bioinfo-pharma.u-strasbg.fr/scPDB/ (accessed on 11 September 2017).

33. Thomsen, R.; Christensen, M.H. MolDock: A new technique for high-accuracy molecular docking. *J. Med. Chem.* **2006**, *49*, 3315–3321. [CrossRef] [PubMed]

34. Setzer, M.S.; Sharifi-Rad, J.; Setzer, W.N. The search for herbal antibiotics: An in-silico investigation of antibacterial phytochemicals. *Antibiotics* **2016**, *5*, 30. [CrossRef] [PubMed]

35. Kryger, G.; Silman, I.; Sussman, J.L. Structure of acetylcholinesterase complexed with E2020 (Aricept®): Implications for the design of new anti-Alzheimer drugs. *Structure* **1999**, *7*, 297–307. [CrossRef]

36. Dabaghian, F.; Azadi, A.; Setooni, M.; Zarshenas, M.M. An overview on multi-ingredient memory enhancers and anti-Alzheimer's formulations from traditional Persian pharmacy. *Trends Pharm. Sci.* **2017**, *3*, 215–220.

37. Hosseinkhani, A.; Sahragard, A.; Namdari, A.; Zarshenas, M.M. Botanical sources for Alzheimer's: A review on reports from traditional Persian medicine. *Am. J. Alzheimer's Dis. Other Dement.* **2017**, *32*, 429–437. [CrossRef] [PubMed]

38. Zaker, S.R.; Beheshti, S.; Aghaie, R.; Noorbakhshnia, M. Effect of olibanum on a rat model of Alzheimer's disease induced by intracerebroventricular injection of streptozotocin. *Physiol. Pharmacol.* **2015**, *18*, 477–489.

39. Beheshti, S.; Aghaie, R. Therapeutic effect of frankincense in a rat model of Alzheimer's disease. *Avicenna J. Phytomed.* **2016**, *6*, 468–475. [PubMed]

40. Mahboubi, M.; Taghizadeh, M.; Talaei, S.A.; Firozeh, S.M.T.; Rashidi, A.A.; Tamtaji, O.R. Combined administration of *Melissa officinalis* and *Boswellia serrata* extracts in an animal model of memory. *Iran. J. Psychiatry Behav. Sci.* **2016**, *10*, e681. [CrossRef] [PubMed]

41. Tajadini, H.; Saifadini, R.; Choopani, R.; Mehrabani, M.; Kamalinejad, M.; Haghdoost, A.A. Herbal medicine Davaie Loban in mild to moderate Alzheimer's disease: A 12-week randomized double-blind placebo-controlled clinical trial. *Complement. Ther. Med.* **2015**, *23*, 767–772. [CrossRef] [PubMed]

42. Aghajani, M.; Taghizadeh, M.; Maghaminejad, F.; Rahmani, M. Effect of frankincense extract and lemon balm extract co-supplementation on memory of the elderly. *Complement. Med. J. Fac. Nurs. Midwifery* **2017**, *7*, 1968–1977.

43. Ismail, S.M.; Aluru, S.; Sambasivarao, K.R.S.; Matcha, B. Antimicrobial activity of frankincense of *Boswellia serrata*. *Int. J. Curr. Microbiol. Appl. Sci.* **2014**, *3*, 1095–1101.

44. Patel, N.B.; Patel, K.C. Antibacterial activity of *Boswellia serrata* Roxb. ex Colebr. ethanomedicinal plant against Gram negative UTI pathogens. *Life Sci. Leafl.* **2014**, *53*, 79–88.

45. El Kichaoui, A.; Abdelmoneim, A.; Elbaba, H.; El Hindi, M. The antimicrobial effects of *Boswellia carterii*, *Glycyrrhiza glabra* and *Rosmarinus officinalis* some pathogenic microorganisms. *IUG J. Nat. Stud.* **2017**, *25*, 208–213.

46. Michie, C.A.; Cooper, E. Frankincense and myrrh as remedies in children. *J. R. Soc. Med.* **1991**, *84*, 602–605. [PubMed]

47. Abdallah, E.M.; Khalid, A.S.; Ibrahim, N. Antibacterial activity of oleo-gum resins of *Commiphora molmol* and *Boswellia papyrifera* against methicillin resistant *Staphylococcus aureus* (MRSA). *Sci. Res. Essays* **2009**, *4*, 351–356.

48. Khosravi Samani, M.; Mahmoodian, H.; Moghadamnia, A.A.; Poorsattar Bejeh Mir, A.; Chitsazan, M. The effect of frankincense in the treatment of moderate plaque-induced gingivitis: A double blinded randomized clinical trial. *DARU J. Pharm. Sci.* **2011**, *19*, 288–294.

49. Tee, W.; Lambert, J.R.; Dwyer, B. Cytotoxin production by *Helicobacter pylori* from patients with upper gastrointestinal-tract diseases. *J. Clin. Microbiol.* **1995**, *33*, 1203–1205. [PubMed]

50. Lemenih, M.; Teketay, D. Frankincense and myrrh resources of Ethiopia: II. Medicinal and industrial uses. *Ethiop. J. Sci.* **2003**, *26*, 161–172.

51. El-Mekkawy, S.; Meselhy, M.R.; Kusumoto, I.T.; Kadota, S.; Hattori, M.; Namba, T. Inhibitory effects of Egyptian folk medicines on human immunodeficiency virus (HIV) reverse transcriptase. *Chem. Pharm. Bull.* **1995**, *43*, 641–648. [CrossRef] [PubMed]

52. Karplus, M. Vicinal proton coupling in nuclear magnetic resonance. *J. Am. Chem. Soc.* **1963**, *85*, 2870–2871. [CrossRef]

53. Haasnoot, C.A.G.; de Leeuw, F.A.A. M.; Altona, C. The relationship between proton-proton NMR coupling constants and substituent electronegativities—I: An empirical generalization of the Karplus equation. *Tetrahedron* **1980**, *36*, 2783–2792. [CrossRef]

54. Shen, J.; Hilgenbrink, A.R.; Xia, W.; Feng, Y.; Dimitrov, D.S.; Lockwood, M.B.; Amato, R.J.; Low, P.S. Folate receptor-β constitutes a marker for human proinflammatory monocytes. *J. Leukoc. Biol.* **2014**, *96*, 563–570. [CrossRef] [PubMed]

55. Shen, J.; Putt, K.S.; Visscher, D.W.; Murphy, L.; Cohen, C.; Singhal, S.; Sandusky, G.; Feng, Y.; Dimitrov, D.S.; Low, P.S. Assessment of folate receptor-β expression in human neoplastic tissues. *Oncotarget* **2015**, *6*, 14700–14709. [CrossRef] [PubMed]

56. Wibowo, A.S.; Singh, M.; Reeder, K.M.; Carter, J.J.; Kovach, A.R.; Meng, W.; Ratnam, M.; Zhang, F.; Dann, C.E. Structures of human folate receptors reveal biological trafficking states and diversity in folate and antifolate recognition. *Proc. Natl. Acad. Sci. USA* **2013**, *110*, 15180–15188. [CrossRef] [PubMed]

57. Ernst, E. Frankincense: Systematic review. *BMJ* **2008**, *337*, a2813. [CrossRef] [PubMed]

58. Khan, M.A.; Ali, R.; Parveen, R.; Najmi, A.K.; Ahmad, S. Pharmacological evidences for cytotoxic and antitumor properties of boswellic acids from *Boswellia serrata*. *J. Ethnopharmacol.* **2016**, *191*, 315–323. [CrossRef] [PubMed]

59. Iram, F.; Khan, S.A.; Husain, A. Phytochemistry and potential therapeutic actions of Boswellic acids: A mini-review. *Asian Pac. J. Trop. Biomed.* **2017**, *7*, 513–523. [CrossRef]

60. Al-Yasiry, A.R.M.; Kiczorowska, B. Frankincense—Therapeutic properties. *Postepy Hig. Med. Dosw.* **2016**, *70*, 380–391. [CrossRef]

61. Popa, O.M.; Cherciu, M.; Cherciu, L.I.; Dutescu, M.I.; Bojinca, M.; Bojinca, V.; Bara, C.; Popa, L.O. *ERAP1* and *ERAP2* gene variations influence the risk of psoriatic arthritis in Romanian population. *Arch. Immunol. Ther. Exp.* **2016**, *64*, 123–129. [CrossRef] [PubMed]

62. Wang, H.; Syrovets, T.; Kess, D.; Büchele, B.; Hainzl, H.; Lunov, O.; Weiss, J.M.; Scharffetter-Kochanek, K.; Simmet, T. Targeting NF-κB with a natural triterpenoid alleviates skin inflammation in a mouse model of psoriasis. *J. Immunol.* **2009**, *183*, 4755–4763. [CrossRef] [PubMed]

63. Moustafa, F.; Feldman, S.R. A review of phosphodiesterase-inhibition and the potential role for phosphodiesterase 4-inhibitors in clinical dermatology. *Dermatol. Online J.* **2014**, *20*, 22608. [PubMed]

64. Kimmatkar, N.; Thawani, V.; Hingorani, L.; Khiyani, R. Efficacy and tolerability of *Boswellia serrata* extract in treatment of osteoarthritis of knee—A randomized double blind placebo controlled trial. *Phytomedicine* **2003**, *10*, 3–7. [CrossRef] [PubMed]

65. Cavaillon, J.M. Pro- versus anti-inflammatory cytokines: Myth or reality. *Cell. Mol. Biol.* **2001**, *47*, 695–702. [PubMed]

66. Bachurin, S.O.; Bovina, E.V.; Ustyugov, A.A. Drugs in clinical trials for Alzheimer's disease: The major trends. *Med. Res. Rev.* **2017**, *37*, 1186–1225. [CrossRef] [PubMed]

67. Brady, N.; Poljak, A.; Jayasena, T.; Sachdev, P. Natural plant-derived acetylcholinesterase inhibitors: Relevance for Alzheimer's disease. In *Natural Products Targeting Clinically Relevant Enzymes*; Andrade, P.B., Valentão, P., Pereira, D.M., Eds.; Wiley-VCH: Weinheim, Germany, 2017; pp. 297–318.

68. Bürkle, A.; Brabeck, C.; Diefenbach, J.; Beneke, S. The emerging role of poly(ADP-ribose) polymerase-1 in longevity. *Int. J. Biochem. Cell Biol.* **2005**, *37*, 1043–1053. [CrossRef] [PubMed]

69. Bryant, H.E.; Schultz, N.; Thomas, H.D.; Parker, K.M.; Flower, D.; Lopez, E.; Kyle, S.; Meuth, M.; Curtin, N.J.; Helleday, T. Specific killing of BRCA2-deficient tumours with inhibitors of poly(ADP-ribose) polymerase. *Nature* **2007**, *434*, 913–917. [CrossRef] [PubMed]

70. Ratnam, K.; Low, J.A. Current development of clinical inhibitors of poly(ADP-ribose) polymerase in oncology. *Clin. Cancer Res.* **2007**, *13*, 1383–1388. [CrossRef] [PubMed]

71. Xia, W.; Low, P.S. Folate-targeted therapies for cancer. *J. Med. Chem.* **2010**, *53*, 6811–6824. [CrossRef] [PubMed]

72. Low, P.S.; Henne, W.A.; Doorneweerd, D.D. Discovery and development of folic-acid-based receptor targeting for imaging and therapy of cancer and inflammatory diseases. *Acc. Chem. Res.* **2008**, *41*, 120–129. [CrossRef] [PubMed]

73. Miller, T.A.; Witter, D.J.; Belvedere, S. Histone deacetylase inhibitors. *J. Med. Chem.* **2003**, *46*, 5097–5116. [CrossRef] [PubMed]

74. Mottamal, M.; Zheng, S.; Huang, T.L.; Wang, G. Histone deacetylase inhibitors in clinical studies as templates for new anticancer agents. *Molecules* **2015**, *20*, 3898–3941. [CrossRef] [PubMed]

75. Yoshida, M.; Furumai, R.; Nishiyama, M.; Komatsu, Y.; Nishino, N.; Horinouchi, S. Histone deacetylase as a new target for cancer chemotherapy. *Cancer Chemother. Pharmacol.* **2001**, *48*, S20–S26. [CrossRef] [PubMed]

76. Lane, A.A.; Chabner, B.A. Histone deacetylase inhibitors in cancer therapy. *J. Clin. Oncol.* **2009**, *27*, 5459–5468. [CrossRef] [PubMed]

77. Karpozilos, A.; Pavlidis, N. The treatment of cancer in Greek antiquity. *Eur. J. Cancer* **2004**, *40*, 2033–2040. [CrossRef] [PubMed]

78. Hamidpour, R.; Hamidpour, S.; Hamidpour, M.; Shahlari, M. Frankincense (乳香 Rǔ Xiāng; *Boswellia* species): From the selection of traditional applications to the novel phytotherapy for the prevention and treatment of serious diseases. *J. Tradit. Complement. Med.* **2013**, *3*, 221–226. [CrossRef] [PubMed]

79. Frank, M.B.; Yang, Q.; Osban, J.; Azzarello, J.T.; Saban, M.R.; Saban, R.; Ashley, R.A.; Welter, J.C.; Fung, K.M.; Lin, H.K. Frankincense oil derived from *Boswellia carteri* induces tumor cell specific cytotoxicity. *BMC Complement. Altern. Med.* **2009**, *9*, 6. [CrossRef] [PubMed]

80. Forouzandeh, S.; Naghsh, N.; Salimi, S.; Jahantigh, D. Cytotoxic effect of *Boswellia serrata* hydroalcoholic extract on human cervical carcinoma epithelial cell line. *Med. Lab. J.* **2014**, *8*, 7–13.

81. Hakkim, F.L.; Al-Buloshi, M.; Al-Sabahi, J. Frankincense derived heavy terpene cocktail boosting breast cancer cell (MDA-MB-231) death in vitro. *Asian Pac. J. Trop. Biomed.* **2015**, *5*, 824–828. [CrossRef]

82. Eichhorn, T.; Greten, H.J.; Efferth, T. Molecular determinants of the response of tumor cells to boswellic acids. *Pharmaceuticals* **2011**, *4*, 1171–1182. [CrossRef]

83. Agrawal, S.S.; Saraswati, S.; Mathur, R.; Pandey, M. Antitumor properties of Boswellic acid against Ehrlich ascites cells bearing mouse. *Food Chem. Toxicol.* **2011**, *49*, 1924–1934. [CrossRef] [PubMed]

84. Takahashi, M.; Sung, B.; Shen, Y.; Hur, K.; Link, A.; Boland, C.R.; Aggarwal, B.B.; Goel, A. Boswellic acid exerts antitumor effects in colorectal cancer cells by modulating expression of the let-7 and miR-200 microRNA family. *Carcinogenesis* **2012**, *33*, 2441–2449. [CrossRef] [PubMed]

85. Yadav, V.R.; Prasad, S.; Sung, B.; Kannappan, R.; Aggarwal, B.B. Targeting inflammatory pathways by triterpenoids for prevention and treatment of cancer. *Toxins* **2010**, *2*, 2428–2466. [CrossRef] [PubMed]

86. Ranzato, E.; Martinotti, S.; Volante, A.; Tava, A.; Masini, M.A.; Burlando, B. The major *Boswellia serrata* active 3-acetyl-11-keto-β-boswellic acid strengthens interleukin-1α upregulation of matrix metalloproteinase-9 via JNK MAP kinase activation. *Phytomedicine* **2017**, *36*, 176–182. [CrossRef] [PubMed]

87. Seckl, J.R.; Walker, B.R. Minireview: 11β-Hydroxysteroid dehydrogenase type 1—A tissue-specific amplifier of glucocorticoid action. *Endocrinology* **2001**, *142*, 1371–1376. [CrossRef] [PubMed]

88. Morton, N.M.; Paterson, J.M.; Masuzaki, H.; Holmes, M.C.; Staels, B.; Fievet, C.; Walker, B.R.; Flier, J.S.; Mullins, J.J.; Seckl, J.R. Novel adipose tissue-mediated resistance to diet-induced visceral obesity in 11β-hydroxysteroid dehydrogenase type 1-deficient mice. *Diabetes* **2004**, *53*, 931–938. [CrossRef] [PubMed]

89. Hosfield, D.J.; Wu, Y.; Skene, E.J.; Hilgers, M.; Jennings, A.; Snell, G.P.; Aertgeerts, K. Conformational flexibility in crystal structures of human 11β-hydroxysteroid dehydrogenase type I provide insights into glucocorticoid interconversion and enzyme regulation. *J. Biol. Chem.* **2005**, *280*, 4639–4648. [CrossRef] [PubMed]

90. Wan, Z.K.; Chenail, E.; Xiang, J.; Li, H.Q.; Ipek, M.; Bard, J.; Svenson, K.; Mansour, T.S.; Xu, X.; Tian, X.; et al. Efficacious 11β-hydroxysteroid dehydrogenase type I inhibitors in the diet-induced obesity mouse model. *J. Med. Chem.* **2009**, *52*, 5449–5461. [CrossRef] [PubMed]

91. Ahangarpour, A.; Heidari, H.; Fatemeh, R.A.A.; Pakmehr, M.; Shahbazian, H.; Ahmadi, I.; Mombeini, Z.; Mehrangiz, B.H. Effect of *Boswellia serrata* supplementation on blood lipid, hepatic enzymes and fructosamine levels in type2 diabetic patients. *J. Diabetes Metab. Disord.* **2014**, *13*, 29. [CrossRef] [PubMed]

92. Khalili, N.; Fereydoonzadeh, R.; Mohtashami, R.; Mehrzadi, S.; Heydari, M.; Huseini, H.F. Silymarin, olibanum, and nettle, a mixed herbal formulation in the treatment of type II diabetes: A randomized, double-blind, placebo-controlled, clinical trial. *J. Evid. Based Complement. Altern. Med.* **2017**, *22*, 603–608. [CrossRef] [PubMed]

93. Shehata, A.M.; Quintanilla-Fend, L.; Bettio, S.; Singh, C.B.; Ammon, H.P.T. Prevention of multiple low-dose streptozotocin (MLD-STZ) diabetes in mice by an extract from gum resin of *Boswellia serrata* (BE). *Phytomedicine* **2011**, *18*, 1037–1044. [CrossRef] [PubMed]

94. Kavitha, J.V.; Rosario, J.F.; Chandran, J.; Anbu, P.; Bakkiyanathan. Hypoglycemic and other related effects of *Boswellia glabra* in alloxan-induced diabetic rats. *Indian J. Physiol. Pharmacol.* **2007**, *51*, 29–39. [PubMed]

95. Abe, I.; Rohmer, M.; Prestwich, G.D. Enzymatic cyclization of squalene and oxidosqualene to sterols and triterpenes. *Chem. Rev.* **1993**, *93*, 2189–2206. [CrossRef]

96. Nes, W.D. Biosynthesis of cholesterol and other sterols. *Chem. Rev.* **2011**, *111*, 6423–6451. [CrossRef] [PubMed]

97. Huff, M.W.; Telford, D.E. Lord of the rings—The mechanism for oxidosqualene:lanosterol cyclase becomes crystal clear. *Trends Pharmacol. Sci.* **2005**, *26*, 335–340. [CrossRef] [PubMed]

98. Rabelo, V.W.H.; Romeiro, N.C.; Abreu, P.A. Design strategies of oxidosqualene cyclase inhibitors: Targeting the sterol biosynthetic pathway. *J. Steroid Biochem. Mol. Biol.* **2017**, *171*, 305–317. [CrossRef] [PubMed]

99. Lenhart, A.; Reinert, D.J.; Aebi, J.D.; Dehmlow, H.; Morand, O.H.; Schulz, G.E. Binding structures and potencies of oxidosqualene cyclase inhibitors with the homologous squalene-hopene cyclase. *J. Med. Chem.* **2003**, *46*, 2083–2092. [CrossRef] [PubMed]

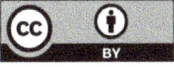

medicines

MDPI

Article

Xanthine Oxidase Inhibitory Potential, Antioxidant and Antibacterial Activities of *Cordyceps militaris* (L.) Link Fruiting Body

Tran Ngoc Quy and Tran Dang Xuan *

Graduate school for International Development and Cooperation, Hiroshima University,
Hiroshima 739-8529, Japan; tnquy@ctu.edu.vn
* Correspondence: tdxuan@hiroshima-u.ac.jp; Tel./Fax: +81-82-424-6927

Received: 10 January 2019; Accepted: 28 January 2019; Published: 29 January 2019

Abstract: Background: *Cordyceps militaris* is a medicinal mushroom and has been extensively used as a folk medicine in East Asia. In this study, the separation of constituents involved in xanthine oxidase (XO) inhibitory, antioxidant and antibacterial properties of *C. militaris* was conducted. **Methods:** The aqueous residue of this fungus was extracted by methanol and then subsequently fractionated by hexane, chloroform, ethyl acetate and water. The ethyl acetate extract possessed the highest XO inhibitory and antioxidant activities was separated to different fractions by column chromatography. Each fraction was then subjected to anti-hyperuricemia, antioxidant and antibacterial assays. **Results:** The results showed that the CM8 fraction exhibited the strongest XO inhibitory activity (the lowest IC_{50}: 62.82 µg/mL), followed by the CM10 (IC_{50}: 68.04 µg/mL) and the CM7 (IC_{50}: 86.78 µg/mL). The level of XO inhibition was proportional to antioxidant activity. In antibacterial assay, the CM9 and CM11 fractions showed effective antibacterial activity (MIC values: 15–25 mg/mL and 10–25 mg/mL, respectively). Results from gas chromatography-mass spectrometry (GC-MS) analyses indicated that cordycepin was the major constituent in the CM8 and CM10 fractions. **Conclusions:** This study revealed that *C. militaris* was beneficial for treatment hyperuricemia although in vivo trials on compounds purified from this medicinal fungus are needed.

Keywords: *Cordyceps militaris*; xanthine oxidase; antioxidant; antibacterial; cordycepin; GC-MS

---

1. Introduction

Species in the genus *Cordyceps* are considered as valuable traditional medicines and other medical applications worldwide, especially in East Asia countries [1,2]. Among them, *Cordyceps militaris* (L.) Link is an ancient medicinal tonic and the most of *C. militaris* nowadays is produced by various modern culture techniques [3]. *C. militaris* exhibited a wide spectrum of clinical health benefits including antifatigue and antistress [4]; anti-inflammatory [5]; antiviral [6]; antifungal and anticancer [7]; HIV-1 protease inhibitory [8]; antioxidant [9]; anti-microbial [10]; inhibition high-fat diet metabolic disorders [11]; immunomodulatory [12]; anti-tumor and anti-metastatic activities [13].

Furthermore, the hot water extract of *C. militaris* has been reported to contain various important bioactive compounds such as cordycepin, adenosine, polysaccharides, fatty acids, mannitol, amino acids, trace elements, ash, fiber and other chemical compositions [7,9,10,14–17]. Many researchers noted that cordycepin (3'-deoxyadenosine) is an important and active metabolite [2,18]. The fermented broth of *C. militaris* obtains clinical effects such as the prevention of alcohol-induced hepatotoxicity [19], inhibitory effects on proliferation and apoptotic cell death for human brain cancer cells [20], inhibitory effects on LPS-induced acute lung injury [21], anti-hyperglycemia [22], anti-tumor and anti-metastatic activities [17]. Adenosine, another bioactive chemical of *C. militaris*, has a number of pharmacological functions such as cardio-protective and therapeutic agents for chronic heart failure, a homeostatic modulator in the central nervous system [16], antioxidant and HIV-1 protease inhibitory [8]. *C. militaris* also exhibited antifungal [23,24], cytotoxic activity [25], antibacterial, anti-tumor agents [13] and plasma glucose reduction [26]. However, the xanthine inhibitory activity of this fungus has not been comprehensively examined.

Nowadays, hyperuricemia, a pre-disposing factor of gout, has been recognized as a lifestyle syndrome that affects the adult population in the developed as well as developing countries [27]. Gout is induced by overproduction or under-excretion of uric acid. It is caused by a high dietary intake of foods containing high amounts of nucleic acids, such as some types of seafood, meats (especially organ meats) and yeasts [28]. Xanthine oxidase (XO) is considered as a cause of hyperuricemia. The acute hyperuricemia can lead to the development of gout, hypertension, diabetes, chronic heart failure, atherosclerosis and hyperlipidemia [29]. Until now, only allopurinol and febuxostat have been clinically approved as XO inhibitors to treat hyperuricemia and gout. However, they also result in many undesirable effects such as hypersensitivity syndrome, hepatitis nephropathy, eosinophilia, vasculitis, fever, and skin rash [30,31].

The discovery of compounds possessing XO inhibitory is necessary to avoid such adverse effects of allopurinol and febuxostat. Yong et al. [29] found that hot water extract of *C. militaris* exhibited significant anti-hyperuricemic action but active components for this activity were not determined. Additionally, the investigation on antibacterial performance of aqueous extracts of *C. militaris* has been proceeded but bioactive compounds from the methanolic extract have not been elaborated [32–35]. Infectious diseases caused by bacteria are still the major reason of illness and death in developing countries [36]. Gastroenteritis and urinary tract infection were predominated by bacteria such as *Escherichia coli*, *Staphylococcus aureus*, *Proteus mirabilis*, and *Bacillus subtilis* [37,38]. Many plant extracts have been found as nutritionally safe and easily degradable source of antibacterial agents against human pathogens [39]. Hence, this study was conducted to investigate the xanthine oxidase inhibitory and determine the correlation to the antioxidant and antibacterial properties of the folk medicine *C. militaris*. The analyses of bioactive constituents from this medicinal mushroom were also conducted.

2. Materials and Methods

2.1. Chemicals

Methanol, hexane, chloroform, ethyl acetate and ethanol were purchased from Junsei Chemical Co., Ltd., Tokyo, Japan. Potassium phosphate monobasic and dibasic, xanthine, xanthine oxidase, allopurinol, and hydrochloric acid were obtained from Sigma-Aldrich Corp., St. Louis, MO, USA. Reagents including 1,1-diphenyl-2-picrylhydrazyl (DPPH), sodium acetate, acetic acid, 2,2′-azinobis (3-ethylbenzothiazoline-6-sulfonic acid) (ABTS), potassium peroxodisulfate, and dibutyl hydroxytoluene (BHT) were supplied by Kanto Chemical Co. Inc., Tokyo, Japan. Four bacteria including *Staphylococcus aureus*, *Escherichia coli*, *Bacillus subtilis*, and *Proteus mirabilis* were provided by Sigma-Aldrich Corp., St. Louis, MO USA. All chemicals used were of analytical grade.

2.2. Plant Materials and Samples Preparation

The dried and sterilized fruiting bodies of *C. militaris* were provided by Truc Anh Company, Bac Lieu city, Vietnam. Fruiting body at green house of Truc Anh Company in the South of Vietnam were harvested and dried by freeze-drying machine (Mactech MSL1000, 15 °C) and packaged on April 18th, 2017. The sample was transferred to the Laboratory of Plant Physiology and Biochemistry, Graduate School for International Development and Cooperation (IDEC), Hiroshima University, Higashi-Hiroshima, Japan for further analysis.

2.3. Preparation of Plant Extract

The whole fruiting body of *C. militaris* was soaked in water for 12 h at room temperature and dried in a convection oven (MOV-212F (U), Sanyo, Japan) at 50 °C for 2 d before pulverized into powder using a grinding machine. The powder (1.0 kg) was immersed in 15 L methanol (MeOH) for two weeks at room temperature. After that, the filtrate from powder-methanol dispersion was concentrated under vacuum at 45 °C using a rotary evaporator (SB-350-EYELA, Tokyo Rikakikai Co., Ltd., Tokyo, Japan) to produce 126.14 g of crude extract. The crude extract was suspended in distilled water (500 mL) and successively fractionated with hexane, chloroform (CHCl$_3$) and ethyl acetate (EtOAc) to produce 10.24, 19.25, 50.21, and 20.17 g extracts, respectively. The extract with the highest xanthine oxidase inhibitory and antioxidant activities was used for further separation by column chromatography.

2.4. Fractionation of Ethyl Acetate Fraction

The EtOAc extract (16.28 g) possessed the highest xanthine oxidase inhibitory and antioxidant on a preliminary test was subjected to a normal-phase of column chromatography (40 mm diameter × 600 mm height, Climbing G2, Mixell, Tokyo, Japan) filled with silica gel (size Å 60, 200–400 mesh particle size, Sigma-Aldrich, Tokyo, Japan). This process yielded 14 fractions by increasing the polarity by MeOH with CHCl$_3$ of the following eluents: CM1 in CHCl$_3$, CM2 in CHCl$_3$:MeOH (9.9:0.1), CM3 in CHCl$_3$:MeOH (9.8:0.2), CM4 in CHCl$_3$:MeOH (9.6:0.4), CM5 in CHCl$_3$:MeOH (9.4:0.6), CM6 in CHCl$_3$:MeOH (9.2:0.8), CM7 in CHCl$_3$:MeOH (9:1), CM8 in CHCl$_3$:MeOH (8.8:1.2), CM9 in CHCl$_3$:MeOH (8.6:1.4), CM10 in CHCl$_3$:MeOH (8.4:1.6), CM11 in CHCl$_3$:MeOH (8:2), CM12 in CHCl$_3$:MeOH (7:3), CM13 in CHCl$_3$:MeOH (1:1), and CM14 in CHCl$_3$:MeOH (4:6).

2.5. Xanthine Oxidase (XO) Inhibitory Activity

The XO inhibitory activity was examined spectrophotometrically in aerobic conditions as described previously [40] with some adjustments. The assay mixture consisted of 50 μL of tests solution (6.25–100.00 μg/mL), 30 μL of 70 mM phosphate buffer (pH = 7.5) and 30 μL of enzyme solution (0.01 units/mL in 70 mM phosphate buffer, pH = 7.5), which were prepared immediately before use. After pre-incubation at 25 °C for 15 min, reaction was initiated by addition of 60 μL of substrate solution (150 μM xanthine in buffer). After that, the assay mixture was incubated at 25 °C for 30 min. The reaction was stopped by adding 25 μL of 1 N hydrochloric acid (HCl) and the absorbance was measured at 290 nm by using a microplate reader (Multiskan™ Microplate Spectrophotometer, Thermo Fisher Scientific, Osaka, Japan). A blank was prepared in similar way but the enzyme solution was accumulated to the assay mixture after the solution of 1 N HCl added. One unit of XO was defined as the amount of enzyme that required to produce 1 μmol of uric acid per min at 25 °C.

The XO inhibitory activity was calculated by this formula (1):

$$\% \text{ Inhibition} = \left\{ \frac{(A - B) - (C - D)}{(A - B)} \right\} \times 100 \tag{1}$$

where A was the activity of the enzyme without test extracts or fractions, B was the control of A without test extracts or fractions and enzyme. C and D were the activities of the test solutions with and without XO. The values of IC$_{50}$ were calculated from the means of the spectrophotometric data of the test trials repeated 5 times. The test solutions were dissolved in DMSO (dimethyl sulfoxide) followed by dilution with buffer. The final concentration of DMSO was less than 0.25%. Allopurinol at 6.25, 12.5, 25, 50, 100 μg/mL dilutions were used as a positive control.

2.6. Antibacterial Activity

The evaluation of antibacterial activity was based on a method described previously [41]. All bacterial strains were cultured in a Luria-Bertani (LB) broth for 24 h at 37 °C. The four bacterial strains employed in this experiment included *Staphylococcus aureus*, *Escherichia coli*, *Bacillus subtilis* and *Proteus mirabilis*. The final population was standardized to be 1.29×10^6 CFU/mL (*S. aureus*), 1.45×10^6 CFU/mL (*E. coli*), 1.63×10^6 CFU/mL (*B. subtilis*) and 2.87×10^6 CFU/mL (*P. mirabilis*). An amount of 0.1 mL of the bacteria suspension was spread over the surface of the solid LB agar medium in Petri dish (9 cm in diameter). After that, filter paper discs (6 mm diameter) loaded with 20 µL of each extract or fraction sample (with a concentration 40 mg/mL in DMSO) were placed on the surface of the LB agar plates. The Petri dishes were incubated at 37 °C for 24 h and then the inhibition zone was measured. Ampicillin and streptomycin were used as the positive controls. The concentrations of the fractions included 1.25, 1.5, 2.5, 5, 10, 20, 25, 30, and 40 mg/mL). The lowest concentration that inhibited the visible bacterial growth was evaluated as minimal inhibitory concentration (MIC). Ampicillin and streptomycin (1.25, 0.625, 0.313, 0.156, 0.078, 0.039, 0.0195, 0.0097, 0.0048, 0.0024, 0.0012, and 0.0006 mg/mL) were used as positive controls. Subsequently, DMSO was used as a negative control.

2.7. Antioxidant Activity

2.7.1. DPPH Radical Scavenging Activity

The antioxidant activity of the extracts and achieved fractions were determined by using 2,2-Diphenyl1-picrylhydrazyl (DPPH) free radical scavenging method as described previously [42] with some adjustments. Briefly, an amount of 100 µL samples was mixed with 50 µL of 0.5 mM DPPH and 100 µL of 0.1 M acetate buffer (pH 5.5). After mixing, the mixtures were maintained in the dark at room temperature for 30 min. The reduction of the DPPH radical was measured at 517 nm using a microplate reader. BHT standard solutions (0.001–0.05 mg/mL) were used as positive controls (2).

$$\text{DPPH radical scavenging activity (\%)} = [\{A_{control} - (A_{sample} - A_{blank\ sample})\}/A_{control}] \times 100 \quad (2)$$

where $A_{control}$ was the absorbance of DPPH solution without samples. A_{sample} was the absorbance of sample with DPPH solution and $A_{blank\ sample}$ was the absorbance of sample without DPPH solution. Lower absorbance showed higher DPPH radical scavenging activity. The IC_{50} (inhibitory concentration) value was determined as the concentration required to decrease the initial DPPH radical concentration by 50%. Therefore, the lower IC_{50} value indicated higher DPPH radical scavenging activity.

2.7.2. ABTS Radical Scavenging Activity

The ABTS radical cation decolorization assay was carried out as an improved ABTS method mentioned noted previously [43] with some modifications. Briefly, the ABTS radical solution was prepared by mixing 7 mM ABTS [2,20-azinobis (3-ethylbenzothiazoline-6-sulfonic acid)] and 2.45 mM potassium persulfate in water. After that, this solution was incubated in the dark at room temperature for 16 h and then diluted with methanol to obtain an absorbance of 0.70 ± 0.05 at 734 nm. An aliquot of 120 µL of the ABTS solution was mixed with 24 µL of samples and the mixture was incubated in the dark at room temperature for 30 min. The absorbance of reaction was recorded at 734 nm using a microplate reader. BHT standard (0.01–0.25 mg/mL) was used as a reference. The percentage inhibition was calculated according to the formula (3):

$$\text{ABTS radical scavenging activity (\%)} = [\{A_{control} - (A_{sample} - A_{blank\ sample})\}/A_{control}] \times 100 \quad (3)$$

The $A_{control}$ was the absorbance of ABTS radical solution without samples. A_{sample} was the absorbance of ABTS radical solution with samples and $A_{blank\ sample}$ was the absorbance of sample without ABTS radical solution. A lower absorbance therefore indicated higher ABTS radical scavenging activity. The IC_{50} (inhibitory concentration) value was calculated as the concentration needed to scavenge 50% of ABTS. As a result, lower IC_{50} value showed higher antioxidant activity.

2.8. Identification of Chemical Constituents by Gas Chromatography-Mass Spectrometry (GC-MS)

A volume of 1 µL aliquot of each *C. militaris* fraction was injected into a GC-MS system (JMS-T100 GCV, JEOL Ltd., Tokyo, Japan). The column employed in this experiment was DB-5MS column (length 30 m, internal diameter 0.25 mm, thickness 0.25 µm) (Agilent Technologies, J & W Scientific

Products, Folsom, CA, USA). The system uses helium as a carrier gas and the split ratio was 5.0/1.0. The temperature program was set up in the GC oven as follows: the initial temperature at 50 °C without hold time, the programmed rate by 10 °C/min up to a final temperature of 300 °C with 20 min for hold time. The injector and detector temperatures were set at 300 °C and 320 °C, respectively. The mass range scanned from 29–800 amu. The peak data set was collected by using the JEOL's GC-MS Mass Center System version 2.65a (JEOL Ltd., Tokyo, Japan) and by comparing detected peaks with National Institute of Standards and Technology (NIST) MS library [44].

2.9. Statistical Analysis

The data were statistically analyzed by one-way ANOVA using the Minitab 16.0 software (Minitab Inc., State College, PA, USA). The significant difference among means were determined by using Fisher's test with the confidence level of 95% ($p < 0.05$). All experiments were carried out in triplicate and expressed as means ± standard deviation (SD).

3. Results

3.1. Xanthine Oxidase Inhibitory Activity of C. militaris Fractions

Xanthine oxidase inhibition, which resulted in a decreased of uric acid production, was measured spectrophotometrically at 290 nm. The ethyl acetate extract (EtOAc extract) showed an xanthine oxidase inhibition by 31.66% at 100 µg/mL concentration, whereas other extracts exhibited negligible inhibitions (Table 1).

Table 1. Xanthine oxidase inhibitory and antioxidant activities of *C. militaris*.

Extracts	% XO Inhibition at 100 µg/mL	Antioxidant Activities	
		DPPH (IC$_{50}$ mg/mL)	ABTS (IC$_{50}$ mg/mL)
Hexane (H)	-	3.07 ± 0.04 [a]	4.45 ± 0.06 [a]
Chloroform (C)	-	1.65 ± 0.15 [b]	2.52 ± 0.19 [b]
Ethyl acetate (E)	31.66 ± 2.86	0.60 ± 0.03 [d]	1.03 ± 0.02 [d]
Aqueous residue (W)	-	1.35 ± 0.07 [c]	1.65 ± 0.07 [c]

Data presented means ± standard deviation (SD). Values in a column with similar letters are not significantly different by Fisher's test ($p < 0.05$). -: not detected.

All of 14 fractions from the EtOAc extract were assessed for their xanthine oxidase inhibitory ability. Of them, eight fractions showed the presence of XO inhibition activity (Table 2). Furthermore, the percentage of XO inhibition of CM8 (52.58%), CM7 (52.72%), CM10 (56.56%), and CM6 (61.70%) fractions were found to be more active than other fractions. The XO inhibition were described by IC$_{50}$ value and the lower IC$_{50}$ indicated the higher XO inhibition activity. Therefore, the CM8 fraction possessed the most potential XO inhibition (IC$_{50}$, 62.82 µg/mL), followed by CM10 (IC$_{50}$, 68.04 µg/mL), CM7 (IC$_{50}$, 86.78 µg/mL), and CM6 (IC$_{50}$, 87.73 µg/mL) fractions. Other fractions exhibited trivial inhibitory activities which were not considerable enough to calculate IC$_{50}$ values.

Table 2. Xanthine oxidase inhibitory activity of EtOAc fractions isolated from *C. militaris*.

Fractions	% XO Inhibition at 100 μg/mL	IC$_{50}$ Value (μg/mL)
CM1	-	-
CM2	-	-
CM3	-	-
CM4	21.88 ± 0.78 [f]	-
CM5	39.57 ± 0.56 [d]	-
CM6	61.70 ± 0.64 [b]	87.73 ± 0.81 [a]
CM7	52.72 ± 0.74 [c]	86.78 ± 1.20 [a]
CM8	52.58 ± 1.55 [c]	62.82 ± 4.48 [b]
CM9	31.12 ± 3.71 [e]	-
CM10	56.56 ± 2.95 [c]	68.04 ± 5.85 [b]
CM11	-	-
CM12	11.92 ± 1.79 [g]	-
CM13	-	-
CM14	-	-
Allopurinol	90.20 ± 6.19 [a]	4.85 ± 2.19 [c]

Data presented means ± standard deviations (SD). Values in a column with similar letters are not significantly different ($p < 0.05$); -: not detected.

3.2. Antioxidant Activities of C. militaris Fractions

The antioxidant activities of *C. militaris* were evaluated using DPPH and ABTS tests, compared with the standard BHT in Figure 1. The antioxidant properties were described by IC$_{50}$ value and the lower IC$_{50}$ indicated the higher radical scavenging activity. Fourteen fractions obtained from *C. militaris* showed various levels of DPPH and ABTS scavenging capacity (Table 1), of which the fraction CM7 presented the strongest antioxidant activity in both DPPH and ABTS assays. Meanwhile, the antioxidant activity of CM5 was the lowest performance in Figure 1.

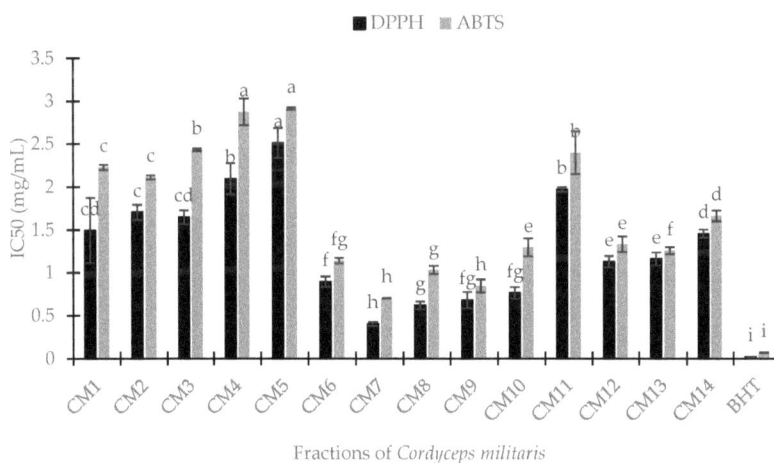

Figure 1. DPPH and ABTS radical scavenging activities of fractions from *C. militaris* and standard antioxidant butylated hydroxytoluene (BHT). Column with similar letters are not significantly different ($p < 0.05$).

In ABTS scavenging activity, the fractions CM7 and CM9 exposed the highest effective activity (IC$_{50}$, 0.702 mg/mL and 0.845 mg/mL, respectively), followed by the CM8 (IC$_{50}$, 1.032 mg/mL) and CM6 (IC$_{50}$, 1.138 mg/mL). In the DPPH assay, the CM8 was also potential but it was statistically similar to that of the CM9 and CM10. Overall, it was found the CM6, CM7, CM8, and CM9 possessed greater antioxidant capacities than other fractions.

3.3. Antibacterial Activities of C. militaris Extracts

The antibacterial activity of *C. militaris* was conducted on two Gram-positive (*B. subtilis* and *S. aureus*) and two Gram-negative (*E. coli* and *P. mirabilis*). Table 3 showed that levels of antibacterial activities versus four bacteria were varied among fractions. Both CM9 and CM11 were the most potential candidates to inhibit the growth of most tested bacteria (MIC, 15–25 mg/mL and 10–25 mg/mL). All fractions showed a lower inhibition than that of streptomycin and ampicillin. Ampicillin and streptomycin provided MIC values of 0.0097–0.039 and 0.078–0.156 mg/mL (Table 3).

Table 3. Antibacterial activity in term of MIC values of EtOAc fractions isolated from *C. militaris*.

Fractions	Minimum Inhibitory Concentration (mg/mL)			
	B. subtilis	*S. auereus*	*E. coli*	*P. mirabilis*
CM1	25	25	30	25
CM2	30	20	25	30
CM3	30	-	30	30
CM4	-	-	-	-
CM5	30	30	30	-
CM6	25	20	-	-
CM7	25	30	25	30
CM8	-	30	20	-
CM9	15	25	25	20
CM10	-	30	30	-
CM11	10	25	15	25
CM12	15	20	20	30
CM13	-	20	-	-
CM14	-	25	-	-
DMSO	-	-	-	-
Ampicillin	0.0195	0.039	0.0097	0.0195
Streptomycin	0.156	0.078	0.156	0.156

-: no inhibition.

3.4. GC-MS of Analysis of C. militaris

Gas chromatographic-mass spectrometry (GC-MS) is a very powerful and reliable analytical technique for identifying the presence of constituents in complex mixtures [45]. The major active components of the principal 14 fractions were detected and identified by GC-MS (Supplementary Materials Figures S1–S14) and summarized in Table 4. Principal constituents from *C. militaris* included cordycepin (3′-deoxyadenosine), hexadecenoic acid and pentadecanal. (Table 4; Supplementary Materials Figures S1–S14).

Cordycepin, appeared as the main compound that was detected in fractions of CM8, CM9 and CM10, while pentadecanal was found in most of fractions (CM3-CM10). Additionally, fatty acids (hexadecanoic acid, methyl hexadecanoate and methyl 2-oxohexadecanoate) were distributed in the CM1, CM2, CM6, CM7, CM11, CM12, CM13 and CM14 fractions. (Table 4; Supplementary Materials Figures S1–S14).

Table 4. Principal compounds identified from different fractions of *C. militaris*.

No.	Major Constituents	Retention Times (min)	Peak Area (%)	Fractions
1	1) Methyl hexadecanoate	16.72	5.95	CM1
	2) Hexadecanoic acid	17.09	17.08	
	3) (9Z,12E)-Octadeca-9,12-dienoic acid	18.73	29.54	
2	1) Methyl hexadecanoate	16.72	2.23	CM2
	2) Hexadecanoic acid	17.11	20.64	
	3) (9Z,12E)-Octadeca-9,12-dienoic acid	18.76	32.16	
	4) (9R,10R,13R,17R)-17-[(E,2R,5R)-5,6-Dimethylhept-3-en-2-yl]-10,13-dimethyl-1,2,9,11,12,15,16,17-octahydrocyclopenta [a] phenanthren-3-one	29.12	6.25	
3	1) Pentadecanal	14.56	16.02	CM3
	2) Methyl 2-oxohexadecanoate	17.41	3.04	
	3) Octadecanal	22.11	34.91	
	4) Dodecanamide	25.55	2.73	
4	1) Pentadecanal	14.56	10.38	CM4
	2) Methyl 2-oxohexadecanoate	17.40	3.20	
	3) Octadecanal	22.11	30.13	
5	1) Pentadecanal	14.56	7.11	CM5
	2) Hexadecanal	15.65	1.30	
	3) Methyl 2-oxohexadecanoate	17.41	3.22	
	4) Octadecanal	22.11	25.85	
6	1) (1R,2R,3S,4R)-3-Deuterio-6,8-dioxabicyclo [3.2.1] octane-2,3,4-triol	11.82	5.65	CM6
	2) Pentadecanal	14.56	53.80	
	3) Hexadecanoic acid	17.07	1.33	
	4) Methyl 2-hydroxyhexadecanoate	20.30	1.25	
	5) Henicosan-1-ol	26.33	1.99	
7	1) (1R,2R,3S,4R)-3-Deuterio-6,8-dioxabicyclo [3.2.1] octane-2,3,4-triol	11.76	1.92	CM7
	2) Pentadecanal	14.52	21.35	
	3) Hexadecanoic acid	17.03	1.75	
	4) Methyl 2-oxohexadecanoate	17.37	1.26	
	5) N-(2-Hydroxyethyl) octanamide	18.77	2.73	
8	1) (1R,2R,3S,4R)-3-Deuterio-6,8-dioxabicyclo [3.2.1] octane-2,3,4-triol	11.76	0.54	CM8
	2) Pentadecanal	14.52	19.79	
	3) 3'-Deoxyadenosine	21.98	55.38	
9	1) Pentadecanal	14.55	19.90	CM9
	2) Methyl 2-oxohexadecanoate	17.40	0.77	
	3) 3'-Deoxyadenosine	21.97	58.04	
10	1) Tetradecanal	13.39	0.83	CM10
	2) Pentadecanal	14.56	45.00	
	3) 3'-Deoxyadenosine	21.95	18.61	
11	1) 2-hydroxybutanedioic acid	6.18	1.89	CM11
	2) Hexadecanoic acid	17.03	1.90	
	3) (11E,13Z)-Octadeca-1,11,13-triene	18.67	0.72	
	4) 1,3-Dihydroxypropan-2-yl hexadecanoate	21.89	3.79	
12	1) Hexadecanoic acid	17.03	1.41	CM12
	2) (11E,13Z)-Octadeca-1,11,13-triene	17.68	1.27	
	3) (1R)-1-Hexadecyl-2,3-dihydro-1H-indene	21.74	2.62	
13	1) Hexadecanoic acid	17.02	4.18	CM13
	2) (11E,13Z)-Octadeca-1,11,13-triene	18.67	15.71	
14	1) N,N-Dimethyl-1-undecanamine	12.06	2.02	CM14
	2) Hexadecanoic acid	17.03	9.95	
	3) (11E,13Z)-Octadeca-1,11,13-triene	18.76	25.50	

4. Discussion

It was reported that the significant increase of gout and hyperuricemia principally caused by the changes in unusual habits of diet and exercise regimen [46]. The food with high content of nucleic acids such as meat and seafood raised the risk of gout disease. Hyperuricemia is a biochemical abnormality or metabolic disorder that results in development of gout and related oxidative stress-related diseases such as cancer, cardiovascular disease and a variety of other disorders [47]. Therefore, the lowering serum uric acid concentration within normal range is important and can be achieved by blocking the biosynthesis of uric acid [27]. Xanthine oxidase (XO) is a form of xanthine oxidoreductase, which has been discovered for decades. Natural XO inhibitors from plants are used in traditional herbal medicines for the treatment of gout or diseases associated with symptoms such as arthritis and inflammation [28]. From this fact, screening of XO inhibitory activity from medicinal plants might be an effective way to find new potential candidates for these major disease treatments. In this study, the xanthine oxidase inhibitory, antioxidant and antibacterial activities of *C. militaris* were determined. It was found that *C. militaris* obtained potent xanthine oxidase inhibitory, antioxidant and antibacterial properties and possessed rich phytochemicals which were characterized by column chromatography and GC-MS analyses (Tables 1–4).

Several previous studies showed that the majority of natural compounds that possessed XO inhibition belonged to lanostanoids [48], flavonoids [31], and phenolics [49]. From GC-MS results, cordycepin appeared as the major bioactive constituents in CM8, CM9, and CM10 fractions separated by column chromatography. Thus it was suggested that this compound may be responsible for the XO inhibition, although the purification of cordycepin as well as other bioactive components and examined for their XO inhibition is apparently required. Earlier researches showed that cordycepin obtained remarkable anti-hyperuricemic action in an in vivo model [50]. Thus, this research highlighted that cordycepin found *C. militaris* played a crucial role in inhibition of XO by an in vitro model. Oxidative stress results in human disease development or an abnormal immune response [9]. Furthermore, it was reported that free radicals caused oxidative damage to biomolecules and are responsible for progression of several diseases such as aging, cancer, inflammatory, diabetes, metabolic disorders, atherosclerosis and cardiovascular diseases [51]. Therefore, xanthine oxidase acted as a biological source of oxygen-derived free radical that led to cell and tissue damage [48]. Obviously, the XO inhibitory activity of *C. militaris* was attributed to their survival strategy to the oxidative stress. For example, several studies showed that polysaccharides from aqueous extracts of *C. militaris* possessed antioxidant properties [33–35] but there was little polysaccharide quantity found in methanolic extracts [25]. Furthermore, the in vitro antioxidant activity was reported to be correlated to cordycepin [21,52] and fatty acids [53]. The considerable amounts of cordycepin and fatty acids observed in CM7, CM8, CM9 and CM10 fractions by this study noticed that these compounds obtained in *C. militaris* might be responsible for significant antioxidant performance (Table 1; Figure 1) as found in previous reports [23,54].

The urinary tract infection and gastroenteritis have become a more serious problem today because of multidrug resistance to *E. coli*, *S. aureus*, *P. mirabilis* and *B. subtilis* infection [37,38]. In recent years, it was documented that methanolic extract of *C. militaris* had potential antibacterial activity [23,25]. To date, thousands of phytochemicals derived from plant extracts with various mechanisms of action have been identified as antibacterial compounds [55]. In this study, cordycepin appeared as the key component antibacterial activity, especially in *E. coli* and *B. subtilis* although further in vitro trial was needed. This study highlighted that *C. militaris* obtained potential substances which may be beneficial for the treatments of gout and bacterial infection. Several previous studies also indicated that fatty acids and the derivative methyl esters exhibited antibacterial activities [53,56]. The fatty acids with a chain length of more than 10 carbon atoms induced lysis of bacterial protoplasts. This mechanism could further distress the expression of bacterial virulence which played an important role in establishing infection [57]. Therefore, the presence of n-hexadecanoic acid (CM12, CM11, CM2, and CM1 fractions), hexadecanoic acid, 2-hydroxy-1-(hydroxymethyl) ethyl ester (CM11), hexadecanoic acid, 2-oxo-, methyl ester (CM9, CM7), hexadecanoic acid, methyl ester and 9,12-octadecadienoic acid methyl ester (Table 4) suggested that these constituents characterized by this study may be responsible for potent antibacterial activity of this medicinal fungus as reported by many previous reports [58,59]. This study has successfully separated fractions from *C. militaris* active on XO inhibitory, antioxidant and antibacterial activities separated by column chromatography and identified potent constituents by

GC-MS analysis. However, the minimum bacteria concentration (MBC) should also be measured to achieve more efficacies on antibacterial activity. It was proposed that there were some compounds other than cordycepin and fatty acids in *C. militaris* can also be potential for pharmaceutical properties and needed further analyses.

5. Conclusions

This is the first study revealed that the medicinal fungus *C. militaris* possessed strong xanthine oxidase inhibition which may be potential for hyperuricemia treatment, although further in vivo trial is required. By employing separative techniques of column chromatography and GC-MS analyses, cordycepin, fatty acids and their derivatives appeared as the major compounds that may be responsible for antioxidant, antibacterial and anti-hyperuricemia activities as observed by this research. Findings of this study highlighted that *C. militaris* is potential to develop foods and drinks potential for treatment of hyperuricemia. Investigation of bioactive constituents purified from *C. militaris* on potent medicinal and pharmaceutical properties of this ancient fungus should be further elaborated.

Supplementary Materials: The following are available online at http://www.mdpi.com/2305-6320/6/1/20/s1, Figure S1: GC-MS spectrum of fraction F1, Figure S2: GC-MS spectrum of fraction F2, Figure S3: GC-MS spectrum of fraction F3–6, Figure S4: GC-MS spectrum of fraction F7–12, Figure S5: GC-MS spectrum of fraction F13–16, Figure S6: GC-MS spectrum of fraction F17–24, Figure S7: GC-MS spectrum of fraction F25–30, Figure S8: GC-MS spectrum of fraction F31–35, Figure S9: GC-MS spectrum of fraction F36–42, Figure S10: GC-MS spectrum of fraction F43–47, Figure S11: GC-MS spectrum of fraction F48–52, Figure S12: GC-MS spectrum of fraction F53–58, Figure S13: GC-MS spectrum of fraction F59–62, Figure S14: GC-MS spectrum of fraction F63–70.

Author Contributions: T.D.X. and T.N.Q. conveyed the idea and carried out experiments. T.D.X. supervised the research and provided critical feedback to the manuscript. T.N.Q. wrote the manuscript and T.D.X. revised the paper. All authors approved the final version of the manuscript.

Funding: This research received no external funding.

Acknowledgments: The authors thanks to the financial support by Hiroshima University and the Ministry of Education and Training of Vietnam under the Hiroshima-VIED to provide a scholarship to Tran Ngoc Quy. Truc Anh Company (Bac Lieu city, Vietnam) was appreciated to kindly provide fruiting body of *Cordyceps militaris*. Thanks are also due to Do Tan Khang, Nguyen Van Quan, Truong Ngoc Minh and Yusuf Andriana for their assistance to this paper's preparation.

Conflicts of Interest: The authors declare no conflict of interest.

References

1. Shrestha, B.; Zhang, W.; Zhang, Y.; Liu, X. The medicinal fungus *Cordyceps militaris*: Research and development. *Mycol. Prog.* **2012**, *11*, 599–614. [CrossRef]
2. Dong, J.Z.; Wang, S.H.; Ai, X.R.; Yao, L.; Sun, Z.W.; Lei, C.; Wang, Y.; Wang, Q. Composition and characterization of cordyxanthins from *Cordyceps militaris* fruit bodies. *J. Funct. Foods* **2013**, *5*, 1450–1455. [CrossRef]
3. Das, S.K.; Matsuda, M.; Sakurai, A.; Sakakibara, M. Medicinal uses of the mushroom *Cordyceps militaris*: Current state and prospect. *Fitoterapia* **2010**, *81*, 961–968. [CrossRef]
4. Koh, J.H.; Kim, K.M.; Kim, J.M.; Song, J.C.; Suh, H.J. Antifatigue and antistress effect of the hot-water fraction from mycelia of *Cordyceps sinensis*. *Biol. Pharm. Bull.* **2003**, *26*, 691–694. [CrossRef] [PubMed]
5. Smiderle, F.R.; Baggio, C.H.; Borato, D.G.; Santana-Filho, A.P.; Sassaki, G.L.; Iacomini, M.; Van Griensven, L.J.L.D. Anti-inflammatory properties of the medicinal mushroom *Cordyceps militaris* might be related to its linear $(1{\rightarrow}3)$-β-D-glucan. *PLoS ONE* **2014**, *9*, e110266. [CrossRef] [PubMed]
6. Ohta, Y.; Lee, J.B.; Hayashi, K.; Fujita, A.; Park, D.K.; Hayashi, T. In vivo anti-influenza virus activity of an immunomodulatory acidic polysaccharide isolated from *Cordyceps militaris* grown on germinated soybeans. *J. Agric. Food Chem.* **2007**, *55*, 10194–10199. [CrossRef]
7. Cho, S.H.; Kang, I.C. The inhibitory effect of cordycepin on the proliferation of cisplatin-resistant A549 lung cancer cells. *Biochem. Biophys. Res. Commun.* **2018**, *498*, 431–436. [CrossRef]

8. Jiang, Y.; Wong, J.H.; Fu, M.; Ng, T.B.; Liu, Z.K.; Wang, C.R.; Li, N.; Qiao, W.T.; Wen, T.Y.; Liu, F. Isolation of adenosine, iso-sinensetin and dimethylguanosine with antioxidant and HIV-1 protease inhibiting activities from fruiting bodies of *Cordyceps militaris*. *Phytomedicine* **2011**, *18*, 189–193. [CrossRef]

9. Liu, J.Y.; Feng, C.P.; Li, X.; Chang, M.C.; Meng, J.L.; Xu, L.J. Immunomodulatory and antioxidative activity of *Cordyceps militaris* polysaccharides in mice. *Int. J. Biol. Macromol.* **2016**, *86*, 594–598. [CrossRef]

10. Zhou, X.; Cai, G.; He, Y.I.; Tong, G. Separation of cordycepin from *Cordyceps militaris* fermentation supernatant using preparative HPLC and evaluation of its antibacterial activity as an NAD$^+$-dependent DNA ligase inhibitor. *Exp. Ther. Med.* **2016**, *12*, 1812–1816. [CrossRef]

11. Kim, S.B.; Ahn, B.; Kim, M.; Ji, H.J.; Shin, S.K.; Hong, I.P.; Kim, C.Y.; Hwang, B.Y.; Lee, M.K. Effect of *Cordyceps militaris* extract and active constituents on metabolic parameters of obesity induced by high-fat diet in C58BL/6J mice. *J. Ethnopharmacol.* **2014**, *151*, 478–484. [CrossRef] [PubMed]

12. Tuli, H.S.; Sharma, A.K.; Sandhu, S.S.; Kashyap, D. Cordycepin: A bioactive metabolite with therapeutic potential. *Life Sci.* **2013**, *93*, 863–869. [CrossRef] [PubMed]

13. Wada, T.; Sumardika, I.W.; Saito, S.; Ruma, I.M.W.; Kondo, E.; Shibukawa, M.; Sakaguchi, M. Identification of a novel component leading to anti-tumor activity besides the major ingredient cordycepin in *Cordyceps militaris* extract. *J. Chromatogr. B Anal. Technol. Biomed. Life Sci.* **2017**, *1061–1062*, 209–219. [CrossRef]

14. Hur, H. Chemical ingredients of *Cordyceps militaris*. *Mycobiology* **2008**, *36*, 233–235. [CrossRef]

15. Zhu, Z.Y.; Liu, F.; Gao, H.; Sun, H.; Meng, M.; Zhang, Y.M. Synthesis, characterization and antioxidant activity of selenium polysaccharide from *Cordyceps militaris*. *Int. J. Biol. Macromol.* **2016**, *93*, 1090–1099. [CrossRef]

16. Chiang, S.S.; Liang, Z.C.; Wang, Y.C.; Liang, C.H. Effect of light-emitting diodes on the production of cordycepin, mannitol and adenosine in solid-state fermented rice by *Cordyceps militaris*. *J. Food Compost. Anal.* **2017**, *60*, 51–56. [CrossRef]

17. Jin, Y.; Meng, X.; Qiu, Z.; Su, Y.; Yu, P.; Qu, P. Anti-tumor and anti-metastatic roles of cordycepin, one bioactive compound of *Cordyceps militaris*. *Saudi J. Biol. Sci.* **2018**, *25*, 991–995. [CrossRef] [PubMed]

18. Masuda, M.; Hatashita, M.; Fujihara, S.; Suzuki, Y.; Sakurai, A. Simple and efficient isolation of cordycepin from culture broth of a *Cordyceps militaris* mutant. *J. Biosci. Bioeng.* **2015**, *120*, 732–735. [CrossRef] [PubMed]

19. Cha, J.Y.; Ahn, H.Y.; Cho, Y.S.; Je, J.Y. Protective effect of cordycepin-enriched *Cordyceps militaris* on alcoholic hepatotoxicity in Sprague-Dawley rats. *Food Chem. Toxicol.* **2013**, *60*, 52–57. [CrossRef]

20. Chaicharoenaudomrung, N.; Jaroonwitchawan, T.; Noisa, P. Cordycepin induces apoptotic cell death of human brain cancer through the modulation of autophagy. *Toxicol. In Vitro* **2018**, *46*, 113–121. [CrossRef]

21. Lei, J.; Wei, Y.; Song, P.; Li, Y.; Zhang, T.; Feng, Q.; Xu, G. Cordycepin inhibits LPS-induced acute lung injury by inhibiting inflammation and oxidative stress. *Eur. J. Pharmacol.* **2018**, *818*, 110–114. [CrossRef] [PubMed]

22. Ma, L.; Zhang, S.; Du, M. Cordycepin from *Cordyceps militaris* prevents hyperglycemia in alloxan-induced diabetic mice. *Nutr. Res.* **2015**, *35*, 431–439. [CrossRef]

23. Reis, F.S.; Barros, L.; Calhelha, R.C.; Ćirić, A.; van Griensven, L.J.L.D.; Soković, M.; Ferreira, I.C.F.R. The methanolic extract of *Cordyceps militaris* (L.) Link fruiting body shows antioxidant, antibacterial, antifungal and antihuman tumor cell lines properties. *Food Chem. Toxicol.* **2013**, *62*, 91–98. [CrossRef]

24. Chen, R.; Jin, C.; Li, H.; Liu, Z.; Lu, J.; Li, S.; Yang, S. Ultrahigh pressure extraction of polysaccharides from *Cordyceps militaris* and evaluation of antioxidant activity. *Sep. Purif. Technol.* **2014**, *134*, 90–99. [CrossRef]

25. Dong, C.H.; Yang, T.; Lian, T. A Comparative study of the antimicrobial, antioxidant and cytotoxic activities of methanol extracts from fruit bodies and fermented mycelia of caterpillar medicinal mushroom *Cordyceps militaris* (Ascomycetes). *Int. J. Med. Mushrooms* **2014**, *16*, 485–495. [CrossRef] [PubMed]

26. Cheng, Y.W.; Chen, Y.I.; Tzeng, C.Y.; Chen, H.C.; Tsai, C.C.; Lee, Y.C.; Lin, J.G.; Lai, Y.K.; Chang, S.L. Extracts of *Cordyceps militaris* lower blood glucose via the stimulation of cholinergic activation and insulin secretion in normal rats. *Phytother. Res.* **2012**, *26*, 1173–1177. [CrossRef] [PubMed]

27. Kapoor, N.; Saxena, S. Xanthine oxidase inhibitory and antioxidant potential of Indian *Muscodor* species. *3 Biotech* **2016**, *6*, 1–6. [CrossRef]

28. Nguyen, M.T.T.; Awale, S.; Tezuka, Y.; Le Tran, Q.; Watanabe, H.; Kadota, S. Xanthine oxidase inhibitory activity of Vietnamese medicinal plants. *Biol. Pharm. Bull.* **2004**, *2*, 1414–1421. [CrossRef]

29. Yong, T.; Zhang, M.; Chen, D.; Shuai, O.; Chen, S.; Su, J.; Chunwei, J.; Delong, F.; Xie, Y. Actions of water extract from *Cordyceps militaris* in hyperuricemic mice induced by potassium oxonate combined with hypoxanthine. *J. Ethnopharmacol.* **2016**, *194*, 403–411. [CrossRef] [PubMed]

30. Liu, F.; Deng, C.; Cao, W.; Zeng, G.; Deng, X.; Zhou, Y. Phytochemicals of *Pogostemon cablin* (Blanco) Benth. aqueous extract: Their xanthine oxidase inhibitory activities. *Biomed. Pharmacother.* **2017**, *89*, 544–548. [CrossRef]

31. Santi, M.D.; Paulino Zunini, M.; Vera, B.; Bouzidi, C.; Dumontet, V.; Abin-Carriquiry, A.; Grougnet, R.; Ortega, M.G. Xanthine oxidase inhibitory activity of natural and hemisynthetic flavonoids from *Gardenia oudiepe* (Rubiaceae) in vitro and molecular docking studies. *Eur. J. Med. Chem.* **2018**, *143*, 577–582. [CrossRef] [PubMed]

32. Zhan, Y.; Dong, C.; Yao, Y. Antioxidant activities of aqueous extract from cultivated fruit-bodies of *Cordyceps militaris* (L.) Link in vitro. *J. Integr. Plant Biol.* **2006**, *48*, 1365–1370. [CrossRef]

33. Yu, R.; Yang, W.; Song, L.; Yan, C.; Zhang, Z.; Zhao, Y. Structural characterization and antioxidant activity of a polysaccharide from the fruiting bodies of cultured *Cordyceps militaris*. *Carbohydr. Polym.* **2007**, *70*, 430–436. [CrossRef]

34. Fengyao, W.; Hui, Y.; Xiaoning, M.; Junqing, J.; Guozheng, Z.; Xijie, G.; Zhongzheng, G. Structural characterization and antioxidant activity of purified polysaccharide from cultured *Cordyceps militaris*. *Afr. J. Microbiol. Res.* **2011**, *5*, 2743–2751. [CrossRef]

35. Chen, X.; Wu, G.; Huang, Z. Structural analysis and antioxidant activities of polysaccharides from cultured *Cordyceps militaris*. *Int. J. Biol. Macromol.* **2013**, *58*, 18–22. [CrossRef] [PubMed]

36. Dzotam, J.K.; Touani, F.K.; Kuete, V. Antibacterial activities of the methanol extracts of *Canarium schweinfurthii* and four other Cameroonian dietary plants against multi-drug resistant Gram-negative bacteria. *Saudi J. Biol. Sci.* **2016**, *23*, 565–570. [CrossRef]

37. Chimnoi, N.; Reuk-ngam, N.; Chuysinuan, P.; Khlaychan, P.; Khunnawutmanotham, N.; Chokchaichamnankit, D.; Thamniyom, W.; Klayraung, S.; Mahidol, C.; Techasakul, S. Characterization of essential oil from *Ocimum gratissimum* leaves: Antibacterial and mode of action against selected gastroenteritis pathogens. *Microb. Pathog.* **2018**, *118*, 290–300. [CrossRef]

38. Mishra, M.P.; Rath, S.; Swain, S.S.; Ghosh, G.; Das, D.; Padhy, R.N. In vitro antibacterial activity of crude extracts of 9 selected medicinal plants against UTI causing MDR bacteria. *J. King Saud Univ. Sci.* **2017**, *29*, 84–95. [CrossRef]

39. Mostafa, A.A.; Al-Askar, A.A.; Almaary, K.S.; Dawoud, T.M.; Sholkamy, E.N.; Bakri, M.M. Antimicrobial activity of some plant extracts against bacterial strains causing food poisoning diseases. *Saudi J. Biol. Sci.* **2018**, *25*, 253–258. [CrossRef]

40. Umamaheswari, M.; AsokKumar, K.; Somasundaram, A.; Sivashanmugam, T.; Subhadradevi, V.; Ravi, T.K. Xanthine oxidase inhibitory activity of some Indian medical plants. *J. Ethnopharmacol.* **2007**, *109*, 547–551. [CrossRef]

41. Fukuta, M.; Xuan, T.D.; Deba, F.; Tawata, S.; Khanh, T.D.; Chung, I.M. Comparative efficacies in vitro of antibacterial, fungicidal, antioxidant and herbicidal activities of momilatones A and B. *J. Plant Interact.* **2007**, *2*, 245–251. [CrossRef]

42. Elzaawely, A.A.; Xuan, T.D.; Tawata, S. Essential oils, kava pyrones and phenolic compounds from leaves and rhizomes of Alpinia zerumbet (Pers.) B.L. Burtt. & R.M. Sm. and their antioxidant activity. *Food Chem.* **2007**, *103*, 486–494. [CrossRef]

43. Mikulic-Petkovsek, M.; Samoticha, J.; Eler, K.; Stampar, F.; Veberic, R. Traditional elderflower beverages: A rich source of phenolic compounds with high antioxidant activity. *J. Agric. Food Chem.* **2015**, *63*, 1477–1487. [CrossRef] [PubMed]

44. Andriana, Y.; Xuan, T.D.; Quan, N.V.; Quy, T.N. Allelopathic potential of *Tridax procumbens* L. on radish and identification of allelochemicals. *Allelopath. J.* **2018**, *43*, 222–238. [CrossRef]

45. Xuan, T.D.; Yulianto, R.; Andriana, Y.; Khanh, T.D. Chemical profile, antioxidant activities and allelopathic potential of liquid waste from germinated brown rice. *Allelopath. J.* **2018**, *45*, 1–12. [CrossRef]

46. Nile, S.H.; Park, S.W. Chromatographic analysis, antioxidant, anti-inflammatory and xanthine oxidase inhibitory activities of ginger extracts and its reference compounds. *Ind. Crops Prod.* **2015**, *70*, 238–244. [CrossRef]

47. Kapoor, N.; Saxena, S. Potential xanthine oxidase inhibitory activity of endophytic *Lasiodiplodia pseudotheobromae*. *Appl. Biochem. Biotechnol.* **2014**, *173*, 1360–1374. [CrossRef]

48. Lin, K.W.; Chen, Y.T.; Yang, S.C.; Wei, B.L.; Hung, C.F.; Lin, C.N. Xanthine oxidase inhibitory lanostanoids from *Ganoderma tsugae*. *Fitoterapia* **2013**, *89*, 231–238. [CrossRef]

49. Gawlik-Dziki, U.; Dziki, D.; Świeca, M.; Nowak, R. Mechanism of action and interactions between xanthine oxidase inhibitors derived from natural sources of chlorogenic and ferulic acids. *Food Chem.* **2017**, *225*, 138–145. [CrossRef]

50. Yong, T.; Chen, S.; Xie, Y.; Chen, D.; Su, J.; Shuai, O.; Jiao, C.; Zuo, D. Cordycepin, a characteristic bioactive constituent in *Cordyceps militaris*, ameliorates hyperuricemia through URAT1 in hyperuricemic mice. *Front. Microbiol.* **2018**, *9*, 1–12. [CrossRef]

51. Ouyang, H.; Hou, K.; Peng, W.; Liu, Z.; Deng, H. Antioxidant and xanthine oxidase inhibitory activities of total polyphenols from onion. *Saudi J. Biol. Sci.* **2017**, *25*, 1509–1513. [CrossRef] [PubMed]

52. Olatunji, O.J.; Feng, Y.; Olatunji, O.O.; Tang, J.; Ouyang, Z.; Su, Z. Cordycepin protects PC12 cells against 6-hydroxydopamine induced neurotoxicity via its antioxidant properties. *Biomed. Pharmacother.* **2016**, *81*, 7–14. [CrossRef] [PubMed]

53. Karimi, E.; Ze Jaafar, H.; Ghasemzadeh, A.; Ebrahimi, M. Fatty acid composition, antioxidant and antibacterial properties of the microwave aqueous extract of three varieties of *Labisia pumila* Benth. *Biol. Res.* **2015**, *48*, 1–6. [CrossRef] [PubMed]

54. Yu, H.M.; Wang, B.S.; Huang, S.C.; Duh, P.D. Comparison of protective effects between cultured *Cordyceps militaris* and natural *Cordyceps sinensis* against oxidative damage. *J. Agric. Food Chem.* **2006**, *54*, 3132–3138. [CrossRef] [PubMed]

55. Barbieri, R.; Coppo, E.; Marchese, A.; Daglia, M.; Sobarzo-Sánchez, E.; Nabavi, S.F.; Nabavi, S.M. Phytochemicals for human disease: An update on plant-derived compounds antibacterial activity. *Microbiol. Res.* **2017**, *196*, 44–68. [CrossRef] [PubMed]

56. Huang, C.B.; Alimova, Y.; Myers, T.M.; Ebersole, J.L. Short- and medium-chain fatty acids exhibit antimicrobial activity for oral microorganisms. *Arch. Oral Biol.* **2011**, *56*, 650–654. [CrossRef]

57. Mohy El-Din, S.M.; El-Ahwany, A.M.D. Bioactivity and phytochemical constituents of marine red seaweeds (*Jania rubens, Corallina mediterranea* and *Pterocladia capillacea*). *J. Taibah Univ. Sci.* **2016**, *10*, 471–484. [CrossRef]

58. Eleazu, C.O. Characterization of the natural products in cocoyam (*Colocasia esculenta*) using GC–MS. *Pharm. Biol.* **2016**, *54*, 2880–2885. [CrossRef]

59. Al-Abd, N.M.; Nor, Z.M.; Mansor, M.; Zajmi, A.; Hasan, M.S.; Azhar, F.; Kassim, M. Phytochemical constituents, antioxidant and antibacterial activities of methanolic extract of *Ardisia elliptica*. *Asian Pac. J. Trop. Med.* **2017**, *7*, 569–576. [CrossRef]

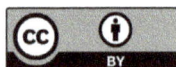

medicines

MDPI

Brief Report

Nutraceutical Characteristics of Ancient *Malus* x *domestica* Borkh. Fruits Recovered across Siena in Tuscany

Roberto Berni [1,2], Claudio Cantini [2], Massimo Guarnieri [1], Massimo Nepi [1], Jean-Francois Hausman [3], Gea Guerriero [3], Marco Romi [1] and Giampiero Cai [1,*]

[1] Department of Life Sciences, University of Siena, I-53100 Siena, Italy; berni10@student.unisi.it (R.B.); massimo.guarnieri@unisi.it (M.G.); massimo.nepi@unisi.it (M.N.); marco.romi@unisi.it (M.R.)
[2] Trees and Timber Institute-National Research Council of Italy (CNR-IVALSA), I-58022 Follonica, Italy; cantini@ivalsa.cnr.it
[3] Environmental Research and Innovation Department, Luxembourg Institute of Science and Technology, L-4362 Esch/Alzette, Luxembourg; jean-francois.hausman@list.lu (J.-F.H.); gea.guerriero@list.lu (G.G.)
* Correspondence: giampiero.cai@unisi.it

Received: 24 January 2019; Accepted: 12 February 2019; Published: 18 February 2019

Abstract: Background: A diet rich in fruits and vegetables contributes to lowering the risk of chronic diseases. The fruits of Malus x domestica are a rich dietary source of bioactive compounds, namely vitamins and antioxidants, with recognized action on human health protection. Tuscany is known for its rich plant biodiversity, especially represented by ancient varieties of fruit trees. Particularly noteworthy are the many ancient Tuscan varieties of apple trees. **Methods:** Sugar quantification via HPLC and spectrophotometric assays to quantify the antioxidant power and total polyphenol content revealed interesting differences in 17 old varieties of Malus x domestica Borkh. recovered in Siena (Tuscany). **Results:** The quantification of antioxidants, polyphenols, and the main free sugars revealed that their content in the old fruits was often superior to the widespread commercial counterparts ('Red Delicious' and 'Golden Delicious'). Such differences were, in certain cases, dramatic, with 8-fold higher values. Differences were also present for sugars and fibers (pectin). Most ancient fruits displayed low values of glucose and high contents of xylitol and pectin. **Conclusions:** The results reported here suggest the possible use of ancient apple varieties from Siena for nutraceutical purposes and draw attention to the valorization of local old varieties.

Keywords: *Malus* x *domestica*; Tuscany; ancient varieties; nutraceutics; antioxidants; polyphenols; sugars; pectin

1. Introduction

The consumption of fruits and vegetables has beneficial effects on human health, as they contribute to lowering the risk of chronic diseases and improve the immune system [1].

The fruits of *Malus* x *domestica* are consumed worldwide [2,3] and are a rich source of phytochemicals (a.k.a. bioactive molecules that are plant metabolites with a biological effect) that contrast oxidative damage and positively impact human health [4]. In particular, polymeric apple proanthocyanidins contribute substantially to limiting lipid peroxidation and, therefore, oxidative stress [5]. Apple oligomeric procyanidins also display anti-cancer properties: they have anti-mutagenic effects, they modulate signal transduction pathways and they may even display epigenetic action [3,6].

The skins of apples contain pentacyclic triterpenes, which have anti-inflammatory effects [2]. Particularly noteworthy is the case of the triterpene-caffeates betulinic acid-3-*cis*-caffeic, betulinic acid-3-*trans*-caffeic and oleanolic acid-3-*trans*-caffeic reported in the suberized skin tissues of the russeted fruits of 'Merton Russet' [7]. The consumption of apple fruits with skins, therefore, results in a higher intake of bioactives, as well as of dietary fibers [8].

The concentration of bioactives varies in function of the apple fruit maturation stage and variety (reviewed by [3]). We have recently reported on the rich repertoire of ancient varieties of both herbaceous and woody plants of Tuscany. In particular, we have shown their nutraceutical values by measuring the content of key bioactive molecules (flavonoids, anthocyanins, carotenoids) [9,10]. Ancient varieties of plants were cultivated in the past but have fallen out of agricultural interest with the progressive development of cultivars meeting specific market needs, e.g., yield/key fruit characteristics such as shape, size and color. Interestingly, such ancient varieties display a high content of bioactive molecules (even superior than commercial counterparts) [9], as well as high adaptability to exogenous stresses [11]. These features make them interesting for agronomical and nutraceutical studies and as a source of interesting genetic characters to be used for breeding purposes.

Many of these ancient varieties have been recovered across Tuscany and, subsequently, included in the regional germplasm bank through law 64/04 (recently reviewed by Berni and co-authors [11]). The province of Siena in Tuscany has recovered many plants thanks to the actions supported by this law, with the aim of protecting and propagating the old local germplasm.

We here investigate the antioxidant power, as well as the polyphenol, free sugar and pectin content of 17 ancient apple fruits representing the biodiversity repertoire of Siena. We provide evidence of their value for nutraceutical applications and promote the valorization, on a local scale, of ancient plants for the diversification of the fruit market and their use in the daily diet as sources of functional molecules.

Locally-grown ancient varieties will contribute to the restoration of regional habitats and exploit local resources, notably the soil (and associated microbial consortia). The products obtained by locally-grown ancient varieties are fully traceable, can be used as functional foods and are obtained with a "0 km" concept [9].

2. Materials and Methods

2.1. Fruit Collection

The fruits of 17 ancient apples (a pool of 3–4 fruits per biological replicate) were harvested during the year 2014 from plants present in the experimental field "Il Campino", a part of the Tuscan regional germplasm bank, localized in Siena (43°18′16″N 11°22′32″E). Fruits were collected at the maximum stage of maturation, i.e., between 30–40 days after flower anthesis. Our study included two commercial varieties 'Red Delicious' and 'Golden Delicious' for comparison. After harvest, fruits were immediately placed at −80 °C to block any metabolic processes. The ancient varieties studied here are: 'Solaio', 'Campo Pianacce', 'Viale Casetta', 'Gialla Pianacce', 'Tre Colli', 'Ancaiano', 'Piatta Cantine', 'Filare Delle Pianacce', 'Tocchi', 'Rossa Casetta', 'Ficareto', 'Rugginosa Delle Pianacce', 'Vecchio Pollaio', 'Strada Pianacce', 'Podere Pianacce', 'Sotto Muro Casetta', 'Casolana', 'Red Delicious', and 'Golden Delicious'.

2.2. Extraction of Antioxidants and Phenolic Compounds

The extraction procedure was performed according to Berni et al. [12] following a previously described method [13]. Fruits were analyzed in three independent biological replicates, as well as three experimental replicates for each variety. Three grams of frozen fruits were added to 9.0 mL of 70% acetone and then homogenized using an Ultra-Turrax®T-25 basic (IKA®-Werke GmbH & Co., IKA, Staufen, Germany). The mixture was then sonicated for 20 min with an Elma Transsonic T 460/H for 20 min and homogenized again to ensure complete tissue lysis. The final mixture was centrifuged for 5 min at 12,000 rpm (centrifuge 5415D, Eppendorf®, Hamburg, Germany) and filtered through a 0.45 μm membrane to remove impurities.

2.3. Evaluation of the Antioxidant Power

The ferric reducing antioxidant power (FRAP) assay was used to determine the antioxidant capacity of the extraction solution [14]. The FRAP assay is a simple, commonly used method to evaluate the antioxidant capacity of plant materials and, in particular, fruits [15,16]. Thaipong and colleagues showed the simplicity, speed and high reproducibility of the FRAP method, as well as the highest Pearson correlation value between total antioxidant compounds and total phenolic molecules [17]. The reduction of ferric to ferrous ions at low pH causes a colored ferrous-tripyridyltriazine (TPTZ) complex. The FRAP reagent was freshly prepared as recently reported in Berni et al. [12] by mixing 2040 µL of sodium acetate 300 mM pH 3.6 to 200 µL of TPTZ 10 nM (Sigma Chemical, St. Louis, MO, USA) and 200 µL of ferric chloride 20 mM. At the end, 20 µL of sample were added to the FRAP reagent and then the solution was incubated for 1 h at 37 °C. The solutions were compared to a previously prepared ferric chloride standard curve measured at 593 nm (UV-Vis instrument Shimadzu UV Visible Recording Spectrophotometer UV 160, Shimadzu, Kyoto, Japan). The values were expressed as micromole (µmol) of Fe^{2+} equivalents per gram of fresh weight (µmol Fe^{2+}/g FW).

2.4. Evaluation of the Phenolic Content

The Folin–Ciocalteu method (F-C method) was performed for the phenolic content determination. The method is described by Berni et al. [12]. Briefly, 0.5 mL of sample was added to 3.0 mL of distilled water and 0.25 mL of F-C reagent (Sigma Chemical, St. Louis, MO, USA). Then, 0.75 mL of saturated sodium carbonate and 0.95 mL distilled water was added to the mixture [18]. The solutions were incubated for 30 min at 37 °C and measured at 765 nm. Results were compared to a previously prepared gallic acid (GA; Sigma chemicals, St. Louis, MO, USA) standard curve. The total phenolic content was expressed as milligrams of gallic acid equivalents per gram of fresh weight (mg GAE/g FW).

2.5. Evaluation of the Sugar Content

For quantification and calibration, a standard solution was prepared by dissolving D(+)-fructose, D(+)-glucose, D(+)-sucrose, and poly-D-galacturonic acid methyl ester (to quantify soluble pectin contents via HPLC, as detailed below) in water (Sigma-Aldrich, St. Louis, MO, USA, HPLC grade) for five different concentration levels, viz. 50, 100, 500, 1000, 2500, and 5000 ppm. The sample preparations and HPLC analyses were performed following the methods described by [19]. Five grams of frozen fruits were dissolved in 10 mL of ultra-pure water, homogenized using an Ultra-Turrax and then sonicated for 20 min. The mixture was homogenized once again and centrifuged at 4 °C at 12,000 rpm for 10 min. The supernatant was filtered through a 0.45 µm membrane and then injected into the HPLC loop. For the soluble sugar analysis, a Waters 600 pump E with refraction index detector 2410 was used. The HPLC analysis was performed isocratically with the column Sugar Pak 1 (S5 µm, 250 mm × 4.6 mm i.d.) in ultra-pure water under the following conditions: flow rate = 1.0 µL/min, data rate = 1 pps, run time = 15 min, gain = 1, column heater temperature = 35 °C, sample temperature = 5 °C, pressure = 50 psi, nebulizer: heating (90%) and injection volume = 20.

2.6. Statistical Analysis

For each extract, three analytical measurements were performed and the final value was calculated as an average for each sample. Three independent biological replicates were obtained from each variety and the values were reported using the standard deviation (SD). A one-way ANOVA with a Tukey's post-hoc test was performed on log2 transformed values with IBM SPSS Statistics v19 (IBM SPSS, Chicago, IL, USA). The Pearson correlation coefficient was calculated using a Pearson correlation coefficient calculator (https://www.socscistatistics.com/tests/pearson/Default2.aspx).

3. Results

3.1. Antioxidant Capacity

The antioxidant capacity values ranged from 97.13 µmol Fe^{2+}/g FW to 5.85 µmol Fe^{2+}/g FW in the ancient apple varieties. The 'Solaio' variety reported the highest antioxidant concentration; also, 'Campo Pianacce' and 'Viale Casetta' varieties showed interesting values (48.79 and 36.29 µmol Fe^{2+}/g FW, respectively, as shown in Table 1). The values obtained for the commercial fruits were 13.51 µmol Fe^{2+}/g FW in 'Red Delicious' and 11.99 µmol Fe^2/g FW in 'Golden Delicious'. Interestingly, 12 out of the 17 ancient varieties studied showed a content of antioxidants that was higher than the commercial ones (Table 1).

Table 1. The table shows the values (±SD) of antioxidants (expressed as µmol Fe^{2+}/g FW) and polyphenols (expressed as mg GAE/g FW) in the ancient and commercial apples studied. Different letters indicate statistically significant differences among values ($p < 0.05$).

Variety Name	Total Antioxidants	Total Polyphenols
Solaio	97.13 ± 4.94^l	8.72 ± 2.46^f
Campo Pianacce	48.79 ± 0.97^k	2.25 ± 0.06^e
Viale Casetta	36.29 ± 3.51^j	1.87 ± 0.04^{de}
Gialla Pianacce	28.34 ± 2.25^{ij}	1.35 ± 0.07^{cde}
Tre Colli	22.87 ± 0.58^{hi}	0.88 ± 0.16^{cde}
Ancaiano	19.90 ± 1.62^{gh}	1.29 ± 0.08^{cde}
Piatta Cantine	18.98 ± 1.12^{fgh}	1.21 ± 0.03^{cde}
Filare Delle Pianacce	18.47 ± 0.55^{fgh}	4.25 ± 0.15^e
Tocchi	18.15 ± 1.45^{fgh}	1.86 ± 0.01^{de}
Rossa Casetta	16.51 ± 0.85^{efg}	0.67 ± 0.07^{abc}
Ficareto	15.55 ± 1.56^{defg}	1.09 ± 0.10^{cde}
Rugginosa Delle Pianacce	14.81 ± 0.16^{cdef}	0.80 ± 0.04^{bcd}
Red Delicious	13.51 ± 0.35^{cde}	0.26 ± 0.01^a
Vecchio Pollaio	13.43 ± 1.74^{cde}	1.10 ± 0.03^{cde}
Strada Pianacce	13.29 ± 0.62^{bcde}	0.66 ± 0.06^{abc}
Golden Delicious	11.99 ± 0.89^{bcd}	0.30 ± 0.01^{ab}
Podere Pianacce	11.35 ± 1.13^{bc}	0.74 ± 0.01^{bcd}
Sotto Muro Casetta	9.98 ± 0.12^b	0.60 ± 0.21^{abc}
Casolana	5.85 ± 1.65^a	0.59 ± 0.20^{abc}

3.2. Total Phenolic Content

The highest polyphenol contents were found in the varieties 'Solaio' and 'Campo Pianacce' (8.72 mg GAE/g FW and 2.25 mg GAE/g FW shown in Table 1).

Interestingly, the commercial varieties showed the lowest values: 0.30 mg GAE/g FW for 'Golden Delicious' and 0.26 mg GAE/g FW for 'Red Delicious' (Table 1). To evaluate the contribution of polyphenols to the total antioxidant capacity, the Pearson correlation coefficient was calculated. It showed a positive correlation ($r = 0.8803$).

3.3. Soluble Sugar and Pectin Contents

As shown in Table 2, the ancient varieties displayed different concentrations, both among themselves and among the commercial ones. As expected, the most prominent soluble sugar in apples was fructose. In the commercial varieties, this sugar was found at the highest concentrations with approximately the same values ('Golden Delicious' 69.14 mg/g FW and 'Red Delicious' 64.46 mg/g FW). Notably, fructose was in high concentrations also in the ancient varieties 'Tre Colli', 'Ficareto' and 'Strada Pianacce' (63.58, 59.14, and 55.29 mg/g FW, respectively; Table 2), while in 'Vecchio Pollaio', and 'Gialla Pianacce', the lowest values were obtained (16.31 and 15.52 mg/g FW;

Table 2). Differently from fructose, the highest values of sucrose were measured in two ancient varieties: 'Casolana' with 61.34 mg/g FW and 'Ficareto' with 53.5 mg/g FW (Table 2).

Table 2. The table shows the values (±SD) of free sugars and pectin (expressed as mg/g FW) in the ancient and commercial apples studied. Different letters indicate significant differences among values ($p < 0.05$).

Variety Name	Glucose	Fructose	Sucrose	Xylitol	Pectins
Solaio	30.72 ± 0.67[l]	48.45 ± 0.26[f]	13.13 ± 0.07[b]	13.70 ± 0.04[k]	19.72 ± 0.06[l]
Campo Pianacce	13.58 ± 0.15[gh]	43.30 ± 0.08[e]	16.96 ± 0.06[c]	3.72 ± 0.05[f]	13.41 ± 0.21[i]
Viale Casetta	31.69 ± 1.57[l]	51.98 ± 0.49[g]	33.36 ± 0.12[i]	13.68 ± 0.04[k]	4.26 ± 0.11[ab]
Gialla Pianacce	17.86 ± 0.28[ij]	15.52 ± 0.32[a]	20.38 ± 0.22[e]	2.61 ± 0.05[d]	4.34 ± 0.07[b]
Tre Colli	17.29 ± 0.34[i]	63.58 ± 0.51[j]	42.35 ± 0.31[l]	6.41 ± 0.32[j]	11.71 ± 0.25[h]
Ancaiano	20.54 ± 0.60[k]	43.59 ± 0.32[e]	20.19 ± 0.08[e]	5.47 ± 0.14[i]	11.86 ± 0.07[h]
Piatta Cantine	19.34 ± 0.34[jk]	49.66 ± 0.20[f]	11.96 ± 0.12[a]	1.01 ± 0.06[a]	9.11 ± 0.12[f]
Filare Delle Pianacce	12.94 ± 0.08[fg]	43.40 ± 0.32[e]	25.03 ± 0.13[f]	4.06 ± 0.09[fg]	13.51 ± 0.05[i]
Tocchi	13.49 ± 0.44[g]	51.68 ± 2.15[g]	41.34 ± 0.20[k]	4.91 ± 0.05[hi]	16.04 ± 0.09[j]
Rossa Casetta	11.93 ± 0.06[f]	51.98 ± 0.62[g]	33.31 ± 0.17[i]	13.79 ± 0.19[k]	4.05 ± 0.16[a]
Ficareto	9.82 ± 0.15[e]	59.14 ± 0.30[i]	53.57 ± 0.31[m]	4.77 ± 0.11[h]	17.06 ± 0.14[k]
Rugginosa Delle Pianacce	14.75 ± 0.16[h]	48.44 ± 0.29[f]	20.21 ± 0.04[e]	4.01 ± 0.07[fg]	12.15 ± 0.16[h]
Red Delicious	30.11 ± 0.42[l]	64.46 ± 0.48[j]	11.81 ± 0.03[a]	1.29 ± 0.09[b]	5.14 ± 0.12[c]
Vecchio Pollaio	8.54 ± 0.08[d]	16.31 ± 0.18[b]	26.55 ± 0.27[h]	3.14 ± 0.07[e]	15.31 ± 0.18[j]
Strada Pianacce	4.50 ± 0.26[b]	55.29 ± 0.29[h]	25.97 ± 0.07[g]	2.10 ± 0.07[c]	10.98 ± 0.16[g]
Golden Delicious	20.44 ± 0.79[k]	69.14 ± 0.36[k]	17.34 ± 0.17[d]	2.31 ± 0.14[c]	6.46 ± 0.26[d]
Podere Pianacce	5.37 ± 0.13[c]	49.68 ± 0.17[f]	32.75 ± 0.10[i]	2.27 ± 0.04[c]	17.38 ± 0.23[k]
Sotto Muro Casetta	9.31 ± 0.26[e]	35.44 ± 0.21[d]	37.63 ± 0.18[j]	4.28 ± 0.31[g]	7.06 ± 0.07[e]
Casolana	1.96 ± 0.09[a]	31.71 ± 0.23[c]	61.34 ± 0.18[p]	3.99 ± 0.03[fg]	9.32 ± 0.18[f]

Concerning glucose, the highest values were measured in 'Viale Casetta' (31.69 mg/g FW), 'Solaio' (30.72 mg/g FW) and 'Red Delicious' (30.11 mg/g FW) and the lowest was observed in 'Casolana' (1.96 mg/g FW). Commercial varieties resulted in much higher concentrations, as compared to most ancient fruits, as reported in Table 2.

The HPLC analysis also showed a high concentration of xylitol in all the varieties studied (Table 2). 'Rossa Casetta', 'Solaio' and 'Viale Casetta' showed the highest xylitol contents (13.79, 13.70, and 13.68 mg/g FW, respectively) and 14 out of 17 ancient varieties displayed higher concentrations, as compared to the commercial counterparts ('Golden Delicious' 2.31 mg/g FW and 'Red Delicious' 1.29 mg/g FW; Table 2).

Finally, the chromatographic method used revealed the presence of fibers in overall high concentration. In particular, pectins were detected. Fourteen out of 17 apple varieties showed higher values than commercial ones, particularly 'Solaio', 'Podere Pianacce' and 'Ficareto' varieties (19.72, 17.38, and 17.06 mg/g FW, respectively; Table 2). 'Rossa Casetta', 'Viale Casetta' and 'Gialla Pianacce' reported instead the lowest values (4.05, 4.26, and 4.34 mg/g FW, respectively; Table 2). The commercial apples 'Red Delicious' and 'Golden Delicious' displayed relatively low values of 5.14 and 6.46 mg/g FW, respectively (Table 2).

4. Discussion

Diet plays an important role in human health: the consumption of specific types of food (fruits and vegetables) has been linked to the prevention of chronic diseases [20]. Functional foods, i.e., those foods that have the added value of exerting a positive effect on health, are rich in nutraceuticals (mainly phytochemicals produced by the plant secondary metabolism, such as the phenylpropanoid pathway), which contribute towards mitigating problems related with, e.g., the gastrointestinal tract [21] and prevent chronic diseases, such as type 2 diabetes [22]. The consumption of functional foods improves the antioxidant and anti-inflammatory responses of the organism and helps fight cardiovascular diseases and cancer [21].

We here report on the nutraceutical content of 17 ancient apples from the province of Siena in Tuscany and compare the values obtained with those measured in two commercial varieties. Twelve of the 17 ancient fruits displayed antioxidant capacity values that were higher than the commercial apples (Table 1) and, interestingly, a high Pearson coefficient was calculated when correlating the antioxidant capacity with the total polyphenol contents. Polyphenols were found in higher quantities in all the ancient apples here studied (Table 1).

The results presented show that the ancient apples from Siena have a remarkably interesting antioxidant potential, which motivates their use as functional foods. As we recently discussed, the valorization of ancient regional varieties grown by exploiting the local soil (and associated microbiota) can greatly contribute to boosting the regional economy and favors the manufacture of fully traceable products with a minimal C footprint [9]. The recovery of such historical fruit tree species diversifies, at a local level, the consumers' choice of fruits and also contributes to the restoration of regional habitats.

Our results are even more interesting if one considers the data about the sugars and fibers. While the commercial fruits displayed among the highest glucose levels, some ancient varieties from Siena, such as 'Strada Pianacce' and 'Casolana', had extremely low values (Table 2).

Carbohydrates are the main source of energy for the human body. They are, therefore, an essential component of the diet, but a high intake can lead to various problems and diseases, such as hyperglycemia and diabetes.

The apple fruit can provide sugars for about 12–18% of its weight [23]. Therefore, determining the sugar classes contained is relevant for nutraceutics. The dominant sugar is fructose and its concentrations were higher in the commercial fruits due to the culture conditions used (e.g., specific fertilization regimes) to meet market demands of yield.

The overall lower presence of glucose in the ancient fruits indicates a potential value of the Tuscan apples in hypoglycemic diets. The higher presence of xylitol in the ancient fruits confirms this, since this sugar has a much lower glycemic index than sucrose and is metabolized independently of insulin [24].

A further element in favor of the use of ancient Tuscan apples as functional foods is the content of fibers (pectins): a diet rich in fibers has been associated with a reduced risk of colorectal cancer [25]. Pectins are interesting for their gelling and emollient properties and they are useful in the regulation of intestinal functions, by preventing the reabsorption of bile acids, thus favoring their elimination [26].

The regional cultivation of ancient plants represents an innovative agricultural strategy relying on the exploitation of local natural resources and has a beneficial agronomical impact from an ecological standpoint. In order to cope with the progressive land loss observed in the last years [27] due to the inexorable industrialization, plant varieties thriving in environments with minimal human input (i.e., fertilization, irrigation) are important resources [9,11].

In terms of sustainable agricultural development, wild lands with minimal human intervention preserve the local microbiota which developed in equilibrium with the local microhabitat and soil properties. Ancient plants have established a perfect synergistic relationship with the local microbiota and soil and such a condition is likely contributing to the higher resilience to exogenous stresses observed in these varieties.

Drought is a major environmental stress compromising agricultural production worldwide and affecting the yield of crops. It is known that non-commercial plant varieties, such as landraces, show enhanced drought tolerance (recently reviewed in [11]), thereby attracting much interest in terms of optimized agricultural programs relying on less water input.

Last but not least, the high content of antioxidants of ancient plant varieties [9,12] can determine a higher resistance to biotic stresses, thanks to the enhanced production of phenolics or terpenoids, which have a protective effect against pests. This can favor a decrease in the use of pesticides. Therefore, an agricultural management based on the cultivation of locally adapted ancient varieties contributes not only to the preservation of the local biodiversity, but has also a beneficial ecological impact, since less water and pesticides may be used.

5. Conclusions

Our study confirms and strengthens the previously reported data on the nutraceutical value of ancient Tuscan plant varieties. We provide here a case study on apples and show that the ancient fruits recovered across the province of Siena represent a rich source of phenolics with antioxidant activity, fibers and sugars with low glycemic index, notably xylitol. Their use in food products, either fresh or processed, is interesting and such ancient apple fruits are an alternative (and in the case of some varieties here analyzed) superior source of nutraceuticals and fibers. Future studies should aim at characterizing, at a molecular level, the genes/enzymes acting in secondary metabolic pathways in such ancient apple varieties.

Author Contributions: R.B. and G.G. wrote the manuscript, analyzed the data, performed the statistical analyses, and prepared the tables. M.R. and G.C. designed the experiments. R.B. and M.G. performed the analyses. J.-F.H, C.C., M.N., and G.C. revised the text.

Funding: This research received no external funding.

Acknowledgments: The authors are grateful to the Tuscany Region and the National Research Council (CNR-Italy) for support. RB is grateful to the Tuscany Region for financial support through the fellowship "Pegaso".

Conflicts of Interest: The authors declare no conflict of interest.

References

1. Chi, C.; Giri, S.S.; Jun, J.W.; Kim, H.J.; Yun, S.; Kim, S.G.; Park, S.C. Immunomodulatory Effects of a Bioactive Compound Isolated from *Dryopteris crassirhizoma* on the Grass Carp *Ctenopharyngodon idella*. *J. Immunol. Res.* **2016**, *2016*. [CrossRef] [PubMed]
2. Andre, C.M.; Greenwood, J.M.; Walker, E.G.; Rassam, M.; Sullivan, M.; Evers, D.; Perry, N.B.; Laing, W.A. Anti-Inflammatory Procyanidins and Triterpenes in 109 Apple Varieties. *J. Agric. Food Chem.* **2012**, *60*, 10546–10554. [CrossRef] [PubMed]
3. Francini, A.; Sebastiani, L. Phenolic Compounds in Apple (*Malus* x *domestica* Borkh.): Compounds Characterization and Stability during Postharvest and after Processing. *Antioxidants* **2013**, *2*, 181–193. [CrossRef] [PubMed]
4. Boyer, J.; Liu, R.H. Apple phytochemicals and their health benefits. *Nutr. J.* **2004**, *3*, 5. [CrossRef] [PubMed]
5. Vanzani, P.; Rossetto, M.; Rigo, A.; Vrhovsek, U.; Mattivi, F.; D'Amato, E.; Scarpa, M. Major Phytochemicals in Apple Cultivars: Contribution to Peroxyl Radical Trapping Efficiency. *J. Agric. Food Chem. (ACS Publications)* **2005**, *53*, 3377–3382. [CrossRef] [PubMed]
6. Gerhauser, C. Cancer Chemopreventive Potential of Apples, Apple Juice, and Apple Components. *Planta Med.* **2008**, *74*, 1608–1624. [CrossRef] [PubMed]
7. Andre, C.M.; Larsen, L.; Burgess, E.J.; Jensen, D.J.; Cooney, J.M.; Evers, D.; Zhang, J.; Perry, N.B.; Laing, W.A. Unusual immuno-modulatory triterpene-caffeates in the skins of russeted varieties of apples and pears. *J. Agric. Food Chem.* **2013**, *61*, 2773–2779. [CrossRef]
8. Sagar, N.A.; Pareek, S.; Sharma, S.; Yahia, E.M.; Lobo, M.G. Fruit and Vegetable Waste: Bioactive Compounds, Their Extraction, and Possible Utilization-Sagar-2018. *Compr. Rev. Food Sci. Food Saf.* **2018**, *17*, 512–531. [CrossRef]
9. Berni, R.; Romi, M.; Cantini, C.; Hausman, J.-F.; Guerriero, G.; Cai, G. Functional molecules in locally-adapted crops: The case study of tomatoes, onions and sweet cherry fruits from Tuscany in Italy. *Front. Plant Sci.* **2018**, *9*, 1983. [CrossRef]
10. Hyson, D.A. A Comprehensive Review of Apples and Apple Components and Their Relationship to Human Health12. *Adv. Nutr.* **2011**, *2*, 408–420. [CrossRef]
11. Berni, R.; Cantini, C.; Romi, M.; Hausman, J.-F.; Guerriero, G.; Cai, G. Agrobiotechnology Goes Wild: Ancient Local Varieties as Sources of Bioactives. *Int. J. Mol. Sci.* **2018**, *19*, 2248. [CrossRef] [PubMed]
12. Berni, R.; Romi, M.; Parrotta, L.; Cai, G.; Cantini, C. Ancient Tomato (*Solanum lycopersicum* L.) Varieties of Tuscany Have High Contents of Bioactive Compounds. *Horticulturae* **2018**, *4*, 51. [CrossRef]

13. Henríquez, C.; Almonacid, S.; Chiffelle, I.; Valenzuela, T.; Araya, M.; Cabezas, L.; Simpson, R.; Speisky, H. Determination of antioxidant capacity, total phenolic content and mineral composition of different fruit tissue of five apple cultivars grown in Chile. *Chil. J. Agric. Res.* **2010**, *70*, 523–536. [CrossRef]

14. Benzie, I.F.; Strain, J.J. The ferric reducing ability of plasma (FRAP) as a measure of "antioxidant power": The FRAP assay. *Anal. Biochem.* **1996**, *239*, 70–76. [CrossRef] [PubMed]

15. Alothman, M.; Bhat, R.; Karim, A.A. Antioxidant capacity and phenolic content of selected tropical fruits from Malaysia, extracted with different solvents. *Food Chem.* **2009**, *115*, 785–788. [CrossRef]

16. Fu, L.; Xu, B.-T.; Xu, X.-R.; Qin, X.-S.; Gan, R.-Y.; Li, H.-B. Antioxidant capacities and total phenolic contents of 56 wild fruits from South China. *Molecules* **2010**, *15*, 8602–8617. [CrossRef] [PubMed]

17. Thaipong, K.; Boonprakob, U.; Crosby, K.; Cisneros-Zevallos, L.; Hawkins Byrne, D. Comparison of ABTS, DPPH, FRAP, and ORAC assays for estimating antioxidant activity from guava fruit extracts. *J. Food Compos. Anal.* **2006**, *19*, 669–675. [CrossRef]

18. Singleton, V.L.; Rossi, J.A. Colorimetry of total phenolics with phosphomolybdic-phosphotungstic acid reagents. *Am. J. Enol. Vitic.* **1965**, *16*, 144–158.

19. Ouchemoukh, S.; Schweitzer, P.; Bachir Bey, M.; Djoudad-Kadji, H.; Louaileche, H. HPLC sugar profiles of Algerian honeys. *Food Chem.* **2010**, *121*, 561–568. [CrossRef]

20. Boeing, H.; Bechthold, A.; Bub, A.; Ellinger, S.; Haller, D.; Kroke, A.; Leschik-Bonnet, E.; Müller, M.J.; Oberritter, H.; Schulze, M.; et al. Critical review: Vegetables and fruit in the prevention of chronic diseases. *Eur. J. Nutr.* **2012**, *51*, 637–663. [CrossRef]

21. Cencic, A.; Chingwaru, W. The role of functional foods, nutraceuticals, and food supplements in intestinal health. *Nutrients* **2010**, *2*, 611–625. [CrossRef] [PubMed]

22. Alkhatib, A.; Tsang, C.; Tiss, A.; Bahorun, T.; Arefanian, H.; Barake, R.; Khadir, A.; Tuomilehto, J. Functional Foods and Lifestyle Approaches for Diabetes Prevention and Management. *Nutrients* **2017**, *9*, 1310. [CrossRef] [PubMed]

23. Lu, R.; Guyer, D.E.; Beaudry, R.M. Determination of firmness and sugar content of apples using near-infrared diffuse reflectance1. *J. Texture Stud.* **2000**, *31*, 615–630. [CrossRef]

24. Brunzell, J.D. Use of fructose, xylitol, or sorbitol as a sweetener in diabetes mellitus. *Diabetes Care* **1978**, *1*, 223–230. [CrossRef] [PubMed]

25. Kunzmann, A.T.; Coleman, H.G.; Huang, W.-Y.; Kitahara, C.M.; Cantwell, M.M.; Berndt, S.I. Dietary fiber intake and risk of colorectal cancer and incident and recurrent adenoma in the Prostate, Lung, Colorectal, and Ovarian Cancer Screening Trial12. *Am. J. Clin. Nutr.* **2015**, *102*, 881–890. [CrossRef] [PubMed]

26. Garcia-Diez, F.; Garcia-Mediavilla, V.; Bayon, J.E.; Gonzalez-Gallego, J. Pectin Feeding Influences Fecal Bile Acid Excretion, Hepatic Bile Acid and Cholesterol Synthesis and Serum Cholesterol in Rats. *J. Nutr.* **1996**, *126*, 1766–1771.

27. Tscharntke, T.; Klein, A.M.; Kruess, A.; Steffan-Dewenter, I.; Thies, C. Landscape perspectives on agricultural intensification and biodiversity–ecosystem service management. *Ecol. Lett.* **2005**, *8*, 857–874. [CrossRef]

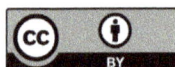

medicines

MDPI

Article

Antioxidant, Cytotoxic, and Antimicrobial Activities of *Glycyrrhiza glabra* L., *Paeonia lactiflora* Pall., and *Eriobotrya japonica* (Thunb.) Lindl. Extracts

Jun-Xian Zhou, Markus Santhosh Braun, Pille Wetterauer, Bernhard Wetterauer and Michael Wink *

Institute of Pharmacy and Molecular Biotechnology, Heidelberg University, Im Neuenheimer Feld 364, 69120 Heidelberg, Germany; junxian.zhou@stud.uni-heidelberg.de (J.-X.Z.); m.braun@uni-heidelberg.de (M.S.B.); p.wetterauer@uni-heidelberg.de (P.W.); bernhard.wetterauer@urz.uni-heidelberg.de (B.W.)
* Correspondence: wink@uni-heidelberg.de; Tel.: +49-(0)6221-544884

Received: 27 February 2019; Accepted: 27 March 2019; Published: 30 March 2019

Abstract: Background: The phytochemical composition, antioxidant, cytotoxic, and antimicrobial activities of a methanol extract from *Glycyrrhiza glabra* L. (Ge), a 50% ethanol (in water) extract from *Paeonia lactiflora* Pall. (Pe), and a 96% ethanol extract from *Eriobotrya japonica* (Thunb.) Lindl. (Ue) were investigated. **Methods:** The phytochemical profiles of the extracts were analyzed by LC-MS/MS. Antioxidant activity was evaluated by scavenging 2,2-diphenyl-1-picrylhydrazyl (DPPH) and 2,2′-azino-bis (3-ethylbenzothiazoline-6-sulphonic acid) (ABTS) radicals and reducing ferric complexes, and the total phenolic content was tested with the Folin–Ciocalteu method. Cytotoxicity was determined with a 3-(4,5-dimethylthiazol-2-yl)-2,5-diphenyltetrazolium bromide (MTT) assay in murine macrophage RAW 264.7 cells. Antimicrobial activity of the three plant extracts was investigated against six bacterial strains with the broth microdilution method. **Results:** Only Pe showed high antioxidant activities compared to the positive controls ascorbic acid and (−)-epigallocatechin gallate (EGCG) in DPPH assay; and generally the antioxidant activity order was ascorbic acid or EGCG > Pe > Ue > Ge. The three plant extracts did not show strong cytotoxicity against RAW 264.7 cells after 24 h treatment with IC_{50} values above 60.53 ± 4.03 μg/mL. Ue was not toxic against the six tested bacterial strains, with minimal inhibitory concentration (MIC) values above 5 mg/mL. Ge showed medium antibacterial activity against *Acinetobacter bohemicus*, *Kocuria kristinae*, *Micrococcus luteus*, *Staphylococcus auricularis*, and *Bacillus megaterium* with MICs between 0.31 and 1.25 mg/mL. Pe inhibited the growth of *Acinetobacter bohemicus*, *Micrococcus luteus*, and *Bacillus megaterium* at a MIC of 0.08 mg/mL. **Conclusions:** The three extracts were low-cytotoxic, but Pe exhibited effective DPPH radical scavenging ability and good antibacterial activity; Ue did not show antioxidant or antibacterial activity; Ge had no antioxidant potential, but medium antibacterial ability against five bacteria strains. Pe and Ge could be further studied for their potential to be developed as antioxidant or antibacterial candidates.

Keywords: TCM; phytochemistry; LC-MS/MS; antioxidant activity; ABTS; DPPH; FRAP; ascorbic acid; EGCG; total phenolics; antimicrobial activity

1. Introduction

Traditional Chinese medicine (TCM) has a history of thousands of years in China. The first professional TCM book was Shen Nong's Chinese Materia Medica written in the Eastern Han Dynasty (AD 25–220), but before that time, people already had records of plants used as medicines. With time and the development of their practical uses, the types of traditional medicines and books about them increased gradually. TCM and the secondary metabolites of TCM plants, such as the anti-malarial drug artemisinin, have been used to treat various diseases and become more and more popular in the world, based on modern pharmacological studies [1]. In vitro antioxidant activities of extracts of TCM plants have been widely studied and the strong antioxidant activity of many TCM plants has been found to be due to high phenolic contents (flavonoids, phenolic acids, lignans, tannins, coumarins, etc.) [2,3].

Aerobic metabolism is important for most cells to produce energy. This process generates free oxygen radicals or reactive oxygen species (ROS). Excessive generation of ROS may lead to oxidative chain reactions and thus an imbalance of oxidants and antioxidants in the body, and can cause molecular damage and several health conditions [4–6]. For example, ROS can oxidize the purine base guanosine, leading to 8-oxoguanosine; if not repaired, this transformation can lead to mutations and proteins with impaired functions. Antioxidants (present in cells or acquired via food or medicinal plants) can delay or inhibit the oxidative reactions or scavenge initiating radicals, thus limiting the oxidative damage [7,8]. The role of antioxidants can be determined by their interaction with oxidative free radicals [9]. A diversity of antioxidants is produced in plants, and phenolics constitute a major antioxidant group in many medicinal and food plants [10,11].

Glycyrrhiza glabra is one of the most frequently used traditional medicine in China and Europe since long ago [12,13]; *Paeonia lactiflora* is often used together with *G. glabra* to enhance the therapeutic effect, for example, in the prescription "Shaoyaogancaotang" [14,15]; one of the main secondary metabolite in *Eriobotrya japonica*, the triterpene ursolic acid, has a similar structure as 18β glycyrrhetinic acid, which is a major secondary metabolite in *G. glabra*. So, the three plant extracts were studied in order to compare their pharmacological effects. The species have been introduced before in Reference [16].

A methanol extract of *Glycyrrhiza glabra* (Ge), a 50% ethanol (in water) extract of *Paeonia lactiflora* (Pe), and a 96% ethanol extract of *Eriobotrya japonica* (Ue) were studied for their antioxidant activity as well as cytotoxicity and antimicrobial activity. The solvents for the extraction were optimized according to the literature [17–19]. Few studies on the antioxidant activity of these species had been conducted, or only one kind of antioxidant assay was applied; and it would also be interesting to study the antibacterial capacity of the species on different bacteria to broaden their future application. Our study may help to evaluate the therapeutic potential of the species.

The phytochemical composition of the extracts was studied by LC-MS/MS and largely confirmed from other laboratories (shown in Tables S1–S4 in the Supplementary Materials). We employed three different assays (DPPH, ABTS, and Ferric Reduction Antioxidant Potential (FRAP) assay) to examine the potential antioxidant activity of the three plant extracts, the Folin–Ciocalteu method to determine the total phenolic contents, and a MTT assay to determine a possible cytotoxicity against murine macrophage RAW 264.7 cells. Antimicrobial activity of the three plant extracts against gram-negative (*E. coli* XL1-Blue MRF′, *Acinetobacter bohemicus*) and gram-positive (*Kocuria kristinae*, *Micrococcus luteus*, *Staphylococcus auricularis*, and *Bacillus megaterium*) bacteria was analyzed using standard broth microdilution assays.

2. Materials and Methods

2.1. Plant Materials and Plant Extraction

The origins of the three TCM plants, and the extraction processes of Ge, Pe, and Ue have previously been described [16].

2.2. Reagents and Chemicals

Ascorbic acid and ferric chloride were purchased from AppliChem (Darmstadt, Germany), and gallic acid from Ferak Berlin (Berlin, Germany). Formic acid and Folin–Ciocalteu were obtained from Merck (Darmstadt, Germany), ampicillin from Panreac AppliChem (Darmstadt, Germany), and acetonitrile, 2,2-diphenyl-1-picrylhydrazyl (DPPH), 2,4,6-tris(2-pyridyl)-s-triazine

(TPTZ), 2,2'-azino-bis (3-ethylbenzothiazoline-6-sulphonic acid) (ABTS), Trolox, (−)-epigallocatechin gallate (EGCG), doxorubicin, ciprofloxacin, and 3-(4,5-dimethylthiazol-2-yl)-2,5-diphenyltetrazolium bromide (MTT) from Sigma-Aldrich (Darmstadt, Germany). The reference substances paeoniflorin and ursolic acid were obtained from Baoji Herbest Bio-Tech (Baoji, China).

2.3. Cell Lines and Bacterial Strains

Murine macrophage cell line RAW 264.7 was a gift from PD Dr. Katharina Kubatzky (Medical Microbiology and Hygiene, Heidelberg University, Heidelberg, Germany). *Acinetobacter bohemicus* DSM 102855, *Kocuria kristinae* DSM 20032 (formerly known as *Micrococcus kristinae*), *Micrococcus luteus* DSM 20030 (synonym *Micrococcus lysodeikticus*), *Staphylococcus auricularis* DSM 20609, and *Bacillus megaterium* DSM 32 were purchased from the German Collection of Microorganisms and Cell Cultures (DSMZ, Braunschweig, Germany). *E. coli* XL1-Blue MRF' is a cloning strain from Stratagene (Heidelberg, Germany).

2.4. LC-MS/MS Analysis

For Ge, the LC-MS/MS analysis was performed on a Thermo Finnigan LCQ Advantage ion trap mass spectrometer (Thermo Finnigan, San Jose, CA, USA) with an ESI source, coupled to a Thermo Scientific Accela HPLC system (MS pump plus, autosampler, and PDA detector plus) (Thermo, San Jose, CA, USA) with an EC 150/2 Nucleodur 100-3 C18ec column (Macherey-Nagel, Düren, Germany). A gradient of water and acetonitrile (ACN) with 0.1% formic acid each for ESI+ and ESI-mode was applied from 20% to 80% ACN in 20 min at 20 °C. The flow rate was 0.3 mL/min. The injection volume was about 25 μL. The MS was operated with a capillary voltage of 10 V (ESI+) or −10 V (ESI-), source temperature of 240 °C, and high purity nitrogen as a sheath and auxiliary gas at a flow rate of 70 and 10 (arbitrary units), respectively.

For Pe and Ue, the LC-MS/MS analysis was performed on a Finnigan LCQ-Duo ion trap mass spectrometer with an ESI source (ThermoQuest, San Jose, CA, USA), coupled to a Thermo Scientific Accela HPLC system (MS pump plus, autosampler, and PDA detector plus) (Thermo, San Jose, CA, USA) with an EC 150/3 Nucleodur 100-3 C18ec column (Macherey-Nagel, Düren, Germany). A gradient of water and ACN with 0.1% formic acid each was applied for Pe from 5% to 40% ACN in 100 min at 30 °C and for Ue from 5% to 80% ACN in 60 min and to 95% in another 30 min at 30 °C. The flow rate was 0.5 mL/min. The injection volume was about 20 μL. The MS was operated with a capillary voltage of 10 V (ESI+) or -10 V (ESI-), source temperature of 240 °C, and high purity nitrogen as a sheath and auxiliary gas at a flow rate of 80 and 40 (arbitrary units), respectively.

In all measurements, the ions were detected in a mass range of 50–2000 m/z. A collision energy of 35% was used in MS/MS for fragmentation. Data acquisitions and analyses were executed by XcaliburTM 2.0.7 software (Thermo Scientific, Karlsruhe, Germany). For compound determination in Ge, the positive and negative modes were used, and for Pe and Ue only the negative mode.

2.5. DPPH Radical Scavenging Assay

The stable free radical DPPH•, shows a deep violet color in solutions and has a strong absorption at 517 nm. When an odd electron is paired off by an antioxidant, the deep violet color disappears. The decrease in absorption is a measure for antioxidant activity [20]. The procedure was modified from Brand-Williams et al. [21]. In a 96-well plate, 100 μL of 0.2 mM DPPH• in methanol was added to 100 μL serial-diluted plant extracts and allowed to react for 30 min in darkness at ambient temperature. Ascorbic acid and EGCG were used as positive controls. The absorption was read spectrophotometrically at 517 nm with a Tecan Nano Quant infinite M200 PRO Plate Reader (Tecan, Männedorf, Switzerland). Results are expressed as EC_{50} (the concentration where 50% of the DPPH radical is inhibited). The calculation equation is:

$$\% \text{ inhibition} = (AB - AE)/AB \times 100$$

where AB and AE are the absorptions in the absence and presence, respectively, of antioxidant substances (plant extracts).

2.6. Assay of Trolox-Equivalent Antioxidant Capacity (TEAC)/ABTS assay

The ABTS radical (ABTS+•) shows a blue-green color and displays absorption at 734 nm. When a pre-formed free radical ABTS+• reacts with electrons donated by an antioxidant, the color and absorption are decreased and compared with that of the standard antioxidant compound Trolox, a water-soluble vitamin E analog [22]. The procedure is according to Pietta et al. [23]. In total, 7 mM ABTS was mixed with 2.45 mM potassium persulfate in de-ionized water and the mixture was put in darkness at ambient temperature for 12–16 h to make the ABTS+• stock solution. The ABTS+• stock solution was diluted with water to obtain the working solution, which should have an absorption of 0.7 ($\pm$ 0.02) at 734 nm. In 96-well plates, 250 µL of ABTS+• working solution was added to 50 µL serial-diluted plant extracts or Trolox. Trolox (0–40 µM) in 100% ethanol was used to make a standard curve. The plates were incubated at 37 °C in darkness for 6 min and the absorption was read at 734 nm with Tecan Nano Quant infinite M200 PRO Plate Reader. Ascorbic acid and EGCG were used as positive controls. Results were compared with Trolox and expressed as TEAC (Trolox equivalents in mM Trolox/mM test substance).

2.7. Assay of the Ferric Reduction Antioxidant Potential (FRAP)

In the FRAP assay, the trivalent ferric ion complex (Fe^{3+} - TPTZ) is reduced by reducing agents or antioxidants under acidic conditions, to a complex of divalent ferrous ion (Fe^{2+} - TPTZ), which shows a blue color and has a peak of absorption at 593 nm [24]. The procedure was performed according to Benzie et al. [25]. Briefly, the FRAP reagent was prepared by mixing 10 mM of TPTZ in 40 mM of hydrogen chloride, 300 mM of acetate buffer (pH 3.6), and 20 mM of ferric chloride in water at a ratio of 1:10:1. In 96-well plates, 175 µL FRAP reagent solution was added to 25 µL serial-diluted substances or ferrous sulfate standards in water. The plates were incubated at 37 °C in darkness for 7 min and the absorption was measured at 593 nm with Tecan Nano Quant infinite M200 PRO Plate Reader. The results are expressed by comparison with the standard ferrous ion to obtain the ferrous equivalent, FE (mmol Fe^{2+}/g test substance).

2.8. Total Phenolic Content Tested by the Folin–Ciocalteu Method

The colorimetric Folin–Ciocalteu method was modified from Swain et al. [26]. The final product from the reaction of the Folin–Ciocalteu method shows a blue color and can be recorded at 750 nm [27]. In total, 100 µL of Folin–Ciocalteu reagent was added to 20 µL of the plant extracts and the standard gallic acid in methanol in a 96-well plate. After 5 min, 80 µL of 7.5% sodium carbonate was added to each well. The plate was allowed to stand in darkness at ambient temperature for 2 h before the absorption was read at 750 nm with Tecan Nano Quant infinite M200 PRO Plate Reader. The standard curve was made with gallic acid (final concentration 0–40 µg/mL). The total phenolic content was compared with gallic acid to obtain the GAE (gallic acid equivalents in mg gallic acid/g test substance).

2.9. Cell Culture and Cytotoxicity Assay

RAW 264.7 cells were cultured in DMEM supplemented with 10% FBS, 100 U/mL penicillin-streptomycin and 2 mM L-glutamine, and incubated at 37 °C with 5% CO_2. The MTT assay was modified from Mosmann [28]. A density of 6×10^4 RAW 264.7 cells was seeded in a 96-well plate and incubated at 37 °C for 24 h. Different concentrations of a substance dissolved in media were added to the cells for an 24 h incubation. The media were removed, and media containing 0.5% MTT were added into every well and further incubated for 2–4 h at 37 °C. Finally, after centrifuging the plate at 400 rpm for 10 min, the absorption was read at 570 nm with the Tecan Nano Quant infinite M200 PRO Plate Reader. The chemotherapeutic agent doxorubicin was used as a positive control.

2.10. Determination of Minimum Inhibitory Concentrations (MIC) and Minimum Bactericidal Concentrations (MBC) by Broth Microdilutions

Broth microdilution was carried out in accordance with CLSI [29]. The plant extract was dissolved in DMSO and then serial diluted with MHB from 10 mg/mL to 0.0048 mg/mL in triplicate in a 96-well plate. The final concentration of DMSO in the test did not exceed 5%. The bacterial suspensions were added to the plate to yield 5×10^5 cfu/mL. The plates were incubated at 37 °C for 20 h. The lowest concentration of plant extract in the well with no visible turbidity was considered the MIC. To determine the minimum bactericidal concentration, 3 µL of suspensions from the clear wells were spread out on an LB agar plate and incubated at 37 °C until sufficient growth was obtained. The lowest concentration that reduced the number of viable cells of the initial inoculum to <0.1% was regarded as the MBC. MHB media, 5% DMSO, ampicillin, ciprofloxacin, and bacterial suspensions were used as controls, respectively.

2.11. Statistical Analysis

Data analysis was carried out with GraphPad Prism 6 (Graphpad Software, San Diego, CA, USA), and SigmaPlot®11.0 (Systat Software, San Jose, CA, USA). Results were expressed as the mean ± SD. Statistical significance was evaluated using t-test and significance was set at $p < 0.05$. All experiments were performed independently at least three times.

3. Results

3.1. LC-MS/MS Analysis of Glycyrrhiza glabra Extract

As we can see from Figure 1 and Table 1, several secondary metabolites have been identified by LC-MS/MS analysis from *Glycyrrhiza glabra*, among which glycyrrhizic acid and (iso)liquiritin apioside isomers are the most abundant compounds.

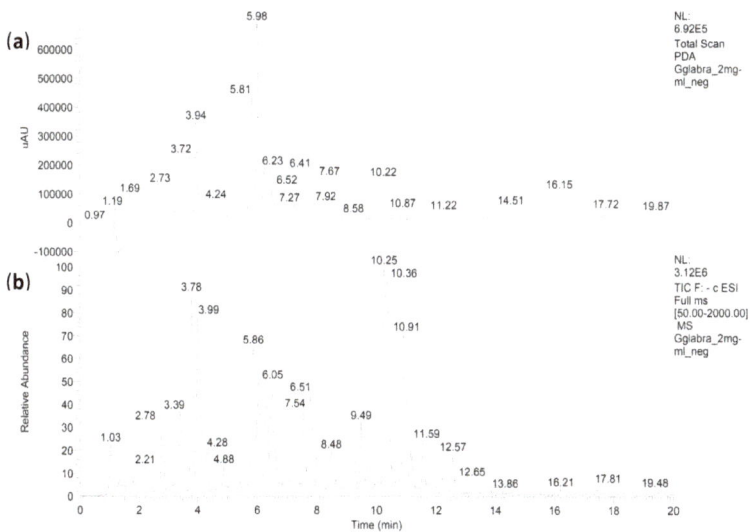

Figure 1. The photodiode array chromatogram (PDA) (**a**) and the total ion current (TIC) (**b**) of the *G. glabra* extract. The compounds listed in Table 1 correspond to the retention times of the TIC.

Table 1. Retention times (RT), MS data, and tentatively identified compounds in the *G. glabra* extract.

RT (min)	[M-H]⁻ (m/z)	MS/MS (m/z) from [M-H]⁻	[M-H]⁺ m/z	MS/MS (m/z) from [M+H]⁺	PDA λmax [nm]	Tentative Identification	References
2.78	563.29	353.19; **443.13**; **473.12**; 503.16	565.07	409.11; **427.05**; 445.06; 457.03; 481.05; **499.03**; **511.04**; **528.96**; **546.95**	217; 274; 334	rhamnoliquiritin	[30]
3.39	577.31	353.21; 383.21; 439.18; 457.14; 473.19; 503.09; 559.26	579.18	423.07; 441.03; **525.04**; **542.95**; **560.91**	217; 272; 331	isoviolanthin	[30,31]
3.78	549.59	**255.12**; 297.14; **429.11**	551.11	388.11	217; 270; 314	liquiritin apioside isomer	[30,32]
			257.21	136.97; 146.94; 238.98		source fragment	
			419.13	**256.94**; 296.73; 364.73; 399.87		source fragment	
3.99	549.43	**255.09**; 297.17; 417.23; **429.12**	551.16	313.29; 388.11	227; 276; 311	liquiritin apioside isomer	[30,32]
			419.05	257.01		source fragment	
			257.21	136.96; 147.03; 238.97		source fragment	
4.28	417.26	n.d.	418.94	257.01	217; 276; 309	liquiritin	[30,32]
			257.17	136.96; 147.03; 238.97		source fragment	
5.86	549.43	n.d.	551.13	n.d.	219; 360	isoliquiritin apioside isomer	[30,32]
6.05	549.36	n.d.	551.14	n.d.	220; 365; 380	isoliquiritin apioside isomer	[30,32]
6.28	695.42	531.22; 549.17	431.13	269.10	218; 262; 307	licorice glycoside isomer	[30]
6.51	695.33	531.18; 549.18	697.26	668.04	220; 282; 316	licorice glycoside isomer	[30]
	725.29	255.32; 416.95; **531.21**; **549.18**	727.21	549.09; 726.16		licorice glycoside isomer	[30]
6.59	417.16	255.09	419.15	257.01	217; 297; 371	isoliquiritin	[30,32]
7.54	983.63	820.91	985.43	n.d.	216	licorice saponin A3	[30,32,33]
7.78	695.30	n.d.	697.1	516.49	218; 325; 362	licorice glycoside isomer	[30]
	725.28	n.d.	727.03	549.09; 726.16		licorice glycoside isomer	[30]
9.49	837.52	530.89; 661.45	839.24	663.02; 761.61	215	licorice saponin G2	[30,32,33]
	1675.47	837.42	-	-		dimer	
10.25	821.75	351.07; 759.49	823.31	n.d.	217; 250	glycyrrhizic acid	[30,32,33]
	1643.72	821.6	1645.69	n.d.		dimer	
10.91	821.67	n.d.	823.31	n.d.	217; 245	probably saponin	pers. com. PW
11.19	821.54	351.12	823.13	n.d.	216; 369	probably saponin	pers. com. PW
11.59	822.91	**351.06**; 646.57; 803.97	825.15	n.d.	216	licorice saponin J2	[30,32,33]
16.17	407.15	n.d.	409.07	203.03; 204.98; 247.05; 363.06; 391.00	217; 280	3-hydroxyglabrol	[30]
17.81	391.28	n.d.	393.08	204.97; 337.00	216; 282	glabrol	[30]
	782.92	n.d.				dimer	

n.d. not detectable. Fragments shown in bold are the main fragments.

3.2. LC-MS/MS Analysis of Paeonia lactiflora Extract

As shown in Figure 2 and Table 2, several compounds have been identified in the *Paeonia lactiflora* extract by LC-MS/MS analysis. Among them, paeoniflorin, galloylpaeoniflorin isomer, probably oxypaeoniflorin, and compounds related to pentagalloyl glucose and to benzoyloxypaeoniflorin are the abundant secondary metabolites.

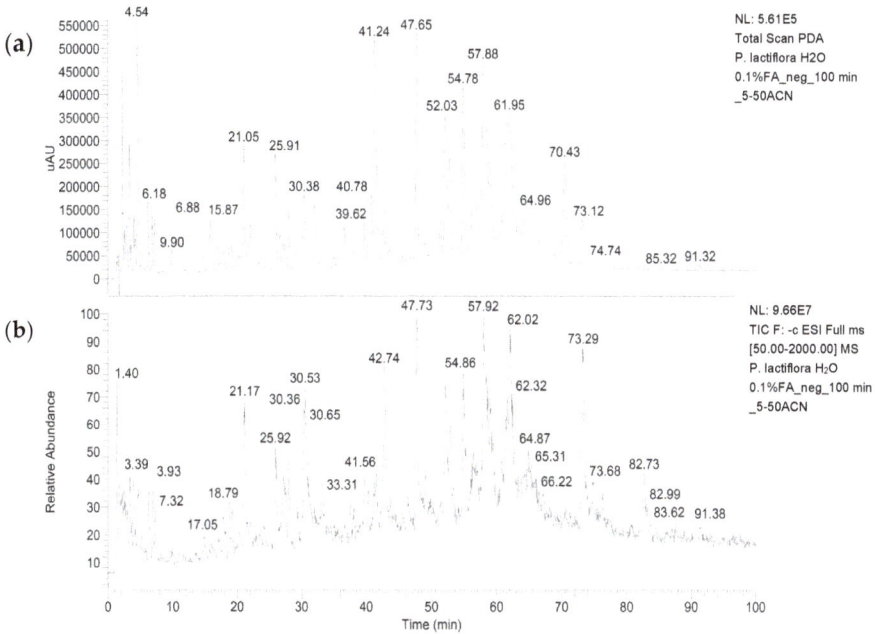

Figure 2. The photodiode array chromatogram (PDA) (**a**) and the total ion current (TIC) (**b**) of the *P. lactiflora* extract. The compounds listed in Table 2 correspond to the retention times of the TIC.

Table 2. Retention times (RT), MS data, and tentatively identified compounds in the *P. lactiflora* extract.

RT (min)	[M-H]$^-$ (m/z)	MS/MS (m/z)	PDA λmax (nm)	Tentative Identification	References
4.63	169.11	**125.22**; 126.38; 169.12	250	gallic acid	[34]
	338.62	**169.12**; 253.11; 291.91; 320.43; 339.05		gallic acid [2M-CO$_2$-H]$^-$	pers. com. BW
6.27	493.26*	169.18; 241.14; 283.26; 313.13; **331.04**; **403.13**	230; 273	galloylsucrose isomer	[35]
	986.96	Nl			
6.97	493.24*	211.22; **271.12**; 313.16; **331.04**; 384.22; 433.14; 475.58	230; 273	galloylsucrose isomer	[35]
	986.98	Nl			
7.32	493.19*	169.25; 271.45; **313.17**; 331.04; 389.98; 449.02	230; 274	galloylsucrose isomer	[35]
	986.88	Nl			

Table 2. *Cont.*

RT (min)	[M-H]⁻ (m/z)	MS/MS (m/z)	PDA λmax (nm)	Tentative Identification	References
9.68	483.19	150.90; **169.14**; 193.34; 223.18; 271.10; 295.22; **313.12**; **331.11**; 426.15	230; 273	digalloyl glucose	[36]
21.17	495.22	177.12; 299.13; **333.19**; 387.11; 447;06; **465.17**; 477.11	227; 253	probably oxypaeoniflorin	[37]
27.50	525.03	196.34; 213.42; 283.35; 317.24; 357.38; 391.56; 435.70; 475.77; **479.07**; 524.58	221; 237; 273	albiflorin	[38]
29.28	197.17	124.32; 141.56; 153.01; **169.18**; **197.16**	231; 272	probably ethyl gallate	[36]
	394.72	-			
30.14	635.1	207.31; 234.79; 313.09; 358.75; **465.13**; 483.14; 524.23; 566.84; 589.17	233; 276	trigalloyl glucose	[36]
30.53	449.04	**165.01**; 179.34; 205.10; 261.31; 282.87; 309.03; **326.95**; 398.60; 431.13	243; 274	peaoniflorin [M-CH₂O-H]⁻	Standard
	479.04	149.09; 177,10; 248.83; 267.08; 309.08; **326.98**; 355.61; **356.96**; 432.93; **449.16**; 460.71; 477.94		paeoniflorin [M-H]⁻	[36,39]
	525.01	176.88; 282.89; 327.09; 356.85; **449.01**; 476.31; **478.83**; 494.01; 506.96		paeoniflorin [M+HCOOH-H]⁻	[37,38]
32.08	463.24	**301.30**; 343.04; 394.94; 445.33; 463.25	253; 361; 280	visculdulin I 2′-glycoside	[38]
39.69	787.17**	295.17; 447.22; 465.33; 483.29; **617.32**; **635.17**	232; 277	probably tetragalloyl glucose isomer	[36]
40.29	611.22	301.30; **343.35**; 385.33; 427.35; **445.21**	232; 272		
40.93	477.22	160.70; 300.45; 315.12; 357.02; 408.88	227; 253; 360	probably related to isorhamnetin 7-O-glucoside	[36]
41.36	301.31	145.14; 185.44; 229.47; 257.47; **301.33**	249; 367		
	509.10	202.99; 254.25; 314.06; 372.80; 440.82; **463.22**; 480.12			
	787.13**	295.23; 403.40; 465.43; 530.46; 573.46; **617.18**; **635.14**; 679.31; 719.88		probably tetragalloyl glucose isomer	[36]
42.74	631.25	271.16; 313.23; 399.30; 465.30; 479.28; 491.23; 509.22; 585.17; **613.18**	234; 274	gallylpaeoniflorin isomer	[35–37,39,40]
47.77	939.11	277.04; 341.21; 385.21; 447.13; 511.35; 573.25; 599.15; **617.19**; 725.13; **769.12**; **787.03**	234; 269	probably related to pentagalloyl glucose	[36]
48.49	615.18	239.29; 263.04; **281.22**; 401.27; **431.23**; **447.22**; 459.26; **477.22**; 495.21; 567.13; **585.16**; **597.17**	232; 275	mudanpioside H	[36]
61.98	599.26	241.29; 281.46; 333.31; 385.39; 403.06; 429.22; 447.51; 459.42; **477.31**; **569.17**; 581,12	233; 274	probably related to benzoyloxypaeoniflorin	[39]
	1394.92	599.23; 937.97; 970.98; **1090.82**; 1126.36; **1165.39**; **1241.78**; 1257.75; 1309.67; **1318.90**; 1336.64			
73.24	628.99	552.66; 582.88	239; 274	probably related to benzoylpaeoniflorin	[37,39]
	1212.42	876.29; 1067.88			

* isomers; ** related; nl: neutral loss. Fragments shown in bold are the main fragments.

3.3. LC-MS/MS Analysis of Eriobotrya japonica Extract

As shown in Figure 3 and Table 3, several main compounds (ursolic acid and nerolidol-trirhamnopyranosyl-glucopyranoside or loquatifolin A or 6,7-trans-nerolidol-trirhamnopyranosyl-glucopyranoside, etc.,) have been identified in the *Eriobotrya japonica* extract by LC-MS/MS analysis.

Table 3. Retention times (RT), MS data, and tentatively identified compounds in the *E. japonica* extract.

RT (min)	[M-H]⁻ (m/z)	MS/MS (m/z)	PDA λmax (nm)	Tentative Identification	References
11.05	352.96	110.40; 143.67; **179.20**; **191.20**; 284.50; 312.26	234; 295; 325	probably chlorogenic acid	[41]
17.18 (16.48–17.26)	420.95	259.61; **301.23**; **331.19**; 343.20; 352.64; 360.36; **375.14**; 385.20; 392.55; 403.15		n.c.	
	463.17	151.00; 179.09; 190.34; 221.17; 255.30; 271.50; **300.25**; **301.16**; 325.03; 343.10; 373.35; 400.93; 418.54; 445.14	234; 347	hyperoside or isoquercetin isomers	[42,43]
	547.19	220.44; 292.64; **310.81**; 384.91; 437.90; 478.82; **500.58**; 515.88		n.c.	
	593.04	255.34; **284.19**; 327.19; 411.21; **429.21**; 447.18; 473.09; 565.32		n.c.	
	855.43	417.31; 545.16; **563.31**; 691.43; **709.34**; 735.38; 864.27		n.c.	
	901.14	299.82; 439.19; 610.71; 721.14; 763.80; 854.33; 914.59		n.c.	
28.12	821.37	511.74; **529.60**; 657.60; **675.39**; 721.14; 766.16	221; 234; 280	(trans)nerolidol-trirhamnopyranosyl-glucopyranoside or loquatifolin A	[44] (compound 1 or 4)
	867.12	596.27; 675.92; 690.31; 721.42; 740.66; 786.99; 815.64; 820.05; 833.88		n.c.	
	1688.98	551.69; 696.87; **719.35**; 821.28; **865.28**; 881.05; **1275.89**; 1396.00; 1541.66		n.c.	
29.11	807.37	529.33; 661.43; **675.31**	217; 234; 280	unknown new compound	[44] (compound 2)
	853.02	350.34; 454.48; 503.33; 649.33; 731.12; 784.53; 809.49; 839.42; 853.53		n.c.	
31.52	675.31	204.97; 307.09; **383.17**; 467.33; **529.20**; 574.81	221; 234; 283; 312	nerolidol-dirhamnopyranosyl-glucopyranoside	[44] (compound 3 or 5)
	721.21	490.37; 597.16; **675.29**		[M+HCOO-H]⁻ of 675.31 [M-H]⁻	[44]
33.12-33.67	967.47	309.10; 351.25; 395.15;437.27; 511.25; **529.48**; 579.22; 639.41; **657.34**; **675.47**; 717.98; **743.29**; 761.35; **803.44**; **821.38**; 848.32; 865.41; 922.75; 945.31	334; 289; 323	n.c.	
	997.51	381.23; 467.03; 511.14; **529.05**; 543.22; 567.25; 603.04; **657.15**; **675.18**; 697.48; 721.08; 773.26; **803.34**; **821.36**; 833.47; 915.25; 938.24		probably nerolidol–rhamnopyranosyl–rhamnopyranosyl–(4-trans-feruloyl)–rhamnopyranosyl–glucopyranoside	[45]
	1065.21	405.44; 513.91; 579.73; 675.96; 1020.72; 1033.32; 1041.27; 1057.41; 1067.28		n.c.	
50.02	633.52	339.61; 469.47; 487.39; **513.48**; 571.44; **589.50**; 615.47; 633.50	219; 235; 310	probably 3-*O*-*p*-coumaroyltormetic acid	[46]
	1267.27	1102.55		n.c.	
62.90	523.39	-	219; 235; 281	Usolic acid (monomer adduct)*	Standard
	933.70	408.37; **455.50**; 500.98; 584.57; 745.53; 870.99; 933.70		Usolic acid [2M + Na⁺ -2H⁺]⁻	Standard
	1411.83	455.52; 501.44; **933.71**; 1302.93; 1377.25; 1410.15		Usolic acid [3M + 2Na⁺ -3H⁺]⁻	Standard
	1885.16	934.78; 1391.11; **1406.28**; 1447.24; 1608.90; 1743.24; 1855.24		Usolic acid [4M + 3Na⁺ -4H⁺]⁻	Standard

All further mass peaks were assumed to be chlorophyll related, because of absorption maxima of 408 nm and higher. n.c.: not classifiable. Fragments shown in bold are the main fragments.* Ursolic acid shows, instead of its monomer ion (m/z 455.50 [M-H⁺]⁻), an unknown adduct combination (X) with m/z 523.39 [M+X-H⁺]⁻ and forms additional dimer, trimer, and tetramer adducts with Na⁺ ions.

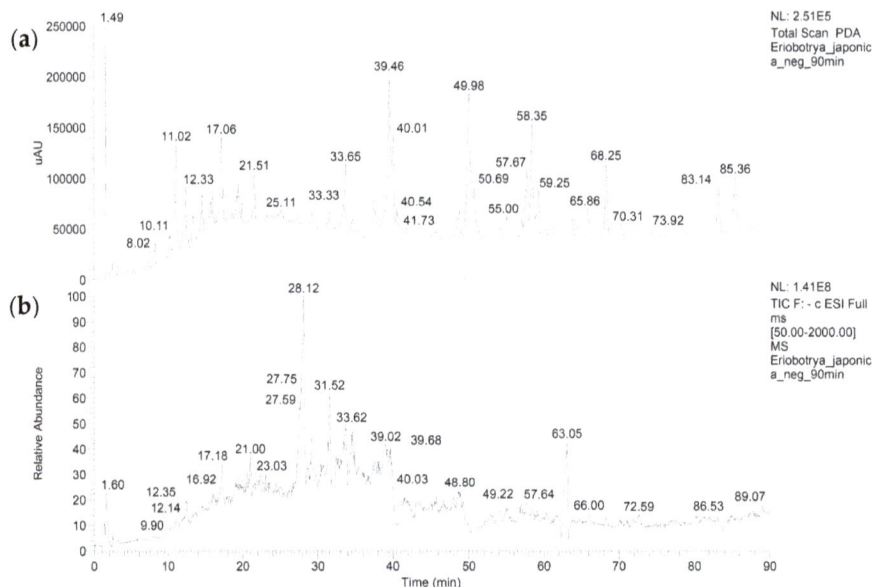

Figure 3. The photodiode array chromatogram (PDA) (**a**) and the total ion current (TIC) (**b**) of the *E. japonica*. The compounds listed in Table 3 correspond to the retention times of the TIC.

3.4. Antioxidant Activities and Total Phenolic Contents

The antioxidant activity of the three plant extracts was determined and compared with the known antioxidants ascorbic acid and EGCG. Results are shown in Table 4. The standard curve of Trolox in the ABTS test, ferrous sulfate in FRAP, and gallic acid equivalents in the total phenol test are provided in supplementary Figure S1. The positive control ascorbic acid showed the lowest EC_{50}, i.e., the highest scavenging effect in DPPH assay. Pe had an EC_{50} value close to ascorbic acid, but slightly higher, meaning it had a slightly weaker antioxidant effect than ascorbic acid; however, this effect was not significant in ABTS and FRAP assays. Ge and Ue did not show stark antioxidant capacity in the three assays. The total phenolic contents analyzed by the Folin–Ciocalteu method are shown as GAE (the phenolic content in 1 g dried sample is equivalent to the amount of gallic acid in mg). The more phenolics in the plant extract, the stronger its antioxidant activity. Pe contained more total phenolics than the Ue and Ge.

Table 4. The in vitro antioxidant capacity and total phenolic content of the plant extracts.

Plant Extracts	DPPH EC_{50} (µg/mL)	TEAC (mM Trolox/mM)	FE (mmol Fe^{2+}/g)	GAE (mg gallic acid/g)
Ascorbic acid	2.31 ± 0.01	6363.67 ± 32.37	$14,268.44 \pm 66.18$	-
EGCG	9.20 ± 1.18	$15,708.35 \pm 54.72$	$25,318.57 \pm 114.83$	-
Glycyrrhiza glabra extract	116.17 ± 0.55	672.19 ± 5.06	477.42 ± 13.00	34.19 ± 2.07
Paeonia lactiflora extract	5.15 ± 0.05	2567.26 ± 32.83	3504.07 ± 51.07	323.19 ± 10.19
Eriobotrya japonica extract	35.50 ± 1.99	758.63 ± 5.23	1464.28 ± 8.32	131.32 ± 12.33

-: not tested; TEAC: Trolox equivalents in mM Trolox/mM test substance; FE: ferrous equivalents in mmol Fe^{2+}/g test substance; GAE: gallic acid equivalents in mg gallic acid/g test substance.

3.5. Cytotoxicity

The potential cytotoxicity (IC_{50} values) of the three plant extracts in RAW 264.7 cells were assessed. The three plant extracts showed concentration-dependent inhibition of cell growth (data not shown), and they were not cytotoxic (with IC$_{50 \text{ values}}$ between 60 and 100 μg/mL) compared to the positive control doxorubicin and EGCG.

3.6. Antimicrobial Activity

The MIC and MBC of the three plant extracts against two gram-negative (*E. coli* XL1-Blue MRF' and *Acinetobacter bohemicus*) and four gram-positive bacteria (*Kocuria kristinae*, *Micrococcus luteus*, *Staphylococcus auricularis*, and *Bacillus megaterium*) are presented in Table 5. At the concentrations tested, the three plant extracts varied considerably in their antimicrobial activity against the six bacterial strains. Ue restrained the growth of bacteria at or above 5 or 10 mg/mL. Ge showed intermediate antibacterial activity against all bacterial species (MIC between 0.31 mg/mL and 1.25 mg/mL), except *E. coli* XL1-Blue MRF' (MIC > 10 mg/mL). On the other hand, Pe inhibited the growth of *Acinetobacter bohemicus*, *Micrococcus luteus*, and *Bacillus megaterium* at 0.08 mg/mL (Table 5). The control groups (5% DMSO and bacterial suspensions) showed normal bacterial growth, meaning that the solvents did not inhibit bacterial growth in any case.

Table 5. Minimum inhibitory concentration (MIC) and minimum bactericidal concentration (MBC) of the three plant extracts.

Bacteria	MIC MBC	Ampicillin (μg/mL)	Ciprofloxacin (μg/mL)	*Glycyrrhiza glabra* Extract (mg/mL)	*Paeonia lactiflora* Extract (mg/mL)	*Eriobotrya japonica* Extract (mg/mL)
E. coli XL1-Blue MRF'	MIC	8	0.03	>10	2.5	10
	MBC	16	0.06	-	5	-
Acinetobacter bohemicus	MIC	2	0.03	1.25	0.08	5
	MBC	8	0.05	2.5	1.25	10
Kocuria kristinae	MIC	0.13	0.13	0.63	1.25	>10
	MBC	0.25	0.5	1.25	2.5	-
Micrococcus luteus	MIC	0.25	0.5	0.31	0.08	10
	MBC	2	2	1.25	0.63	-
Staphylococcus auricularis	MIC	0.5	0.06	0.63	1.25	5
	MBC	4	0.13	1.25	>10	10
Bacillus megaterium	MIC	0.25	0.06	0.31	0.08	10
	MBC	1	0.13	0.63	0.31	-

-: not detectable.

4. Discussion

Pe has a relatively high DPPH• scavenging activity, which is comparable to that of ascorbic acid. This finding is in agreement with Lee et al. and Bae et al. [47,48]. Ge and Ue extracts were weaker antioxidants in DPPH, ABTS, and FRAP assays. The results of Ge are in agreement with literature data, in which the main plant secondary metabolites (PSMs) liquiritin, glycyrrhizin, and glycyrrhetinic acid did not scavenge the DPPH• or the effects were not strong [49–51]. We also tested the effect of glycyrrhizin on scavenging DPPH•, but the effect was negligible (data not shown).

Plant polyphenols usually exhibit good antioxidant properties [11,52–55]. In detail, the specific structure of polyphenols enables them to donate hydrogen, delocalize electrons, quench singlet oxygen, and react with free radicals [56,57]. *E. japonica,* the leaves of which contain polyphenols, was found to possess a high degree of antioxidant activity and the radical scavenging activity of its seed extract increased with the polyphenol content [58,59]. The difference of the antioxidant activity of *E. japonica* between our results and the literature may be due to different solvents of the plant extracts. The three methods used employ different mechanisms, but the reducing capacity of the three plant extracts showed the same trend in the three assays (ascorbic acid or EGCG > Pe > Ue > Ge). Pe contained the most phenolics and therefore showed probably the strongest antioxidant activity.

Our previous study examined the cytotoxicity of the three plant extracts in the drug-resistant cancer cell line CEM/ADR 5000 and Caco-2 compared to the sensitive cancer cell line CCRF-CEM and HCT-116. The three plant extracts did not show strong cytotoxicity compared to the positive control doxorubicin in sensitive and resistant cell lines [16]. This time, we showed that the three plant extracts were not cytotoxic against a murine macrophage RAW 264.7 cell line, either. These results verify that the traditional usage of these plants is safe and pave the way for their future usage.

Plant extracts and essential oils have been widely studied and used as antimicrobial agents in the last decades [11,60]. The MBC of the three plant extracts is usually two to four times that of MIC, suggesting a dose-dependent effect on bacteria. The ratio of some MBC to MIC is >4, suggesting the bacteriostatic effect of the plant extracts on the bacteria. Few antimicrobial studies of the leaf extract of *E. japonica* have been conducted and it did not show toxicity against the six bacterial strains here. The *G. glabra* extract showed antimicrobial activity in some other bacterial strains [61–65] and medium effect against five bacterial strains in this study. The *P. lactiflora* extract was reported to exhibit antibacterial and antiviral activity [66,67]; its antibacterial effect was strong on some bacteria species here. The secondary metabolites in plants, such as saponins, phenolic compounds (e.g., flavonoids or tannins), essential oils, and monoterpenes, contribute to their antimicrobial capacity [11,68–70]. Wang reviewed the finding that one triterpene (18β-glycyrrhetinic acid) and four flavonoids (licochalcone A, licochalcone E, glabridin, and liquiritigenin) underlie the antimicrobial activity in *G. glabra* [71]. Low concentrations of the PSMs in *G. glabra*, such as glycyrrhizic acid, 18β-glycyrrhetinic acid, liquiritigenin, and isoliquiritigenin, were also tested in the six species, but the effect was not significant (data not shown), suggesting that these PSMs did not contribute to the medium antibacterial activity of *G. glabra*. However, polyphenols can interact with proteins in cells, because they possess several phenolic OH groups, which allow them to make hydrogen and ionic bonds with amino groups in proteins. When important bacterial proteins are affected, an antimicrobial effect can occur [72]. The strong antibacterial effect of Pe was probably due to its phenolic content. Correspondingly, the same principle might also explain the antibacterial activity of Ge and Ue. The mechanism of antimicrobial activity of *P. lactiflora* root and *E. japonica* leaves was reported to be disruption of protein and cell-wall synthesis [73]. More studies are needed to elucidate the potential of the three plant extracts as antimicrobial agents and the possible mechanisms.

5. Conclusions

Our results show that the three extracts of TCM plants are low-toxic, but biologically active, which would explain their wide usage in traditional medicine. Especially Pe and Ge, should be studied further for their potential to be developed as antioxidant food supplements or antibacterial drugs.

Supplementary Materials: The following are available online at http://www.mdpi.com/2305-6320/6/2/43/s1, Figure S1: The standard curves in the TEAC, FRAP, and Folin–Ciocateu assays shown as absorption vs. concentration, Table S1: Secondary metabolites in *Glycyrrhiza glabra*, Table S2: Secondary metabolites in *Peonia lactiflora*, Table S3: Secondary metabolites in *Paeonia veitchii*, Table S4: Secondary metabolites in *Eriobotrya japonica*.

Author Contributions: Conceptualization, J.-X.Z. and M.W.; methodology, J.-X.Z., M.S.B., P.W., and B.W.; writing—original draft preparation, J.-X.Z., P.W., and B.W.; writing—review and editing, J.-X.Z., M.S.B., P.W., B.W., and M.W. Supervision, M.W.

Funding: We acknowledge financial support by Deutsche Forschungsgemeinschaft within the funding programme Open Access Publishing, by the Baden-Württemberg Ministry of Science, Research and the Arts and by Ruprecht-Karls-Universität Heidelberg.

Acknowledgments: We kindly thank Mariana Roxo for introducing J.-X.Z. to the antioxidant assay methods. We also thank Douglas Fear for checking the English.

Conflicts of Interest: The authors declare no conflict of interest.

References

1. Gao, Z. Artemisinin anti-malarial drugs in China. *Acta Pharm. Sin. B* **2016**, *6*, 115–124. [CrossRef]
2. Chan, S.; Li, S.; Kwok, C.; Benzie, I.; Szeto, Y.; Guo, D.; He, X.; Yu, P. Antioxidant activity of Chinese medicinal herbs. *Pharm. Biol.* **2008**, *46*, 587–595. [CrossRef]
3. Liao, H.; Banbury, L.K.; Leach, D.N. Antioxidant activity of 45 Chinese herbs and the relationship with their TCM characteristics. *Evid. Based Complement. Alternat. Med.* **2008**, *5*, 429–434. [CrossRef]
4. Kaushik, A.; Jijta, C.; Kaushik, J.J.; Zeray, R.; Ambesajir, A.; Beyene, L. FRAP (Ferric reducing ability of plasma) assay and effect of *Diplazium esculentum* (Retz) Sw. (a green vegetable of North India) on central nervous system. *Indian J. Nat. Prod. Resour.* **2012**, *3*, 228–231.
5. Dudonné, S.; Vitrac, X.; Coutière, P.; Woillez, M.; Mérillon, J. Comparative study of antioxidant properties and total phenolic content of 30 plant extracts of industrial interest using DPPH, ABTS, FRAP, SOD, and ORAC Assays. *J. Agric. Food Chem.* **2009**, *57*, 1768–1774. [CrossRef]
6. Antolovich, M.; Prenzler, P.D.; Patsalides, E.; McDonald, S.; Robards, K. Methods for testing antioxidant activity. *Analyst* **2002**, *127*, 183–198. [CrossRef]
7. Gutteridge, J.M.C. Biological origin of free radicals, and mechanisms of antioxidant protection. *Chem. Biol. Interact.* **1994**, *91*, 133–140. [CrossRef]
8. Irshad, Md.; Zafaryab, Md.; Singh, M.; Rizvi, M.M.A. Comparative analysis of the antioxidant activity of *Cassia fistula* extracts. *Int. J. Med. Chem.* **2012**, *2012*, 157125. [CrossRef]
9. Mambro, V.M.D.; Fonseca, M.J.V. Assays of physical stability and antioxidant activity of a topical formulation added with different plant extracts. *J. Pharm. Biomed. Anal.* **2005**, *37*, 287–295. [CrossRef]
10. Vaya, J.; Belinky, P.A.; Aviram, M. Antioxidant constituents from licorice roots: Isolation, structure elucidation and antioxidative capacity toward LDL oxidation. *Free Radic. Biol. Med.* **1997**, *23*, 302–313. [CrossRef]
11. Van Wyk, B.E.; Wink, M. *Medicinal Plants of the World*, 2nd ed.; Briza: Pretoria, South Africa, 2017.
12. Shibata, S. A drug over the millennia: Pharmacognosy, chemistry, and pharmacology of licorice. *Yakugaku Zasshi* **2000**, *120*, 849–862. [CrossRef] [PubMed]
13. Fiore, C.; Eisenhut, M.; Ragazzi, E.; Zanchin, G.; Armanini, D. A history of the therapeutic use of liquorice in Europe. *J. Ethnopharmacol.* **2005**, *99*, 317–324. [CrossRef]
14. Wang, W.; Wang, C.; Gu, S.; Cao, Q.; Lv, Y.; Gao, J.; Wang, S. Pharmacokinetic studies of the significance of herbaceous compatibility of peony liquorice decoction. *World Sci. Technol.* **2009**, *11*, 382–387. [CrossRef]
15. Zhang, B.; Liu, Q. Experimental study on the prescription of Shaoyao Gancao Decoction. *Chin. Tradit. Pat. Med.* **2012**, *34*, 1354–1358. (In Chinese)
16. Zhou, J.; Wink, M. Reversal of multidrug resistance in human colon cancer and human leukemia cells by three plant extracts and their major secondary metabolites. *Medicines* **2018**, *5*, 123. [CrossRef]
17. Duan, T.; Yu, M.; Liu, C.; Ma, C.; Wang, W.; Wei, S. Simultaneous determination of glycyrrhizic acid, liquiritin and fingerprint of licorice by RP-HPLC. *Chin. Tradit. Pat. Med.* **2006**, *28*, 161–165. (In Chinese)
18. Yu, D.; Gu, X.; Zhang, C.; Chen, C.; Ma, Y. Comparison of different extracting processes for paeoniflorin in Paeoniae Radix Alba. *Chin. J. Exp. Tradit. Med. Formul.* **2013**, *19*, 49–51.
19. Xiang, Y.; Yang, X.; Yang, G.; Huang, W. Extraction and isolation of ursolic acid from the leaves of *Eriobotrya japonica*. *Herald Med.* **2005**, *12*, 1105–1106. (In Chinese)
20. Blois, M.S. Antioxidant determinations by the use of a stable free radical. *Nature* **1958**, *181*, 1199–1200. [CrossRef]
21. Brand-Williams, W.; Cuvelier, M.E.; Berset, C. Use of a free radical method to evaluate antioxidant activity. *Lebensmittel-Wissenschaft und -Technologie* **1995**, *28*, 25–30. [CrossRef]
22. Miller, N.J.; Rice-Evans, C.A. Factors influencing the antioxidant activity determined by the ABTS radical cation assay. *Free Radic. Res.* **1996**, *26*, 195–199. [CrossRef]
23. Pietta, P.; Simonetti, P.; Gardana, C.; Mauri, P. Trolox equivalent antioxidant capacity (TEAC) of *Ginkgo biloba* flavonol and *Camellia sinensis* catechin metabolites. *J. Pharm. Biomed. Anal.* **2000**, *23*, 223–226. [CrossRef]
24. Liu, T.Z.; Chin, N.; Kiser, M.D.; Bigler, W.N. Specific spectrophotometry of ascorbic acid in serum or plasma by use of ascorbate oxidase. *Clin. Chem.* **1982**, *28*, 2225–2228.
25. Benzie, I.F.F.; Strain, J.J. The ferric reducing ability of plasma (FRAP) as a measure of "antioxidant power": The FRAP assay. *Anal. Biomed.* **1996**, *239*, 70–76. [CrossRef]
26. Swain, T.; Hillis, W.E. The phenolic constituents of *Prunus domestica*. *J. Sci. Food Agric.* **1959**, *10*, 63–68. [CrossRef]

27. Singleton, V.L.; Orthofer, R.; Lamuela-Raventós, R.M. Analysis of total phenols and other oxidation substrates and antioxidants by means of Folin-Ciocalteu reagent. *Methods Enzymol.* **1999**, *299*, 152–178. [CrossRef]

28. Mosmann, T. Rapid colorimetric assay for cellular growth and survival: Application to proliferation and cytotoxicity assays. *J. Immunol. Methods* **1983**, *65*, 55–63. [CrossRef]

29. CLSI. *Methods for Dilution Antimicrobial Susceptibility Tests for Bacteria That Grow Aerobically; Approved Standard*, 9th ed.; CLSI document M07-A9; Clinical and Laboratory Standards Institute: Wayne, PA, USA, 2012.

30. Farag, M.A.; Porzel, A.; Wessjohann, L.A. Comparative metabolite profiling and fingerprinting of medicinal licorice roots using a multiplex approach of GC-MS, LC-MS and 1D NMR techniques. *Phytochemistry* **2012**, *76*, 60–72. [CrossRef]

31. Ye, Z.; Dai, J.; Zhang, C.; Lu, Y.; Wu, L.; Gong, A.G.W.; Xu, H.; Tsim, K.W.K.; Wang, Z. Chemical differentiation of *Dendrobium officinale* and *Dendrobium devonianum* by using HPLC fingerprints, HPLC-ESI-MS, and HPTLC analyses. *Evid. Based Complement. Alternat. Med.* **2017**. [CrossRef]

32. Link, P.; Wetterauer, B.; Fu, Y.; Wink, M. Extracts of *Glycyrrhiza uralensis* and isoliquiritigenin counteract amyloid-β toxicity in *Caenorhabditis elegans*. *Planta Med.* **2015**, *81*, 357–362. [CrossRef]

33. Montoro, P.; Maldini, M.; Russo, M.; Postorino, S.; Piacente, S.; Pizza, C. Metabolic profiling of roots of liquorice (*Glycyrrhiza glabra*) from different geographical areas by ESI/MS/MS and determination of major metabolites by LC-ESI/MS and LC-ESI/MS/MS. *J. Pharm. Biomed. Anal.* **2011**, *54*, 535–544. [CrossRef]

34. Song, R.; Xu, L.; Zhang, Z.; Tian, Y.; Xu, F.; Dong, H. Determination of gallic acid in rat plasma by LC-MS-MS. *Chroma* **2010**, *71*, 1107–1111. [CrossRef]

35. Niu, Y.; Wang, S. Analysis on chemical constituents in Danggui-Shaoyao-San by LC-Q-TOF-MS and LC-IT-MS^n. *Chin. Tradit. Herb. Drugs* **2014**, *45*, 1056–1062. (In Chinese) [CrossRef]

36. Li, F.; Zhang, B.; Wei, X.; Song, C.; Qiao, M.; Zhang, H. Metabolic profiling of Shu-Yu capsule in rat serum based on metabolic fingerprinting analysis using HPLC-ESI-MS^n. *Mol. Med. Rep.* **2016**, *13*, 4191–4204. [CrossRef]

37. Wu, X.; Wu, M.; Chen, X.; Zhang, H.; Ding, L.; Tian, F.; Fu, X.; Qiu, F.; Zhang, D. Rapid characterization of the absorbed chemical constituents of Tangzhiqing formula following oral administration using UHPLC-Q-TOF-MS. *J. Sep. Sci.* **2018**, *41*, 1025–1038. [CrossRef]

38. Ye, M.; Liu, S.; Jiang, Z.; Lee, Y.; Tilton, R.; Cheng, Y. Liquid chromatography/mass spectrometry analysis of PHY906, a Chinese medicine formulation for cancer therapy. *Rapid Commun. Mass Spectrom.* **2007**, *21*, 3593–3607. [CrossRef]

39. Shi, Y. Chemical constituents with anti-allergic activity from red peony root and a horticultural cultivar of *Paeonia lactiflora* and monoterpenoids profiles of peony related species. Ph.D. Thesis, University of Toyama, Toyama, Japan, March 2016.

40. Dong, H.; Liu, Z.; Song, F.; Yu, Z.; Li, H.; Liu, S. Structural analysis of monoterpene glycosides extracted from *Paeonia lactiflora* Pall. using electrospray ionization Fourier transform ion cyclotron resonance mass spectrometry and high-performance liquid chromatography/electrospray ionization tandem mass spectrometry. *Rapid Commun. Mass Spectrom.* **2007**, *21*, 3193–3199. [CrossRef]

41. Gao, J.; Zhang, J.; Qu, Z.; Zhou, H.; Tong, Y.; Liu, D.; Yang, H.; Gao, W. Study on the mechanisms of the bronchodilator effects of Folium Eriobotryae and the selected active ingredient on isolated gunea pig tracheal strips. *Pharm. Biol.* **2016**, *54*, 2742–2752. [CrossRef]

42. Zhou, C.; Liu, Y.; Su, D.; Gao, G.; Zhou, X.; Sun, L.; Ba, X.; Chen, X.; Bi, K. A sensitive LC-MS-MS method for simultaneous quantification of two structural isomers, hyperoside and isoquercitrin: Application to pharmacokinetic studies. *Chroma* **2011**, *73*, 353–359. [CrossRef]

43. Lin, Y.; Xu, W.; Huang, M.; Xu, W.; Li, H.; Ye, M.; Zhang, X.; Chu, K. Qualitative and quantitative analysis of phenolic acids, flavonoids and iridoid glycosides in yinhua kanggan tablet by UPLC-QqQ-MS/MS. *Molecules* **2015**, *20*, 12209–12228. [CrossRef]

44. Zhao, L.; Chen, J.; Yin, M.; Ren, B.; Li, W. Analysis of sesquiterpene glycosides from loquat leaves by UPLC-Q-TOF-MS. *Chin. Tradit. Pat. Med.* **2015**, *37*, 1498–1502. (In Chinese)

45. De Tommasi, N.; Aquino, R.; De Simone, F.; Pizza, C. Plant metabolites. New sesquiterpene and ionone glycosides from *Eriobotrya japonica*. *J. Nat. Prod.* **1992**, *55*, 1025–1032. [CrossRef]

46. Wu, L.; Jiang, X.; Huang, L.; Chen, S. Processing technology investigation of loquat (*Eriobotrya japonica*) leaf by ultra-performance liquid chromatography-quadrupole time-of-flight mass spectrometry combined with chemometrics. *PLoS ONE* **2013**, *8*, e64178. [CrossRef]

47. Lee, C.; Kwon, Y.S.; Son, K.H.; Kim, H.P.; Heo, M.Y. Antioxidative constituents from *Paeonia lactiflora*. *Arch. Pharm. Res.* **2005**, *28*, 775–783. [CrossRef] [PubMed]

48. Bae, J.; Kim, C.Y.; Kim, H.J.; Park, J.H.; Ahn, M. Differences in the chemical profiles and biological activities of *Paeonia lactiflora* and *Paeonia obovata*. *J. Med. Food* **2015**, *18*, 224–232. [CrossRef]

49. Cheel, J.; Antwerpen, P.V.; Tumová, L.; Onofre, G.; Vokurková, D.; Zouaoui-Boudjeltia, K.; Vanhaeverbeek, M.; Nève, J. Free radical-scavenging, antioxidant and immunostimulating effects of a licorice infusion (*Glycyrrhiza glabra* L.). *Food Chem.* **2010**, *122*, 508–517. [CrossRef]

50. Kato, T.; Horie, N.; Hashimoto, K.; Satoh, K.; Shimoyama, T.; Kaneko, T.; Kusama, K.; Sakagami, H. Bimodal effect of glycyrrhizin on macrophage nitric oxide and prostaglandin E2 production. *In Vivo* **2008**, *22*, 583–586. [PubMed]

51. Imai, K.; Takagi, Y.; Iwazaki, A.; Nakanishi, K. Radical scavenging ability of glycyrrhizin. *Free Radic. Antioxid.* **2013**, *3*, 40–42. [CrossRef]

52. Bors, W.; Michel, C. Chemistry of the antioxidant effect of polyphenols. *Ann. N. Y. Acad. Sci.* **2002**, *957*, 57–69. [CrossRef] [PubMed]

53. Zahin, M.; Aqil, F.; Ahmad, I. The in vitro antioxidant activity and total phenolic content of four Indian medicinal plants. *J. Pharm. Pharm. Sci.* **2009**, *1*, 88–95.

54. Li, X.; Wu, X.; Huang, L. Correlation between antioxidant activities and phenolic contents of radix *Angelicae sinensis* (Danggui). *Molecules* **2009**, *14*, 5349–5361. [CrossRef] [PubMed]

55. Tosun, M.; Ercisli, S.; Sengul, M.; Ozer, H.; Polat, T.; Ozturk, E. Antioxidant properties and total phenolic content of eight *Salvia* species from Turkey. *Biol. Res.* **2009**, *42*, 175–181. [CrossRef] [PubMed]

56. Proestos, C.; Lytoudi, K.; Mavromelanidou, O.K.; Zoumpoulakis, P.; Sinanoglou, V.J. Antioxidant capacity of selected plant extracts and their essential oils. *Antioxidants* **2013**, *2*, 11–22. [CrossRef] [PubMed]

57. Rice-Evans, C.A.; Miller, N.J.; Paganga, G. Structure-antioxidant activity relationships of flavonoids and phenolic acids. *Free Radic. Biol. Med.* **1996**, *20*, 933–956. [CrossRef]

58. Song, F.; Gan, R.; Zhang, Y.; Xiao, Q.; Kuang, L.; Li, H.B. Total phenolic contents and antioxidant capacities of selected Chinese medicinal plants. *Int. J. Mol. Sci.* **2010**, *11*, 2362–2372. [CrossRef]

59. Yokota, J.; Takuma, D.; Hamada, A.; Onogawa, M.; Yoshioka, S.; Kusunose, M.; Miyamura, M.; Kyotani, S.; Nishioka, Y. Scavenging of reactive oxygen species by *Eriobotrya japonica* seed extract. *Biol. Pharm. Bull.* **2006**, *29*, 467–471. [CrossRef]

60. Hamoud, R.; Sporer, F.; Reichling, J.; Wink, M. Antimicrobial activity of a traditionally used complex essential oil distillate (Olbas® Tropfen) in comparison to its individual essential oil ingredients. *Phytomedicine* **2012**, *19*, 969–976. [CrossRef]

61. Gupta, V.K.; Fatima, A.; Faridi, U.; Negi, A.S.; Shanker, K.; Kumar, J.K.; Rahuja, N.; Luqman, S.; Sisodia, B.S.; Saikia, D.; et al. Antimicrobial potential of *Glycyrrhiza glabra* roots. *J. Ethnopharmacol.* **2008**, *116*, 377–380. [CrossRef]

62. Sedighinia, F.; Afshar, A.S.; Soleimanpour, S.; Zarif, R.; Asili, J.; Ghazvini, K. Antibacterial activity of *Glycyrrhiza glabra* against oral pathogens: An in vitro study. *Avicenna J. Phytomed.* **2012**, *2*, 118–124.

63. Geetha, R.V.; Roy, A. In Vitro evaluation of antibacterial activity of ethanolic root extract of *Glycyrrhiza glabra* on oral microbes. *Int. J. Drug Dev. Res.* **2012**, *4*, 161–165.

64. Aggarwal, H.; Ghosh, J.; Rao, A.; Chhokar, V. Evaluation of root and leaf extracts of *Glycyrrhiza glabra* for antimicrobial activity. *J. Med.Bioeng.* **2015**, *4*, 81–85.

65. Nitalikar, M.M.; Munde, K.C.; Dhore, B.V.; Shikalgar, S.N. Studies of antibacterial activities of *Glycyrrhiza glabra* root extract. *Int. J. PharmTech. Res.* **2010**, *2*, 899–901.

66. Park, K.; Cho, S. Antimicrobial characteristics of *Paeonia lactiflora* Pall. extract tested against food-putrefactive microorganisms. *Korean J. Food Preserv.* **2010**, *17*, 706–711.

67. Boo, K.; Lee, D.; Woo, J.; Ko, S.H.; Jeong, E.; Hong, Q.; Riu, K.Z.; Lee, D. Anti-bacterial and anti-viral activity of extracts from *Paeonia lactiflora* roots. *J. Korean Soc. Appl. Biol. Chem.* **2011**, *54*, 132–135. [CrossRef]

68. Dhanya, K.N.M.; Sidhu, P. The antimicrobial activity of *Azardirachta indica*, *Glycyrrhiza glabra*, *Cinnamum zeylanicum*, *Syzygium aromaticum*, *Accacia nilotica* on *Streptococcus mutans* and *Enterococcus faecalis*—An in vitro study. *Endodontology* **2011**, *23*, 18–25.

69. Sharopov, F.; Braun, M.S.; Gulmurodov, I.; Khalifaev, D.; Isupov, S.; Wink, M. Antimicrobial, antioxidant, and anti-inflammatory activities of essential oils of selected aromatic plants from Tajikistan. *Foods* **2015**, *4*, 645–653. [CrossRef]

70. Youssef, F.S.; Hamoud, R.; Ashour, M.L.; Singab, A.N.; Wink, M. Volatile oils from the aerial parts of *Eremophila maculata* and their antimicrobial activity. *Chem. Biodivers.* **2014**, *11*, 831–841. [CrossRef]
71. Wang, L.; Yang, R.; Yuan, B.; Liu, Y.; Liu, C. The antiviral and antimicrobial activities of licorice, a widely-used Chinese herb. *Acta Pharm. Sin. B* **2015**, *5*, 310–315. [CrossRef]
72. Wink, M. Modes of action of herbal medicines and plant secondary metabolites. *Medicines* **2015**, *2*, 251–286. [CrossRef] [PubMed]
73. Viswanad, V.; Aleykutty, N.A.; Zachariah, S.M.; Prabhakar, V. Antimicrobial potential of herbal medicines. *Int. J. Pharm. Sci. Res.* **2011**, *2*, 1651–1658.

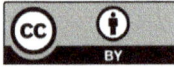

medicines

MDPI

Review

Medicinal Potentialities of Plant Defensins: A Review with Applied Perspectives

Nida Ishaq [1], Muhammad Bilal [2,*] and Hafiz M.N. Iqbal [3,*]

[1] School of Agriculture and Biology, Shanghai Jiao Tong University, Shanghai 200240, China; nidaishaq88@yahoo.com

[2] School of Life Science and Food Engineering, Huaiyin Institute of Technology, Huaian 223003, China

[3] Tecnologico de Monterrey, School of Engineering and Sciences, Campus Monterrey, Ave. Eugenio Garza Sada 2501, CP 64849 Monterrey, N.L., Mexico

* Correspondence: bilaluaf@hotmail.com (M.B.); hafiz.iqbal@itesm.mx (H.M.N.I.);
  Tel.: +52-81-8358-2000 (ext. 5679) (H.M.N.I.)

Received: 31 January 2019; Accepted: 18 February 2019; Published: 19 February 2019

Abstract: Plant-based secondary metabolites with medicinal potentialities such as defensins are small, cysteine-rich peptides that represent an imperative aspect of the inherent defense system. Plant defensins possess broad-spectrum biological activities, e.g., bactericidal and insecticidal actions, as well as antifungal, antiviral, and anticancer activities. The unique structural and functional attributes provide a nonspecific and versatile means of combating a variety of microbial pathogens, i.e., fungi, bacteria, protozoa, and enveloped viruses. Some defensins in plants involved in other functions include the development of metal tolerance and the role in sexual reproduction, while most of the defensins make up the innate immune system of the plants. Defensins are structurally and functionally linked and have been characterized in various eukaryotic microorganisms, mammals, plants, gulls, teleost species of fish, mollusks, insect pests, arachnidan, and crustaceans. This defense mechanism has been improved biotechnologically as it helps to protect plants from fungal attacks in genetically modified organisms (GMO). Herein, we review plant defensins as secondary metabolites with medicinal potentialities. The first half of the review elaborates the origin, structural variations, and mechanism of actions of plant defensins. In the second part, the role of defensins in plant defense, stress response, and reproduction are discussed with suitable examples. Lastly, the biological applications of plant defensins as potential antimicrobial and anticancer agents are also deliberated. In summary, plant defensins may open a new prospect in medicine, human health, and agriculture.

Keywords: defensins; secondary metabolites; plant defense; antimicrobial and anticancer activity; medicine; innate immunity

---

1. Introduction

In nature, plants are continuously confronted with attacks from pests and other microbial pathogens such as fungi and bacteria. In addition, plants also suffer and face harsh environmental conditions of salt and drought stress. To overcome these stresses, plants have established a very complex mechanism to protect themselves from pests, pathogens, and fungal attacks [1]. Besides, many other defense factors including polyacetylenes, phenolics, alkaloids, terpenoids, and hydrogen peroxide are also generated to circumvent these kinds of occurrences. Along with the above-described chemicals, plants also released an array of defensins and defensin-related proteins [2,3].

Plant defensins are cysteine-rich highly stable peptides of 4–45 amino acid residues, comprising a part of the immune system that can present antifungal, antibacterial, or proteinase inhibitory activity. These peptides display a conserved three-dimensional structure containing α-helix and triple-stranded β-sheet stabilized into a compact structure through disulfide linkages [4]. This structure resembles defense peptides in insects and mammals, revealing a common historic origin. Moreover, only one class, namely defensins, seems to be conserved between invertebrates, plants, and vertebrates (Figure 1) [5]. Nowadays, it is revealed that the ubiquitous presence of these peptides among the plant kingdom play a noteworthy role in the innate immune system of plants. Plants that express defensins are highly resilient to fungal attacks and show augmented growth and development [6]. Active against a variety of human and fungal pathogens, these proteins have a potential use in therapeutics, medicines, as well as agriculture. As plant defensins play a very important role in defending plants against pathogenic microorganisms and other insects, they also interfere with the plant cells along with fungal cells. Some defensins can destroy microorganisms in 15–90 min by their disruptive actions on the cytoplasmic membrane.

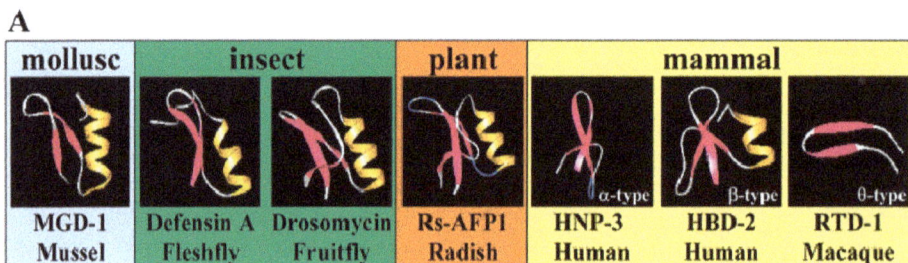

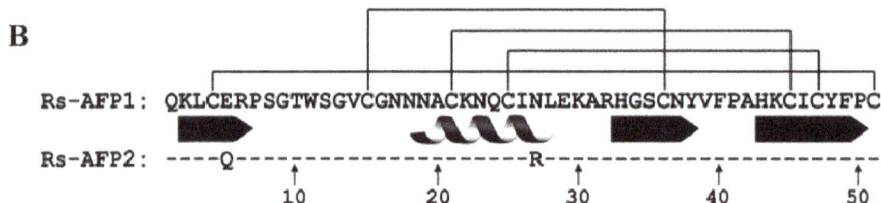

Figure 1. (**A**) Three-dimensional structure of defensins of plant, invertebrate (insect and mollusk), and vertebrate (mammalian) origin. Structures were downloaded from the protein data bank (http://www.rcsb.org/pdb; PDB accession ID numbers: MGD-1: 1FJN, defensin A: 1ICA, drosomycin: 1MYN, Rs-AFP1: 1AYJ, HNP-3: 1DFN, HBD-2: 1FD3, RTD-1: 1HVZ). Pictures were generated using Rasmol software. The α-helices and β-sheets are shown in yellow and red, respectively. (**B**) The amino acid sequence of mature Rs-AFP1 and 2. Dashes indicate identical amino acid residues. Connecting lines between cysteine residues represent disulfide bonds, while the spiral and arrows indicate the location of the α-helix and β-strands, respectively. Adapted from Thomma et al. [5], with permission from Springer Nature. Copyright (2002) Springer-Verlag.

2. Origin of Defensins

At the start of the 1990s, numerous cationic plants with cysteine-abundance antimicrobial peptides were investigated. At first, plant defensins were reported in the seed products associated with whole wheat (*Triticum turgidum*) as well as barley (*Hordeum vulgare*) [7,8]. Initially, these peptides were categorized as a novel and detached member of the thionin family because of their resemblance in amino acid sequence, molecular weight, and the number of cysteines [7–9]. Nevertheless, subsequent research revealed significant variations within the arrangement of the disulfide bridge, showing no relationship between these two peptide families [10]. Broekaert et al. [11] renamed these types of peptides as plant defensins after evaluating their functional and structural similarities to formerly identified antimicrobial peptides (AMPs) found in mammals and insects. Defensins are structurally as well as functionally linked defense peptides that have been characterized in various eukaryotic microorganisms, as well as in mammals, plants, gulls, teleost species of fish, mollusks, insect pests, arachnidan, and crustaceans, in addition to fungi [11–16]. Phylogenetic studies indicated that these kinds of peptides share a common antecedent as tested among mollusk, arthropod, mammal, and bird defensins [17]. This prediction was usually reported because of the common interspecies conservation at different levels of peptide structures. The unique cysteine residue and the useful interspecies conservation affirmed that particular defensins present a common evolution. Depending on these types of results, the polyphyletic source associated with defensin peptides was uncertain. Through in silico studies, Zhu [18] revealed the existence of defensin-like peptides in *Anaeromyxobacter dehalogenans*, *Myxobacteria*, and *Stigmatella aurantiaca*. Despite the scarcity of details regarding antimicrobial activities, it is likely that these peptides characterize an antique method of defense inside prokaryotes that were transferred to the particular eukaryotic family during their progression [6]. In consonance with this particular perspective, six new groups of AMPs have been recognized in fungi. These families comprise 25 members containing defensins related to plant, insect, and invertebrate defensins [19]. This discovery provided insight into the resemblance of a bacterial peptide to two fungal defensin-like peptides, revealing that a bacterial antecedent contributed to these defensin molecules [19].

3. Structure of Defensins

Plant defensins exhibit a highly conserved three-dimensional structural conformation comprised of one α-helix and three β-strands in antiparallel position. In addition, the arrangement of the amino acid sequence is also well conserved because of the occurrence of 6–8 cysteine residues constituting 3–4 disulfide interactions in the following order: Cys1–Cys8, Cys2–Cys5, Cys3–Cys6, and Cys4–Cys7 [20]. Nonetheless, plant defensins with five disulfide bridges have also been identified. The presence of an additional disulfide bond positioned after the α-helix and the primary β-sheet does not influence the typical three-dimensional structural organization of the defensins [21]. Moreover, the literature survey also revealed plant defensins with alternate structural organizations, including defensins from *Petunia hybrida* (PhD1 and PhD2), *Nicotiana alata* (NaD1), and ZmESR6 obtained from evolving maize kernels. These kinds of defensins comprise an additional acidic C-terminal pro-domain with still unknown functionalities. However, De Coninck and colleagues [22] reported its involvement in vacuolar targeting and circumventing damaging consequences caused by the basicity of the defensin. The sequence arrangement of plant defensins amino acids is not a conservative sequence, except the cysteines and a glycine located in the second β-sheet [23]. Figure 2 shows the three-dimensional structural conformation of six antifungal defensins from plants [3].

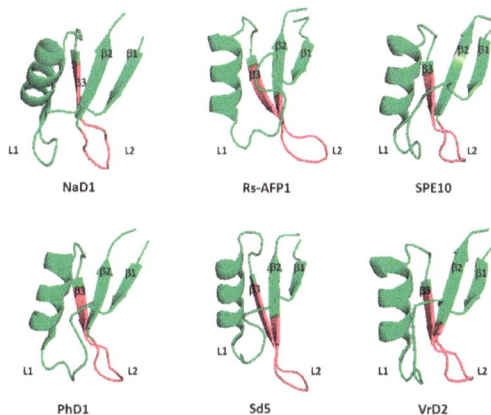

Figure 2. Three-dimensional structural conformation of six antifungal plant defensins (adopted from Lacerda et al. [3], an open-access article distributed under the terms of the Creative Commons Attribution License (CC BY)).

4. Mode of Action

A representation of the proposed action mechanisms of the plant defensins is shown in Figure 3 [24]. Indeed, the mechanism of antifungal defensins is most likely subject to electrostatic interactions in the middle of peptides and hyphal films, prompting a disturbance by a fast instigation of K$^+$ efflux and Ca$^+$ uptake and preventing parasitic growth. Notably, two major scientific hypotheses—the carpet model and the pore model—have been speculated to elucidate the action mechanism of antimicrobial defensin peptides. According to both models, defensins preferentially interrelate with negatively charged structures of pathogens' cell membrane, resulting in increased membrane permeability and cell leakage followed by necrotic cell death. The carpet model explicates the pore formation of several peptides into the cell membrane, whereas the pore model demonstrates the formation of oligomers of those peptides, which then produce numerous pores into the membrane [3]. On the contrary, several reports have hypothesized an alternative mechanism of action of defensins without damaging the cell membrane of pathogens. In this hypothesis, these defense peptides are internalized into the intracellular environment, leading to elevated ion penetrability by reacting with the membrane phospholipids [25,26]. Therefore, they can also increase the generation of reactive oxygen species (ROS) and trigger apoptosis or intracellular programmed cell death [25,26]. The location of positively charged amino acids at loops or β-sheet regions has been reported to be useful for antifungal potentiality, suggesting that the interaction of positively charged Rs-AFP1 peptide with fungal pathogens might occur through electrostatic interfaces [27]. Some other reports focused on the structural assessments of plant defensins also recognized the significance of positively charged amino acid residues (located at the loop region) for antifungal activities, as well as working as a specificity factor against a range of pathogenic fungi [28]. Sagaram et al. [29] reported the presence of amino acid residues at the γ-core motif of MtDef4 as a crucial antifungal tool and specificity factor towards numerous pathogens. The mutagenesis studies of the RGFRRR region from MtDef4 revealed that the replacement of Arg and Phe at positions 4 and 3, respectively (positively charged hydrophobic residues), with Ala residues led to a significant deterioration of antifungal activity [29].

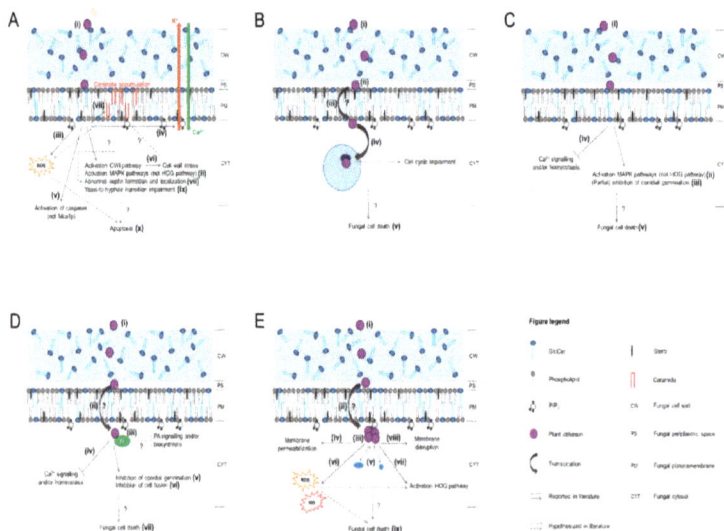

Figure 3. Schematic overview of the proposed mechanisms of action of the plant defensins. (**A**) RsAFP1 and RsAFP2; (**B**) Psd1; (**C**) MsDef1; (**D**) MtDef4; (**E**) NaD1. Reprinted from Vriens et al. [24], an open-access article distributed under the terms and conditions of the Creative Commons Attribution license (http://creativecommons.org/licenses/by/3.0/). Copyright (2014) the authors, Licensee MDPI, Basel, Switzerland.

5. Role of Defensins in Plant Defense

The protective role of defensin peptides in the protection of plants has been well described. Many reports have revealed that defensins are an essential component of the plant inherent immunity [30]. De Beer and Vivier [31] isolated four defensin genes (Hc-AFP1–4) with homology and clustered closest to defensins isolated from other Brassicaceae species. The same study also used propidium iodide assays to reveal the anti-fungal potential of all newly isolated defensin genes against *Botrytis cinerea*. A light microscopy analysis confirmed that the anti-fungal activity was related to an increase in membrane permeabilization (Figure 4) [31]. In summary, most of the plant defensins exhibited a constitutive expression pattern with upregulation following pathogens attacks, injuries, and abiotic stresses. Defensins are widely distributed and identified in flowers, tubers, leaves, pods, and seeds, where these peptides play a significant protective role during seed germination and seedling development [32]. Besides, plant defensins are also found in different tissues such as stomata, xylem, stomata, and parenchyma cells, and other peripheral regions [33]. Interestingly, plant defensins presented broad-spectrum antimicrobial activities, and some reports described the production of transgenic plants with the constitutive expression of foreign defensins. Therefore, these transgenic plants possess multiple biological potentialities, such as antibacterial, antifungal, and insecticidal activities, protein synthesis inhibition, inhibitors of digestive enzymes, and abiotic stress and heavy metal resistance [6,34]. Due to their potential biological activities, these defensins are categorized as promiscuous proteins. For instance, different homologous forms of a family of defensins isolated from *V. unguiculata* may present antibacterial and antifungal activities, as well as enzyme inhibition [35]. Though they display numerous biological activities, the antimicrobial role of plant defensins is predominantly noticed against a range of pathogenic fungi.

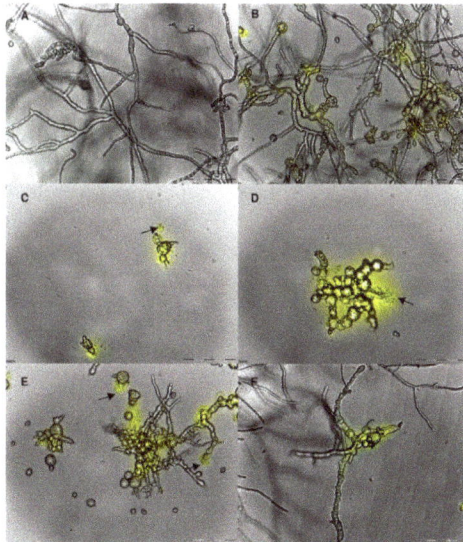

Figure 4. Combined overlay of the light microscopical analysis at 20× magnification and the cell permeabilization assay conducted on *B. cinerea* grown in the presence of Hc-AFPs for 48 h at 23 °C. (**A**) Control, (**B**) Hc-AFP1 25 µg/mL, (**C** and **D**) Hc-AFP2 15 µg/mL, (**E**) Hc-AFP3 25 µg/mL, (**F**) Hc-AFP4 18 µg/mL. The yellow fluorescence indicates a compromised membrane and the black arrows indicate structures that are leaking their cellular content into the surrounding medium. Adapted from De Beer and Vivier [31], an open-access article distributed under the terms of the Creative Commons Attribution License (http://creativecommons.org/licenses/by/2.0). Copyright (2011) the authors, licensee BioMed Central Ltd.

6. Peptides Involved in the Stress Response

Metal ions at higher concentrations are known to retard plant growth and development. Higher concentrations stimulate the generation of ROS such as free radicals, leading to oxidative stress. Plants exhibit defensive strategies such as cellular-free metal content (i.e., metal prohibition, cell wall binding, chelation, and sequestration), and governing cellular responses (i.e., anti-oxidative defense and the repair of stress-damaged proteins to cope with diverse types of these toxic metals) [36]. However, the synthesis of explicit chelators followed by metal complexes sequestration is of prime significance to restrict concentrations of free metals. As a key component of the metal-scavenging system, glutathione is a peptide that controls the metal ions uptake in response to ROS in plants due to its high affinity to metals [37]. The biosynthesis of glutathione (GSH) and its contribution in chelation–redox control are schematically shown in Figure 5 [37]. In addition, it acts as an important precursor of phytochelatins (PCs) that form complexes with heavy metals, which can then easily be accommodated into vacuoles. It has been observed that these PCs are effective in retaining high levels of metals in tobacco and other plants. These are also involved in the transport of metals. PCs are synthesized under specific conditions of plant growth and development. The activity of glutamylcysteine synthase, phytochelatin synthase, and serine acetyltransferase enzymes determine their synthesis and the binding capacity of metals to different sites [37].

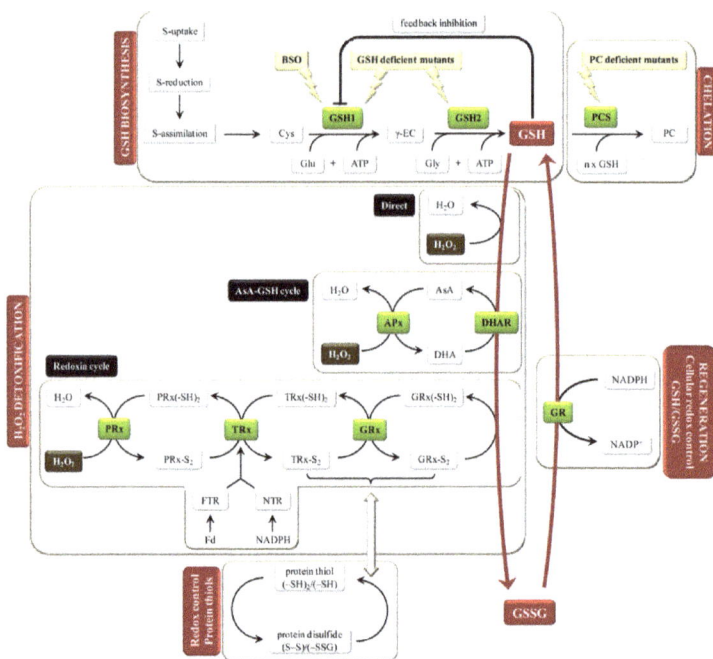

Figure 5. A schematic illustration of glutathione (GSH) biosynthesis and its involvement in chelation and redox control. Adapted from Jozefczak et al. [37], an open-access article distributed under the terms and conditions of the Creative Commons Attribution license (http://creativecommons.org/licenses/by/3.0/). Copyright (2012) the authors; licensee Molecular Diversity Preservation International, Basel, Switzerland.

7. Involvement of Peptides in Reproduction

SCR/SP11 (S locus cysteine-rich) is a peptide of 15 units. It consists of eight cysteine residues and its structure resembles that of defensins. Its structure is helpful in interaction with sigma kinase.

LAT52, a member of this family, is important in developing a connection between stigma and pollen, which enhances hydration and the sprouting of the pollen tube. Another type of peptide, LTPs, were found to exhibit the same function in pollen growth when studied in *Arabidopsis thaliana*. These are slightly larger at 70 units. Therefore, these are not subjected to proteolysis and secreted like other peptides. In *Liliumlongi florum*, peptide SCA (stigma/style cysteine-rich adhesin) is involved in the attachment of pollens. This peptide works in association with chemocyanin and exhibits chemotropic behavior towards the pollen tube. It is a plant cyanin, which contains Cu as a binder. A defensin named LURE, which has been found to contain this cysteine, acts in defense and reproduction in *Torenia fournieri* L. Here, this defensin functions as a chemoattractant for pollens. In maize, it is secreted by synergid cells and helps in the release of sperms from pollens. LURE contains disulfide bonds that assure attachment of egg with sperm. It is actively released upon the approach of sperms in the ovary. ZmTLA1 is a peptide found in maize. Its nature is hydrophobic and it acts as a proteolipid. It is present in protoplast and actively takes part in the maturation of pollens [38].

8. Biological Functionalities of Plant Defensins

Different plant defensins possess multiple biological functionalities due to the huge variations in amino acid sequences on the surface loops. Notable functions include antibacterial activity, the inhibition of protein formation, α-amylase and trypsin enzyme interference, heavy metals resistance, and plant growth, development, and sexual reproduction [7,39–42]. Among these functions, antifungal activity is the most common function and is a well-characterized function of plant defensins.

8.1. Plant Defensins—Antimicrobial Activity

In the early 1990s, Terras and colleagues [43] revealed that the antimicrobial activity of plant defensins was predominantly investigated against fungal pathogens. Nevertheless, some bacterial strains particularly belonging to the Gram-positive group were also detected to be suppressed by plant defensins, but the activity was less pronounced as compared to fungi. The growth of Gram-positive bacteria inhibited by plant defensins include *Bacillus subtilis*, *Bacillus cereus*, *Bacillus megaterium*, *Curtobacterium flaccumfaciens*, *Clavibacter michiganensis*, *Staphylococcus aureus*, *Staphylococcus epidermidis*, *Sarcina lutea*, and *Mycobacterium phlei*. Amongst the Gram-negative bacterial strains tried in inhibition bioassays were *Agrobacterium tumefaciens*, *Agrobacterium rhizogens*, *Agrobacterium radiobacter*, *Azospirillum brasilense*, *Alcaligenes eutrophus*, *Erwinia carotovora*, *Escherichia coli*, *Proteus vulgaris*, *Pseudomonas aeruginosa*, *Pseudomonas synrigae*, *Pseudomonas cichorii*, *Pseudomonas fluorescens*, *Pseudomonas lachrymans*, and *Salmonella typhimurium* [43–50]. Antibacterial activity is the most important characteristic of the vertebrate *trans*-defensins; however, it is less common in the *cis*-defensins family peptides from plants. In *trans*-defensins, disulfides orient in opposite directions and link to different secondary structure elements. Meanwhile, in *cis*-defensins, disulfides orient to the same cysteine-stabilized α-helix. Except for fabatins from the broad bean, *Vicia faba* has a profound inhibitory potential towards Gram-negative *Pseudomonas aeruginosa* and is moderately active against *Enterococcus hirae* and *Escherichia coli*. Notably, they have bacteria-specific activity, and thus exhibit no activity against *Candida albicans* or *Saccharomyces cerevisiae* [51]. In contrary, defensins from other *Fabaceae* members such as Ct-AMP1 from *Clitoria terna* and VaD1 from azuki bean are active against bacteria as well as fungal species [45]. As compared to lipid II binding by vertebrate defensins, plant defensins commonly carry out their antibacterial activity by binding to other lipids, i.e., phospholipids and fungus-specific sphingolipids [52,53]. Unlike bacteria, fungal pathogens are a more common risk faced by plants; this explains the prevalence of antifungal defensins over defensins with antibacterial activity. Several reports have shown the inhibition in growth of an array of fungal species by incubation with plant peptides. These strains and phytopathogens include *Aspergillus niger*, *Saccharomyces cerevisiae*, *Neurospora crassa*, *Alternaria solani*, *Alternaria brassicola*, *Cladosporium sphaerospermum*, *Fusarium oxysporum*, *Cladosporium colocasiae*, *Colletotrichum lindemuthianum*, *Fusarium decemcellulare*, *Fusarium culmorum*, *Fusarium graminearum*, *Fusarium verticillioides*, *Nectria haematococca*, *Penicillium expansum*,

Penicillium digitatum, Rhizoctonia solani, Septoria tritici, Trichoderma viride, Verticilium alboatrum, and *Verticillium dahliae* [45,54–60]. The suppressive activity and required concentration of defensin for inhibition varies and depends on specific fungal pathogens and the plant defensin. Some potential antimicrobial mechanisms of plant defensin-based AMPs or host defense peptides (HDPs) are shown in Figure 6.

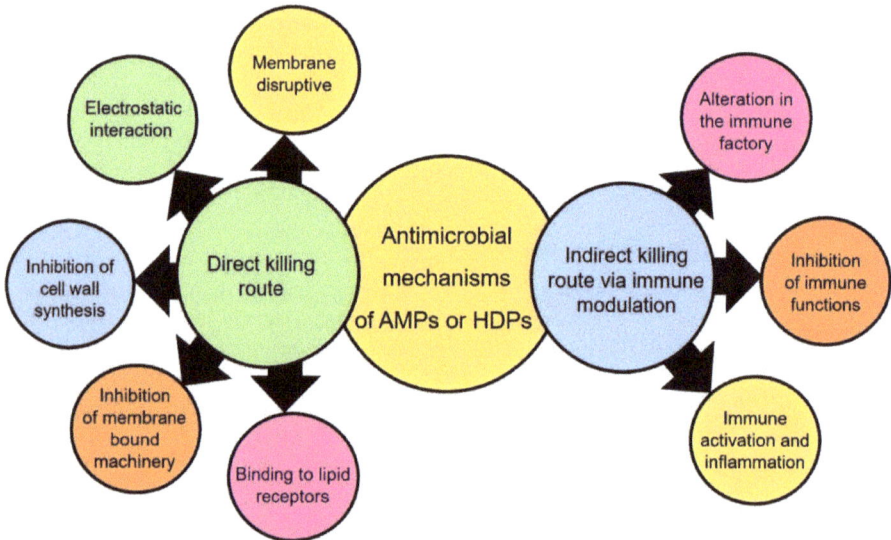

Figure 6. Potential antimicrobial mechanisms of plant defense-based antimicrobial peptides (AMPs) or host defense peptides HDPs.

8.2. Plant Defensins—Anticancer Activity

Cancer is one of the prevalent causes of worldwide mortality, with approximately 8.2 million deaths in 2012 [61]. In spite of progress made in cancer treatment, conventional chemotherapy presents the serious disadvantage of broad-spectrum toxicity. The use of AMPs appeared as a unique and alternative family of anticancer agents to overcome the drawbacks of chemotherapeutic drugs [62,63]. Defensin-like peptides and plant defensins, in addition to their antimicrobial activities, also possess potential anticancer and cytotoxicity effects [63]. Wong and Ng [64] reported the first plant defensin, sesquin from *Vigna sesquipedalis*, which showed anticancer activity and repressed the growth of leukemia M1 and MCF-7 cell lines. Later on, the same research group found a limenin defensin from *Phaseolus limensis* that caused 30% and 60% proliferation inhibition of L1210 and M1 leukemia cells, respectively [65]. Lunatusin, another anticancer defensin obtained from *Phaseolus lunatus* seeds, suppressed the propagation of MCF-7 cancer cell lines. However, the cell-free inhibitory activity of lunatusin in the reticulocytes system of rabbit indicates its cytotoxicity towards normal cell types and tissues [66]. Subsequently, many reports have identified a number of different plant defensins with great potential to inhibit the multiplication of colon and breast cancer cell lines without exhibiting any cytotoxic effects on normal types. For example, Lin and colleagues [67] identified a defensin from *Phaseolus vulgaris* that potentially suppressed the growth of various cancer cells such as MCF-7, HepG2, HT-29, and Sila without affecting human erythrocytes or embryonic liver cells under the identical conditions. The proliferation of L1210 and HL60 cells was inhibited by a coccinin defensin peptide from *Phaseolus coccineus*, but it did not exhibit any cytotoxic influence on the propagation of mouse spleen cells [68]. Likewise, *Phaseolus coccineus*-derived phaseococcin possessed profound inhibitory activity against L1210 and HL60 cells without affecting the normal proliferation of rabbit reticulocytes or mouse splenocytes [69]. Without any effect on immortalized bovine endothelial cells, the complete inhibition of HeLa cells viability was achieved by γ-thionin defensin from *Capsicum chinense* [70]. Generally, the mechanism of anticancer activity of plant defensins is poorly elucidated. Though a study by Lobo et al. [71] unveiled the only mechanism of action speculated to date, experimental studies are still necessary for further corroboration. Indeed, antimicrobial peptides have been found to possess an amphipathic three-dimensional structural organization, with one positively charged hydrophilic face and another hydrophobic portion of the molecule. Notably, these charged faces of the plant defensin molecules constitute an initial electrostatic binding with structures of opposite charge on the surface of the pathogenic microorganisms [34]. This speculation is substantiated by charged structures on the surface of microorganisms/mammalian cells and charged amino acids [72–74]. The hydrophobic portion following the initial binding is moved near the cell membrane, resulting in the lysis of the membrane. In contrast to normal cells, mammalian cancer cells exhibit a greater negative surface charge because of their high transmembrane potential and the aberrant expression of sialic acid. As a result, these cancer cells have an electrophoretic influence on antimicrobial peptides and thus attract them towards the membrane [75,76]. The interaction between defensing peptides and cancer cells presenting abnormal sphingolipids related to tumor development is another alternative mechanism of action, but lacks practical validation [34].

9. Concluding Remarks and Future Prospects

Increasing pathogen resistance to conventional antibiotics and inadequate health treatment options have intensified the development of new treatment approaches to overcome these challenges. In these scenarios, cationic plant peptides are very important for many biotechnological and medicinal purposes owing to their broad-spectrum biological activities. These plant defensins can also be produced in the eukaryotic host by heterologous expression due to non-toxic effects to mammalian cells. Notably, these defensin peptides from many plants such as *Abutilon indicum* can be used to treat many kinds of infectious diseases such as tuberculosis, piles, and liver disorders. Moreover, they can also be used to cure a variety of cancers. In addition, antifungal defensin-based agro-bioproducts are expected to be targeted as an essential means to improve crop productivity in the near future. Given the accelerated development of peptide libraries, bioinformatics, proteomics, and agriculture biotechnology strategies, these plant defensins could emerge as novel antimicrobial or anticancer drugs for a myriad of medical applications.

Author Contributions: Conceptualization, M.B. and H.M.N.I.; Literature Review, N.I. and M.B.; Writing—Original Draft Preparation, N.I.; Editing, M.B. and H.M.N.I.; Submission and Correspondence, M.B. and H.M.N.I.; APC Funding Acquisition, H.M.N.I.

Funding: This research received no external funding. The APC (ID: medicines-448499) was funded by MDPI, St. Alban-Anlage 66, 4052 Basel, Switzerland.

Acknowledgments: The literature facilities provided by the representative institutes/universities are gratefully acknowledged.

Conflicts of Interest: The authors declare no conflict of interest.

References

1. Gachomo, E.W.; Seufferheld, M.J.; Kotchoni, S.O. Melanization of appressoria is critical for the pathogenicity of *Diplocarpon rosae*. *Mol. Biol. Rep.* **2010**, *37*, 3583–3591. [CrossRef] [PubMed]
2. Van Loon, L.C.; Rep, M.; Pieterse, C.M.J. Significance of inducible defense-related proteins in infected plants. *Ann. Rev. Phytopathol.* **2006**, *44*, 135–162. [CrossRef]
3. Lacerda, A.; Vasconcelos, É.A.R.; Pelegrini, P.B.; Grossi-de-Sa, M.F. Antifungal defensins and their role in plant defense. *Front. Microbial.* **2014**, *5*, 116. [CrossRef]
4. Zhu, S.; Gao, B.; Tytgat, J. Phylogenetic distribution, functional epitopes and evolution of the CSab superfamily. *Cell Mol. Life Sci.* **2005**, *62*, 2257–2269. [CrossRef]
5. Thomma, B.P.; Cammue, B.P.; Thevissen, K. Plant defensins. *Planta* **2002**, *216*, 193–202. [CrossRef] [PubMed]

6.	de Carvalho, A.O.; Gomes, V.M. Plant defensins—Prospects for the biological functions and biotechnological properties. *Peptides* **2009**, *30*, 1007–1020. [CrossRef]

7.	Colilla, F.J.; Rocher, A.; Mendez, E. gamma-purothionins: Amino acid sequence of two polypeptides of a new family of thionins from wheat endosperm. *FEBS Lett.* **1990**, *270*, 191–194. [CrossRef]

8.	Mendez, E.; Moreno, A.; Colilla, F.; Pelaez, F.; Limas, G.G.; Mendez, R.; Soriano, F.; Salinas, M.; de Haro, C. Primary structure and inhibition of protein synthesis in eukaryotic cell-free system of a novel thionin, g-hordothionin, from barley endosperm. *Eur. J. Biochem.* **1990**, *194*, 533–539. [CrossRef] [PubMed]

9.	Pelegrini, P.B.; Franco, O.L. Plant g-thionins: Novel sinsites on the mechanisms of actions of a multi-functional class of defense proteins. *Int. J. Biochem. Cell Biol.* **2005**, *37*, 2239–2253. [CrossRef]

10.	Bruix, M.; Gonzalez, C.; Santoro, J.; Soriano, F.; Rocher, A.; Mendez, E.; Rico, M. 1H-NMR studies on the structure of a new thionin from barley endosperm. *Biopolymers* **1995**, *36*, 751–763. [CrossRef]

11.	Broekaert, W.F.; Terras, F.R.G.; Cammue, B.P.A.; Osborn, R.W. Plant Defensins—Novel antimicrobial peptides as components of the host-defense system. *Plant Physiol.* **1995**, *108*, 1353–1358. [CrossRef] [PubMed]

12.	Cociancich, S.; Goyffon, M.; Bontems, F.; Bulet, P.; Bouet, F.; Menez, A.; Hoffmann, J. Purification and characterization of a scorpion defensin, a 4 kDa antibacterial peptide presenting structural similarities with insect defensis and scorpion toxins. *Biochem. Biophys. Res. Commun.* **1993**, *194*, 17–22. [CrossRef] [PubMed]

13.	Saito, T.; Kawabata, S.; Shigenaga, T.; Takayenoki, Y.; Cho, J.; Nakajima, H.; Hirat, M.; Iwanaga, S. A novel big defensin identified in horseshoe crab hemocytes: Isolation, amino acid sequence, and antibacterial activity. *J. Biochem.* **1995**, *117*, 1131–1137. [CrossRef]

14.	Charlet, M.; Chernysh, S.; Philippe, H.; Hetru, C.; Hoffmann, J.A.; Bulet, P. Isolation of several cysteine-rich antimicrobial peptides from the blood of a mollusc, *Mytilus edulis*. *J. Biol. Chem.* **1996**, *271*, 21808–21813. [CrossRef] [PubMed]

15.	Mygind, P.H.; Fischer, R.L.; Schnorr, K.M.; Hansen, M.T.; So¨nksen, C.P.; Ludvigsen, S.; Raventós, D.; Buskov, S.; Christensen, B.; De Maria, L.; et al. Plectasin is a peptide antibiotic with therapeutic potential from a saprophytic fungus. *Nature* **2005**, *437*, 975–980. [CrossRef]

16.	Zou, J.; Mercier, C.; Koussounadis, A.; Secombes, C. Discovery of multiple beta defensing like homologues in teleost fish. *Mol. Immunol.* **2007**, *44*, 638–647. [CrossRef]

17.	Sugiarto, H.; Yu, P.-L. Avian antimicrobial peptides: The defense role of bdefensins. *Biochem. Biophys. Res. Commun.* **2004**, *323*, 721–727. [CrossRef]

18.	Zhu, S. Evidence for myxobacterial origin of eukaryotic defensins. *Immunogenetics* **2007**, *59*, 949–954. [CrossRef] [PubMed]

19.	Zhu, S. Discovery of six families of fungal defensin-like peptides provides insights into origin and evolution of the CSab defensins. *Mol. Immunol.* **2008**, *45*, 828–838. [CrossRef]

20.	Lay, F.T.; Anderson, M.A. Defensins–components of the innate immune system in plants. *Curr. Protein Pept. Sci.* **2005**, *6*, 85–101. [CrossRef]

21.	Janssen, B.J.C.; Schirra, H.J.; Lay, F.T.; Anderson, M.A.; Craik, D.J. Structure of Petunia hybrid defensing 1, a novel plant defensen with five disulfide bonds. *Biochemistry* **2003**, *42*, 8214–8222. [CrossRef] [PubMed]

22.	De Coninck, B.; Cammue, B.P.A.; Thevissen, K. Modes of antifungal action and in planta functions of plant defensins and defensin-like peptides. *Fungal Biol. Rev.* **2013**, *26*, 109–120. [CrossRef]

23.	Vander Weerden, N.; Anderson, M.A. Plant defensins: Commons fold, multiple functions. *Fungal Biol. Rev.* **2013**, *26*, 121–131. [CrossRef]

24.	Vriens, K.; Cammue, B.; Thevissen, K. Antifungal plant defensins: Mechanisms of action and production. *Molecules* **2014**, *19*, 12280–12303. [CrossRef]

25.	Hegedus, N.; Marx, F. Antifungal proteins: More than antimicrobials? *Fungal Biol. Rev.* **2013**, *26*, 132–145. [CrossRef]

26.	Wilmes, M.; Cammuer, B.P.A.; Sahl, H.-G.; Thevisse, K. Antibiotic activities of host defense peptides: More to it than lipid bilayer perturbation. *Nat. Prod. Rep.* **2011**, *28*, 1350–1358. [CrossRef] [PubMed]

27.	Fant, F.; Vranken, W.; Broekaert, W.; Borremans, F. Determination of the three-dimensional solution structure of *Raphanus sativus* antifungal protein 1 by 1HNMR. *J. Mol. Biol.* **1998**, *279*, 257–270. [CrossRef]

28.	Lay, F.T.; Schirra, H.J.; Scalon, M.J.; Anderson, M.A.; Craik, D.J. The three-dimensional solution structure of NaD1, a new floral defensin from *Nicotiana alata* and its application to a homology model of the crop defense protein alfAFP. *J. Mol. Biol.* **2003**, *325*, 175–188. [CrossRef]

29. Sagaram, U.S.; Pandurangi, R.; Karu, J.; Smith, T.J.; Shah, D.M. Structure-activity determinants in antifungal plant defensins MsDef1 and MtDef4 with different modes of action against *Fusarium graminearum*. *PLoS ONE* **2011**, *6*, e18550. [CrossRef] [PubMed]

30. Selitrennikoff, C.P. Antifungal proteins. *App. Environ. Microbiol.* **2001**, *67*, 2883–2894. [CrossRef]

31. de Beer, A.; Vivier, M.A. Four plant defensins from an indigenous South African *Brassicaceae* species display divergent activities against two test pathogens despite high sequence similarity in the encoding genes. *BMC Res. Notes* **2011**, *4*, 459. [CrossRef] [PubMed]

32. Garcia-Olmedo, F.; Molina, A.; Alamillo, J.M.; Rodriguez-Palenzuela, P. Plant defense peptides. *Biopolymers* **1998**, *47*, 479–491. [CrossRef]

33. Chen, K.-C.; Lin, C.-Y.; Chung, M.-C.; Kuan, C.C.; Sung, H.Y.; Tsou, S.C.S.; Kuo, G.; Chen, C.-S. Cloning and characterization of a cDNA encoding an antimicrobial protein from mung bean seeds. *Bot. Bull. Acad. Sin.* **2002**, *43*, 251–259.

34. de Oliveira Carvalho, A.; Moreira Gomes, V. Plant defensins and defensin-like peptides-biological activities and biotechnological applications. *Curr. Pharm. Des.* **2011**, *7*, 4270–4293. [CrossRef]

35. Franco, O.L. Peptide promiscuity: An evolutionary concept for plant defense. *FEBS Lett.* **2011**, *585*, 995–1000. [CrossRef] [PubMed]

36. Hall, J.L. Cellular mechanisms for heavy metal detoxification and tolerance. *J. Exp. Bot.* **2002**, *53*, 1–11. [CrossRef] [PubMed]

37. Jozefczak, M.; Remans, T.; Vangronsveld, J.; Cuypers, A. Glutathione is a key player in metal-induced oxidative stress defenses. *Int. J. Mol. Sci.* **2012**, *13*, 3145–3175. [CrossRef] [PubMed]

38. Yount, N.Y.; Yeaman, M.R. Multidimensional signatures in antimicrobial peptides. *Proc. Natl. Acad. Sci. USA* **2004**, *101*, 7363–7368. [CrossRef]

39. Méndez, E.; Rocher, A.; Calero, M.; Girbés, T.; Citores, L.; Soriano, F. Primary structure of omega-hordothionin, a member of a novel family of thionins from barley endosperm, and its inhibition of protein synthesis in eukaryotic and prokaryotic cell-free systems. *Eur. J. Biochem.* **1996**, *239*, 67–73. [CrossRef]

40. Mirouze, M.; Sels, J.; Richard, O.; Czernic, P.; Loubet, S.; Jacquier, A.; François, I.E.; Cammue, B.; Lebrun, M.; Berthomieu, P. A putative novel role for plantd efensins: A defensin from the zinc hyper-accumulating plant, Arabidopsis halleri, confers zinc tolerance. *Plant J.* **2006**, *47*, 329–342. [CrossRef]

41. Ferreira, R.B.; Monteiro, S.A.R.A.; Freitas, R.; Santos, C.N.; Chen, Z.; Batista, L.M.; Teixeira, A.R. The role of plant defence proteins in fungal pathogenesis. *Mol. Plant Pathol.* **2007**, *8*, 677–700. [CrossRef] [PubMed]

42. Parisi, K.; Shafee, T.M.; Quimbar, P.; van der Weerden, N.L.; Bleackley, M.R.; Anderson, M.A. The evolution, function and mechanisms of action for plant defensins. *Semin. Cell. Dev. Biol.* **2018**, in press. [CrossRef] [PubMed]

43. Terras, F.R.G.; Schoofs, H.M.E.; De Bolle, M.F.C.; Van Leuven, F.; Rees, S.B.; Vanderleyden, J.; Cammue, B.P.; Broekaert, W.F. Analysis of two novel classes of plant antifungal proteins from radish (*Raphanus sativus* L.) seeds. *J. Biol. Chem.* **1992**, *267*, 15301–15309. [PubMed]

44. Fujimuram, M.; Ideguchi, M.; Minami, Y.; Watanabe, K.; Tadera, K. Purification, characterization and sequencing of novel antimicrobial peptides Tu-AMP1 and Tu-AMP2 from bulbs of tulip (*Tulipa gesneriana* L.). *Biosci. Biotechnol. Biochem.* **2004**, *68*, 571–577. [CrossRef] [PubMed]

45. Chen, G.-H.; Hsu, M.-P.; Tan, C.-H.; Sung, H.-Y.; Kuo, C.G.; Fan, M.-J.; Chen, H.-M.; Chen, S.; Chen, C.-S. Cloning and characterization of a plant defensin VaD1 from azuki bean. *J. Agric. Food Chem.* **2005**, *53*, 982–988. [CrossRef] [PubMed]

46. Wong, J.H.; Ng, T.B. Vulgarinin, a broad-spectrum antifungal peptide from haricot beans (*Phaseolus vulgaris*). *IJBCB* **2005**, *37*, 1626–1632. [CrossRef] [PubMed]

47. Franco, O.L.; Murad, A.M.; Leite, J.R.; Mendes, P.A.M.; Prates, M.V.; Bloch, C., Jr. Identification of a cowpea g-thionin with bactericidal activity. *FEBS J.* **2006**, *273*, 3489–3497. [CrossRef] [PubMed]

48. Wong, J.H.; Zhang, X.Q.; Wang, H.X.; Ng, T.B. Amitogenic defensin from white cloud beans (*Phaseolus vulgaris*). *Peptides* **2006**, *27*, 2075–2081. [CrossRef] [PubMed]

49. Huang, G.-J.; Lai, H.-C.; Chang, Y.-S.; Sheu, M.-J.; Lu, T.-L.; Huang, S.-S.; Lin, Y.H. Antimicrobial, dehydroascorbate reductase, and monodehydroascorbate reductase activities of defensin from sweet potato [Ipomoea batatas (L.) Lam. 'tainong 57'] storage roots. *J. Agric. Food Chem.* **2008**, *56*, 2989–2995. [CrossRef]

50. van der Weerden, N.L.; Lay, F.T.; Anderson, M.A. The plant defensin, NaD1, enters the cytoplasm of *Fusarium oxysporum* hyphae. *J. Biol. Chem.* **2008**, *283*, 14445–14452. [CrossRef]

51. Zhang, Y.; Lewis, K. Fabatins: New antimicrobial plant peptides. *FEMS Microbiol. Lett.* **1997**, *149*, 59–64.

52. Thevissen, K.; Cammue, B.P.A.; Lemaire, K.; Winderickx, J.; Dickson, R.C.; Lester, R.L.; Ferket, K.K.A.; Van Even, F.; Parret, A.H.A.; Broekaert, W.F. A gene-encoding sphingolipid biosynthesis enzyme determines the sensitivity of *Saccharomyces cerevisiae* to an antifungal plant defensin from dahlia (*Dahlia merckii*). *Proc. Natl. Acad. Sci. USA* **2000**, *97*, 9531–9536. [CrossRef] [PubMed]

53. Poon, I.K.; Baxter, A.A.; Lay, F.T.; Mills, G.D.; Adda, C.G.; Payne, J.A.; Phan, T.K.; Ryan, G.F.; White, J.A.; Veneer, P.K. Phosphoinositide-mediated oligomerization of a defensin induces cell lysis. *Elife* **2014**, *3*, e01808. [CrossRef] [PubMed]

54. Park, H.C.; Kang, Y.H.; Chun, H.J.; Koo, J.C.; Cheong, Y.H.; Kim, C.Y.; Kim, M.C.; Chuang, W.S.; Kim, J.C.; Yoo, J.H.; et al. Characterization of a stamen-specific cDNA encoding a novel plant defensin in Chinese cabbage. *Plant Mol. Biol.* **2002**, *50*, 59–69. [CrossRef] [PubMed]

55. Ye, X.Y.; Ng, T.B. A new antifungal peptide from rice beans. *J. Peptide Res.* **2002**, *60*, 81–87. [CrossRef]

56. Wisniewski, M.E.; Bassett, C.L.; Artlip, T.S.; Webb, R.P.; Janisiewicz, W.J.; Norelli, J.L.; Goldway, M.; Droby, S. Characterization of a defensin in bark and fruit tissues of peach and antimicrobial activity of a recombinant defensin in the yeast, Pichia pastoris. *Physiol. Plant* **2003**, *119*, 563–572. [CrossRef]

57. Vriens, K.; Peigneur, S.; De Coninck, B.; Tytgat, J.; Cammue, B.P.; Thevissen, K. The antifungal plant defensin AtPDF2. 3 from Arabidopsis thaliana blocks potassium channels. *Sci. Rep.* **2016**, *6*, 32121. [CrossRef]

58. Olli, S.; Kirti, P.B. Cloning, characterization and antifungal activity of defensing Tfgd1 from *Trigonella foenum-graecum* L. *J. Biochem. Mol. Biol.* **2006**, *39*, 278–283.

59. Solis, J.; Medrano, G.; Ghislain, M. Inhibitory effect of a defensin gene from the Andean crop maca (*Lepidium meyenii*) against Phytophthora infestans. *J. Plant Physiol.* **2007**, *164*, 1071–1082. [CrossRef]

60. Finkina, E.I.; Shramova, E.I.; Tagaev, A.A.; Ovchinnikova, T.V. A novel defensin from the lentil Lens culinaris seeds. *Biochem. Biophys. Res. Commun.* **2008**, *371*, 860–865. [CrossRef]

61. Ferlay, J.; Soerjomataram, I.; Dikshit, R.; Eser, S.; Mathers, C.; Rebelo, M.; Parkin, D.M.; Forman, D.; Bray, F. Cancer incidence and mortality worldwide: Sources, methods and major patterns in GLOBOCAN 2012. *Int. J. Cancer* **2015**, *136*, E359–E386. [CrossRef] [PubMed]

62. Al-Benna, S.; Shai, Y.; Jacobsen, F.; Steinstraesser, L. Oncolytic activities of host defense peptides. *Int. J. Mol. Sci.* **2011**, *12*, 8027–8051. [CrossRef] [PubMed]

63. Guzmán-Rodríguez, J.J.; Ochoa-Zarzosa, A.; López-Gómez, R.; López-Meza, J.E. Plant antimicrobial peptides as potential anticancer agents. *BioMed Res. Int.* **2015**. [CrossRef] [PubMed]

64. Wong, J.H.; Ng, T.B. Sesquin, a potent defensin-like antimicrobial peptide from ground beans with inhibitory activities toward tumor cells and HIV-1 reverse transcriptase. *Peptide* **2005**, *26*, 1120–1126. [CrossRef] [PubMed]

65. Wong, J.H.; Ng, T.B. Limenin, a defensin-like peptide with multiple exploitable activities from shelf beans. *J. Peptide Sci.* **2006**, *12*, 341–346. [CrossRef]

66. Wong, J.H.; Ng, T.B. Lunatusin, a trypsin-stable antimicrobial peptide from Lima beans (*Phaseolus lunatus* L.). *Peptides* **2005**, *26*, 2086–2092. [CrossRef] [PubMed]

67. Lin, P.; Wong, J.H.; Ng, T.B. A defensin with highly potent antipathogenic activities from the seeds of purple pole bean. *Biosci. Rep.* **2010**, *30*, 101–109. [CrossRef] [PubMed]

68. Ngai, P.H.K.; Ng, T.B. Coccinin, an antifungal peptide with antiproliferative and HIV-1 reverse transcriptase inhibitory activities from large scarlet runner beans. *Peptides* **2004**, *25*, 2063–2068. [CrossRef]

69. Ngai, P.H.K.; Ng, T.B. Phaseococcin, an antifungal protein with antiproliferative and anti-HIV-1 reverse transcriptase activities from small scarlet runner beans. *Biochem. Cell Biol.* **2005**, *83*, 212–220. [CrossRef]

70. Anaya-Lopez, J.L.; Lopez-Meza, J.E.; Baizabal-Aguirre, V.M.; Cano-Camacho, H.; Ochoa-Zarzosa, A. Fungicidal and cytotoxic activity of a *Capsicum chinense* defensin expressed by endothelial cells. *Biotechnol. Lett.* **2006**, *28*, 1101–1108. [CrossRef]

71. Lobo, D.S.; Pereira, I.B.; Fragel-Madeira, L.; Medeiros, L.N.; Cabral, L.M.; Faria, J.; Bellio, M.; Campos, R.C.; Linden, R.; Kurtenbach, E. Antifungal *Pisum sativum* defensin 1 interacts with *Neurospora crassa* cyclin F related to the cell cycle. *Biochemistry* **2007**, *46*, 987–996. [CrossRef] [PubMed]

72. Almeida, M.S.; Cabral, K.M.S.; Kurtenbach, E.; Almeida, F.C.L.; Valente, A.P. Solution structure of *Pisum sativum* defensin 1 by high resolution NMR: Plant defensins, identical backbone with different mechanisms of action. *J. Mol. Biol.* **2002**, *315*, 749–757. [CrossRef] [PubMed]

73. Monk, B.C.; Harding, D.R.K. Peptides motifs for cell-surface intervention. *Biodrugs* **2005**, *19*, 261–278. [CrossRef] [PubMed]

74. Liu, Y.-J.; Cheng, C.-S.; Lai, S.-M.; Hsu, M.-P.; Chen, C.-S.; Lyu, P.-C. Solution structure of the plant defensin *Vr*D1 from mung bean and its possible role in insecticidal activity against bruchids. *Proteins* **2006**, *63*, 777–786. [CrossRef] [PubMed]

75. Dobrzyska, I.; Szachowicz-Petelska, B.; Sulkowski, S.; Figaszewski, Z. Changes in electric charge and phospholipids composition in human colorectal cancer cells. *Mol. Cell Biochem.* **2005**, *276*, 113–119. [CrossRef] [PubMed]

76. Fuster, M.M.; Esko, J.D. The sweet and sour of cancer: Glycans as novel therapeutic targets. *Nat. Rev. Cancer* **2005**, *5*, 526–542. [CrossRef]

medicines

MDPI

Review

Cannabis and Its Secondary Metabolites: Their Use as Therapeutic Drugs, Toxicological Aspects, and Analytical Determination

Joana Gonçalves [1,†], Tiago Rosado [1,†], Sofia Soares [1,†], Ana Y. Simão [1,†], Débora Caramelo [1,†], Ângelo Luís [1,†], Nicolás Fernández [2,†], Mário Barroso [3], Eugenia Gallardo [1] and Ana Paula Duarte [1,*]

[1] Centro de Investigação em Ciências da Saúde, Faculdade de Ciências da Saúde da Universidade da Beira Interior (CICS-UBI), 6200-506 Covilhã, Portugal; janitagoncalves@hotmail.com (J.G.); tiagorosadofful@hotmail.com (T.R.); sofia_soares_26@hotmail.com (S.S.); anaaysa95@gmail.com (A.Y.S.); deboracaramela50@gmail.com (D.C.); afluis27@gmail.com (Â.L.); egallardo@fcsaude.ubi.pt (E.G.)

[2] Universidad de Buenos Aires, Facultad de Farmacia y Bioquímica, Cátedra de Toxicología y Química Legal, Laboratorio de Asesoramiento Toxicológico Analítico (CENATOXA). Junín 956 7mo piso. Ciudad Autónoma de Buenos Aires (CABA), Buenos Aires C1113AAD, Argentina; nfernandez@ffyb.uba.ar

[3] Serviço de Química e Toxicologia Forenses, Instituto de Medicina Legal e Ciências Forenses - Delegação do Sul, 1169-201 Lisboa, Portugal; mario.j.barroso@inmlcf.mj.pt

*   Correspondence: apduarte@fcsaude.ubi.pt; Tel.: +35-127-532-9002

†   These authors contributed equally to this work.

Received: 31 January 2019; Accepted: 18 February 2019; Published: 23 February 2019

Abstract: Although the medicinal properties of *Cannabis* species have been known for centuries, the interest on its main active secondary metabolites as therapeutic alternatives for several pathologies has grown in recent years. This potential use has been a revolution worldwide concerning public health, production, use and sale of cannabis, and has led inclusively to legislation changes in some countries. The scientific advances and concerns of the scientific community have allowed a better understanding of cannabis derivatives as pharmacological options in several conditions, such as appetite stimulation, pain treatment, skin pathologies, anticonvulsant therapy, neurodegenerative diseases, and infectious diseases. However, there is some controversy regarding the legal and ethical implications of their use and routes of administration, also concerning the adverse health consequences and deaths attributed to marijuana consumption, and these represent some of the complexities associated with the use of these compounds as therapeutic drugs. This review comprehends the main secondary metabolites of *Cannabis*, approaching their therapeutic potential and applications, as well as their potential risks, in order to differentiate the consumption as recreational drugs. There will be also a focus on the analytical methodologies for their analysis, in order to aid health professionals and toxicologists in cases where these compounds are present.

Keywords: cannabis; cannabinoids; therapeutics; toxicology; analytical determination; legalization

1. Introduction

The secondary metabolism of plants plays an important role in their survival in its environment. Secondary metabolites are able to attract pollinators, to defend plants against predators and diseases, and for that reason have been exploited for biopharmaceutical purposes. The secondary metabolites are also present in great amounts in the so-called food plants, conferring them taste, color, and scent. Moreover, numerous plant secondary metabolites such as alkaloids, anthocyanins, flavonoids, quinones, lignans, steroids, and terpenoids have found commercial applications, namely as drugs, dye, flavor, fragrance, and insecticides [1].

Cannabis sativa L. (*Cannabinaceae*), also known as marijuana or hemp, belongs to a group of herbaceous shrubs 1 to 2 m in height, and is widely distributed in temperate and tropical areas. Three species are usually recognized: *Cannabis sativa*, *Cannabis indica*, and *Cannabis ruderalis* (the latter may be included under *C. sativa*), and all may be treated as subspecies of a single species, *C. sativa*. The plant is accepted as being native from Central Asia. Several preparations of *C. sativa* including marijuana, hashish, charas, dagga, and bhang, are estimated to be consumed by 200–300 million people around the world [2], being the most popular illicit drug of the 21st century according to the United Nation Office on Drugs and Crime (UNODC) [3].

Cannabis has been cultivated widely in the world for its achene fruits (often wrongly referred to as seeds), which are rich in oils and other phytonutrients, and are frequently used as human food or animal feedstuff, as well as for its fibers, for traditional medicine and spiritual purposes as therapeutic and hallucinogenic drug [2,4]. *Cannabis* is one of the most consumed drugs worldwide, together with legal drugs such as tobacco, alcohol, and caffeine.

Cannabis plants contain more than 545 known compounds. In addition to phytocannabinoids (which are C_{21} terpenophenolic, or C_{22} for the carboxylated forms, compounds with physiological and often psychotogenic effects, possessing monoterpene and alkylresorcinol moieties in their molecules [4–6]), they include alkanes, sugars, nitrogenous compounds (such as spermidine alkaloids or muscarine), flavonoids, non-cannabinoid phenols, phenylpropanoids, steroids, fatty acids, approximately 140 different terpenes that are predominantly monoterpenes such as β-myrcene, α- and β-pinene, α-terpinolene, but also sesquiterpenes including β-caryophyllene, di- and triterpenes, as well as various other common compounds [4,5].

Out of over 100 cannabinoids identified so far, the most potent in terms of psychoactive activity is *trans*-Δ-9-tetrahydrocannabinol (THC) [7]. Four stereoisomers of THC exist, but only the (−)-trans isomer occurs naturally. Two structurally related substances (Δ9-tetrahydrocannabinol-2-oic acid and Δ9-tetrahydrocannabinol-4-oic acid - THCA) are usually also present, sometimes in large amounts. The heat of combustion during smoking converts partly THCA to THC. One isomer which is also active (Δ8-THC) occurs in much smaller amounts. Other related compounds include cannabidiol (CBD) and cannabinol (CBN), the latter particularly in aged samples, and presenting pharmacological effects different than those attributed to THC (Figure 1). All these compounds are collectively known as cannabinoids and, unlike many other psychoactive substances, are not nitrogenous bases [8]. Individual cannabinoids are being developed and identified in *Cannabis* strains, and their effects on symptoms of illnesses suffered by patients are being studied. The main types of natural cannabinoids belong to the families of the cannabigerol-type, cannabichromene-type, cannabidiol-type, cannabinodiol-type, tetrahydrocannabinol-type, cannabinol-type, cannabitriol-type, cannabielsoin-type, isocannabinoids, cannabicyclol-type, cannabicitran-type, and cannabichromanone-type [9].

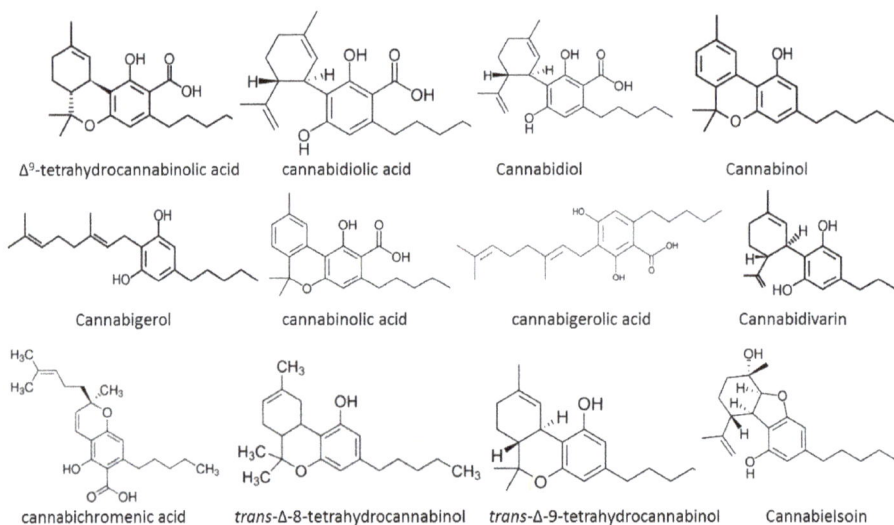

Figure 1. Some natural cannabinoids from the cannabis plant.

THC has been used as an anti-vomiting drug in cancer chemotherapy and as an appetite stimulant, especially for AIDS patients [2]. On the other hand, CBD, the isomer of THC, has no psychotropic effect. However, it possesses a variety of other pharmacological activities [2], namely, it reduces aggressive behavior in the L-pyroglutamate-treated rat, spontaneous dyskinesias in the dystonic rat, and turning behavior in the 6-hydroxyldopamine-treated rat caused by apomorphine [2]. Cannabichromene and related compounds possess anti-inflammatory, anti-fungal, and anti-microbial activities [2]. Therefore, cannabinoids are considered to be promising agents for the treatment of several types of diseases [2].

Based on the content of the psychoactive constituent THC, the chemotypes of *C. sativa* include the drug type (marijuana, 1.0–20% THC), intermediate type (0.3–1.0% THC), and fiber type (hemp, <0.3% THC) [10,11]. The drug type is regarded as an illicit drug of abuse and its cultivation is prohibited in most nations due to the psychotropic effect [10]. While the fiber type (hemp), cultivated as a source of textiles and food, is legal in several countries [10].

Cannabinoids are synthesized and stored predominantly in glandular trichomes, hair-like epidermal protrusions densely concentrated in the bracts and flowers of cannabis plants [12]. Various strategies have been pursued to extract and deliver the pharmacological agents from cannabis. The use of chemical solvents such as petroleum ether or ethanol are likely to leave unwanted residues, whereas extractants such as olive or coconut oil provide a more organic alternative [12].

The therapeutic potential and applications of those compounds, as well as their potential risks, in order to differentiate from recreational consumption will be discussed below. In addition, a focus on the analytical methodologies for their analysis will be presented.

2. Modes of Use in Recreational and Therapeutic Situations, Pharmacokinetics, and Pharmacodynamics

Despite the increasing interest that cannabinoids have aroused, their pharmacokinetics and pharmacodynamics are not yet fully understood, limiting the work of researchers [13]. Regarding the cannabinoids with therapeutic applications, the information about these concepts is even less abundant [13]. The pharmacokinetics of these compounds are strongly related to their route of administration [14–16]. The route of consumption of cannabinoids most commonly used is the airways. Smoking is more common for recreational consumption, while the vaporized form is used for both recreational and therapeutic purposes [13]. However, the trends of consumption of cannabis as recreational use change quickly, namely with the advent of new synthetic substances, as synthetic cannabinoids [17].

The use of the respiratory tract as a form of consumption allows a rapid and efficient passage from the lungs to the brain [18]. Plasma concentrations of THC and CBD are detected within a few seconds of inhalation, reaching their maximum 3 to 10 min after consumption [19–22]. In a study by Kauert et al. [23], it was found that the maximum concentrations of serum THC after smoking cigarettes with about 18.2 mg and 36.5 mg of cannabinoids were 48 µg/L and 79 µg/L, respectively. The bioavailability of CBD is about 31% and ranges from 10% to 35% for THC [20,21]. The large range of variation is due not only to the variability within subjects, but also to inhalation time, number, interval, and duration of puffs, inhalation volume, and particle size [15,24]. The inhaled device also interferes with these values because when using tobacco, part of the active compound present in the cigarette is destroyed by pyrolysis (about 23% to 30%) [25]. There are also losses at the end of the cigarette and second-hand smoke since they are not consumed [25]. It should be emphasized that the bioavailability values vary between smokers and non-smokers. Studies by Lindgren et al. [26] and by Azorloza et al. [27] allowed to verify that the bioavailability of THC in smokers (23% to 27%) is superior to the bioavailability in non-smokers (10% to 14%).

Another common way to consume cannabinoids, both therapeutic and recreational, is oral administration in the form of capsules, food or cannabis-infused drink [18]. This route has the advantage of not forming harmful compounds during consumption, as it happens when smoked [18]. By oral consumption, both THC and CBD have reduced bioavailability (less than 20%), since they are highly lipophilic [28–30]. In a study by Ohlsson et al. [31] a bioavailability of $6 \pm 3\%$ was obtained for the ingestion of 20 mg of THC in a chocolate biscuit. However, in another study by Wall et al. [32], after ingestion of cannabinoids in gelatine capsules, the bioavailability obtained was 10% to 20%. Absorption is variable, as the compounds are degraded either in the stomach or in the intestines [33]. In areas where pH is low, isomerizations and protonations may occur, resulting in substituted CBDs [33]. This route of administration causes extensive hepatic metabolism to the ingested compounds, with maximum plasma concentrations of THC and CBD being reached between 1 h and 2 h after the consumption [13,20]. Nevertheless, there are studies where these same concentrations were only reached at 4 h [34] and 6 h [26,35] after consumption. In 2015, Ahmed et al. [36] administered orally 0.75 mg and 1.5 mg in elderly patients, with a maximum concentration of 0.41 µg/L and 1 µg/L, respectively. However, in another study, where 20 mg of cannabinoids were administered orally in daily users, the maximum concentrations obtained were 16.5 µg/L [37].

One variation of oral administration is the use of oromucosal delivery. This route of administration is mainly used for therapeutic applications [13]. Absorption occurs rapidly through the buccal mucosa, reaching higher plasma concentrations when compared to the oral route of administration [13]. Sublingual administration is also common for therapeutic use [20]. By using this route of administration, first-pass hepatic metabolism is avoided [18]. In a phase II study where THC was administered, it was possible to measure plasma concentrations of 14 µg/L [38].

The dermal administration of cannabinoids is a pathway that has been used for therapeutic purposes [20]. The application of compounds in the skin also avoids the first pass metabolism [18]. Cannabinoids have a hydrophobic nature, limiting its diffusion through the skin [13]. Studies on human skin have shown that CBD crosses the skin barrier more easily than THC, since it is more lipophilic [39,40]. Another study in guinea pigs showed that the plasma concentration of THC was 4.4 ng/mL at 1.4 h and was maintained for more than 48 h [41]. There are also studies in which the ways of improving the bioavailability of cannabinoids using this route of administration have been explored [20,40,42].

Other less common routes that have been investigated for therapeutic purposes are rectal and ophthalmic [20]. During rectal administration, the bioavailability of cannabinoids is very discrepant, depending on the composition of the suppository [20]. A THC hemisuccinate suppository was the one with the highest bioavailability (13.5%) in monkeys [43]. In a study by Brenneisen et al. [44], where

THC plasma concentrations were evaluated, it was found that after administration of 2.5 to 5 mg of THC, peak plasma concentrations ranged from 1.1 to 4.1 ng/mL and were reached between 2 h and 8 h, respectively. Regarding the ophthalmic route, there is a much smaller number of studies. A study in rabbits showed very different bioavailability values (6% to 40%). It was also possible to verify that maximum plasma concentrations were reached after 1 h of administration [45].

After absorption, the cannabinoids decrease their concentration in the plasma, as they are distributed rapidly by the tissues [18]. This distribution is based on the physical-chemical properties of cannabinoids and the degree of the tissue irrigation [13,20]. Also, individual characteristics, such as body composition and health status, can influence this process [46]. Thus, cannabinoids distribute more rapidly through more irrigated tissues, such as the brain, lung, heart and liver [13,47,48]. Distribution volumes are estimated approximately 3.4 L/kg for THC and 32 L/kg for CBD [21,49]. Due to their lipophilicity, these compounds have high affinity for adipose tissue, and their chronic consumption can lead to accumulation in that tissue with subsequent redistribution [13,20].

In the particular case of cannabinoid consumption during pregnancy, THC crosses the placenta rapidly and can reach the foetus [30,50]. Studies have revealed that maternal blood THC concentrations were very close to the concentrations found in foetal blood, although foetal blood concentrations were lower [20]. Chronic cannabinoid consumption also leads to accumulation of THC in breast milk [20]. A human study showed that the concentration of THC in breast milk was higher than the concentration of the same compound in plasma [51]. In this way, it was verified that a child in the stage of breast-feeding consumes daily between 0.01 and 0.1 mg of THC, for each one or two cigarettes of cannabis that the mother smokes [20].

The metabolism of THC is mainly at the hepatic level and involves phase I reactions: aliphatic hydroxylations, oxidation of alcohols to ketones and acids, β-oxidation and degradation of the pentyl lateral chain, epoxides, decarboxylations, and conjugations [18,20,52]. Microsomal reactions involve cytochrome P450 (CYP) complex enzymes [53,54]. In humans the CYP2C9, CYP2C19, and CYP3A4 subfamilies are responsible for the metabolism of THC in the liver [13,20,55]. However, extrahepatic metabolism also occurs in tissues expressing CYP450 complex enzymes, such as the brain, small intestine, heart, and lung [13,20]. More than 100 THC metabolites were identified, which are mostly mono-hydroxylated compounds [20,25]. In humans, C-11 is the most attacked site, being the major metabolites 11-hydroxy-THC (11–OH–THC, active) and 11-carboxy-THC (THC–COOH, inactive) (Figure 2) [20,21,52,56]. Huestis et al. [57] detected peak concentrations of 11–OH–THC only 13 min after the onset of smoking. Subsequently, these metabolites undergo glucuronidation as a phase II reaction, or, less commonly, conjugation with amino acids, fatty acids, sulphate and glutathione [13,18,20]. These reactions are catalysed by UGT1A9 and UGT1A10 in the case of 11–OH–THC and UGT1A1 and UGT1A3 in the case of THC-COOH [30]. Also, C-8 and C-9 are attacked, but in a smaller scale [18,20].

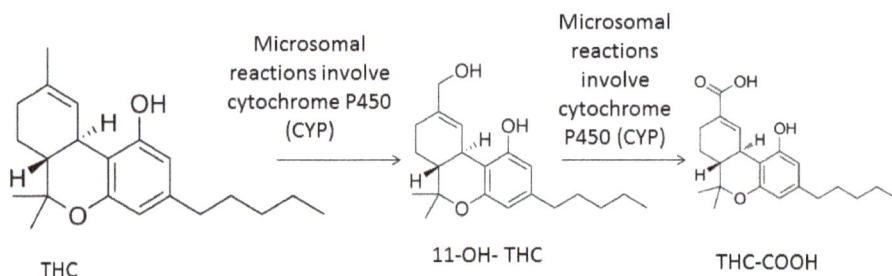

Figure 2. Main metabolites of THC.

The metabolism of CBD and CBN is similar to that of THC [18,20]. Concerning CBD, it also occurs at the hepatic level and is firstly performed by the CYP2C19 and CYP3A4 subfamilies and subsequently by the CYP1A1, CYP1A2, CYP2C9, and CYP2D6 subfamilies [13,58]. Oxidation reactions occur at C-9 and the lateral chain, but a part of this compound is excreted unchanged [18]. As regards CBN, a primary metabolite is formed by hydroxylation of C-9 to form an additional aromatic ring [18]. Thus, this compound is metabolized more slowly and less extensively than THC [59].

After metabolism, the plasma concentrations of cannabinoids and their metabolites gradually decrease. In a study by Huestis et al. [22], the concentration of 0.5 µg/L of THC in the plasma took between 3 h and 12 h to be reached after smoking a cigarette with 16 mg of THC. When consuming a dose of 34 mg, the same concentration took between 6 and 27 h to be reached. In the same study, THC-COOH was detected between 2 and 7 days at the lowest dose and between 3 and 7 days after administration of the highest dose [22]. The elimination half-life of THC is not easy to calculate because it is influenced by the balance between plasma and adipose tissue, which is a time-consuming process [13,20]. Also, CBD presents a great variation as regards its half-life time. In a study by Consroe et al. [60], it was possible to verify that after daily oral intake of CBD, elimination half-life ranged from 2 to 50 days. In another work by Ohlsson et al. [21] a mean elimination half-life of 31 ± 4 h after inhalation of CBD was reported.

Cannabinoids after being metabolized are excreted for days [61]. Typically, between 80% and 90% of the THC consumed is excreted as carboxylate and hydroxylate metabolites [18,62,63]. Approximately 5% of the acid metabolites are eliminated unchanged, 20% to 35% are excreted in the urine, and between 65% and 80% are eliminated in the faeces [25,32,48]. The major excreted glucuronic metabolite is THC–COOH glucuronide. However, its free form (THC–COOH) is also excreted through the urine [34,64,65]. On the other hand, the predominantly excreted form in faeces is 11–OH–THC [18,63]. The elimination of CBD is similar to the one of THC [20]. About 16% of the metabolites of this compound are excreted via urine in 72 h [20]. However, in the case of CBD a high amount is excreted unchanged in the faeces [20].

Concerning the mechanism of action, the effects of cannabinoids occur through agonism in specific receptors [20]. These receptors are part of the endocannabinoid system, which plays important roles in the development of the central nervous system (CNS), synaptic plasticity, and also in the response to both external and endogenous aggressions. This system is constituted not only by cannabinoid receptors, but by endogenous cannabinoids (endocannabinoids) and the enzymes responsible for their synthesis and degradation as well [66]. Two cannabinoid receptors are identified, CB1 and CB2 [67]. Other entities, as the transient receptor potential (TRP) channels, and peroxisome proliferator activated receptors (PPARs) are also engaged by some cannabinoid's compounds. The endocannabinoid system also plays an important role in different diseases, for instance in epilepsia. CB1 and CB2 receptors are coupled to inhibitory G proteins, which when activated inhibit adenylate cyclase, inhibiting the conversion of AMP to cyclic-AMP [20]. CB1 receptors are found mainly in the central and peripheral nervous system and also in some peripheral organs and tissues (e.g., leukocytes, spleen, endocrine glands, heart and areas of the reproductive, urinary and gastrointestinal systems) [67]. CB2 receptors are mainly located at the level of the immune system (tonsils, spleen, and leukocytes) and hematopoietic cells, which are of great interest for therapeutic purposes [20,30]. The affinity presented by cannabinoids is different for each type of receptor [20]. THC has affinity for both types of receptors, behaving as a partial agonist of both, yet it is more effective for CB1 type [13,20,68]. It is through this link that THC exerts its psychoactive and analgesic effects [13]. Cannabidiol has low affinity for both types of receptors [69,70]. It has been described that this compound exerts its activity through non-cannabinoid receptors [30,69]. This evidence was verified in a study by Laprairie et al. [69] where CBD was found to modulate CB1R receptors by binding to an allosteric site. TRP channels are located mostly on cell-membranes, and many of them are responsible for mediating several physiological responses, for instance pain, temperature, tastes, pressure, and vision. These channels interact with other proteins, and often form signalling complexes, for which the exact pathways of which are not known [71]. TRP channels, particularly TRPV1, which is located in dorsal root and trigeminal ganglia, brain, peripheral nerve ends, skin, bladder, pancreas and testis, are activated by the endocannabinoid anandamide under certain conditions [72]. On the other hand, PPARs are a group of nuclear receptor proteins that act as transcription factors that regulate gene expression. They play crucial roles in the regulation of cell differentiation, development, metabolism, and tumorigenesis of higher organisms. The different isoforms of PPARs (α, β, and γ) are activated by some cannabinoids, as has been shown in reporter gene assays, binding studies, selective antagonists and knockout studies. Some cannabinoid-induced effects follow the activation of these isoforms, mainly PPARα and γ, including analgesic, neuroprotective, neuronal function modulation, anti-inflammatory, metabolic, anti-tumor, gastrointestinal and cardiovascular effects. This activation often occurs in conjunction with the activation of the more traditional target sites of action, namely the CB1 and CB2 receptors and the TRPV1 ion channel. Some of the effects of inhibitors of endocannabinoid degradation or transport are also mediated by PPARs [73].

3. Secondary and Toxic Effects, Dependence, and Tolerance

Cannabis smokers usually inhale deeply and hold their breath to maximize THC absorption in the lungs, in order to achieve the desired effects. These effects appear within a few minutes time interval, and one of the most common is euphoria. The sensations of relaxation and pleasure are the main reason for young people to take cannabis, but the intensity of the "high" depends on the dose, mode of administration and the user's prior experience with cannabis or other drugs (for example, tobacco smokers have more experience compared to people who have never smoked). Besides the known euphoria and therapeutic effects, there are several authors that report effects on memory and cognition, motor function, reaction time, and psychomotor performance. A state of physical inertia with ataxia, dysarthria, and incoordination are some symptoms that can last for a few hours, as well as an increased speed of thought. The time distortion along with poor psychomotor performance for certain tasks can be explained by memory lapses. Physically, the immediate effect that cannabis users present is the increase in blood pressure, which may account for changes in the heart rate. Taking into account the effects usually associated with cannabis consumption, a major concern nowadays is the ability to drive motor vehicles under the influence of such substances. In fact, cannabis use is a major risk for road accidents, even more because it is often used concomitantly with other drugs, such as alcohol; in addition, the effects of both drugs on the psychomotor impairment are additive [74,75].

Regarding acute toxicity, there is no supporting evidence that cannabinoid consumption may induce overdose and/or death situations [76]. However, coma situations have been described in case of ingestion by children [74].

The chronic effects of cannabis are characterized by their complexity, and the literature reports that cannabis users are usually affected in several organic systems (immune, respiratory, gastrointestinal, cardiovascular, and reproductive). Concerning the cardiovascular system, besides the negative effects on the oxygen delivery, smoking cannabis contributes to the increase of carboxyhaemoglobin and heart effort. As mentioned above, elevated blood pressure may lead to strokes in patients with cerebrovascular disease, or to exacerbations in case of hypertensive patients [75]. In contrast, chronic cannabis smokers develop bronchitis and emphysema symptoms, as well as abnormalities in the large airways and poor function of the lungs. Another factor which may contribute to respiratory complications is that cannabis is usually smoked together with tobacco, increasing the risks of lung cancer and other diseases. Regarding the reproductive system, men are affected by a reduction in the number of spermatozoids and decreased sperm mobility, facing the risk of infertility, while in women the effects caused by cannabis-smoking mothers during their pregnancy are not very clear. It is assumable that during the pregnancy, as a result of exposure of the fetus in the uterus, the use of cannabis produces an increased risk of birth defects [74]. Concerning the role of CB2 receptors on the immunosuppressive actions, high doses or concentrations of THC may induce effects on the immunologic system, such as stimulation of the lymphocytes proliferation, enhanced production of interleukin-2, and macrophage function [77]. Cannabis use has also been correlated to the onset of some psychotic episodes. Despite being uncommon, some studies have associated these episodes to heavy cannabis users, in which large doses of THC produced delusions, hallucinations, and paranoid ideations. This so-called "cannabis psychosis" has been reported to cause an exacerbation of the symptoms of mental illness, like schizophrenia. The frequent use and the rising potency of cannabis suggest that young people may have their first-episode of psychosis earlier than usual [74,78].

Other disorders related with mood and anxiety have been part of the complications of long-term use of cannabis. Bipolar disorder, panic attacks, and severe anxiety are some effects caused by this chronic cannabis use [79].

Tolerance to cannabis is usually associated to effects as antinociception, anticonvulsant activity, loss of locomotor activity, and hypotension caused by repeated doses of THC and other psychoactive cannabinoids. Tolerance to most drugs normally occurs in two ways, either by changes in pharmacokinetics or by variations in pharmacodynamics. In the case of cannabinoids tolerance develops by changes in pharmacodynamics, once there is evidence that the receptors play an important role [77]. Tolerance can affect mood, memory, psychomotor performance, sleep, heart rate, arterial pressure and body temperature, among other symptoms. In several studies the cognitive effects of tolerance were identified, but not much attention was paid to psychopathological effects [74]. These studies play a decisive role in what concerns the therapeutic use of cannabis, which may promote certain problems if drug consumption originates serious manifestations. Furthermore, there is frequent development of tolerance in conjunction with dependence and withdrawal symptoms.

Dependence and withdrawal symptoms are characterized by a strong desire to reuse the substance and a defective control over its use, and these are indicators that a person is undergoing a drug dependency. Abstinence symptoms occur when there is an interruption in drug use and adverse effects appear due to this abrupt reduction of use [80].

For many years, it was common to claim that cannabis did not present dependence, since there was no evidence of tolerance or withdrawal syndrome, particularly when compared to other drugs.

However, it was observed in some studies that the withdrawal syndrome of cannabis had some similarities to those of alcohol and opioid withdrawal states. Some of the effects related to this dependence include anxiety, irritability, insomnia, muscle tremor, anorexia, and increased reflexes [74,75]. In recent surveys [81], a substantial proportion of people who show dependence are long-term cannabis users, with 57% from 243 users qualified for lifetime DSM-III-R and ICD-10 cannabis dependence diagnoses. On the other hand, Anthony et al. [82] estimated that few persons who had ever used cannabis met the criteria DSM-III-R for dependence on this drug at some time in their lives, which suggests that some chronic cannabis users can develop cannabis dependence syndrome. In fact, most authors claim that long-term cannabis use has been associated with a decline in cognitive functions, which seemingly can be reversed, however, after a few days of abstinence [9,83,84].

Budney et al. [85] reported a comparison of three possible treatments based on motivational strategies. However, it is still not clear what treatment must be provided, if some, for dependent cannabis users that cannot stop using despite of knowing the adverse effects.

Despite the controversy regarding dependence, relative to other drugs of abuse, cannabis is usually associated with minimal withdrawal symptoms, but with the development of tolerance instead.

4. Prevalence and Control Status

High-risk drug use is one of the five key indicators of the European Monitoring Centre for Drugs and Drug Addiction (EMCDDA) for monitoring in Europe. This type of indicator is an important tool for consumption trends, as well as for drug categorization. As mentioned above, cannabis is the most consumed drug worldwide, which is due in part to the ease of acquisition and to the low prevalence of dependence situations. In the last report of the EMCDDA, in 2017, the drug accounted for 74% of an overall estimate of 1.5 million offences. Cannabis is also the most commonly used illicit drug in Europe, and its prevalence is about five times higher than that of other drugs. It is estimated that 17.2 million young adults (aged 15–34 years) have used cannabis in the last year across the European Union, while 87.6 million will use it throughout life (aged 15–64 years). The trends in use also vary between countries. In surveys performed from around 2017, the prevalence rates in the previous year in the age range of 15 to 34 range from 3.5% in Hungary to 21.5% in France [86,87]. Based on surveys of the general population, it is estimated that around 1% of European adults are daily or almost daily users of cannabis, meaning that they have consumed this drug in 20 or more days from the previous month. About 37% of these people are older consumers, aged 35-64, with about three-quarters of them being male [86–89].

Concerning regulation issues, cannabis and cannabis resin are both listed in Schedules I and IV of the United Nations 1961 Single Convention on Narcotic Drugs [90]. The debate concerning laws aiming at prohibiting or permitting the use of this drug worldwide has gained new fuel since 2012, as the supply and use of recreational cannabis in Uruguay and some states of the US (and more recently in Canada). Legislative proposals aiming at legalizing cannabis have raised important concerns on the eventual increase in its use, and consequently the related harms, and possibilities related to the ways in which cannabis for non-medical purposes could be regulated to mitigate these concerns have raised. Indeed, the use of cannabis-based products as medicine to treat certain conditions is not prohibited by international law. Also, and according to UN conventions, the use of any drug under international control should be limited to those situations involving medical and scientific purposes.

The system of controls which is deemed necessary in the case that a country decides to allow cultivation of cannabis not intended for industrial or horticultural purposes is described under Article 28 of the 1961 Convention, while the 1971 Convention controls specifically THC. In Europe, THC may be included in capsules, cannabis extract may be used as a mouth spray, and dried cannabis flowers may be used for vaporizing or making cannabis tea, all of those uses in the case of authorized medicines [86]. By contrast, smoking cannabis for medical purposes is not authorized at all, which is due on the one hand to the fact that there are many strains of cannabis plants, and each one of them has the capability of producing a wide range of chemicals. In addition, the range and concentration of chemicals may also vary within one plant, and it depends for instance on light levels during growth or maturity at harvest. Therefore, these factors should have to be strictly controlled to allow the prescriber and/or the pharmacist to be able to judge the content and as such deliver the needed chemicals for a particular patient. On the other hand, inhaling smoke from burning plant material can hardly be considered a healthy method for the delivery of substances to the bloodstream, as harmful tars and particles will be inhaled as well. Also, when the chemicals have no psychoactive activity, for instance as occurs with CBD, it is difficult for the user to know accurately the dose. There is no harmonized EU law on cannabis use, and each country may deal with drug offences differently [86]. Indeed, while many countries have adopted decriminalization and have turned the simple possession of drugs a non-criminal offense, others have preconize much more severe penalties, and the mere possession of even small amounts of drug can lead to several years in prison [91].

The evolution of the cannabis market, triggered by recent developments on the American continent concerning its legalization in some jurisdictions, entails new policy challenges, as a rapid development of a commercial market for cannabis has emerged. Consequently, innovations concerning the preparations under which the drug is available (for instance highly potent strains of cannabis, vaping liquids, and edible products) or in delivery systems for its consumption. In some jurisdictions, the legal market for recreational drugs has been accompanied by regulations that allow access to cannabis for medical and therapeutic purposes. Other important policy issues in this area include questions on what constitutes appropriate treatment for cannabis-related disorders, how to ensure policy synergies with tobacco control strategies, and what constitutes a harm reduction approach which is effective with this regard. The prevalence of cannabis use in Europe remains high in historical terms, and recent increases have been observed in some EU Member States. The potency of the drug, which has risen sharply in the last decade, also reaches high levels, whether it is cannabis resin or herbaceous cannabis. Beyond public health issues, there are concerns about what will be the impact of this large illicit market on community safety and how it might even be funding organized crime. Taking into account the several involved issues, defining what constitutes the most appropriate response to cannabis use is a task of growing complexity and importance [86,87].

5. Therapeutic Indications

The use of preparations derived from *Cannabis sativa* in medicine has a long history. However, this use has largely declined in the twentieth century, and its consumption for medical purposes was limited when cannabis was included in the United Nations Single Convention on Narcotic Drugs in 1961, and classified as not presenting known medical uses. Notwithstanding, there has been a reappearance of patient interest in using these drugs for the treatment of a variety of medical conditions, including chronic and cancer pain, depression, anxiety disorders, sleep disturbances and neurological disorders in the past 20 years, since their symptoms were reportedly improved by using cannabis.

This increased interest of patients in using cannabis medically was accompanied by a renewed interest of scientists on the potential medical use of several of the plant's constituents. This occurred after the discovery in the early 1990s of a cannabinoid system in the human organism, which has been associated to the control of important biological functions, such as cognition, memory, pain, sleep and immune functioning. However, the early classification of cannabis as a drug with no medical use has made it difficult to adequately conduct clinical research on the matter. In the mid-1990s the medical use of cannabis for people with a variety of illnesses, such as chronic pain, terminal cancer and multiple sclerosis was legalized in several states of the USA, which was afterwards followed by many other states. In 1999, Canada introduced a program involving medical cannabis, which has expanded thereafter. In fact, since the early 2000s, several other countries have implemented the medical use of cannabis under specified conditions, for instance Israel (2001), the Netherlands (2003), Switzerland (2011), Czech Republic (2013), Chile (2015), Australia (2016), Norway (2016), Peru (2017), Germany (2017) and more recently Thailand (2018) among others legislated to allow the medical use of cannabis under specified conditions.

Most EU countries now allow, or are considering allowing, the medical use of cannabis or cannabinoids in some form [86,92]. "Sativex®", containing approximately equal quantities of THC and CBD is the most recognized product marketed in a number of European countries. This product, which is administered by spraying inside the cheek or under the tongue, has been authorized in 17 EU Member States (Austria, Belgium, Czech Republic, Denmark, Finland, France, Germany, Ireland, Italy, Luxembourg, Netherlands, Poland, Portugal, Slovakia, Spain, Sweden, United Kingdom) and Norway for the treatment of muscle spasticity in patients with multiple sclerosis. Other products available in Europe are Marinol (Dronabinol), containing synthetic THC, which is used in cancer treatment, AIDS and multiple sclerosis; and Cesamet™ (Nabilone), containing a synthetic analog to THC, used for cancer treatment. However, national approaches vary widely in terms of both the products allowed and the regulatory frameworks governing their provision [92].

Other countries have however more restrictive laws, allowing only the use of certain cannabis-derived pharmaceutical products, such as Sativex®, Marinol or Epidiolex® (CBD). In the United States, 33 states and the District of Columbia have legalized the medical use of cannabis, but at the federal level its use remains prohibited for all purposes [93,94]. In the following lines, a more comprehensive review will be made on the uses of cannabis to treat medical conditions. This search was made based on the PubMed and Google Scholar databases using the following search strings: "cannabis insomnia"; "cannabis and anxiety"; "cannabis and post-traumatic stress disorder"; "cannabis and fibromyalgia"; "cannabis and pain management"; "cannabis and appetite treatment", "cannabinoids and dermatology or skin therapy", "cannabinoids and glaucoma", "cannabinoids and infections therapy", "cannabis and epilepsy", "cannabis and Tourette syndrome", "cannabis and Parkinson disease", "cannabis and Alzheimer disease", "cannabis and multiple sclerosis", " cannabis and nausea and/or vomiting".

This section summarizes the evidences on the properties of cannabis and cannabinoids from systematic reviews of random controlled clinical trials. A particular challenge in interpreting the evidences is that several different cannabis products and preparations have often been used and may have contained several different active ingredients.

5.1. Pain Management

Pain management is a problem of general interest and a public health issue, which increasingly attracts the attention of several countries that consider the use of cannabis in cases of acute or chronic pain. It can be said that legal and political decisions influence the habits of cannabis use in these situations. Since the early 2000s, several studies have been published on the advantages and limitations of cannabis implementation in the therapy of patients with persistent pain. In recent years there has been an increase in the number of studies and reviews conducted in this area.

As an example, the study by Bigand et al. [95] aimed at analyzing health outcomes of adults using opioids for pain with the addition of cannabis use, evaluating the beneficial or non-beneficial effects of this. One-hundred-and-fifty patients aged between 19 and 85 years prescribed with opiates for the treatment of persistent pain, including pain correlated to cancer, were included in this study. The management of physiological symptoms was considered by patients to be a major benefit of cannabis use, and most reported the relieve of symptoms, namely pain, insomnia and nausea, anxiety, depression, and stress. Negative symptoms such as weight gain, red eyes, dry mouth, nausea, fast heart, lack of concentration, poor memory, drowsiness, apathy, lack of motivation, and more serious symptoms such as increased anxiety, paranoia, seizures and anaphylaxis due to allergic reaction were reported as well. The authors of this study concluded that legalizing cannabis for medical and recreational use brings more knowledge to both patients and health professionals who become more aware of the effects of cannabis on pain-related symptoms, thus enabling open communication, more treatment options, and greater safety for patients.

By the end of 2017, Armour et al. [96] conducted an online study of endometriosis in the female population of Australia between the ages of 18 and 45. Current medical treatments do not generally provide sufficient pain relief or have intolerable side effects, and this research aimed to determine the prevalence of use of common forms of self-management. Four hundred and eighty-four responses were considered as valid. The authors concluded that women using cannabis and hemp/CBD oil reported these substances among the most well-evaluated in terms of effectiveness in reducing pain. However, as the number of women using it was small and the results were self-reported, clinical trials are needed in this area to determine any possible role of legally-obtained medicinal cannabis in the management of endometriosis.

The pain of rheumatic patients is one of the reasons to consider using medicinal cannabis as an alternative treatment to the implemented therapies, such as opioids. Fitzcharles et al. [97] compiled the Canadian legislation and the studies conducted on the effects of medicinal cannabis in these patients, and have concluded that patients should be provided with health professionals that have the best evidence-based information on the beneficial effects as well as on cannabis damage, facilitating dialogue between patients and physicians, in an attempt to reduce drug-related harms, not only to patients but also to society. However, clinical trials of medicinal cannabis in these patients have not yet been conducted, and the beneficial evidence for pharmaceutical cannabinoids in fibromyalgia, osteoarthritis, rheumatoid arthritis, and back pain are insufficient. On the other hand, there is evidence of a high risk of harm. They have also concluded that medical cannabis can provide relief for some patients and short-term risks such as psychomotor effects, appetite changes, dizziness, mood effects, and more serious effects such as disorientation and psychosis may even be anticipated. It is also known that cannabis should not be smoked because the inhalation of combustible products carries a bronchial risk; however, long-term risks have not yet been determined.

Palace et al. [98] developed a state program with safe and controlled administration of medical cannabis to resident patients diagnosed with chronic pain, neuropathy or Parkinson's disease. These authors concluded that the elderly who used medicinal cannabis demonstrated significant decreases in the use of prescription drugs, mainly the use of opioids, and medicinal cannabis should be seen as an additional clinical option to relief the symptoms. As in the previously described studies, they concluded that with the acceptance and diffusion of this knowledge, more health professionals could help patients to benefit and request this alternative therapy. These authors stated that the available medicinal cannabis formulations contained a standardized dose of CBD with little or no THC; this is capable of eliminating psychoactive effects in the elderly, improving the safety profile in chronic pain treatment.

Shin et al. [99] have reviewed the available literature on the use of cannabis and cannabinoids in the treatment of cancer pain, such as breast cancer, lymphoma, and cervical cancer. As the number of studies on the efficacy of these compounds is limited, it becomes challenging and difficult to give a definite recommendation for a certain practice. Although evidence is scarce, they is enough to justify more research on the use of cannabis in cancer, and this process is facilitated in cases of legislation changes concerning its consumption. Limitations such as the small number of patients in the study, abstinence, withdrawal due to negative side effects, and use of different pain scales were found. The authors concluded that some of the studies reported that THC is more effective than the placebo, but other studies have found THC to be no more effective than placebo, making it difficult to find agreement on its use for treatment.

More recently, Campbell et al. [100] have delineated the currently available evidence on cannabis and medicinal cannabis for the treatment of non-oncologic chronic pain, such as neuropathic pain, multiple sclerosis-related pain and visceral pain, which are among the most important reasons for research in the use of these compounds. These authors concluded that there are several limitations that need to be studied because the patients' perceptions regarding the efficacy of cannabinoids in cases of pain are not included in the existing evidence. This makes it important to manage patients' expectations and to better understand what the potential side effects are, as these can limit the drug's use. It is accepted that in most of these studies a combined dose of THC and CBD was used, with little proof of the benefits that other cannabis-based medicines have in neuropathic pain.

Noteworthy is the work developed by Perron et al. [101], who intended to describe abstinence patterns of cannabis in a large sample of patients who used medical cannabis, in order to test the association between withdrawal symptoms and functioning. Participants in this study were adults over 21 years of age interested in having or maintaining medical certification for the use of cannabis for the treatment of chronic pain. Two-thirds of the patients reported at least one symptom of moderate or severe abstinence and the most frequently observed symptom was difficult sleep, which was followed by anxiety, irritability and appetite disturbances. Abstinence symptoms occurred at significantly higher rates for patients with poor mental functioning compared to patients with high mental functioning. In addition, there was no visible association between physical functioning and withdrawal symptoms. The authors concluded that these abstinence symptoms were highly prevalent in patients who used medical cannabis at least three times a week. These findings, although limited, may be important for patients and may assist health professionals in deciding which therapies to apply, and therefore a more effective intervention, as they become better aware of the negative consequences of using medical cannabis. Additional studies will always be necessary, addressing other issues, such as legislation and the differences between countries and how patients may be affected by this.

Cannabinoids may also be used in the treatment of fibromyalgia, namely in the relief of lumbar pain, fatigue and mood disturbances, symptoms which are usually associated to this disease [102,103]. Some researchers have found a correlation between deficiencies in endocannabinoid system and fibromyalgia, and recently published studies have focused on the therapeutic effects of cannabis on it [97,104–106]. Yassin et al. [107] evaluated the improvement of pain and function in situations of patients with fibromyalgia, with the addition of cannabis therapy to the standardized pharmacological analgesic treatment. A cross-over observational study was conducted in which thirty-one patients between 21 and 75 years were observed and treated with the standard therapy (oxycodone hydrochloride, naloxone hydrochloride, and duloxetine) for three months. After that time, patients were able to choose cannabis treatment for six months. The authors concluded that the standardized therapy led to a small improvement when compared to non-treated situations, while the cannabis treatment allowed a significant improvement after three months of implementation and that this improvement was maintained at six months. There was, thus, an advantage of cannabis treatment compared to the medication normally prescribed in a patient with low back pain associated to fibromyalgia. No patient had to discontinue therapy due to adverse events, and most of them have decreased or discontinued standard analgesics consumption. The authors further concluded that additional randomized clinical trials are needed to assess whether the results can be generalized to the general population, as the mechanism of cannabis pain relief associated to this pathology is not defined. Another associated problem is the lack of standardization of the amount of THC/CBD that should be applied. The proportion of THC to CBD recommended in the chronic pain therapeutic in this trial was 1:4.

Pain treatment is undoubtedly the most studied therapeutic indication of cannabis. In general, researchers have found that cannabis-based medicines are probably effective for treating the neuropathic pain and painful spasms usually associated to multiple sclerosis [108], as well as neuropathic pain associated to diabetes, HIV, and other illnesses. However, it is unclear whether or not smoked marijuana is effective in reducing pain in multiple sclerosis [108,109]. Cannabis can be used to treat chronic pain associated to cancer and other causes, and studies generally suggested cannabis-related improvements in chronic pain measures in cancer patients [103,110,111]. Most studies used Sativex® preparations, and have generally shown positive results [111,112].

5.2. Epilepsy

Epilepsy is a disorder from the CNS in which the brain activity becomes abnormal, causing episodes of involuntary movement that may involve a part or the entire body. Globally, an estimated 2.4 million people are diagnosed with epilepsy each year and has an annual cumulative incidence of 67.77 per 100,000 persons [113].

Drug resistance epilepsy is defined as failure to stop all seizures in a patient who had adequate trials of at least two appropriate medications, such as Dravet syndrome and Lennox–Gastaut syndrome, in which it is usual to have both generalized and focal drug-resistant seizures [114].

New medications have been approved in the past two decades, but these have not reduced the proportion of patients with intractable epilepsy [115]. In the last few years enormous interest has been generated by social and news media about the beneficial effects of cannabis products for the treatment of drug-resistant or refractory epilepsy. This is the most recent therapeutic approach for cannabis products, and evidences found in studies using animals will be separated from those obtained in clinical trials aiming at a better systematization of the gathered information.

5.2.1. Evidence in Animal Models and Basic Pharmacological Mechanisms

After centuries of anecdotal reports, there has been an expansion of preclinical trials in order to investigate the pharmacologic potential of various phytocannabinoids as anticonvulsant drugs. These reports evaluate those cannabinoids that do not have psychoactive properties, mainly CBD but also including cannabidivarin and Δ9-tetrahydrocannabivarin.

In the early 1970s, CBD was found to have anticonvulsant properties in experimental animal models. Carlini et al. [116] suggested that 200 mg/kg of CBD significantly protected the mice from the convulsant and lethal effects of leptazol. Furthermore, Consroe et al. [117] suggested that the CBD effects were comparable to those of phenytoin and enhance the anticonvulsant effects of phenobarbital and phenytoin. In subsequent reports, CBD consistently showed anticonvulsant effects in several animal epileptic models including: maximal electroshock test (mES) [118–120]; 6 Hz and subcutaneous metrazol threshold test [120]; pentylenetetrazol [121]; pilocarpine and penicillin models [122].

To date, the antiepileptic mechanism of action of CBD remains unknown. CBD has low affinity for both CB1 and CB2 endocannabinoid receptors and is therefore likely to be exerting its activity via cannabinoid receptor-independent [119,121,123]. In contrast to CB1, CB2 receptors are attractive targets for the development of novel therapeutic approaches, and nowadays it is acknowledged that the anti-inflammatory properties of cannabinoid agonists also involve these last receptors. CB2 receptor activation has proven to decrease the production of proinflammatory molecules in a number of neural cell types, such as rat microglial cells, primary mouse astrocytes, human microglial, and THP-1 cells [124–127]. Other potential mechanisms includes agonist at transient receptor potential (TRP) cation channels (specifically calcium channel modulation) [128]; blocks T-type calcium channels [129]; modulation of serotonin (5-HT_{1A}/5-HT_{2A}) and adenosine (A_1 and A_2) receptors [130,131] and modulation of voltage dependent anion-selective channel protein 1 (VDAC1) [132].

Cannabidivarin (propyl analogue of CBD) is an effective anticonvulsant in a broad range of seizure models [133]. Like CBD, cannabidivarin anticonvulsant properties are not mediated by CB1 receptor and have agonist effects at TRP cation channel [134]. Δ9-tetrahydrocannabivarin, another cannabinoid found in cannabis, exerts some anti-epileptiform effects in vitro and very limited anticonvulsant effects on pentylenetetrazole–induced seizure model. The anticonvulsant properties are consistent with a CB1 receptor–mediated mechanism [135].

Although cannabis has been used medicinally for centuries, it is only within the last few decades that there is accumulated evidence that some cannabinoids have anticonvulsant properties in animal epileptic models. Despite this evidence, the mechanisms by which these compounds exert anti-seizure effects are poorly understood. Identification of mechanisms underlying the anticonvulsant efficacy of cannabinoids is critical to determine other potential treatment options.

5.2.2. Clinical Evidence in Epilepsy

From the 1980s to the last few years, several studies have been conducted, some of them randomized and blinded, that involve the use of isolated CBD as a therapeutic option for epilepsy.

Mechoulam and Carlini [136] treated four patients with CBD (200 mg daily) and five patients with placebo. CBD treatment showed that 75% of the patients had a remarkable improvement in seizures throughout the entire three-month period while none of the placebo patients showed any improvement.

Cunha et al. [137] conducted a trial of fifteen adult patients with focal-onset epilepsies. The patients were given between 200–300 mg of CBD or placebo. Patients treated with CBD, 7/8 reported improvement in seizures; while seven of the patients who received placebo remained unchanged [137].

In contrast, two studies provided a few details (patients with uncontrolled seizures were randomized into either placebo or CBD groups) but suggested little or no difference in seizure frequency between placebo and CBD groups. In Ames 1985, 12 patients institutionalized due to mental retardation with uncontrolled seizures were given three capsules of placebo or 100 mg of CBD [138]. The other trial was an unpublished abstract from a conference. Twelve patients were treated with a single-blind placebo for six months followed by double-blind 300 mg of CBD or placebo in a cross-over trial lasting an additional 12 months [138].

Insufficient preclinical and clinical data have intersected with a need for more effective therapies for drug resistance epilepsy, which created a demand for CBD-based treatments. Recently, there has been a surge in clinical trials investigating the additive effects of highly purified CBD treatment (Epidiolex®; GW Pharmaceuticals) to daily antiepileptic drugs (AEDs) regimens in both children and adults [139–144].

In an open-label interventional trial, 214 patients (aged 1–30) with severe, intractable, childhood-onset, treatment resistant epilepsy, were given oral CBD at 2–5 mg/kg/day, then up-titrated until intolerance or to a maximum dose (25 or 50 mg/kg/day) for 12 weeks. Add-on treatment with CBD led to a clinically meaningful reduction in seizure frequency and had an adequate tolerability and safety profile [141].

Devinsky et al. [142] reported results on both efficacy and safety data on patients who received Epidiolex® as part of their daily regimen for at least 14 weeks. In this double-blind, placebo-controlled trial, 120 children and young adults with drug-resistant Dravet syndrome, were randomly assigned in a 1:1 ratio to receive CBD oral solution (dose escalated up to 20 mg/kg/day) or placebo. This trial showed that CBD resulted in a greater reduction in convulsive–seizure frequency than placebo. The median frequency of convulsive seizures per month decreased from 12.4 to 5.9 with CBD, in comparison with a decrease from 14.9 to 14.1 with placebo. At least a 50% reduction in convulsive seizure frequency was 43% with CBD (27% with placebo) and 5% of patients became seizure-free (0% with placebo) [142].

In 2018, a series of trials showed the long-term safety and efficacy of CBD in children and adults with treatment-resistant epilepsies. An update on an expanded access program provided the safety outcomes up to 144 weeks and efficacy up to 96 weeks in more than 600 patients. Results from this ongoing expanded access program supported that add-on CBD may be an efficacious long-term treatment option for treatment-resistant epilepsies. CBD treatment was associated with 51% and 48% reductions in median monthly convulsive and total seizures respectively after 12 weeks. Reductions were similar among visit windows through 96 weeks of treatment and CBD was generally well tolerated [139].

In addition, Devinsky et al. [143] presented an interim analysis of the safety and efficacy from 264 patients with Dravet syndrome treated with long-term CBD (mean modal dose 21 mg/kg/day, median treatment 274 days). In this open-label extension trial, CBD treatment had an acceptable safety profile. Sustained reductions in convulsive and total seizures were observed through 48 weeks and 85% of patientscaregivers reported improvements in overall condition [143].

In two additional randomized, double-blind, placebo-controlled trials, CBD treatment at a dose of 10 mg or 20 mg per kilogram per day was associated with greater reductions in the frequencies of seizures among children and adults with the Lennox–Gastaut syndrome [140,144].

Adverse events that occurred more frequently in the CBD treatment with the concomitant AEDs included diarrhea, vomiting, fatigue, pyrexia, somnolence, and abnormal results on liver-function tests [139–144].

Some effects of CBD may relate to interactions with other AED [145]. CBD inhibits cytochrome P450 (CYP2C19) and produces an increase in plasma concentrations of N-desmethylclobazam (active metabolite) [146]. In patients taking clobazam and CBD who experience bothersome sedation, a reduction of the clobazam (or CBD) dose may be considered.

In these trials [139–144], abnormal liver function test results were noted in participants taking concomitant valproate, suggesting a CBD-valproate interaction. CBD had no effect on systemic levels of valproate, which suggests that the interaction may be pharmacodynamics [147].

Based on the results obtained in these clinical trials, in June 2018, the US Food and Drug Administration (FDA) approved Epidiolex®; for the treatment of seizures associated with Lennox–Gastaut syndrome or Dravet syndrome in patients two years of age or older.

Recently, there has been a growing interest in using of CBD-enriched cannabis oil (medical cannabis) for the treatment of drug-resistance epilepsy. One case (called Charlotte case) that received a lot of media attention, reported a little girl who showed substantial decreased seizures when she started therapy with a high concentration of CBD/THC cannabis oil. Charlotte was given a low dose of a sublingual preparation of a cannabis extract and slowly increased the extract dose, keeping the THC content sufficiently low to avoid psychotropic effects. For the first time, Charlotte experienced seven consecutive days without a single seizure. With a baseline frequency of 300 convulsions per week, Charlotte had a >90% reduction in seizures [148].

Several online forum surveys have been performed examining the effects of medical cannabis for intractable pediatric epilepsy. In a telephone/Internet survey, 84% of parents who had administered CBD-enriched cannabis to 19 children with epilepsy (Dravet syndrome, Doose syndrome, Lennox–Gastaut syndrome and idiopathic epilepsy) reported substantial reductions in seizures frequency [149].

Another online parental survey focused on perceived efficacy, dosage, and tolerability of medical cannabis in 117 children with epilepsy syndrome (infantile spasms, Lennox–Gastaut syndrome, and other). The perceived efficacy and tolerability were similar across etiologic subgroups, with 85% of them reporting some reduction in seizure frequency and 14% reporting complete seizure freedom. The median duration and the median dosage of CBD exposure were 6.8 months and 4.3 mg/kg/day, respectively [150].

Finally, Press et al. [151] presented a retrospective review of children and adolescents (*n* = 75) with various epileptic encephalopathies who were given oral cannabis extracts. Thirteen percent of patients reported to have a reduction in seizure frequency (>50% in response). The responder rate varied based on epilepsy syndrome: Dravet 23%, Doose 0%, and Lennox–Gastaut syndrome 88.9% [151].

Other beneficial effects reported in these three studies included increased alertness, better mood, and improved sleep [149–151]. In addition, Hussain et al. [150] reported improvements in language and motor skills when using CBD. The few side effects reported included increased appetite, somnolence/fatigue, and an increase in seizure frequency [149–151].

The limitations of the online surveys are of paramount importance and introduce the possibility for numerous sources of confounding: bias selection patients, lack of placebo controls, unblinded self-assessment of efficacy/tolerability, inconsistency of CBD concentration and inaccuracy in the identification of patients' epilepsy syndromes.

Three publications on clinical trials appeared between 2016 and 2018 evaluating the efficacy and safety of medical cannabis for the treatment of refractory epilepsy. An observational longitudinal study suggested that adding CBD-enriched cannabis extract to the treatment regimen of patients with refractory epilepsy may result in a significant reduction in seizure frequency according to parental reports [152]. Fifty-seven children and adolescents (1–20 years) with epilepsy of various etiologies were treated with cannabis oil extract (CBD/THC ratio of 20:1) for at least three months. A dose of 2–5 mg/kg/day (divided into three daily doses) was added to the baseline antiepileptic regimen and the dosage was incremented until intolerance (THC did not exceed 0.15–1.35 mg/kg/day). Of the 46 patients included in the efficacy analysis, 43.5% had a seizure reduction >50%; 22% had a reduction of 50–75%; 30% had a reduction of 75–99%; and 4% were seizure-free [152].

The second report was a prospective open-label trial that described safe dose, tolerability, and efficacy of a cannabis oil containing CBD/THC ratio of 50:1 in children with Dravet syndrome. Nineteen participants completed the 20-week intervention. Mean dose achieved was 13.3 mg/kg/day of CBD (range 7–16 mg/kg/day) and 0.27 mg/kg/day of THC (range 0.14–0.32 mg/kg/day). Cannabis oil treatment resulted in a significant reduction in motor seizures of 70.6%, improvement in quality of life and reduction in electroencephalogram spike activity [153].

The last report was a retrospective study describing the effect of medicinal cannabis on children and adolescents with intractable epilepsy. Seventy-four patients started the treatment (CBD/THC ratio of 20:1) for at least three months (average six months). CBD dose ranged from 1 to 20 mg/kg/day and THC dosage did not exceed 0.5 mg/kg/day. Most of the patients (89%) reported a reduction in seizure frequency (18% reported 75–100% reduction; 34% reported 50–75% reduction, 12% reported 25–50% reduction, and 26% reported <25% reduction) [154].

CBD-enriched medical cannabis is shaping up to be a very promising anticonvulsant option, with favorable safety profile. For a clearer judgment of the potential therapeutic effects, the risks and legality of a cannabis oil, it is important to know its exact composition. Consistent formulation through strict methodology will allow to assess the synergism of other phytocannabinoids as well as other compounds such as flavonoids and terpenoids.

5.3. Neurodegenerative Disorders: Parkinson's Disease, Alzheimer's Disease, and Multiple Sclerosis

5.3.1. Parkinson's Disease

Parkinson's Disease (PD) is a progressive neurodegenerative disorder characterized clinically by symptoms such as bradykinesia, rigidity, tremor, and postural instability. These symptoms are produced by brain dopaminergic denervation at the striatum level and progressive death of dopaminergic neurons in the pars compacta of the substantia nigra. Parkinson's Disease is multifaceted with disparate etiologies, a range of clinical symptoms and variations in pathology [155]. Scientific evidence indicates that immunological pathways are important in the pathophysiology of PD [156].

The impact cannabis has on motor and nonmotor symptoms of PD may be modulated by the dopaminergic, serotonergic, adrenergic, and neuroprotective properties of cannabinoids. The CB1 receptor is one of the most abundant receptors in the CNS. The CB1 receptor is highly expressed in the basal ganglia, the brain structures primarily affected in PD [157]. This specific localization of CB1 may explain the effect of cannabinoids on cognitive and motor activity. The CB2 receptors are expressed primarily in peripheral immunocompetent cells and lymphoid organs but are also expressed in the CNS [158]. The CB2 receptors have been found to modulate microglia activation and may play a role in neuroinflammation/neuroprotection [159], since as mentioned above, their activation has proven to decrease the production of proinflammatory molecules in a number of neural cell types.

Furthermore, pre-clinical research demonstrated that cannabinoids prevent neuronal damage into the nigra pars compacta in rodents probably by its antioxidant activity, possibly associated a CB receptor-independent [160]. In an additional study Peres et al. [161] reported that CBD's antioxidant and anti-inflammatory actions would attenuate reserpine-induced motor and cognitive impairments in an experimental model.

In animal models of PD, the levels of CB1 receptors appear to be downregulated in the substantia nigra and the globus pallidus at early phases (12 months of age). By contrast, CB1 receptors showed an elevation in the same areas when animals were analyzed at older ages [162]. Together, these studies suggest a complex link between the pathophysiology of PD and changes in the endocannabinoid system.

The results of clinical trials examining the role of cannabinoids in the treatment of PD are mixed. A first preliminary clinical open pilot study reported that CBD treatment (100–600 mg/day CBD in capsules with sesame oil vehicle) for six weeks in PD patients, improved dystonia in all patients (n = 5) in a range from 20 to 50%. However, in two patients CBD treatment at doses over 300 mg/day exacerbated the hypokinesia and resting tremor. Side effects included hypotension, dry mouth, psychomotor slowing, lightheadedness, and sedation [163].

An open-label pilot study reported that CBD in flexible dose (started with an oral dose of 150 mg/day) for 4 weeks in six patients with psychosis in PD, improved the psychotic symptoms [164].

In another trial, 21 PD patients were randomized to placebo, CBD 75mg/day or CBD 300 mg/day for six weeks. No significant changes were found between CBD and placebo in scores obtained with Unified PD Rating Scale (motor and general symptoms score) and possible neuroprotective effects. However, in the PD Questionnaire (well-being and quality of life) significant differences were found between the total score of the placebo and CBD 300 mg/day groups. No serious adverse events were reported [165].

Many studies examining the efficacy of cannabis in PD are limited to questionnaires and observation in patients actively consuming marijuana either recreational or prescribed. These observational/questionnaires uncontrolled studies suggest that cannabis could improve motor symptoms. In some studies, patients who consumed cannabis reported improvements in some of the symptoms of the PD: tremor, bradykinesia, rigidity, problems with sleep and pain [166–170]. In other study, five patients with idiopathic PD found no benefit for tremor following a single administration of smoked cannabis (1 g. cigarette containing 2.9 % THC) [171].

Unfortunately, a few randomized double-blind clinical trials have been carried out with cannabis on people with PD. A crossover study in 19 PD patients demonstrated that an oral cannabis extract (1.25 mg CBD and 2.5 mg THC and per capsule, maximum daily dose 0.25 mg/kg THC) was well tolerated and had no pro- or antiparkinsonian action [172].

At present, a phase II randomized, open-label, double-blind trial, is underway to evaluate the tolerability, safety and dose-finding of cannabis oil for pain in PD. Mixed cannabis oil preparation consisting of three differing formulations of THC and CBD (proportions of THC and CBD in the following ratios: 18:0.2; 10:10; 1:20) will be administered to a total of 15 assigned patients randomly to one of the three groups. Estimated primary completion date will be available in December 2019 [173].

5.3.2. Alzheimer's Disease

A widely accepted theory underlying the pathophysiology of Alzheimer's disease (AD) is the deposition of amyloid-β protein in specific brain regions leading to localized neuroinflammatory responses and accumulation of intra-cellular neurofibrillary tangles. These events result in neuronal cell death with accompanying loss of functional synapses and changes in neurotransmitter levels [174].

Pre-clinical studies suggest that the endocannabinoid system protects against neuronal cell death, oxidative stress, and inflammation, events associated with the development of AD. In-vitro experiments determined that THC could bind and competitively inhibit the enzyme acetylcholinesterase as well as prevent acetylcholinesterase-induced amyloid-β protein aggregation [175]. Several mechanisms have been suggested to explain CBD neuroprotection: reduction of oxidative stress and anti-apoptotic effects [176], inhibition Aβ-induced tau protein hyperphosphorylation which leads to the formation of neurofibrillary tangles [177], decrease in amyloid-β production and amyloid-β induced neurodegeneration by inhibition of inducible nitric oxide synthase (iNOS) and interleukin-1β protein expression [178].

Long-term CBD treatment (CBD 20 mg/kg/day for 8 months) in a transgenic model of AD, prevented social recognition deficit (not associated with any changes in amyloid load or oxidative damage). This study revealed a subtle impact of CBD on neuroinflammation, cholesterol and dietary phytosterol retention [179].

Clinical evidence indicates that dronabinol (synthetic form of THC) and medical cannabis may have some benefit in treatment of behavioral and psychological symptoms of dementia.

There were two open-label prospective studies [180,181], two randomized double-blind placebo-controlled repeated crossover trials [182,183], a double-blind placebo-controlled crossover design [184], a placebo-controlled trial [185] and one retrospective study [186]. Five reports used dronabinol [180,182,184–186] and two reports used medical cannabis [181,183]. Three studies were 2 weeks in duration [180,182,185], one trial was 17 (mean) days long [186], another study was 4 weeks in duration [181] and two trials were 12 weeks in duration [183,184].

The dose of dronabinol were 2.5 mg/day [180,182,184,185] and one study used dronabinol at 7.03 mg/day (mean) [186], one trial used THC up to 3 mg/day [183], and one used maximal dose of 15 mg/day [181].

Six studies indicated that symptoms improved with the use of cannabinoids: reduction of nocturnal motor activity and agitation [180,182,185], decreased of delusions, agitation/aggression, irritability, apathy, sleep and caregiver distress [181,184], decreased of aberrant vocalization, motor agitation, aggressiveness and resisting care [186]. Only one found that there was no benefit to using THC when compared with placebo over a 12-week period at a maximum dose of 3 mg/day [183]. Adverse effects reported with dronabinol were tiredness, sedation, somnolence, confusion, and euphoria for a longer period [184,186].

The limitations of these studies include a small number of participants, short study duration and lack of placebo group. Current data should be considered as preliminary. It would be premature to say that the cannabinoids have any effect on dementia symptoms or progression. Additional double blinded, randomized, placebo-controlled trials are needed to evaluate the efficacy and safety of cannabinoids in AD. In addition, CBD has demonstrated effects in pre-clinical AD models suggesting a deeper investigation to clarify the potential clinical utility of CBD.

5.3.3. Multiple Sclerosis

Multiple sclerosis is a chronic autoimmune, inflammatory neurological disease characterized by demyelination in the CNS caused by inflammatory immune-mediated attacks [187,188]. In 2015 there were more than 2 million people worldwide affected by multiple sclerosis [189] and it is currently incurable [190].

Typical syndromes at presentation include monocular visual loss due to optic neuritis, limb weakness or sensory loss, double vision or ataxia [191]. A progressive clinical course develops in many of the persons affected, eventually leading to impaired mobility and cognition.

Pre-clinical studies suggest that cannabis and individual cannabinoids improve the signs of motor dysfunction in experimental models of multiple sclerosis [192].

Lyman was one of the first to report the effects of THC in animals with autoimmune encephalomyelitis (multiple sclerosis model). In that study, affected animals treated with THC either had no clinical signs of the disorder or showed mild clinical signs with delayed onset. In addition, examination of central nervous system tissue revealed a marked reduction of inflammation [193].

Additional reports have supported and extended these findings demonstrating that THC, but not CBD, ameliorated both tremor and spasticity and reduced the overall clinical severity of the disease [194,195].

Some reports highlight the importance of the CB1 receptor in controlling spasticity, tremor and the neuroinflammatory response in multiple sclerosis [195–197]. Although great evidence suggests cannabinoids exert immunosuppressive effects, it is believed that the neuroprotective properties of cannabinoids may be more relevant than their immunosuppressive characteristics in multiple sclerosis [197–199].

Cannabinoids therapeutic potential has aroused considerable interest in multiple sclerosis treatment. Patients with multiple sclerosis are using or considering using cannabis for a range of symptoms. Recent studies have indicated that there is a wide acceptance of cannabis within the multiple sclerosis community, with 20–60% of MS currently using cannabis, and 50–90% would consider usage if it were legal and more scientific evidence was available [200,201].

In some countries a mixture of cannabinoids (Nabiximols/Sativex®: mixture of THC and CBD in an approximate ratio of 1:1) has been approved for the symptomatic treatment of multiple sclerosis spasticity and neuropathic pain in cases in which previous medication has proved ineffective [202].

Recently, Torres-Moreno et al. [203] conducted a systematic review and meta-analysis to assess the efficacy and tolerability of medicinal cannabinoids by oral or oromucosal administration in the symptomatic treatment (spasticity, pain, and bladder dysfunction) of patients with multiple sclerosis. The medicinal cannabinoids evaluated were nabiximols; oral cannabis extract contains THC and CBD; dronabinol and nabilone.

Nineteen studies involving 3161 patients were identified to have satisfied the eligible criteria (randomized, placebo-controlled, double-blind, and parallel/crossover-designed trials for a minimum length of treatment of 2 weeks). Medicinal cannabinoids produce a limited and mild reduction of subjective spasticity, pain, and bladder dysfunction in patients with multiple sclerosis, but no changes in objectively measured spasticity. In the analysis of subjective spasticity, significant differences were observed with respect to the active treatments of oral cannabis extract and nabiximols. Efficacy in pain of oral cannabis extract and nabilone was also demonstrated, in addition to efficacy in bladder dysfunction for oral cannabis extract.

Variability in the compounds studied also influences the interpretation of tolerability results. In the total adverse events analysis, there was a higher risk of adverse events in nabiximols treatments and a higher risk of withdrawals due to adverse events in nabiximols; oral cannabis extract and dronabinol treatment.

Currently, there is no evidence of reports that evaluate the efficacy of cannabinoids versus other treatments (corticosteroids, anticholinergic agents) in multiple sclerosis. In addition, research into the possible combinations might bring about greater synergy benefits than in an individual form.

Future research should also be aimed at obtaining more conclusive evidence about the efficacy of cannabis or individual cannabinoids against the signs and symptoms of multiple sclerosis, dose and route of administration and at exploring strategies that maximize separation between the beneficial therapeutic effects and the undesirable effects.

5.4. Post-Traumatic Stress Disorder

In the present day, clinicians need to counsel patients with post-traumatic stress disorder (PTSD) who are using or requesting to use cannabis for therapeutic or recreational purposes. For this reason, it is important to understand benefits or potential harms of cannabis in this disorder [204]. O'Neil et al. [205] report that in a general way, there is insufficient evidence regarding the benefits and harms of cannabis preparations for patients with PTSD. A review made by these authors points several trials treating PTSD patients with THC and CBD, randomizing its amounts present in smoked cannabis. The outcomes observed were categorized as changes in the Clinician-Administered PTSD Scale.

However, according to Bitencourt and Takahashi [206], human and animal studies suggest that CBD may offer therapeutic benefits for PTSD, revealing fewer side effects than the pharmacological therapy currently adopted for this disorder. Although with evidence that points to the modulation of the endocannabinoid system, the authors recognize that more studies should be performed for a better understanding of the neurobiological mechanisms. CBD was also studied by Elms et al. [207] who observed that patients taking daily oral CBD over an 8-week period demonstrated an overall decrease in PTSD symptom severity. The authors recognize the good toleration of CBD and that only a minority of patients did report fatigue and gastrointestinal discomfort. Steenkamp et al. [208] report that their clinical and preclinical studies suggest the cannabinoids may offer therapeutic benefits in this disorder, and that the pharmacological enhancement of endocannabinoid system signaling has yielded promising results in rodents, preventing dysfunctional stress-related processes. The authors also recommend future controlled studies in humans for a better evaluation of the relation between PTSD and cannabis.

5.5. Tourette's Syndrome

Tourette's syndrome (TS) is an inherited neuropsychiatric disorder characterized by the presence of multiple motor tics and at least one vocal tic [209]. Although the cause of TS is unknown, current research points to abnormalities in certain brain regions (basal ganglia, frontal lobes, and cortex), the circuits that interconnect these regions, and the neurotransmitters dopamine, serotonin, and norepinephrine [210,211].

Since the central endocannabinoid system is an important modulatory in the brain that influences and controls all important neurotransmitter systems, it can be speculated that TS might be caused by a dysfunction in the central endocannabinoid system. Noteworthy, there is a strong interaction between the dopaminergic and the central endocannabinoid system [212,213], particularly in basal ganglia [214,215]. Therefore, it can also be speculated that cannabinoids may inhibit dopaminergic activity in brain areas associated with motor control resulting in movements such as tics [216].

For many patients with TS, available medications do not help with their symptoms, or cause significant side effects. Cannabinoids have been explored as a treatment for TS since the 1980s. In 1988, for the first time it was suggested that cannabis might be such an alternative treatment option for TS. Sandyk et al. [217] reported three patients who experienced a reduction in motor tics and obsessive-compulsive behavior when smoking cannabis. No side effects occurred, and treatment effect was stable over time and did not decrease [217]. Subsequently, a small number of case studies has been published describing beneficial effects of cannabis in patients with TS. In most of these cases, the authors report about beneficial effects on both tics and psychiatric symptoms and no reports available about severe side effects [218,219].

Later, two clinical trials investigated the effect of oral THC in TS patients. In a double-blind placebo-controlled trial 12 adult patients were randomly treated with oral THC (gelatin capsules at 2.5 and 5.0 mg) or placebo [220]. Patients received a single dose of THC (5; 7.5 or 10 mg) according to their body weight, sex, age, and prior use of cannabis. Motor and vocal tics and obsessive-compulsive behavior were improved in the treatment groups. No side effect or mild transient adverse reaction (headache, nauseas, ataxia, and anxiety) were reported in patients who had received 7.5 or 10 mg of THC [220]. The second report is a randomized, double-blind, placebo-controlled study with 17 patients with TS treated over a 6-week period with up to 10 mg/day of THC [221]. Tic severity and global clinical outcome scores were improved in some patients, while other patients did not benefit from THC treatment. In addition, THC reached effectiveness after a three-week period treatment, which persisted or even increased after more than four weeks. No serious side effects occurred during the study [221].

While these trials have shown promising results, recently Abi-Jaoude et al. [222] conducted a retrospective study of cannabis (smoked or vaporized) effectiveness and tolerability in 19 adult patients with TS. Nine patients had previously participated in trials with one or more pharmaceutical cannabinoid. The frequency of use varied significantly, from frequent usage of small doses throughout the day to daily use for one week followed by three weeks off. The estimated average total daily dose also varied substantially, from less than 0.1–10 g, for a median of 1 g daily. Tic severity decreased by 60% and 94.7% of the patients were at least "very much improved" or "much improved" according to the clinical global impression severity scales. Cannabis was generally well-tolerated, although most participants reported side effects. It is interesting that patients reported to have much greater improvement in their symptoms using inhaled cannabis than using cannabinoid pharmaceuticals (pure oral THC, THC/CBD oromucosal spray, or the oral cannabinoid nabilone) [222].

To date, a double-blind, randomized, crossover pilot trial is underway to assess the efficacy and safety of three vaporized medical cannabis products with different THC and CBD contents, as well as placebo, in adults with TS [223]. Estimated completion date will be available on May 2019.

Based on clinical evidence and preliminary controlled studies, it has been suggested that cannabis-based medication may be a new and promising treatment strategy for patients with TS. Several clinical studies have been initiated to further investigate the efficacy and tolerability of different cannabis-based medications in the treatment of patients with TS including nabiximols (Sativex®) [224], THC (dronabinol) [225,226], and medicinal cannabis [223].

5.6. Nausea and Vomiting

Chemotherapy-induced nausea and vomiting (CINV) is one of the most distressing and common adverse events associated with cancer treatment [227]. The CB1 and CB2 receptors have been found in areas of the brainstem associated with emetogenic control [158,228]. Pre-clinical studies suggest that the anti-nausea and anti-emetic properties of cannabinoids (THC, dronabinol, nabilone) are most related to their actions at CB1 receptors [229–231]. In addition, an in vitro study suggests that Δ9-THC antagonizes the serotonin receptor (5-HT$_3$), a target of standard anti-emetic drugs [232].

Cannabinoids have been used effectively for treating CINV since 1985. In a systematic review, Whiting et al. [103] reported 28 studies (1772 participants) that assessed the use of cannabinoids for nausea and vomiting due to chemotherapy. Fourteen studies assessed nabilone, 3 for dronabinol, 1 for nabiximols, 4 for levonantradol, and 6 for THC. Other specific cannabinoids were not discriminated and individually evaluated. These trials included placebo controlled or used the antiemetics (prochlorperazine, chlorpromazine and domperidone) as comparators. The authors concluded that all trials suggested a greater benefit for cannabinoids than for both comparator and placebo, although the differences did not reach statistical significance in all studies [103].

Dronabinol and nabilone were approved by the FDA in 1985 for the treatment of CINV in patients who have failed to respond adequately to conventional antiemetic treatment [233,234]. The American Society for Clinical Oncology Expert Panel on Antiemetics recently issued updated guidelines and recommended dronabinol and nabilone for the treatment of nausea and vomiting caused by chemotherapy or radiation therapy [235].

Clinical experience remains insufficient for recommendation of cannabis for the treatment of nausea and vomiting caused by chemotherapy or radiation therapy. An uncontrolled pilot study reported that fifty-six patients who had no improvement with standard antiemetic agents were treated with cannabis and 78% demonstrated a positive response to marijuana [236].

Musty et al. [237] reported that patients who used a THC capsule experienced 76–88% relief from nausea and vomiting while those who smoked cannabis showed a 70–100% relief [237]. While a clinical trial comparing ondansetron to smoked cannabis (in doses of 8.4 mg or 16.9 mg THC; 0.30% cannabinol; 0.05% CBD) showed that both doses of Δ^9-THC reduced subjective ratings of queasiness and objective measures of vomiting; however, the effects were very modest compared to ondansetron [238].

The insufficient clinical evidence of medical cannabis combined with the relatively unfavorable side effect profile and the lack of trials comparing cannabinoids with newer antiemetics has limited their clinical utility.

In addition, because medical and legal concerns, the use of medical cannabis and CBD oil is not recommended for management of CINV and is not included in the most recent guidelines for CINV from the Multinational Association of Supportive Care in Cancer (MASCC)/European Society for Medical Oncology (ESMO) and the American Society of Clinical Oncology (ASCO) [235,239].

5.7. Treatment of Loss of Appetite

Weight loss and anorexia can be considered as common secondary side effects of several diseases, such as cancer, and represent a frequent clinical manifestation in patients with human immunodeficiency virus infection (HIV) and advanced acquired immunodeficiency syndrome (AIDS) [102]. This means that when cannabis or its derivatives are implemented, they can improve effects such as pain but can also influence the effect of loss of appetite or weight.

Two systematic reviews were conducted on trials implementing therapies with cannabinoids in patients with HIV and AIDS. Whiting et al. [103] evaluated four randomized controlled trials using dronabinol, with one of them investigating inhaled cannabis as well. These authors concluded that there was some evidence suggesting that cannabinoids were effective in weight gain for patients diagnosed with HIV. Lutge et al. [240] have focused their review on weight and appetite changes in patients with HIV or AIDS in trials in which dronabinol or inhaled cannabis have been implemented. These studies concluded that patient weight increased at higher doses of dronabinol and cannabis and that the median weight also increased with consumption of these compounds when compared to placebo. However, these investigators concluded that evidence on the use of cannabis and cannabinoids in relation to efficacy, safety and changes in appetite and weight were limited and insufficient.

More recently, Badowski and Yanful [241] performed a review where they compiled information on the use of oral dronabinol in controlling anorexia and weight loss in patients with HIV, AIDS and cancer. This natural compound exerts the effects acting directly on the appetite and vomiting control centers, being indicated in adult patients with HIV and AIDS but not being approved in cancer cases. The authors concluded that there is a limitation in the standardized definitions and that anorexia and weight loss can be misjudged when present in these diseases, and dronabinol can be considered as an additional treatment option in patients. Once again, it was also concluded that with legalization, new studies and new research should be carried out to evaluate the efficacy and safety of cannabis and dronabinol in appetite stimulation.

Andries et al. [242] carried out a study with the aim of investigating the effects of dronabinol treatment on weight and eating disorder-related psychopathological personality traits in cases of women with severe and prolonged anorexia nervosa. The study was conducted at a specialist care center for eating disorders, which included twenty-five women over the age of 18 and diagnosed for at least 5 years, where a randomized study was led between dronabinol-placebo and placebo-dronabinol. The authors concluded that although the sample size was low, there was good tolerance to dronabinol therapy during the four weeks of study, which induced significant weight gain, while no serious psychotropic adverse events were observed. They also concluded that this compound administered at low doses can be used as a safe palliative therapy in diagnosed and selected women.

Finally, Scheffler et al. [243] investigated long-term changes in body mass index, among other parameters, in cannabis users compared to non-users. This study included 109 patients who were treated for various levels of schizophrenia from one episode to patients receiving antipsychotics for

12 months. In contrast to the other reported studies, the researchers that during the first year of treatment there was a greater increase in body mass index in cannabis negative cases compared to cannabis positive cases, after adjusting the different parameters. These differences were not adequately explained by differences in sex, age, alcohol or methamphetamine use, dose or duration of treatment. In contrast to the use of acute cannabis that stimulates appetite, it can be hypothesized that chronic cannabis use may have the effect of suppressing appetite and thus avoiding the weight gain of its users and reducing the risk of obesity. However, other factors such as food malpractice and smoking may influence and contribute to these outcomes. The authors emphasize once again the importance of further longitudinal studies to evaluate possible effects varying in dose and composition of cannabis, with genetics and aspects of quotidian life and in determining the mechanisms by which cannabis reduces the weight gain, being unlikely that it will be used for this purpose.

5.8. Cutaneous Treatments and Dermatology

Over the past years, cannabinoids grew interest in the dermatologic area, mostly due to their anti-inflammatory and immunosuppressive properties, as well as its hydrophobic behavior [244]. Some of the research focus on pathologies such as skin cancer and inflammatory skin diseases as contact dermatitis and atopic dermatitis, amongst others [245]. However, according to Theroux and Cropley [246], Piffard was one of the pioneers in this field, leading to further investigation in the present and future, thus suggesting that this theme is not so recent after all. Despite that, the studies covered in this review are recent.

Wilkinson and Williamson [247] conducted a study where the main goal was not only to analyze if phytocannabinoids (THC, CBD and cannabigerol) can inhibit keratinocytes hyper-proliferation (one of the reasons why psoriasis occurs), but also if there is any connection with cannabinoid receptors. In fact, the authors made two important findings. The first is that all cannabinoids tested could indeed inhibit in vitro keratinocytes proliferation. IC_{50} values of maximum inhibition of proliferation for all compounds was reached between 3 and 5 mM, apart from cannabigerol, that was 2.5 and 3 mM. The second is that this mechanism is autonomous from CB1 and CB2 agonist receptors activation. Hence, their hypothesis was that the anti-proliferative effects observed were due to the interaction between cannabinoids and peroxisome proliferator-activated receptor-gamma (PPAR-γ) [247]. The authors observed that cannabigerol and CBD revealed greater potency regarding anti-proliferation, and that the greatest IC_{50} was observed for THC. Still, these results show a potential in using cannabinoids to treat psoriasis.

A different pathology is sebum's excess and acne. In 2015, Ali et al. [248] conducted a clinical trial where they assessed the effects of a 3% cannabis seed extract cream on 11 males who suffered from acne. By applying such formulation on the subjects' right cheek twice a day for 12 weeks, culminated in a reduction of sebum level after 48 h, in contrast to the control (cannabis free formulation) on the left cheek. In addition, results show a decrease in skin erythema. Most importantly, no side effects were observed, which sounds promising for future treatments.

Callaway et al. [249], performed a comparative clinical trial where patients ingested hempseed oil, suggesting this consumption can improve atopic dermatitis. A daily ingestion of 30 mL of the oil showed improvement on skin dryness, irritation, and itchiness, observing a reduction of these symptoms. The group of researchers believes that this results from the high content of polyunsaturated fatty acids present in the hempseed oil. It has been demonstrated that commercial hempseed oil is rich in CBDA, THCA, CBD, THC, CBG, CBN and CBDV [250]. However, Callaway et al., [249] have not studied which of the latter could be responsible for the outcome.

In 2007, a therapeutic clinical trial was carried out in by Eberlein et al. [251] using an endocannabinoid, namely N-palmitoylethanolamine, in a cream used as a regular treatment to assess atopic dermatitis and its symptoms. At the end of the trial, a 58.6% combined score was achieved in what concerns a decline in overall symptoms—erythema, pruritus, and dryness, amongst others.

This comes to prove that it is possible to perceive with studies of this kind, in order to reduce corticosteroids as a route of treatment in diseases as atopic dermatitis.

In a three case-study report, patients autonomously made use of formulations with cannabinoids in its composition, in the form of cream, oil, and spray, in order to treat epidermolysis bullosa, a genetic skin disorder that causes blisters and skin erosion. All three, expressed a decrease of pain and blister's formation, as well as wound healing [252]. This is beneficial, since it avoids the use of other medicines; however, it is necessary to proceed with further investigation, because this observational study did not take enough further conclusions.

Another study and a different pathology—Kaposi sarcoma—was studies and it was proved by Maor et al. [253] that CBD can induce cancer cells' apoptosis, the mechanism is associated to a G protein-coupled receptor that binds to CBD.

Armstrong et al. [254] proved that the induction of autophagy can make THC trigger apoptosis of melanoma cells, leading to loss of carcinogenic cells' viability. Also, by administrating a "Sativex-like" admixture of equivalent quantity of THC and CBD leads to a less harmful environment, since it prevents melanoma from progressing and inhibits tumor growth. This Sativex® formula is provided as a great example to treat metastatic melanoma, nonetheless further studies should be performed in humans [254].

Amongst other herbs, cannabis was included in a study review by Li et al. [255] in which they scrutinized the use of herbs as a medicine for skin cancer. They referred to an in vitro study where anandamide, 2-arachidonoylglycerol, and N-palmitoylethanolamine were used and they observed a reduction of cell viability.

In 2017, Maida et al. [256] observed cases of patients with pyoderma gangrenosum, a case of inflammatory dermatosis in which patients experience extreme and sometimes chronic painful ulcers. In this study, three patients were observed and accepted to be part of the trial. Patient 1 had applied in his wounds an oil (5 mg/mL of THC + 6 mg/mL of CBD), which was commercially acquired. A daily dose of 1 mL of such oil applied to wounds and bandaging made the patient experience relief of pain and skin irritation, which led to stoppage of the use of corticosteroids. Patient 2, used the same oil with different ratios (7 mg/mL of THC + 9 mg/mL of CBD), applying 0.5–1.0 mL to wounds two/three times a day. As a result, patient experienced a reduction of pain symptoms, nonetheless not statistically significant ($p = 0.0720$). Finally, patient 3 used the same oil composition of patient 2 and applied the same amount (0.5–1.0 mL) two times a day. This patient also experienced pain relief [256]. This research brings out new perspectives for cannabis as an analgesic. However, further studies should be performed, since the sample does not permit to take general conclusions.

In general, the obtained results bring hope to the potential of cannabinoids as a therapeutic in dermatology. Still, a lot more needs to be done and more clinical trials should be performed. As said before, researches in this field are becoming more frequent. That is why, several reviews on the topic were performed [245,257,258].

5.9. Infectious Diseases

Pathogenic microorganisms can cause infectious diseases that can spread from one living organism to another, which includes animals and humans. Therefore, there is an urgent need to find solutions to eradicate such diseases. Even though cannabis is being recently investigated as a treatment for many other disorders, when it comes to infections studies they are scarce. In spite of this, there is a case in which CBD was tested as a neuroprotective agent in patients with cerebral malaria [259]. Campos et al. [259], were able to prove in a murine model that CBD can serve as an adjuvant treatment, helping on behavior, relief of anxiety, and improvement of the cognitive function, since the cannabis secondary metabolite promotes recovery of cognitive deficits. In addition, it helped by increasing survival. In any case, these results imply a potential role of cannabinoids as a treatment option, further studies need to be undertaken, to determine cannabinoids' full potential in this field.

Meza and Lehmann [260] hypothesized that the phytocannabinoid betacaryophyllene (BCP) could activate the cannabinoid type 2 receptor (CB2R) (part of the endocannabinoid system) bettering the beginning of hyper-inflammatory phase on patients with sepsis. The CB2R activation allows an immunosuppressive response, which plays a crucial role in such a phase. As result, it is believed that sepsis aggravation will be reduced. Nevertheless, this study is just a proposal, and further studies need to be pursued to achieve solid and accurate results.

As observed, studies correlating cannabis as a potential therapeutic target to treat infections are scarce. More needs to be performed in order to achieve significant conclusions.

5.10. Glaucoma

Glaucoma is often caused by an anomalously high intraocular pressure (IOP) on the eye [261]. This pressure can be controlled, therefore for most treatments the main goal is to decrease it [261].

In 1998, a review performed by Green [262] came into realization that oral or topical cannabinoids administration would be a good option for glaucoma therapy. However, the same did not happen for smoked marijuana. In spite of IOP reduction on smoking marijuana users, its toxic effects surpassed what was supposed to be beneficial. Nonetheless, only THC is mentioned, and the author defended that further investigation regarding cannabinoids should be done.

In 2006, a trial with six participants was conducted by Tomida et al. [263]. Five milligrams of THC was administrated sublingually and had an effect on the reduction of IOP. Contrarily , 40 mg of CBD increased IOP. Overall, studies are promising, regarding sublingual route administration of THC. However, taking into account that TCH mechanisms on reducing IOP is not yet fully understood, further research and studies need to be performed.

A recent study by Miller and colleagues [264] tested two phytocannabinoids on mice. THC and CBD were applied atopically. Results showed that 5 mM of THC reduced IOP at a rate of 30% for at least 8 h. The mechanism is associated with cannabinoid-related receptors (CB1 and GPR18). Diversely, CBD was counterproductive, because it diminished THC effects, which was the opposite desire outcome [264].

Regardless of the few and redundant studies on this topic, it is possible to conclude that topical and oral administration of cannabinoids have a potential to become part of anti-glaucoma treatment, encouraging research to pursue such an agenda in the field.

5.11. Sleep and Anxiety Disorders

The therapeutic use of cannabis to treat insomnia is a bit controversial, since this is one of the symptoms usually associated to the consumption of this substance. However, in recent years some studies have become very relevant in the therapeutic use of cannabis on people who show sleeping problems. Usually, insomnia is defined as a multifaceted disorder, which is caused by stress factors, health problems that patients may suffer or simply by their daily lives [109]. In some research, it is stated that THC is responsible for sleep promotion, as well as CBD, which have both psychoactive and non-psychoactive properties, which suggests a possible interaction on both cannabis components [265]. Nicholson et al. [266] concluded that THC and CBD have distinct activities on sedative and alerting situations, and therefore their combinations apparently would provide better balance on their activity. Furthermore, some authors claimed that cannabis is effective for insomnia treatment showing results that support the idea of cannabis' inducing effects on sleep [267]. Nonetheless, it was also evaluated that the use of cannabis would be associated with poor quality of sleep; these contradictory effects found in several studies depend on the concentration of cannabinoids, dose, and the route of administration of this substance [268].

Discoveries about the increased consumption of cannabis in people with anxiety problems led some authors to investigate a possible reason for this. The fact that people consume the drug to relax (since relaxation is the most common symptom reported from this drug) may explain this situation [269]. Apparently, THC presents two different effects: when at high doses, the anxiogenic symptoms are predominant, while at low doses the anxiolytic effects prevail. CBD also plays an interesting role in this area, producing anxiolytic effects, and when administered orally has the ability to attenuate the anxiogenic effects of THC. Bergamaschi et al. [270] found that patients who suffer social anxiety disorder had less anxiety when a dose of CBD was provided. This suggests that cannabis use as a medication for anxiety disorders is a very appealing subject for further research.

To date, studies that were focused on disorders like the Huntington's or Parkinson's diseases, dystonia, and also on inflammatory bowel diseases (such as the Crohn's disease) have not provided scientists with sufficient evidence supporting the effectiveness of cannabis. This situation occurs also with anxiety-related disorders, such as post-traumatic stress disorder; depressive disorders; sleep disorders; and types of chronic pain not yet included in clinical trials as well. Despite that, some patients suffering from these conditions have reported clinical benefits from using cannabis or cannabinoids.

However, for the great majority of these medical conditions, there is either no evidence of effectiveness from controlled clinical trials, or there is limited evidence from studies rated as susceptible to bias because of small patient samples, poor controls or no comparison between cannabis or cannabinoids with placebo or active drug treatments was made [103,261]. Therefore, medical professionals who treat these conditions may be reluctant to use cannabinoids outside clinical trials in the absence of such evidence. Nonetheless, patients are using cannabis and cannabinoids to treat symptoms of these conditions in countries where they are able to do so. This highlights the need to expand the evidence base by undertaking robust studies that cover the full range of cannabis preparations being used, including addressing the issue raised by some patients who report greater benefit from using the whole plant than from using single extracts of cannabinoids, the so-called entourage effect [92,271].

6. Challenges in the Determination of Secondary Metabolites of Cannabis

A laboratorial analysis to determine cannabis products use or content can be carried out by measuring of a wide number of cannabinoids and possible metabolites [272]. Nowadays, the most commonly searched cannabinoids on a routine analysis involve cannabigerol, cannabigerolic acid, CBD, cannabidiolic acid, THC, THCA, Δ8-THC, tetrahydrocannabivarin, cannabichromene, and CBN, and their presence can be influenced by several factors. These factors can turn into challenges that can result in erroneous interpretations or incorrect results if not taken into consideration. This analytical determination is of importance, since therapeutic and clinical decisions may depend on it and the assessment of patient compliance as well. In addition, it is also important to evaluate whether the consumption was licit or not, or even to know the concentrations of the active ingredients in formulations. Three big challenges are going to be pointed: (1) sample used for determination; (2) sample preparation; and finally (3) analytical instrumentation, covering the major concerns when cannabinoids are to be determined.

6.1. Samples used for Determination

The first big challenge regarding the mentioned cannabinoids is related to the selection of the sample used for their identification and quantification. The analytical field is versatile but requires a careful evaluation according to the main goal of the analysis. The determination of cannabinoids in biological and other specimens has a great importance either in forensic or clinical toxicology, since they are the most widely abused drugs over the world [273]. This analysis can be performed in both biological and non-biological specimens.

6.1.1. Biological Specimens

Blood and urine are historically the elected biological specimens for drug test analysis either in ante-mortem or post-mortem cases [274]. Blood usually identifies a recent drug use and gives an indication of the degree of influence by a drug at the time of collection [272,275]. However, the invasive procedure necessary for its sampling has been pointed as a pitfall. The common alternative is the analysis of urine, applied successfully in workplace drug testing and in abstinence control programs [275–277]. Although the presence of certain drugs of abuse or their metabolites in urine can be interpreted as evidence of relatively recent exposure, this does not apply for cannabis [278].

Currently there is an increasing interest for alternative samples to determine cannabinoids, with focus on less invasive collectors and the acquisition of more information regarding cannabis use [274]. These include other body fluids and tissues such as oral fluid, sweat, and hair , or in case of foetal drug exposure, meconium and umbilical cord [272,274].

Oral fluid collection is easy and non-invasive, and considered by some authors the only body fluid where drug levels would correlate to those in blood [272,275,278–280]. These reasons justified the extensive application of this biological fluid to determine cannabinoids [281–285]. However, the risk of contamination from residual drug in the mouth might not allow this correlation hence this biological specimen has not received broader acceptance to date [272,276]. In addition, its collection may be thwarted by lack of sample available for analysis caused by physiological, or drug itself factors [286]. The presence of food and stimulation techniques might also result in an incorrect quantification of drug presence [286].

The evolution of analytical instrumentation, mainly related to its sensitivity, together with the advances in sweat collection, have made possible the determination of drugs in this specimen [285]. The detection of THC in sweat was reported for the first time in 1990 [287] and later detected in sweat wipes drivers under influence [288,289]. In the past, the scientific community has questioned this matrix's usefulness since there was a variation between individuals in the amount of sweat they excreted, and the first trials to determine the presence of xenobiotics applied patches that occluded the skin resulting in skin problems (e.g., irritation, alteration of the steady-state, pH, and infections) [274]. More recently, non-occlusive patches are being applied which use an absorbent cellulose pad, being able to detect drug use shortly before the patch was applied and lasting up to seven days [272,275]. Nevertheless, THC is a neutral molecule, unlike the majority of other drugs of abuse, and for this reason, its diffusion is expected to be slower and low amounts are usually detected (ng/patch) [289].

The hair drug analysis has become widespread in recent years and thus has become increasingly important [272,290–292]. The analysis provides long-term information on drug use over a time period as long as the length of the hair allows (weeks, months, or even years), something that does not occur with other biological matrices [290,292,293]. However, this specimen also presents its pitfalls. One must consider the cosmetic treatments of hair or ethnicity (black or brown hair tend to accumulate more basic-type drugs, due to higher levels of eumelanin) [272]. These factors may lead to an incorrect interpretation of results. In hair, THC was proven to be detected in greater concentrations when compared to THC–COOH, usually the target metabolite to identify cannabis use. This metabolite, although inactive, has a long half-life, but the concentrations found in hair are very low (e.g., sub-picogram per mg range) due to the very poor hair incorporation rate, and sometimes not detectable at all even when extremely sensitive analytical methods are used [294,295]. This may be a problem, since the detection of this metabolite in hair is mandatory to distinguish active consumption from external contamination. In this sense, only sophisticated analytical methods are capable of THC–COOH determination, such as: GC-MS with negative chemical ionisation (NCI) after derivatization with fluorinated reagents; special GC techniques (large injection volume or bi-dimensional-GC); GC-MS/MS; LC-MS, and MS^2 [290]. In addition, external contamination of THCA has been reported, due to manipulation of cannabis material and side stream smoke [290]. Also, there is evidence of formation of THC resulting from decarboxylation of THCA when alkaline hair digestion at elevated temperatures was applied in sample preparation [290]. Furthermore, the phase I metabolites of THC undergo phase II, forming corresponding glucuronides, and although THC–COOH-glucuronide has been already characterised in hair, the same has not been reported for 11–OH–THC glucuronide [290].

Regarding maternal and neonatal biological specimens, the identification and quantification of drugs and their metabolites offer an objective and reliable approach. Among these specimens, meconium has been widely employed to identify foetal drug exposure during the 3rd trimester [275,296,297]. The main metabolite of THC, THC–COOH, has been reported as the most abundant metabolite detected in meconium samples [298]. The collection of meconium from diapers is also considered non-invasive, which is a big advantage when we are dealing with new-borns, nevertheless some pitfalls have also been pointed, such as the fact that meconium can be expelled prior to, or during, delivery and become unavailable for analysis [299]. In addition, the meconium may not be expelled for days to weeks after birth, and it is often of limited quantity [299]. The determination of cannabinoids in this matrix may be possible without hydrolysing the sample because it has been proven that hydrolysis increases the positivity identification rate [300]. Hydrolysis is known for allowing glucuronides cleavage increasing the free analytes concentration [300].

An alternative to meconium regarding foetal drug exposure is the umbilical cord tissue. This specimen is available immediately at birth, for all neonates, and a large amount of tissue is usually available for the analysis [299]. The cannabis data in this sample is scarce and not much information is available on metabolite profile [297].

6.1.2. Non-Biological Specimens

The remarkable pharmacological activity of psychoactive cannabinoids makes drug-type *Cannabis sativa* one of the most researched medicinal plant [301]. However, to the pharmaceutical industry, only two phenotypes are taken in consideration, one being the drug-type cannabis, rich in THC, and used for medicinal or recreational purposes, and other is fibre-type cannabis which is known for being rich in non-psychoactive cannabinoids [302]. The chemical composition of cannabis strains is limited, there is a variability within the plants, interaction of the environment of production, all factors that still require to be carefully monitored [303]. One has to consider that there are a large number of compounds and due to the necessity for standardized treatment in patients (composition and dosage), the use of cannabis should be standardized [304]. Regarding pharmaceutical products, for hemp oil, a great variability was observed for the two samples analysed, although the main component detected was CBD [301]. The authors of this study also point that a decarboxylation process of cannabidiolic acid into CBD might happen for hemp oil and extract during the extraction or during storage over time [301].

In addition, around the world different forms of cannabis products such as, fibres, oils, resins, dried inflorescences, and leaves are consumed [303]. The recent surge in the sale of cannabis-based consumer products has also increased the challenge for sample types required for analysis. These include foods, candies, beverages, topicals, vapes/eliquids, and oral supplements in various forms [305].

6.2. Sample Preparation

In any analytical protocol, the sample preparation is crucial in order to achieve accurate and reliable results [273]. The complex nature of the sample matrices, mentioned above, in which cannabinoids may be present, does not allow them to be directly introduced into the analytical instrument [306]. These challenges start with the matrix homogenization and continue through the analyte extraction, clean-up to remove unwanted interferences and derivatization [273].

The traditional liquid–liquid extraction (LLE) and solid-phase extraction (SPE) are commonly the most widely used techniques on a routine cannabinoid determination [272,290,297–299,307–310]. The most common solvent applied in LLE of cannabinoids is mixture of hexane:ethyl acetate on proportions of 9:1 [272,298,307,311] although 1:1 is also mentioned [309]. Other organic solvents might be applied in this technique, such as acetonitrile [310], but the extractions may not reveal as efficient. Regarding SPE, the reported sorbents include mainly mixed mode and cation exchange ones such as Oasis MCX [300], Chromabond HR-XA [290], Strata X-C [281,297], CleanScreen [285],

Isolute HCX [312], and specific THC sorbents, such as, CEREX HPSPE THC [299]. These conventional sample preparation techniques result, overall, in great cannabinoids recoveries, nevertheless, several drawbacks have been pointed in the most recent years, namely, difficulty in automation, its complicated and time-consuming processes, and the large amounts of sample and organic solvents that they usually require [313].

The mentioned drawbacks have nowadays been overcome by modern microextraction techniques [273,314,315]. Jain and Singh (2016) [273] have made and excellent and extensive review on these miniaturized procedures applied to cannabinoids determination. Among the most common techniques are solid-phase microextraction (SPME) [316–322] solid-phase dynamic extraction (SPDE) [323,324], microextraction by packed sorbents (MEPS) [325,326], and dispersive liquid–liquid microextraction (DLLME) [327] among others. These techniques focus on reducing the time of sample preparation and the amounts of organic solvents. Moreover, also trying to reduce the amount of biological specimen required, it reveals advantages such as, low-cost operation, possibility to couple online with analytical instruments and good extraction efficiencies [273,314,315,328].

Regarding the cannabis plants and its commercial products such as pharmaceutical formulations, one should also consider the challenge of maceration and homogenization. As mentioned above, there should be a careful standardization of the method used for cannabis extraction as it is highly important for the introduction of this plant as therapeutic drug [304]. Several extraction solvents have been applied for this purpose. They include ethanol, methanol, chloroform, hexane, petroleum ether, and mixtures of them but in these reports recovery rates are scarce [329].

Moran et al. [304] have reported polar solvents as the best suitable to extract cannabinoids, whereas it is most adequate to extract all active compounds with a mixture of polar and non-polar solvents, such as n-hexane and ethanol. These authors focus on FDA regulations that limit the levels of n-hexane in pharmaceutical products, but this can be surpassed by the usage of a more polar solvent such as heptane [304]. On the contrary, Richins [303] uses a less polar solvent, acetone, justifying it as an excellent option for THC with the advantage of extracting fewer sugars and polysaccharides than methanol does. Gul et al. [330] used a mixture of methanol and chloroform (9: 1, v/v) in sample preparation reporting recovery rates above 90% to major components but in the case of cannabigerolic acid, cannabigerol, and Δ8-THC the recovery rates were lower than 85%.

6.3. Analytical Instrumentation

Several analytical methods have been applied to determine cannabinoids in a wide range of matrices. The rising expansion on cannabis market has resulted in a constant development of quantitative analytical methods for their major compounds [305]. Cannabinoids can be detected using immunoassays (EMIT®, ELISA, fluorescence polarization, radioimmunoassay), which are usually adopted as a preliminary method in a systematic toxicological analysis (STA). Nevertheless, these can result in false negative and false positive reports which might be consequence of structurally related drugs recognized by the antibodies, adulterants affecting pH, detergents, and other surfactants [331]. In this sense, it is common procedure to confirm by chromatographic techniques any positive result given by the immunoassay [331]. The most common use gas chromatography (GC) coupled to mass spectrometry (GC/MS) [272,285,310–312] or flame ionization detector (GC/FID) [303] and liquid chromatography (LC) coupled to mass spectrometry (LC/MS) [301,302,332] or ultraviolet detector (LC/UV) [250,302,305,333]. Nevertheless, GC methods are recognized for its difficulty to identify and quantify acidic cannabinoids such as cannabigerolic acid, cannabidiolic acid, and THCA because they are decarboxylated into their neutral forms during analysis [329,334]. This decarboxylation of cannabinoid acids can be avoided if previously derivatized [335]. Cardenia et al. [335] tested different derivatization procedures with silylation and esterification (diazomethane-mediated), reagents and solvents (pyridine or ethyl acetate), and observed that methylation caused an increase in the signal-to-noise ratio of all carboxylic compounds, except for cannabigerolic acid. In comparison to the GC, the LC appears as a suitable tool to analyze the native composition of the cannabis plant [329].

Another challenge related with the analytical instrumentation is their ability to determine these cannabinoids when present in low concentrations. LC coupled to tandem mass spectrometry (LC–MS/MS) using electrospray ionization (ESI) or atmospheric pressure chemical ionization (APCI) is considered nowadays by many authors as the method of choice when drugs of abuse are to be determined, mainly because of the elevated signal-to-noise ratio and selectivity presented [336,337]. For an accurate mass measurement LC coupled with time-of-flight (TOF) MS [299] or hybrid linear ion-trap-Orbitrap (LTQ-Orbitrap) MS [308,338] have been successfully applied to determine cannabinoids [336]. These accurate mass analytical instruments can reveal themselves of crucial importance, together with in vivo assays, for the determination of unknown metabolites.

7. Conclusions and Future Perspectives

There is still much to know concerning the effects of most chemical components of cannabis, their efficacy, whether or not patients are responding to the treatment, defining the correct doses, which is the best way of administration, and the side effects. Notwithstanding, the scientific community is becoming more and more interested in studying new therapeutic possibilities of cannabis, despite the fact that there is no scientific evidence supporting its adequate use for most situations.

Cannabis legalization for medical purposes is still a barrier that needs to be overcome, since in most cases legislation is ambiguous and insufficient to allow regulated access for use in medical situations. Its recreational use concerns authorities, as it is the most consumed drug worldwide; indeed, 200–300 million consumers are estimated around the world. Besides the high number of consumers, in several countries, maximum historical figures were achieved, and there have been several changes in trafficking, with the appearance of high-potency strains of cannabis, edible products, and e-liquids, innovations in the forms of available drug and delivery systems for consumption, which nowadays represent sources of concern for authorities. There is no doubt that further studies are needed to ascertain whether or not the potential benefits compensate the risks, namely in terms of the long-term adverse effects, which are still barely known.

Author Contributions: J.G. was responsible for articles search and writing of the manuscript concerning modes of use, the pharmacodynamics, and pharmacokinetic section. T.R. was responsible for research and writing the manuscript concerning the analytical methodologies section and revising the manuscript. S.S. was responsible for research and writing the manuscript concerning the therapeutic uses section, namely the uses of cannabis in pain and loss of appetite. A.Y.S. was responsible for research and writing the manuscript concerning the therapeutic uses section, namely the uses of cannabis in infection diseases, glaucoma. D.C. was responsible for research and writing of the manuscript concerning the secondary and toxic effects section, dependence, and tolerance, as well anxiety and insomnia. Â.L. was responsible for ressearch and writing of the manuscript concerning the secondary metabolites section and revising the manuscript. N.F. was responsible for research and writing of the manuscript concerning the therapeutic uses section, namely the uses in epilepsy, neurodegenerative disorders, and other uses. The authors J.G., T.R., S.S., A.Y.S., D.C., Â.L. and N.F. contributed equally to this paper. M.B. was responsible for research and writing the section of legal aspects and prevalence, and revising the manuscript. E.G. was responsible for designing the study, writing the section on the therapeutic uses of cannabis, organization and revising the manuscript. A.P.D. was responsible for designing the study, organization and revising the manuscript.

Funding: This research was funded by FEDER funds through the POCI-COMPETE 2020-Operational Programme Competitiveness and Internationalisation in Axis I-Strengthening research, technological development and innovation, grant number "Project POCI-01-0145-FEDER-007491" and National Funds by FCT-Fundação para a Ciência e a Tecnologia, grant number "Project UID/Multi/00709/2013". S. Soares and J. Gonçalves acknowledge Program Santander-Totta Universidades in the form of a fellowship grant number "Bolsa BID/UBI-Santander Universidades/2018". Â. Luís acknowledges the contract in the scientific area of Microbiology (Scientific Employment) financed by FCT.

Conflicts of Interest: The authors declare that they have no conflict of interest or financial involvement regarding this submission.

References

1. Verpoorte, R.; Contin, A.; Memelink, J. Biotechnology for the production of plant secondary metabolites. *Phytochem. Rev.* **2002**, *1*, 13–25. [CrossRef]
2. Sirikantaramas, S.; Taura, F.; Morimoto, S.; Shoyama, Y. Recent Advances in *Cannabis sativa* Research: Biosynthetic Studies and Its Potential in Biotechnology. *Curr. Pharm. Biotechnol.* **2007**, *8*, 237–243. [CrossRef] [PubMed]
3. Cohen, K.; Weinstein, A. The effects of cannabinoids on executive functions: Evidence from cannabis and synthetic cannabinoids—A systematic review. *Brain Sci.* **2018**, *8*, 40. [CrossRef] [PubMed]
4. Solymosi, K.; Kofalvi, A. Cannabis: A Treasure Trove or Pandora's Box? *Mini Rev. Med. Chem.* **2017**, *17*, 1223–1291. [CrossRef] [PubMed]
5. ElSohly, M.A.; Radwan, M.M.; Gul, W.; Chandra, S.; Galal, A. Phytochemistry of *Cannabis sativa* L. *Prog. Chem. Org. Nat. Prod.* **2017**, *103*, 1–36. [PubMed]
6. Andre, C.M.; Hausman, J.-F.; Guerriero, G. *Cannabis sativa*: The Plant of the Thousand and One Molecules. *Front. Plant Sci.* **2016**, *7*, 19. [CrossRef] [PubMed]
7. Bonini, S.A.; Premoli, M.; Tambaro, S.; Kumar, A.; Maccarinelli, G.; Memo, M.; Mastinu, A. *Cannabis sativa*: A comprehensive ethnopharmacological review of a medicinal plant with a long history. *J. Ethnopharmacol.* **2018**, *227*, 300–315. [CrossRef] [PubMed]
8. Brenneisen, R. Chemistry and Analysis of Phytocannabinoids and Other Cannabis Constituents—Marijuana and the Cannabinoids. In *Marijuana and the Cannabinoids*; ElSohly, M.A., Ed.; Humana Press: Totowa, NJ, USA, 2007; pp. 17–49. ISBN 978-1-59259-947-9.
9. El Sohly, M.A. (Ed.) *Marijuana and the Cannabinoids*; Humana Press: Totowa, NJ, USA, 2017; ISBN 9781588294562.
10. Guo, T.T.; Zhang, J.C.; Zhang, H.; Liu, Q.C.; Zhao, Y.; Hou, Y.F.; Bai, L.; Zhang, L.; Liu, X.Q.; Liu, X.Y.; et al. Bioactive spirans and other constituents from the leaves of *Cannabis sativa* f. sativa. *J. Asian Nat. Prod. Res.* **2017**, *19*, 793–802. [CrossRef] [PubMed]
11. Appendino, G.; Chianese, G.; Taglialatela-Scafati, O. Cannabinoids: Occurrence and Medicinal Chemistry. *Curr. Med. Chem.* **2011**, *18*, 1085–1099. [CrossRef] [PubMed]
12. Grof, C.P.L. Cannabis, from plant to pill. *Br. J. Clin. Pharmacol.* **2018**, *84*, 2463–2467. [CrossRef] [PubMed]
13. Lucas, C.J.; Galettis, P.; Schneider, J. The pharmacokinetics and the pharmacodynamics of cannabinoids. *Br. J. Clin. Pharmacol.* **2018**, *84*, 2477–2482. [CrossRef] [PubMed]
14. Newmeyer, M.N.; Swortwood, M.J.; Barnes, A.J.; Abulseoud, O.A.; Scheidweiler, K.B.; Huestis, M.A. Free and Glucuronide Whole Blood Cannabinoids' Pharmacokinetics after Controlled Smoked, Vaporized, and Oral Cannabis Administration in Frequent and Occasional Cannabis Users: Identification of Recent Cannabis Intake. *Clin. Chem.* **2016**, *62*, 1579–1592. [CrossRef] [PubMed]
15. Solowij, N.; Broyd, S.J.; van Hell, H.H.; Hazekamp, A. A protocol for the delivery of cannabidiol (CBD) and combined CBD and Δ9-tetrahydrocannabinol (THC) by vaporisation. *BMC Pharmacol. Toxicol.* **2014**, *15*, 58. [CrossRef] [PubMed]
16. Johansson, E.; Norén, K.; Sjövall, J.; Halldin, M.M. Determination of Δ1-tetrahydrocannabinol in human fat biopsies from marihuana users by gas chromatography-mass spectrometry. *Biomed. Chromatogr.* **1989**, *3*, 35–38. [CrossRef] [PubMed]
17. Rosado, T.; Gonçalves, J.; Luís, Â.; Malaca, S.; Soares, S.; Vieira, D.N.; Barroso, M.; Gallardo, E. Synthetic cannabinoids in biological specimens: A review of current analytical methods and sample preparation techniques. *Bioanalysis* **2018**, *10*, 1609–1623. [CrossRef] [PubMed]
18. Huestis, M.A. Pharmacokinetics and Metabolism of the Plant Cannabinoids, Δ9-Tetrahydrocannibinol, Cannabidiol and Cannabinol. In *Cannabinoids*; Pertwee, R.G., Ed.; Springer: Berlin/Heidelberg, Germany, 2005; pp. 657–690. ISBN 978-3-540-26573-3.
19. Toennes, S.W.; Ramaekers, J.G.; Theunissen, E.L.; Moeller, M.R.; Kauert, G.F. Comparison of cannabinoid pharmacokinetic properties in occasional and heavy users smoking a marijuana or placebo joint. *J. Anal. Toxicol.* **2008**, *32*, 470–477. [CrossRef] [PubMed]
20. Grotenhermen, F. Pharmacokinetics and Pharmacodynamics of Cannabinoids. *Clin. Pharmacokinet.* **2003**, *42*, 327–360. [CrossRef] [PubMed]

21. Ohlsson, A.; Lindgren, J.E.; Andersson, S.; Agurell, S.; Gillespie, H.; Hollister, L.E. Single-dose kinetics of deuterium-labelled cannabidiol in man after smoking and intravenous administration. *Biomed. Environ. Mass Spectrom.* **1986**, *13*, 77–83. [CrossRef] [PubMed]

22. Huestis, M.A.; Henningfield, J.E.; Cone, E.J. Blood cannabinoids. I. Absorption of THC and formation of 11-OH-THC and THCCOOH during and after smoking marijuana. *J. Anal. Toxicol.* **1992**, *16*, 276–282. [CrossRef] [PubMed]

23. Kauert, G.F.; Ramaekers, J.G.; Schneider, E.; Moeller, M.R.; Toennes, S.W. Pharmacokinetic Properties of 9-Tetrahydrocannabinol in Serum and Oral Fluid. *J. Anal. Toxicol.* **2007**, *31*, 288–293. [CrossRef] [PubMed]

24. Martin, J.H.; Schneider, J.; Lucas, C.J.; Galettis, P. Exogenous Cannabinoid Efficacy: Merely a Pharmacokinetic Interaction? *Clin. Pharmacokinet.* **2018**, *57*, 539–545. [CrossRef] [PubMed]

25. Goullé, J.-P.; Saussereau, E.; Lacroix, C. Pharmacocinétique du delta-9-tétrahydrocannabinol (THC). *Ann. Pharm. Françaises* **2008**, *66*, 232–244. [CrossRef] [PubMed]

26. Lindgren, J.E.; Ohlsson, A.; Agurell, S.; Hollister, L.; Gillespie, H. Clinical effects and plasma levels of delta 9-tetrahydrocannabinol (delta 9-THC) in heavy and light users of cannabis. *Psychopharmacology* **1981**, *74*, 208–212. [CrossRef] [PubMed]

27. Azorlosa, J.L.; Heishman, S.J.; Stitzer, M.L.; Mahaffey, J.M. Marijuana smoking: Effect of varying delta 9-tetrahydrocannabinol content and number of puffs. *J. Pharmacol. Exp. Ther.* **1992**, *261*, 114–122. [PubMed]

28. Agurell, S.; Carlsson, S.; Lindgren, J.E.; Ohlsson, A.; Gillespie, H.; Hollister, L. Interactions of delta 1-tetrahydrocannabinol with cannabinol and cannabidiol following oral administration in man. Assay of cannabinol and cannabidiol by mass fragmentography. *Experientia* **1981**, *37*, 1090–1092. [CrossRef] [PubMed]

29. Eichler, M.; Spinedi, L.; Unfer-Grauwiler, S.; Bodmer, M.; Surber, C.; Luedi, M.; Drewe, J. Heat Exposure of *Cannabis sativa* Extracts Affects the Pharmacokinetic and Metabolic Profile in Healthy Male Subjects. *Planta Med.* **2012**, *78*, 686–691. [CrossRef] [PubMed]

30. Grant, K.S.; Petroff, R.; Isoherranen, N.; Stella, N.; Burbacher, T.M. Cannabis use during pregnancy: Pharmacokinetics and effects on child development. *Pharmacol. Ther.* **2018**, *182*, 133–151. [CrossRef] [PubMed]

31. Ohlsson, A.; Lindgren, J.-E.; Wahlen, A.; Agurell, S.; Hollister, L.E.; Gillespie, H.K. Plasma delta-9-tetrahydrocannabinol concentrations and clinical effects after oral and intravenous administration and smoking. *Clin. Pharmacol. Ther.* **1980**, *28*, 409–416. [CrossRef] [PubMed]

32. Wall, M.E.; Sadler, B.M.; Brine, D.; Taylor, H.; Perez-Reyes, M. Metabolism, disposition, and kinetics of delta-9-tetrahydrocannabinol in men and women. *Clin. Pharmacol. Ther.* **1983**, *34*, 352–363. [CrossRef] [PubMed]

33. Garrett, E.R.; Hunt, C.A. Physicochemical Properties, Solubility, and Protein Binding of Δ9-Tetrahydrocannabinol. *J. Pharm. Sci.* **1974**, *63*, 1056–1064. [CrossRef] [PubMed]

34. Law, B.; Mason, P.A.; Moffat, A.C.; Gleadle, R.I.; King, L.J. Forensic aspects of the metabolism and excretion of cannabinoids following oral ingestion of cannabis resin. *J. Pharm. Pharmacol.* **1984**, *36*, 289–294. [CrossRef] [PubMed]

35. Frytak, S.; Moertel, C.G.; Rubin, J. Metabolic studies of delta-9-tetrahydrocannabinol in cancer patients. *Cancer Treat. Rep.* **1984**, *68*, 1427–1431. [PubMed]

36. Ahmed, A.I.A.; van den Elsen, G.A.H.; Colbers, A.; Kramers, C.; Burger, D.M.; van der Marck, M.A.; Olde Rikkert, M.G.M. Safety, pharmacodynamics, and pharmacokinetics of multiple oral doses of delta-9-tetrahydrocannabinol in older persons with dementia. *Psychopharmacology* **2015**, *232*, 2587–2595. [CrossRef] [PubMed]

37. Schwilke, E.W.; Schwope, D.M.; Karschner, E.L.; Lowe, R.H.; Darwin, W.D.; Kelly, D.L.; Goodwin, R.S.; Gorelick, D.A.; Huestis, M.A. Delta9-tetrahydrocannabinol (THC), 11-hydroxy-THC, and 11-nor-9-carboxy-THC plasma pharmacokinetics during and after continuous high-dose oral THC. *Clin. Chem.* **2009**, *55*, 2180–2189. [CrossRef] [PubMed]

38. Leuschner, J.T.; Harvey, D.J.; Bullingham, R.E.; Paton, W.D. Pharmacokinetics of delta 9-tetrahydrocannabinol in rabbits following single or multiple intravenous doses. *Drug Metab. Dispos.* **1986**, *14*, 230–238. [PubMed]

39. Challapalli, P.V.; Stinchcomb, A.L. In vitro experiment optimization for measuring tetrahydrocannabinol skin permeation. *Int. J. Pharm.* **2002**, *241*, 329–339. [CrossRef]

40. Stinchcomb, A.L.; Valiveti, S.; Hammell, D.C.; Ramsey, D.R. Human skin permeation of Δ^8-tetrahydrocannabinol, cannabidiol and cannabinol. *J. Pharm. Pharmacol.* **2004**, *56*, 291–297. [CrossRef] [PubMed]

41. Valiveti, S.; Hammell, D.C.; Earles, D.C.; Stinchcomb, A.L. In vitro/in vivo correlation studies for transdermal Δ8-THC development. *J. Pharm. Sci.* **2004**, *93*, 1154–1164. [CrossRef] [PubMed]

42. Touitou, E.; Fabin, B.; Dany, S.; Almog, S. Transdermal delivery of tetrahydrocannabinol. *Int. J. Pharm.* **1988**, *43*, 9–15. [CrossRef]

43. Elsohly, M.A.; Stanford, D.F.; Harland, E.C.; Hikal, A.H.; Walker, L.A.; Little, T.L.; Rider, J.N.; Jones, A.B. Rectal Bioavailability of Δ-9-Tetrahydrocannabinol from the Hemisuccinate Ester in Monkeys. *J. Pharm. Sci.* **1991**, *80*, 942–945. [CrossRef] [PubMed]

44. Brenneisen, R.; Egli, A.; Elsohly, M.A.; Henn, V.; Spiess, Y. The effect of orally and rectally administered delta 9-tetrahydrocannabinol on spasticity: A pilot study with 2 patients. *Int. J. Clin. Pharmacol. Ther.* **1996**, *34*, 446–452. [PubMed]

45. Chiang, C.W.; Barnett, G.; Brine, D. Systemic absorption of delta 9-tetrahydrocannabinol after ophthalmic administration to the rabbit. *J. Pharm. Sci.* **1983**, *72*, 136–138. [CrossRef] [PubMed]

46. Lucas, C.; Galettis, P.; Song, S.; Solowij, N.; Reuter, S.; Schneider, J.; Martin, J. Cannabinoid Disposition After Human Intraperitoneal Use: An Insight Into Intraperitoneal Pharmacokinetic Properties in Metastatic Cancer. *Clin. Ther.* **2018**, *40*, 1442–1447. [CrossRef] [PubMed]

47. Gaston, T.E.; Friedman, D. Pharmacology of cannabinoids in the treatment of epilepsy. *Epilepsy Behav.* **2017**, *70*, 313–318. [CrossRef] [PubMed]

48. Hunt, C.; Jones, R. Tolerance and disposition of tetrahydrocannabinol in man. *J. Pharmacol. Exp. Ther.* **1980**, *215*, 35–44. [PubMed]

49. Huestis, M.A. Human Cannabinoid Pharmacokinetics. *Chem. Biodivers.* **2007**, *4*, 1770–1804. [CrossRef] [PubMed]

50. Blackard, C.; Tennes, K. Human Placental Transfer of Cannabinoids. *N. Engl. J. Med.* **1984**, *311*, 797. [PubMed]

51. Perez-Reyes, M.; Wall, M.E. Presence of Δ^9-Tetrahydrocannabinol in Human Milk. *N. Engl. J. Med.* **1982**, *307*, 819–820. [PubMed]

52. Agurell, S.; Halldin, M.; Lindgren, J.E.; Ohlsson, A.; Widman, M.; Gillespie, H.; Hollister, L. Pharmacokinetics and metabolism of delta 1-tetrahydrocannabinol and other cannabinoids with emphasis on man. *Pharmacol. Rev.* **1986**, *38*, 21–43. [PubMed]

53. Matsunaga, T.; Iwawaki, Y.; Watanabe, K.; Yamamoto, I.; Kageyama, T.; Yoshimura, H. Metabolism of delta 9-tetrahydrocannabinol by cytochrome P450 isozymes purified from hepatic microsomes of monkeys. *Life Sci.* **1995**, *56*, 2089–2095. [CrossRef]

54. Narimatsu, S.; Watanabe, K.; Matsunaga, T.; Yamamoto, I.; Imaoka, S.; Funae, Y.; Yoshimura, H. Cytochrome P-450 isozymes involved in the oxidative metabolism of delta 9-tetrahydrocannabinol by liver microsomes of adult female rats. *Drug Metab. Dispos.* **1992**, *20*, 79–83. [PubMed]

55. Watanabe, K.; Matsunaga, T.; Yamamoto, I.; Funae, Y.; Yoshimura, H. Involvement of CYP2C in the metabolism of cannabinoids by human hepatic microsomes from an old woman. *Biol. Pharm. Bull.* **1995**, *18*, 1138–1141. [CrossRef] [PubMed]

56. Widman, M.; Halldin, M.; Martin, B. In vitro metabolism of tetrahydrocannabinol by rhesus monkey liver and human liver. *Adv. Biosci.* **1979**, *22–23*, 101–103.

57. Huestis, M.A.; Cone, E.J. Differentiating new marijuana use from residual drug excretion in occasional marijuana users. *J. Anal. Toxicol.* **1998**, *22*, 445–454. [CrossRef] [PubMed]

58. Zendulka, O.; Dovrtělová, G.; Nosková, K.; Turjap, M.; Šulcová, A.; Hanuš, L.; Juřica, J. Cannabinoids and Cytochrome P450 Interactions. *Curr. Drug Metab.* **2016**, *17*, 206–226. [CrossRef]

59. Harvey, D.J.; Martin, B.R.; Paton, W.D.M. Identification and measurement of cannabinoids and their in vivo metabolites in liver by gas chromatography-mass spectrometry. *Marihuana Biol. Eff.* **1979**, 45–62. [CrossRef]

60. Consroe, P.; Laguna, J.; Allender, J.; Snider, S.; Stern, L.; Sandyk, R.; Kennedy, K.; Schram, K. Controlled clinical trial of cannabidiol in Huntington's disease. *Pharmacol. Biochem. Behav.* **1991**, *40*, 701–708. [CrossRef]

61. Maurer, H.H.; Sauer, C.; Theobald, D.S. Toxicokinetics of Drugs of Abuse: Current Knowledge of the Isoenzymes Involved in the Human Metabolism of Tetrahydrocannabinol, Cocaine, Heroin, Morphine, and Codeine. *Ther. Drug Monit.* **2006**, *28*, 447–453. [CrossRef] [PubMed]

62. Halldin, M.M.; Widman, M.; Bahr, C.V.; Lindgren, J.E.; Martin, B.R. Identification of in vitro metabolites of delta 1-tetrahydrocannabinol formed by human livers. *Drug Metab. Dispos.* **1982**, *10*, 297–301. [PubMed]

63. Harvey, D.J. Absorption, Distribution, and Biotransformation of the Cannabinoids. In *Marihuana and Medicine*; Nahas, G.G., Sutin, K.M., Harvey, D., Agurell, S., Pace, N., Cancro, R., Eds.; Humana Press: Totowa, NJ, USA, 1999; pp. 91–103. ISBN 978-1-59259-710-9.

64. Kelly, P.; Jones, R.T. Metabolism of tetrahydrocannabinol in frequent and infrequent marijuana users. *J. Anal. Toxicol.* **1992**, *16*, 228–235. [CrossRef] [PubMed]

65. Alburges, M.E.; Peat, M.A. Profiles of Δ^9-Tetrahydrocannabinol Metabolites in Urine of Marijuana Users: Preliminary Observations by High Performance Liquid Chromatography-Radioimmunoassay. *J. Forensic Sci.* **1986**, *31*, 12302J. [CrossRef]

66. Lu, H.C.; Mackie, K. An Introduction to the Endogenous Cannabinoid System. *Biol. Psychiatry* **2016**, *79*, 516–525. [CrossRef] [PubMed]

67. Pertwee, R.G. Pharmacology of cannabinoid CB1 and CB2 receptors. *Pharmacol. Ther.* **1997**, *74*, 129–180. [CrossRef]

68. Pertwee, R.G. Pharmacology of cannabinoid receptor ligands. *Curr. Med. Chem.* **1999**, *6*, 635–664. [PubMed]

69. Laprairie, R.B.; Bagher, A.M.; Kelly, M.E.M.; Denovan-Wright, E.M. Cannabidiol is a negative allosteric modulator of the cannabinoid CB $_1$ receptor. *Br. J. Pharmacol.* **2015**, *172*, 4790–4805. [CrossRef] [PubMed]

70. McCarberg, B.H.; Barkin, R.L. The Future of Cannabinoids as Analgesic Agents: A Pharmacologic, Pharmacokinetic, and Pharmacodynamic Overview. *Am. J. Ther.* **2007**, *14*, 475–483. [CrossRef] [PubMed]

71. Di Marzo, L.; De Petrocellis, V. Endocannabinoids as Regulators of Transient Receptor Potential (TRP)Channels: A Further Opportunity to Develop New Endocannabinoid-Based Therapeutic Drugs. *Curr. Med. Chem.* **2010**, *17*, 1430–1449. [CrossRef] [PubMed]

72. Zygmunt, P.M.; Petersson, J.; Andersson, D.A.; Chuang, H.; Sørgård, M.; Di Marzo, V.; Julius, D.; Högestätt, E.D. Vanilloid receptors on sensory nerves mediate the vasodilator action of anandamide. *Nature* **1999**, *400*, 452. [CrossRef] [PubMed]

73. O'Sullivan, S.E. An update on PPAR activation by cannabinoids. *Br. J. Pharmacol.* **2016**, *173*, 1899–1910. [CrossRef] [PubMed]

74. Ashton, C.H. Adverse effects of cannabis and cannabinoids. *Br. J. Anaesth.* **1999**, *83*, 637–649. [CrossRef] [PubMed]

75. Hall, W. The health and psychological effects of cannabis use. *Curr. Issues Crim. Just.* **1994**, *6*, 208. [CrossRef]

76. Degenhardt, L.; Hall, W. Extent of illicit drug use and dependence, and their contribution to the global burden of disease. *Lancet* **2012**, *379*, 55–70. [CrossRef]

77. Ameri, A. The effects of cannabinoids on the brain. *Prog. Neurobiol.* **1999**, *58*, 315–348. [CrossRef]

78. Fergusson, D.M.; Horwood, L.J.; Swain-Campbell, N.R. Cannabis dependence and psychotic symptoms in young people. *Psychol. Med.* **2003**, *33*, 15–21. [CrossRef] [PubMed]

79. De Aquino, J.P.; Sherif, M.; Radhakrishnan, R.; Cahill, J.D.; Ranganathan, M.; D'Souza, D.C. The Psychiatric Consequences of Cannabinoids. *Clin. Ther.* **2018**, *40*, 1448–1456. [CrossRef] [PubMed]

80. Swift, W.; Hall, W.; Teesson, M. Characteristics of DSM-IV and ICD-10 cannabis dependence among Australian adults: Results from the National Survey of Mental Health and Wellbeing. *Drug Alcohol Depend.* **2001**, *63*, 147–153. [CrossRef]

81. Swift, W.; Hall, W.; Didcott, P.; Reilly, D. Patterns and correlates of cannabis dependence among long-term users in an Australian rural area. *Addiction* **1998**, *93*, 1149–1160. [CrossRef] [PubMed]

82. Anthony, J.C.; Warner, L.A.; Kessler, R.C. Comparative Epidemiology of Dependence on Tobacco, Alcohol, Controlled Substances, and Inhalants: Basic Findings From the National Comorbidity Survey. *Exp. Clin. Psychopharmacol.* **1994**, *2*, 244–268. [CrossRef]

83. Solowij, N. Do cognitive impairments recover following cessation of cannabis use? *Life Sci.* **1995**, *56*, 2119–2126. [CrossRef]

84. Pope, H.G., Jr.; Gruber, A.J.; Hudson, J.I.; Huestis, M.A.; Yurgelun-Todd, D. Cognitive Measures in Long-Term Cannabis Users. *J. Clin. Pharmacol.* **2002**, *42*, 41S–47S. [CrossRef]

85. Budney, A.J.; Higgins, S.T.; Radonovich, K.J.; Novy, P.L. Adding voucher-based incentives to coping skills and motivational enhancement improves outcomes during treatment for marijuana dependence. *J. Consult. Clin. Psychol.* **2000**, *68*, 1051–1061. [CrossRef] [PubMed]

86. European Monitoring Centre for Drugs and Drug Adiction. Cannabis Legislation in Europe. Available online: http://www.emcdda.europa.eu/system/files/publications/4135/TD0217210ENN.pdf (accessed on 22 January 2019).

87. European Monitoring Centre for Drugs and Drug Adiction. 2018 European Drug Report. Available online: http://www.emcdda.europa.eu/system/files/publications/8585/20181816_TDAT18001PTN_PDF.pdf (accessed on 11 January 2019).

88. Serviço de intervenção nos comportamentos aditivos e nas dependências. Relatório Anual 2016 A Situação do País em Matéria de Drogas e Toxicodependências. Available online: file://turing/users2\$/saude/depcmed/mega/Desktop/RelatorioAnual_2016_A_SituacaoDoPaisEmMateriaDeDrogas_e_Toxicodependencias.pdf (accessed on 17 January 2019).

89. European Monitoring Centre for Drugs and Drug Addiction. ESPAD Report 2015: Results from the European School Survey Project on Alcohol and Other Drugs. Available online: http://www.espad.org/sites/espad.org/files/ESPAD_report_2015.pdf (accessed on 17 January 2019).

90. United Nations. The Single Convention on Narcotic Drugs. Available online: File:///C:/Users/Administrator/Desktop/convention_1961_en.pdf (accessed on 18 January 2019).

91. Powell, B. The 7 Countries With The Strictest Weed Laws. Available online: https://www.medicalmarijuana.com.au/medical-marijuana/cannabis/the-7-countries-with-the-strictest-weed-laws (accessed on 17 January 2019).

92. European Monitoring Centre for Drugs and Addiction. Medical Use of Cannabis and Cannabinoids: Questions and Answers for Policymaking. Available online: http://www.emcdda.europa.eu/publications/rapid-communications/medical-use-of-cannabis-and-cannabinoids-questions-and-answers-for-policymaking_en (accessed on 22 January 2019).

93. National Alliance for Model State Drug Laws Use of Marijuana for Medicinal Purposes: Map of State Laws. Available online: http://www.namsdl.org/Maps/UseofMarijuanaforMedicinalPurposes-MapofStateLaws-1_10_2017-FINAL.pdf (accessed on 21 January 2019).

94. National Conference of State Legislatures. Marijuana Overview. Available online: http://www.ncsl.org/research/civil-and-criminal-justice/marijuana-overview.aspx (accessed on 18 January 2019).

95. Bigand, T.; Anderson, C.L.; Roberts, M.L.; Shaw, M.R.; Wilson, M. Benefits and Adverse Effects of Cannabis use among Adults with Persistent Pain. *Nurs. Outlook* **2018**. [CrossRef] [PubMed]

96. Armour, M.; Sinclair, J.; Chalmers, K.J.; Smith, C.A. Self-management strategies amongst Australian women with endometriosis: A national online survey. *BMC Complement. Altern. Med.* **2019**, *19*, 17–24. [CrossRef] [PubMed]

97. Fitzcharles, M.-A.; Zahedi Niaki, O.; Hauser, W.; Hazlewood, G.; the Canadian Rheumatology Association. Position Statement: A Pragmatic Approach for Medical Cannabis and Patients with Rheumatic Diseases. *J. Rheumatol.* **2019**, *46*, 181120. [CrossRef] [PubMed]

98. Palace, Z.J.; Reingold, D.A. Medical Cannabis in the Skilled Nursing Facility: A Novel Approach to Improving Symptom Management and Quality of Life. *J. Am. Med. Dir. Assoc.* **2019**, *20*, 94–98. [CrossRef] [PubMed]

99. Shin, S.; Mitchell, C.; Mannion, K.; Smolyn, J.; Meghani, S.H. An Integrated Review of Cannabis and Cannabinoids in Adult Oncologic Pain Management. *Pain Manag. Nurs.* **2018**. [CrossRef] [PubMed]

100. Campbell, G.; Stockings, E.; Nielsen, S. Understanding the evidence for medical cannabis and cannabis-based medicines for the treatment of chronic non-cancer pain. *Eur. Arch. Psychiatry Clin. Neurosci.* **2019**. [CrossRef] [PubMed]

101. Perron, B.E.; Holt, K.R.; Yeagley, E.; Ilgen, M. Mental health functioning and severity of cannabis withdrawal among medical cannabis users with chronic pain. *Drug Alcohol Depend.* **2019**, *194*, 401–409. [CrossRef] [PubMed]

102. National Academies of Sciences Engineering and Medicine. Therapeutic Effects of Cannabis and Cannabinoids. In *The Health Effects of Cannabis and Cannabinoids: The Current State of Evidence and Recommendations for Research*; National Academies Press: Washington, DC, USA, 2017; pp. 94–97.

103. Whiting, P.F.; Wolff, R.F.; Deshpande, S.; Di Nisio, M.; Duffy, S.; Hernandez, A.V.; Keurentjes, J.C.; Lang, S.; Misso, K.; Ryder, S.; et al. Cannabinoids for Medical Use: A Systematic Review and Meta-analysis. *J. Am. Med. Assoc.* **2015**, *313*, 2456–2473. [CrossRef] [PubMed]

104. Habib, G.; Artul, S. Medical Cannabis for the Treatment of Fibromyalgia. *JCR J. Clin. Rheumatol.* **2018**, *24*, 255–258. [CrossRef] [PubMed]

105. Habib, G.; Avisar, I. The Consumption of Cannabis by Fibromyalgia Patients in Israel. *Pain Res. Treat.* **2018**, *2018*, 7829427. [CrossRef] [PubMed]

106. van de Donk, T.; Niesters, M.; Kowal, M.A.; Olofsen, E.; Dahan, A.; van Velzen, M. An experimental randomized study on the analgesic effects of pharmaceutical-grade cannabis in chronic pain patients with fibromyalgia. *Pain* **2018**, in press. [CrossRef] [PubMed]

107. Yassin, M.; Robinson, D. Effect of Adding Medical Cannabis Treatment (MCT) to Analgesic Treatment in Patients with Low Back Pain related to Fibromyalgia: An Observational Cross-over Single Center Study. *Int. J. Anesthesiol. Pain Med.* **2017**, *3*, 1–8. [CrossRef]

108. Koppel, B.S.; Brust, J.C.M.; Fife, T.; Bronstein, J.; Youssof, S.; Gronseth, G.; Gloss, D. Systematic review: Efficacy and safety of medical marijuana in selected neurologic disorders. *Neurology* **2014**, *82*, 1556–1563. [CrossRef] [PubMed]

109. Klumpers, L.E.; Thacker, D.L. A Brief Background on Cannabis: From Plant to Medical Indications. *J. AOAC Int.* **2018**. [CrossRef] [PubMed]

110. Jett, J.; Stone, E.; Warren, G.; Cummings, K.M. Cannabis Use, Lung Cancer, and Related Issues. *J. Thorac. Oncol.* **2018**, *13*, 480–487. [CrossRef] [PubMed]

111. Johnson, J.R.; Burnell-Nugent, M.; Lossignol, D.; Ganae-Motan, E.D.; Potts, R.; Fallon, M.T. Multicenter, Double-Blind, Randomized, Placebo-Controlled, Parallel-Group Study of the Efficacy, Safety, and Tolerability of THC:CBD Extract and THC Extract in Patients with Intractable Cancer-Related Pain. *J. Pain Symptom Manag.* **2010**, *39*, 167–179. [CrossRef] [PubMed]

112. Portenoy, R.K.; Ganae-Motan, E.D.; Allende, S.; Yanagihara, R.; Shaiova, L.; Weinstein, S.; McQuade, R.; Wright, S.; Fallon, M.T. Nabiximols for opioid-treated cancer patients with poorly-controlled chronic pain: A randomized, placebo-controlled, graded-dose trial. *J. Pain* **2012**, *13*, 438–449. [CrossRef] [PubMed]

113. Fiest, K.M.; Sauro, K.M.; Wiebe, S.; Patten, S.B.; Kwon, C.-S.; Dykeman, J.; Pringsheim, T.; Lorenzetti, D.L.; Jetté, N. Prevalence and incidence of epilepsy: A systematic review and meta-analysis of international studies. *Neurology* **2017**, *88*, 296–303. [CrossRef] [PubMed]

114. Schuele, S.U.; Lüders, H.O. Intractable epilepsy: Management and therapeutic alternatives. *Lancet Neurol.* **2008**, *7*, 514–524. [CrossRef]

115. Brodie, M.J.; Barry, S.J.E.; Bamagous, G.A.; Norrie, J.D.; Kwan, P. Patterns of treatment response in newly diagnosed epilepsy. *Neurology* **2012**, *78*, 1548–1554. [CrossRef] [PubMed]

116. Carlini, E.A.; Leite, J.R.; Tannhauser, M.; Berardi, A.C. Cannabidiol and *Cannabis sativa* extract protect mice and rats against convulsive agents. *J. Pharm. Pharmacol.* **1973**, *25*, 664–665. [CrossRef] [PubMed]

117. Consroe, P.; Wolkin, A. Cannabidiol–antiepileptic drug comparisons and interactions in experimentally induced seizures in rats. *J. Pharmacol. Exp. Ther.* **1977**, *201*, 26–32. [PubMed]

118. Consroe, P.; Benedito, M.A.C.; Leite, J.R.; Carlini, E.A.; Mechoulam, R. Effects of cannabidiol on behavioral seizures caused by convulsant drugs or current in mice. *Eur. J. Pharmacol.* **1982**, *83*, 293–298. [CrossRef]

119. Wallace, M.J.; Wiley, J.L.; Martin, B.R.; DeLorenzo, R.J. Assessment of the role of CB1 receptors in cannabinoid anticonvulsant effects. *Eur. J. Pharmacol.* **2001**, *428*, 51–57. [CrossRef]

120. Jones, N.; Hill, T.; Stott, C.; Wright, S. Assessment of the anticonvulsant effects and tolerability of GW Pharmaceuticals' cannabidiol in the anticonvulsant screening program. In Proceedings of the American Epilepsy Society Annual Meeting, Philadelphia, PA, USA, 3–7 December 2015; pp. 4–8.

121. Jones, N.A.; Hill, A.J.; Smith, I.; Bevan, S.A.; Williams, C.M.; Whalley, B.J.; Stephens, G.J. Cannabidiol displays antiepileptiform and antiseizure properties in vitro and in vivo. *J. Pharmacol. Exp. Ther.* **2010**, *332*, 569–577. [CrossRef] [PubMed]

122. Jones, N.A.; Glyn, S.E.; Akiyama, S.; Hill, T.D.M.; Hill, A.J.; Weston, S.E.; Burnett, M.D.A.; Yamasaki, Y.; Stephens, G.J.; Whalley, B.J.; et al. Cannabidiol exerts anti-convulsant effects in animal models of temporal lobe and partial seizures. *Seizure* **2012**, *21*, 344–352. [CrossRef] [PubMed]

123. Thomas, A.; Baillie, G.L.; Phillips, A.M.; Razdan, R.K.; Ross, R.A.; Pertwee, R.G. Cannabidiol displays unexpectedly high potency as an antagonist of CB1 and CB2 receptor agonists in vitro. *Br. J. Pharmacol.* **2007**, *150*, 613–623. [CrossRef] [PubMed]

124. Puffenbarger, R.A.; Boothe, A.C.; Cabral, G.A. Cannabinoids inhibit LPS-inducible cytokine mRNA expression in rat microglial cells. *Glia* **2000**, *29*, 58–69. [CrossRef]

125. Facchinetti, F.; Del Giudice, E.; Furegato, S.; Passarotto, M.; Leon, A. Cannabinoids ablate release of TNFα in rat microglial cells stimulated with lypopolysaccharide. *Glia* **2003**, *41*, 161–168. [CrossRef] [PubMed]

126. Molina-Holgado, E.; Vela, J.M.; Arévalo-Martín, A.; Almazán, G.; Molina-Holgado, F.; Borrell, J.; Guaza, C. Cannabinoids Promote Oligodendrocyte Progenitor Survival: Involvement of Cannabinoid Receptors and Phosphatidylinositol-3 Kinase/Akt Signaling. *J. Neurosci.* **2002**, *22*, 9742–9753. [CrossRef] [PubMed]

127. Benito, C.; Tolón, R.M.; Pazos, M.R.; Núñez, E.; Castillo, A.I.; Romero, J. Cannabinoid CB2 receptors in human brain inflammation. *Br. J. Pharmacol.* **2008**, *153*, 277–285. [CrossRef] [PubMed]

128. Bisogno, T.; Hanus, L.; De Petrocellis, L.; Tchilibon, S.; Ponde, D.E.; Brandi, I.; Moriello, A.S.; Davis, J.B.; Mechoulam, R.; Di Marzo, V. Molecular targets for cannabidiol and its synthetic analogues: Effect on vanilloid VR1 receptors and on the cellular uptake and enzymatic hydrolysis of anandamide. *Br. J. Pharmacol.* **2001**, *134*, 845–852. [CrossRef] [PubMed]

129. Ross, H.R.; Napier, I.; Connor, M. Inhibition of recombinant human T-type calcium channels by Delta9-tetrahydrocannabinol and cannabidiol. *J. Biol. Chem.* **2008**, *283*, 16124–16134. [CrossRef] [PubMed]

130. Russo, E.B.; Burnett, A.; Hall, B.; Parker, K.K. Agonistic Properties of Cannabidiol at 5-HT1a Receptors. *Neurochem. Res.* **2005**, *30*, 1037–1043. [CrossRef] [PubMed]

131. Liou, G.I.; Auchampach, J.A.; Hillard, C.J.; Zhu, G.; Yousufzai, B.; Mian, S.; Khan, S.; Khalifa, Y. Mediation of Cannabidiol Anti-inflammation in the Retina by Equilibrative Nucleoside Transporter and A2A Adenosine Receptor. *Investig. Ophthalmol. Vis. Sci.* **2008**, *49*, 5526–5531. [CrossRef] [PubMed]

132. Rimmerman, N.; Ben-Hail, D.; Porat, Z.; Juknat, A.; Kozela, E.; Daniels, M.P.; Connelly, P.S.; Leishman, E.; Bradshaw, H.B.; Shoshan-Barmatz, V.; et al. Direct modulation of the outer mitochondrial membrane channel, voltage-dependent anion channel 1 (VDAC1) by cannabidiol: A novel mechanism for cannabinoid-induced cell death. *Cell Death Dis.* **2013**, *4*, e949. [CrossRef] [PubMed]

133. Hill, A.J.; Mercier, M.S.; Hill, T.D.M.; Glyn, S.E.; Jones, N.A.; Yamasaki, Y.; Futamura, T.; Duncan, M.; Stott, C.G.; Stephens, G.J.; et al. Cannabidivarin is anticonvulsant in mouse and rat. *Br. J. Pharmacol.* **2012**, *167*, 1629–1642. [CrossRef] [PubMed]

134. Hill, T.D.M.; Cascio, M.-G.; Romano, B.; Duncan, M.; Pertwee, R.G.; Williams, C.M.; Whalley, B.J.; Hill, A.J. Cannabidivarin-rich cannabis extracts are anticonvulsant in mouse and rat via a CB1 receptor-independent mechanism. *Br. J. Pharmacol.* **2013**, *170*, 679–692. [CrossRef] [PubMed]

135. Hill, A.J.; Weston, S.E.; Jones, N.A.; Smith, I.; Bevan, S.A.; Williamson, E.M.; Stephens, G.J.; Williams, C.M.; Whalley, B.J. Δ9-Tetrahydrocannabivarin suppresses in vitro epileptiform and in vivo seizure activity in adult rats. *Epilepsia* **2010**, *51*, 1522–1532. [CrossRef] [PubMed]

136. Mechoulam, R.; Carlini, E.A. Toward drugs derived from cannabis. *Naturwissenschaften* **1978**, *65*, 174–179. [CrossRef] [PubMed]

137. Cunha, J.M.; Carlini, E.A.; Pereira, A.E.; Ramos, O.L.; Pimentel, C.; Gagliardi, R.; Sanvito, W.L.; Lander, N.; Mechoulam, R. Chronic Administration of Cannabidiol to Healthy Volunteers and Epileptic Patients. *Pharmacology* **1980**, *21*, 175–185. [CrossRef] [PubMed]

138. Gloss, D.; Vickrey, B. Cannabinoids for epilepsy. *Cochrane Database Syst. Rev.* **2012**, *6*, CD009270.

139. Szaflarski, J.P.; Bebin, E.M.; Comi, A.M.; Patel, A.D.; Joshi, C.; Checketts, D.; Beal, J.C.; Laux, L.C.; De Boer, L.M.; Wong, M.H.; et al. Long-term safety and treatment effects of cannabidiol in children and adults with treatment-resistant epilepsies: Expanded access program results. *Epilepsia* **2018**, *59*, 1540–1548. [CrossRef] [PubMed]

140. Thiele, E.A.; Marsh, E.D.; French, J.A.; Mazurkiewicz-Beldzinska, M.; Benbadis, S.R.; Joshi, C.; Lyons, P.D.; Taylor, A.; Roberts, C.; Sommerville, K.; et al. Cannabidiol in patients with seizures associated with Lennox-Gastaut syndrome (GWPCARE4): A randomised, double-blind, placebo-controlled phase 3 trial. *Lancet* **2018**, *391*, 1085–1096. [CrossRef]

141. Devinsky, O.; Marsh, E.; Friedman, D.; Thiele, E.; Laux, L.; Sullivan, J.; Miller, I.; Flamini, R.; Wilfong, A.; Filloux, F.; et al. Cannabidiol in patients with treatment-resistant epilepsy: An open-label interventional trial. *Lancet Neurol.* **2016**, *15*, 270–278. [CrossRef]

142. Devinsky, O.; Cross, J.H.; Laux, L.; Marsh, E.; Miller, I.; Nabbout, R.; Scheffer, I.E.; Thiele, E.A.; Wright, S. Trial of Cannabidiol for Drug-Resistant Seizures in the Dravet Syndrome. *N. Engl. J. Med.* **2017**, *376*, 2011–2020. [CrossRef] [PubMed]

143. Devinsky, O.; Nabbout, R.; Miller, I.; Laux, L.; Zolnowska, M.; Wright, S.; Roberts, C. Long-term cannabidiol treatment in patients with Dravet syndrome: An open-label extension trial. *Epilepsia* **2019**, *60*, 294–302. [CrossRef] [PubMed]

144. Devinsky, O.; Patel, A.D.; Cross, J.H.; Villanueva, V.; Wirrell, E.C.; Privitera, M.; Greenwood, S.M.; Roberts, C.; Checketts, D.; VanLandingham, K.E.; et al. Effect of Cannabidiol on Drop Seizures in the Lennox–Gastaut Syndrome. *N. Engl. J. Med.* **2018**, *378*, 1888–1897. [CrossRef] [PubMed]

145. Gaston, T.E.; Bebin, E.M.; Cutter, G.R.; Liu, Y.; Szaflarski, J.P. Interactions between cannabidiol and commonly used antiepileptic drugs. *Epilepsia* **2017**, *58*, 1586–1592. [CrossRef] [PubMed]

146. Geffrey, A.L.; Pollack, S.F.; Bruno, P.L.; Thiele, E.A. Drug–drug interaction between clobazam and cannabidiol in children with refractory epilepsy. *Epilepsia* **2015**, *56*, 1246–1251. [CrossRef] [PubMed]

147. Devinsky, O.; Patel, A.D.; Thiele, E.A.; Wong, M.H.; Appleton, R.; Harden, C.L.; Greenwood, S.; Morrison, G.; Sommerville, K.; Group, G.P.A.S. Randomized, dose-ranging safety trial of cannabidiol in Dravet syndrome. *Neurology* **2018**, *90*, e1204–e1211. [CrossRef] [PubMed]

148. Maa, E.; Figi, P. The case for medical marijuana in epilepsy. *Epilepsia* **2014**, *55*, 783–786. [CrossRef] [PubMed]

149. Porter, B.E.; Jacobson, C. Report of a parent survey of cannabidiol-enriched cannabis use in pediatric treatment-resistant epilepsy. *Epilepsy Behav.* **2013**, *29*, 574–577. [CrossRef] [PubMed]

150. Hussain, S.A.; Zhou, R.; Jacobson, C.; Weng, J.; Cheng, E.; Lay, J.; Hung, P.; Lerner, J.T.; Sankar, R. Perceived efficacy of cannabidiol-enriched cannabis extracts for treatment of pediatric epilepsy: A potential role for infantile spasms and Lennox–Gastaut syndrome. *Epilepsy Behav.* **2015**, *47*, 138–141. [CrossRef] [PubMed]

151. Press, C.A.; Knupp, K.G.; Chapman, K.E. Parental reporting of response to oral cannabis extracts for treatment of refractory epilepsy. *Epilepsy Behav.* **2015**, *45*, 49–52. [CrossRef] [PubMed]

152. Hausman-Kedem, M.; Menascu, S.; Kramer, U. Efficacy of CBD-enriched medical cannabis for treatment of refractory epilepsy in children and adolescents—An observational, longitudinal study. *Brain Dev.* **2018**, *40*, 544–551. [CrossRef] [PubMed]

153. McCoy, B.; Wang, L.; Zak, M.; Al-Mehmadi, S.; Kabir, N.; Alhadid, K.; McDonald, K.; Zhang, G.; Sharma, R.; Whitney, R.; et al. A prospective open-label trial of a CBD/THC cannabis oil in dravet syndrome. *Ann. Clin. Transl. Neurol.* **2018**, *5*, 1077–1088. [CrossRef] [PubMed]

154. Tzadok, M.; Uliel-Siboni, S.; Linder, I.; Kramer, U.; Epstein, O.; Menascu, S.; Nissenkorn, A.; Yosef, O.B.; Hyman, E.; Granot, D.; et al. CBD-enriched medical cannabis for intractable pediatric epilepsy: The current Israeli experience. *Seizure* **2016**, *35*, 41–44. [CrossRef] [PubMed]

155. Mhyre, T.R.; Boyd, J.T.; Hamill, R.W.; Maguire-Zeiss, K.A. Parkinson's disease. *Subcell. Biochem.* **2012**, *65*, 389–455. [PubMed]

156. Zipp, F.; Aktas, O. The brain as a target of inflammation: Common pathways link inflammatory and neurodegenerative diseases. *Trends Neurosci.* **2006**, *29*, 518–527. [CrossRef] [PubMed]

157. Benarroch, E. Endocannabinoids in basal ganglia circuits Implications for Parkinson disease. *Neurology* **2007**, *69*, 306–309. [CrossRef] [PubMed]

158. Van Sickle, M.D.; Duncan, M.; Kingsley, P.J.; Mouihate, A.; Urbani, P.; Mackie, K.; Stella, N.; Makriyannis, A.; Piomelli, D.; Davison, J.S.; et al. Identification and functional characterization of brainstem cannabinoid CB2 receptors. *Science* **2005**, *310*, 329–332. [CrossRef] [PubMed]

159. Nunez, E.; Benito, C.; Tolon, R.M.; Hillard, C.J.; Griffin, W.S.T.; Romero, J. Glial expression of cannabinoid CB2 receptors and fatty acid amide hydrolase are beta amyloid–linked events in Down's syndrome. *Neuroscience* **2008**, *151*, 104–110. [CrossRef] [PubMed]

160. Lastres-Becker, I.; Molina-Holgado, F.; Ramos, J.A.; Mechoulam, R.; Fernández-Ruiz, J. Cannabinoids provide neuroprotection against 6-hydroxydopamine toxicity in vivo and in vitro: Relevance to Parkinson's disease. *Neurobiol. Dis.* **2005**, *19*, 96–107. [CrossRef] [PubMed]

161. Peres, F.F.; Levin, R.; Suiama, M.A.; Diana, M.C.; Gouvêa, D.A.; Almeida, V.; Santos, C.M.; Lungato, L.; Zuardi, A.W.; Hallak, J.E.C. Cannabidiol prevents motor and cognitive impairments induced by reserpine in rats. *Front. Pharmacol.* **2016**, *7*, 343. [CrossRef] [PubMed]

162. García-Arencibia, M.; García, C.; Kurz, A.; Rodríguez-Navarro, J.A.; Gispert-Sánchez, S.; Mena, M.A.; Auburger, G.; de Yébenes, J.G.; Fernández-Ruiz, J. Cannabinoid CB 1 receptors are early downregulated followed by a further upregulation in the basal ganglia of mice with deletion of specific park genes. In *Birth, Life and Death of Dopaminergic Neurons in the Substantia Nigra*; Springer: New York, NY, USA, 2009; pp. 269–275.

163. Consroe, P.; Sandyk, R.; Snider, S.R. Open label evaluation of cannabidiol in dystonic movement disorders. *Int. J. Neurosci.* **1986**, *30*, 277–282. [CrossRef] [PubMed]

164. Zuardi, A.W.; Crippa, J.A.S.; Hallak, J.E.C.; Pinto, J.P.; Chagas, M.H.N.; Rodrigues, G.G.R.; Dursun, S.M.; Tumas, V. Cannabidiol for the treatment of psychosis in Parkinson's disease. *J. Psychopharmacol.* **2009**, *23*, 979–983. [CrossRef] [PubMed]

165. Chagas, M.H.N.; Zuardi, A.W.; Tumas, V.; Pena-Pereira, M.A.; Sobreira, E.T.; Bergamaschi, M.M.; dos Santos, A.C.; Teixeira, A.L.; Hallak, J.E.C.; Crippa, J.A.S. Effects of cannabidiol in the treatment of patients with Parkinson's disease: An exploratory double-blind trial. *J. Psychopharmacol.* **2014**, *28*, 1088–1098. [CrossRef] [PubMed]

166. Venderová, K.; Růžička, E.; Vořišek, V.; Višňovský, P. Survey on cannabis use in Parkinson's disease: Subjective improvement of motor symptoms. *Mov. Disord.* **2004**, *19*, 1102–1106. [CrossRef] [PubMed]

167. Balash, Y.; Schleider, L.B.-L.; Korczyn, A.D.; Shabtai, H.; Knaani, J.; Rosenberg, A.; Baruch, Y.; Djaldetti, R.; Giladi, N.; Gurevich, T. Medical Cannabis in Parkinson Disease: Real-Life Patients' Experience. *Clin. Neuropharmacol.* **2017**, *40*, 268–272. [CrossRef] [PubMed]

168. Lotan, I.; Treves, T.A.; Roditi, Y.; Djaldetti, R. Cannabis (medical marijuana) treatment for motor and non–motor symptoms of Parkinson disease: An open-label observational study. *Clin. Neuropharmacol.* **2014**, *37*, 41–44. [CrossRef] [PubMed]

169. Kindred, J.H.; Li, K.; Ketelhut, N.B.; Proessl, F.; Fling, B.W.; Honce, J.M.; Shaffer, W.R.; Rudroff, T. Cannabis use in people with Parkinson's disease and Multiple Sclerosis: A web-based investigation. *Complement. Ther. Med.* **2017**, *33*, 99–104. [CrossRef] [PubMed]

170. Shohet, A.; Khlebtovsky, A.; Roizen, N.; Roditi, Y.; Djaldetti, R. Effect of medical cannabis on thermal quantitative measurements of pain in patients with Parkinson's disease. *Eur. J. Pain* **2017**, *21*, 486–493. [CrossRef] [PubMed]

171. Frankel, J.P.; Hughes, A.; Lees, A.J.; Stern, G.M. Marijuana for parkinsonian tremor. *J. Neurol. Neurosurg. Psychiatry* **1990**, *53*, 436. [CrossRef] [PubMed]

172. Carroll, C.B.; Bain, P.G.; Teare, L.; Liu, X.; Joint, C.; Wroath, C.; Parkin, S.G.; Fox, P.; Wright, D.; Hobart, J. Cannabis for dyskinesia in Parkinson disease: A randomized double-blind crossover study. *Neurology* **2004**, *63*, 1245–1250. [CrossRef] [PubMed]

173. Clinicaltrials.gov Cannabis Oil for Pain in Parkinson's Disease. Available online: https://clinicaltrials.gov/ct2/show/NCT03639064 (accessed on 20 January 2019).

174. Wang, J.; Gu, B.J.; Masters, C.L.; Wang, Y.-J. A systemic view of Alzheimer disease—Insights from amyloid-β metabolism beyond the brain. *Nat. Rev. Neurol.* **2017**, *13*, 612. [CrossRef] [PubMed]

175. Eubanks, L.M.; Rogers, C.J.; Beuscher IV, A.E.; Koob, G.F.; Olson, A.J.; Dickerson, T.J.; Janda, K.D. A molecular link between the active component of marijuana and Alzheimer's disease pathology. *Mol. Pharm.* **2006**, *3*, 773–777. [CrossRef] [PubMed]

176. Iuvone, T.; Esposito, G.; Esposito, R.; Santamaria, R.; Di Rosa, M.; Izzo, A.A. Neuroprotective effect of cannabidiol, a non-psychoactive component from *Cannabis sativa*, on β-amyloid-induced toxicity in PC12 cells. *J. Neurochem.* **2004**, *89*, 134–141. [CrossRef] [PubMed]

177. Esposito, G.; De Filippis, D.; Maiuri, M.C.; De Stefano, D.; Carnuccio, R.; Iuvone, T. Cannabidiol inhibits inducible nitric oxide synthase protein expression and nitric oxide production in β-amyloid stimulated PC12 neurons through p38 MAP kinase and NF-κB involvement. *Neurosci. Lett.* **2006**, *399*, 91–95. [CrossRef] [PubMed]

178. Esposito, G.; Scuderi, C.; Savani, C.; Steardo Jr., L.; De Filippis, D.; Cottone, P.; Iuvone, T.; Cuomo, V.; Steardo, L. Cannabidiol in vivo blunts β-amyloid induced neuroinflammation by suppressing IL-1β and iNOS expression. *Br. J. Pharmacol.* **2007**, *151*, 1272–1279. [CrossRef] [PubMed]

179. Cheng, D.; Spiro, A.S.; Jenner, A.M.; Garner, B.; Karl, T. Long-term cannabidiol treatment prevents the development of social recognition memory deficits in Alzheimer's disease transgenic mice. *J. Alzheimer's Dis.* **2014**, *42*, 1383–1396. [CrossRef] [PubMed]

180. Walther, S.; Mahlberg, R.; Eichmann, U.; Kunz, D. Delta-9-tetrahydrocannabinol for nighttime agitation in severe dementia. *Psychopharmacology* **2006**, *185*, 524–528. [CrossRef] [PubMed]

181. Shelef, A.; Barak, Y.; Berger, U.; Paleacu, D.; Tadger, S.; Plopsky, I.; Baruch, Y. Safety and efficacy of medical cannabis oil for behavioral and psychological symptoms of dementia: An-open label, add-on, pilot study. *J. Alzheimer's Dis.* **2016**, *51*, 15–19. [CrossRef] [PubMed]

182. Walther, S.; Schüpbach, B.; Seifritz, E.; Homan, P.; Strik, W. Randomized, controlled crossover trial of dronabinol, 2.5 mg, for agitation in 2 patients with dementia. *J. Clin. Psychopharmacol.* **2011**, *31*, 256–258. [CrossRef] [PubMed]

183. van den Elsen, G.A.H.; Ahmed, A.I.A.; Verkes, R.-J.; Feuth, T.; van der Marck, M.A.; Rikkert, M.G.M.O. Tetrahydrocannabinol in behavioral disturbances in dementia: A crossover randomized controlled trial. *Am. J. Geriatr. Psychiatry* **2015**, *23*, 1214–1224. [CrossRef] [PubMed]

184. Volicer, L.; Stelly, M.; Morris, J.; McLAUGHLIN, J.; Volicer, B.J. Effects of dronabinol on anorexia and disturbed behavior in patients with Alzheimer's disease. *Int. J. Geriatr. Psychiatry* **1997**, *12*, 913–919. [CrossRef]

185. Mahlberg, R.; Walther, S. Actigraphy in agitated patients with dementia. *Z. Gerontol. Geriatr.* **2007**, *40*, 178–184. [CrossRef] [PubMed]

186. Woodward, M.R.; Harper, D.G.; Stolyar, A.; Forester, B.P.; Ellison, J.M. Dronabinol for the treatment of agitation and aggressive behavior in acutely hospitalized severely demented patients with noncognitive behavioral symptoms. *Am. J. Geriatr. Psychiatry* **2014**, *22*, 415–419. [CrossRef] [PubMed]

187. Calabresi, P.A. Diagnosis and management of multiple sclerosis. *Am. Fam. Phys.* **2004**, *70*, 1935–1944.

188. Hauser, S.L.; Goodwin, D.S. Multiple sclerosis and other demyelinating diseases. In *Harrison's Principles of Internal Medicine*; Fauci, A.S., Braunwald, E., Kasper, D.L., Hauser, S., Eds.; McGraw-Hill Medical: New York, NY, USA, 2008; pp. 2611–2621.

189. Global, regional, and national burden of neurological disorders during 1990–2015: A systematic analysis for the Global Burden of Disease Study 2015. *Lancet. Neurol.* **2017**, *16*, 877–897. [CrossRef]

190. Comi, G.; Radaelli, M.; Soelberg Sorensen, P. Evolving concepts in the treatment of relapsing multiple sclerosis. *Lancet* **2017**, *389*, 1347–1356. [CrossRef]

191. Brownlee, W.J.; Hardy, T.A.; Fazekas, F.; Miller, D.H. Diagnosis of multiple sclerosis: Progress and challenges. *Lancet* **2017**, *389*, 1336–1346. [CrossRef]

192. Pertwee, R.G. Cannabinoids and multiple sclerosis. *Mol. Neurobiol.* **2007**, *36*, 45–59. [CrossRef] [PubMed]

193. Lyman, W.D.; Sonett, J.R.; Brosnan, C.F.; Elkin, R.; Bornstein, M.B. Delta 9-tetrahydrocannabinol: A novel treatment for experimental autoimmune encephalomyelitis. *J. Neuroimmunol.* **1989**, *23*, 73–81. [CrossRef]

194. Baker, D.; Pryce, G.; Croxford, J.L.; Brown, P.; Pertwee, R.G.; Huffman, J.W.; Layward, L. Cannabinoids control spasticity and tremor in a multiple sclerosis model. *Nature* **2000**, *404*, 84–87. [CrossRef] [PubMed]

195. Maresz, K.; Pryce, G.; Ponomarev, E.D.; Marsicano, G.; Croxford, J.L.; Shriver, L.P.; Ledent, C.; Cheng, X.; Carrier, E.J.; Mann, M.K.; et al. Direct suppression of CNS autoimmune inflammation via the cannabinoid receptor CB1 on neurons and CB2 on autoreactive T cells. *Nat. Med.* **2007**, *13*, 492–497. [CrossRef] [PubMed]

196. Pryce, G.; Baker, D. Control of spasticity in a multiple sclerosis model is mediated by CB1, not CB2, cannabinoid receptors. *Br. J. Pharmacol.* **2007**, *150*, 519–525. [CrossRef] [PubMed]

197. Croxford, J.L.; Pryce, G.; Jackson, S.J.; Ledent, C.; Giovannoni, G.; Pertwee, R.G.; Yamamura, T.; Baker, D. Cannabinoid-mediated neuroprotection, not immunosuppression, may be more relevant to multiple sclerosis. *J. Neuroimmunol.* **2008**, *193*, 120–129. [CrossRef] [PubMed]

198. Baker, D.; Jackson, S.J.; Pryce, G. Cannabinoid control of neuroinflammation related to multiple sclerosis. *Br. J. Pharmacol.* **2007**, *152*, 649–654. [CrossRef] [PubMed]

199. Sanchez, A.J.; Garcia-Merino, A. Neuroprotective agents: Cannabinoids. *Clin. Immunol.* **2012**, *142*, 57–67. [CrossRef] [PubMed]

200. Cofield, S.S.; Salter, A.R.; Tyry, T.; Mcneal, S.; Cutter, G.R.; Marrie, R.A.; Fox, R.J. Current Marijuana Usage By MS Status and Disability in the NARCOMS Registry. *Int. J. Mult. Scler. Care* **2015**, *17* (Suppl. S1), 1–9.

201. Chong, M.S.; Wolff, K.; Wise, K.; Tanton, C.; Winstock, A.; Silber, E. Cannabis use in patients with multiple sclerosis. *Mult. Scler.* **2006**, *12*, 646–651. [CrossRef] [PubMed]

202. GW Pharmaceuticals Plc. Sativex® (Delta-9-Tetrahydrocannibinol and Cannabidiol in the EU) (Nabiximols in the USA). Available online: https://www.gwpharm.com/healthcare-professionals/sativex/patient-information (accessed on 20 January 2019).

203. Torres-Moreno, M.C.; Papaseit, E.; Torrens, M.; Farré, M. Assessment of Efficacy and Tolerability of Medicinal Cannabinoids in Patients With Multiple Sclerosis: A Systematic Review and Meta-analysisAssessment of Efficacy and Tolerability of Cannabinoids in Patients With Multiple SclerosisAssessment of Efficacy a. *JAMA Netw. Open* **2018**, *1*, e183485. [CrossRef] [PubMed]

204. Kansagara, D.; O'Neil, M.; Nugent, S.; Freeman, M.; Low, A.; Kondo, K.; Elven, C.; Zakher, B.; Motu'apuaka, M.; Paynter, R. *Benefits and Harms of Cannabis in Chronic Pain or Post-Traumatic Stress Disorder: A Systematic Review*; Department of Veterans Affairs: Washington, DC, USA, 2017.

205. O'neil, M.E.; Nugent, S.M.; Morasco, B.J.; Freeman, M.; Low, A.; Kondo, K.; Zakher, B.; Elven, C.; Motu'apuaka, M.; Paynter, R. Benefits and harms of plant-based cannabis for posttraumatic stress disorder: A systematic review. *Ann. Intern. Med.* **2017**, *167*, 332–340. [CrossRef] [PubMed]

206. Bitencourt, R.M.; Takahashi, R.N. Cannabidiol as a therapeutic alternative for post-traumatic stress disorder: From bench research to confirmation in human trials. *Front. Neurosci.* **2018**, *12*, 502. [CrossRef] [PubMed]

207. Elms, L.; Shannon, S.; Hughes, S.; Lewis, N. Cannabidiol in the Treatment of Post-Traumatic Stress Disorder: A Case Series. *J. Altern. Complement. Med.* **2018**. [CrossRef] [PubMed]

208. Steenkamp, M.M.; Blessing, E.M.; Galatzer-Levy, I.R.; Hollahan, L.C.; Anderson, W.T. Marijuana and other cannabinoids as a treatment for posttraumatic stress disorder: A literature review. *Depress. Anxiety* **2017**, *34*, 207–216. [CrossRef] [PubMed]

209. Fahn, S.; Bruun, R.D.; Caine, E.; Cohen, D.J.; Comings, D.E.; Como, P.G.; Conneally, P.M.; Gancher, S.T.; Goetz, C.; Golden, G.S.; et al. Definitions and Classification of Tic Disorders. *Arch. Neurol.* **1993**, *50*, 1013–1016.

210. Gerard, E.; Peterson, B.S. Developmental processes and brain imaging studies in Tourette syndrome. *J. Psychosom. Res.* **2003**, *55*, 13–22. [CrossRef]

211. Mink, J.W. Neurobiology of basal ganglia circuits in Tourette syndrome: Faulty inhibition of unwanted motor patterns? *Adv. Neurol.* **2001**, *85*, 113–122. [PubMed]

212. Mechoulam, R.; Parker, L.A. The Endocannabinoid System and the Brain. *Annu. Rev. Psychol.* **2013**, *64*, 21–47. [CrossRef] [PubMed]

213. Abrahamov, A.; Abrahamov, A.; Mechoulam, R. An efficient new cannabinoid antiemetic in pediatric oncology. *Life Sci.* **1995**, *56*, 2097–2102. [CrossRef]

214. Giuffrida, A.; Parsons, L.H.; Kerr, T.M.; de Fonseca, F.R.; Navarro, M.; Piomelli, D. Dopamine activation of endogenous cannabinoid signaling in dorsal striatum. *Nat. Neurosci.* **1999**, *2*, 358–363. [CrossRef] [PubMed]

215. Di Marzo, V.; Hill, M.P.; Bisogno, T.; Crossman, A.R.; Brotchie, J.M. Enhanced levels of endogenous cannabinoids in the globus pallidus are associated with a reduction in movement in an animal model of Parkinson's disease. *FASEB J.* **2000**, *14*, 1432–1438. [PubMed]

216. Müller-Vahl, K.R. Cannabinoids reduce symptoms of Tourette's syndrome. *Expert Opin. Pharmacother.* **2003**, *4*, 1717–1725. [CrossRef] [PubMed]

217. Sandyk, R.; Awerbuch, G. Marijuana and Tourette's syndrome. *J. Clin. Psychopharmacol.* **1988**, *8*, 444–445. [CrossRef] [PubMed]

218. Hemming, M.; Yellowlees, P.M. Effective treatment of Tourette's syndrome with marijuana. *J. Psychopharmacol.* **1993**, *7*, 389–391. [CrossRef] [PubMed]

219. Müller-Vahl, K.R.; Kolbe, H.; Schneider, U.; Emrich, H.M. Cannabinoids: Possible role in patho-physiology and therapy of Gilles de la Tourette syndrome. *Acta Psychiatr. Scand.* **1998**, *98*, 502–506. [CrossRef] [PubMed]

220. Müller-Vahl, K.; Schneider, U.; Koblenz, A.; Jöbges, M.; Kolbe, H.; Daldrup, T.; Emrich, H. Treatment of Tourette's Syndrome with Δ^9-Tetrahydrocannabinol (THC): A Randomized Crossover Trial. *Pharmacopsychiatry* **2002**, *35*, 57–61. [CrossRef] [PubMed]

221. Muller-Vahl, K.R.; Schneider, U.; Prevedel, H.; Theloe, K.; Kolbe, H.; Daldrup, T.; Emrich, H.M. Delta 9-Tetrahydrocannabinol (THC) is Effective in the Treatment of Tics in Tourette Syndrome. *J. Clin. Psychiatry* **2003**, *64*, 459–465. [CrossRef] [PubMed]

222. Abi-Jaoude, E.; Chen, L.; Cheung, P.; Bhikram, T.; Sandor, P. Preliminary Evidence on Cannabis Effectiveness and Tolerability for Adults With Tourette Syndrome. *J. Neuropsychiatry Clin. Neurosci.* **2017**, *29*, 391–400. [CrossRef] [PubMed]

223. ClinicalTrials.gov Safety and Efficacy of Cannabis in Tourette Syndrome. Available online: https://clinicaltrials.gov/ct2/show/NCT03247244. (accessed on 20 January 2019).

224. ClinicalTrials.gov CANNAbinoids in the Treatment of TICS (CANNA-TICS)—Full Text View—ClinicalTrials.gov. Available online: https://clinicaltrials.gov/ct2/show/NCT03087201?term=cannabis&cond=Tourette+Syndrome (accessed on 20 January 2019).

225. ClinicalTrials.gov Efficacy of a Therapeutic Combination of Dronabinol and PEA for Tourette Syndrome—Full Text View—ClinicalTrials.gov. Available online: https://clinicaltrials.gov/ct2/show/NCT03066193?term=THC&cond=Tourette+syndrome (accessed on 20 January 2019).

226. ClinicalTrials.gov A Study to Examine the Efficacy of a Therapeutic THX-110 for Tourette Syndrome—Full Text View—ClinicalTrials.gov. Available online: https://clinicaltrials.gov/ct2/show/NCT03651726?term=THC&cond=Tourette+syndrome (accessed on 20 January 2019).

227. Navari, R.M. Pharmacological Management of Chemotherapy-Induced Nausea and Vomiting. *Drugs* **2009**, *69*, 515–533. [CrossRef] [PubMed]

228. Hornby, P.J. Central neurocircuitry associated with emesis. *Am. J. Med.* **2001**, *111*, 106–112. [CrossRef]

229. Darmani, N.A.; Janoyan, J.J.; Crim, J.; Ramirez, J. Receptor mechanism and antiemetic activity of structurally-diverse cannabinoids against radiation-induced emesis in the least shrew. *Eur. J. Pharmacol.* **2007**, *563*, 187–196. [CrossRef] [PubMed]

230. Parker, L.A.; Rock, E.M.; Limebeer, C.L. Regulation of nausea and vomiting by cannabinoids. *Br. J. Pharmacol.* **2011**, *163*, 1411–1422. [CrossRef] [PubMed]

231. Darmani, N.A. The cannabinoid CB1 receptor antagonist SR 141716A reverses the antiemetic and motor depressant actions of WIN 55, 212-2. *Eur. J. Pharmacol.* **2001**, *430*, 49–58. [CrossRef]

232. Barann, M.; Molderings, G.; Brüss, M.; Bönisch, H.; Urban, B.W.; Göthert, M. Direct inhibition by cannabinoids of human 5-HT3A receptors: Probable involvement of an allosteric modulatory site. *Br. J. Pharmacol.* **2002**, *137*, 589–596. [CrossRef] [PubMed]

233. US Food and Drug Administration. *MARINOL (Dronabinol) Capsules, for Oral Use*; US Food and Drug Administration: Silver Spring, MD, USA, 2017.

234. US Food and Drug Administration. *Cesamet FDA Approval*; US Food and Drug Administration: Silver Spring, MD, USA, 2006.

235. Hesketh, P.J.; Kris, M.G.; Basch, E.; Bohlke, K.; Barbour, S.Y.; Clark-Snow, R.A.; Danso, M.A.; Dennis, K.; Dupuis, L.L.; Dusetzina, S.B.; et al. Antiemetics: American Society of Clinical Oncology Clinical Practice Guideline Update. *J. Clin. Oncol.* **2017**, *35*, 3240–3261. [CrossRef] [PubMed]

236. Vinciguerra, V.; Moore, T.; Brennan, E. Inhalation marijuana as an antiemetic for cancer chemotherapy. *N. Y. State J. Med.* **1988**, *88*, 525–527. [PubMed]

237. Musty, R.E.; Rossi, R. Effects of Smoked Cannabis and Oral Δ9-Tetrahydrocannabinol on Nausea and Emesis After Cancer Chemotherapy: A Review of State Clinical Trials. *J. Cannabis Ther.* **2001**, *1*, 29–56. [CrossRef]

238. Söderpalm, A.H. V.; Schuster, A.; de Wit, H. Antiemetic efficacy of smoked marijuana: Subjective and behavioral effects on nausea induced by syrup of ipecac. *Pharmacol. Biochem. Behav.* **2001**, *69*, 343–350. [CrossRef]

239. Roila, F.; Feyer, P.; Hesketh, P.J.; Jordan, K.; Olver, I.; Rapoport, B.L.; Roscoe, J.; Walsh, D.; Warr, D.; van der Wetering, M.; et al. 2016 MASCC and ESMO guideline update for the prevention of chemotherapy- and radiotherapy-induced nausea and vomiting and of nausea and vomiting in advanced cancer patients. *Ann. Oncol.* **2016**, *27*, v119–v133. [CrossRef] [PubMed]

240. Lutge, E.E.; Gray, A.; Siegfried, N. The medical use of cannabis for reducing morbidity and mortality in patients with HIV/AIDS. *Cochrane Database Syst. Rev.* **2013**, *30*, CD005175. [CrossRef] [PubMed]

241. Badowski, M.E.; Yanful, P.K. Dronabinol oral solution in the management of anorexia and weight loss in AIDS and cancer. *Ther. Clin. Risk Manag.* **2018**, *14*, 643–651. [CrossRef] [PubMed]

242. Andries, A.; Frystyk, J.; Flyvbjerg, A.; Støving, R.K. Dronabinol in severe, enduring anorexia nervosa: A randomized controlled trial. *Int. J. Eat. Disord.* **2014**, *47*, 18–23. [CrossRef] [PubMed]

243. Scheffler, F.; Kilian, S.; Chiliza, B.; Asmal, L.; Phahladira, L.; du Plessis, S.; Kidd, M.; Murray, R.M.; Di Forti, M.; Seedat, S.; et al. Effects of cannabis use on body mass, fasting glucose and lipids during the first 12months of treatment in schizophrenia spectrum disorders. *Schizophr. Res.* **2018**, *199*, 90–95. [CrossRef] [PubMed]

244. Marks, D.H.; Friedman, A. The Therapeutic Potential of Cannabinoids in Dermatology. *Skin Ther. Lett.* **2018**, *23*, 1–5.

245. Mounessa, J.S.; Siegel, J.A.; Dunnick, C.A.; Dellavalle, R.P. The role of cannabinoids in dermatology. *J. Am. Acad. Dermatol.* **2017**, *77*, 188–190. [CrossRef] [PubMed]

246. Theroux, Z.; Cropley, T. Cannabis and Dr Piffard—A Century Ahead of the Curve. *JAMA Dermatol.* **2016**, *152*, 972. [CrossRef] [PubMed]

247. Wilkinson, J.D.; Williamson, E.M. Cannabinoids inhibit human keratinocyte proliferation through a non-CB1/CB2 mechanism and have a potential therapeutic value in the treatment of psoriasis. *J. Dermatol. Sci.* **2007**, *45*, 87–92. [CrossRef] [PubMed]

248. Ali, A.; Akhtar, N. The safety and efficacy of 3% Cannabis seeds extract cream for reduction of human cheek skin sebum and erythema content. *Pak. J. Pharm. Sci.* **2015**, *28*, 1389–1395. [PubMed]

249. Callaway, J.; Schwab, U.; Harvima, I.; Halonen, P.; Mykkänen, O.; Hyvönen, P.; Järvinen, T. Efficacy of dietary hempseed oil in patients with atopic dermatitis. *J. Dermatolog. Treat.* **2005**, *16*, 87–94. [CrossRef] [PubMed]

250. Citti, C.; Pacchetti, B.; Vandelli, M.A.; Forni, F.; Cannazza, G. Analysis of cannabinoids in commercial hemp seed oil and decarboxylation kinetics studies of cannabidiolic acid (CBDA). *J. Pharm. Biomed. Anal.* **2018**, *149*, 532–540. [CrossRef] [PubMed]

251. Eberlein, B.; Eicke, C.; Reinhardt, H.-W.; Ring, J. Adjuvant treatment of atopic eczema: Assessment of an emollient containing N-palmitoylethanolamine (ATOPA study). *J. Eur. Acad. Dermatol. Venereol.* **2008**, *22*, 73–82. [CrossRef] [PubMed]

252. Chelliah, M.P.; Zinn, Z.; Khuu, P.; Teng, J.M.C. Self-initiated use of topical cannabidiol oil for epidermolysis bullosa. *Pediatr. Dermatol.* **2018**, *35*, e224–e227. [CrossRef] [PubMed]

253. Maor, Y.; Yu, J.; Kuzontkoski, P.M.; Dezube, B.J.; Zhang, X.; Groopman, J.E. Cannabidiol Inhibits Growth and Induces Programmed Cell Death in Kaposi Sarcoma-Associated Herpesvirus-Infected Endothelium. *Genes Cancer* **2012**, *3*, 512–520. [CrossRef] [PubMed]

254. Armstrong, J.L.; Hill, D.S.; McKee, C.S.; Hernandez-Tiedra, S.; Lorente, M.; Lopez-Valero, I.; Eleni Anagnostou, M.; Babatunde, F.; Corazzari, M.; Redfern, C.P.F.; et al. Exploiting Cannabinoid-Induced Cytotoxic Autophagy to Drive Melanoma Cell Death. *J. Investig. Dermatol.* **2015**, *135*, 1629–1637. [CrossRef] [PubMed]

255. Li, J.Y.; Kampp, J.T. Review of Common Alternative Herbal "Remedies" for Skin Cancer. *Dermatol. Surg.* **2019**, *45*, 58–67. [CrossRef] [PubMed]

256. Maida, V.; Corban, J. Topical Medical Cannabis: A New Treatment for Wound Pain—Three Cases of Pyoderma Gangrenosum. *J. Pain Symptom Manag.* **2017**, *54*, 732–736. [CrossRef] [PubMed]

257. Eagleston, L.R.M.; Kalani, N.K.; Patel, R.R.; Flaten, H.K.; Dunnick, C.A.; Dellavalle, R.P. Cannabinoids in dermatology: A scoping review. *Dermatol. Online J.* **2018**, *24*, 1–17.

258. Milando, R.; Friedman, A. Cannabinoids: Potential Role in Inflammatory and Neoplastic Skin Diseases. *Am. J. Clin. Dermatol.* **2018**, in press. [CrossRef] [PubMed]

259. Campos, A.C.; Brant, F.; Miranda, A.S.; Machado, F.S.; Teixeira, A.L. Cannabidiol increases survival and promotes rescue of cognitive function in a murine model of cerebral malaria. *Neuroscience* **2015**, *289*, 166–180. [CrossRef] [PubMed]

260. Meza, A.; Lehmann, C. Betacaryophyllene—A phytocannabinoid as potential therapeutic modality for human sepsis? *Med. Hypotheses* **2018**, *110*, 68–70. [CrossRef] [PubMed]

261. National Academies of Sciences Engineering and Medicine. *The Health Effects of Cannabis and Cannabinoids: The Current State of Evidence and Recommendations for Research*; The National Academies Press: Washington, DC, USA, 2017.

262. Green, K. Marijuana smoking vs cannabinoids for glaucoma therapy. *Arch. Ophthalmol.* **1998**, *116*, 1433–1437. [CrossRef] [PubMed]

263. Tomida, I.; Azuara-Blanco, A.; House, H.; Flint, M.; Pertwee, R.G.; Robson, P.J. Effect of Sublingual Application of Cannabinoids on Intraocular Pressure: A Pilot Study. *J. Glaucoma* **2006**, *15*, 349–353. [CrossRef] [PubMed]

264. Miller, S.; Daily, L.; Leishman, E.; Bradshaw, H.; Straiker, A. Δ^9-Tetrahydrocannabinol and Cannabidiol Differentially Regulate Intraocular Pressure. *Investig. Opthalmol. Vis. Sci.* **2018**, *59*, 5904–5911. [CrossRef] [PubMed]

265. Belendiuk, K.A.; Babson, K.A.; Vandrey, R.; Bonn-Miller, M.O. Cannabis species and cannabinoid concentration preference among sleep-disturbed medicinal cannabis users. *Addict. Behav.* **2015**, *50*, 178–181. [CrossRef] [PubMed]

266. Nicholson, A.N.; Turner, C.; Stone, B.M.; Robson, P.J. Effect of Δ-9-tetrahydrocannabinol and cannabidiol on nocturnal sleep and early-morning behavior in young adults. *J. Clin. Psychopharmacol.* **2004**, *24*, 305–313. [CrossRef] [PubMed]

267. Tringale, R.; Jensen, C. Cannabis and insomnia. *Depression* **2011**, *4*, 0–68.

268. Babson, K.A.; Sottile, J.; Morabito, D. Cannabis, Cannabinoids, and Sleep: A Review of the Literature. *Curr. Psychiatry Rep.* **2017**, *19*, 1–12. [CrossRef] [PubMed]

269. Crippa, J.; Zuardi, A.; Mertín-Santos, R.; Bhattacharyya, S.; Atakan, Z.; McGuire, P.; Fusar-Poli, P. Cannabis and anxiety: A critical review of the evidence. *Hum. Psychopharmacol. Clin. Exp.* **2009**, *24*, 515–523. [CrossRef] [PubMed]

270. Bergamaschi, M.M.; Queiroz, R.H.C.; Chagas, M.H.N.; De Oliveira, D.C.G.; De Martinis, B.S.; Kapczinski, F.; Quevedo, J.; Roesler, R.; Schröder, N.; Nardi, A.E.; et al. Cannabidiol reduces the anxiety induced by simulated public speaking in treatment-nave social phobia patients. *Neuropsychopharmacology* **2011**, *36*, 1219–1226. [CrossRef] [PubMed]

271. Russo, E.B. Taming THC: Potential cannabis synergy and phytocannabinoid-terpenoid entourage effects. *Br. J. Pharmacol.* **2011**, *163*, 1344–1364. [CrossRef] [PubMed]

272. Gambelunghe, C.; Fucci, N.; Aroni, K.; Bacci, M.; Marcelli, A.; Rossi, R. Cannabis Use Surveillance by Sweat Analysis. *Ther. Drug Monit.* **2016**, *38*, 634–639. [CrossRef] [PubMed]

273. Jain, R.; Singh, R. Microextraction techniques for analysis of cannabinoids. *TrAC Trends Anal. Chem.* **2016**, *80*, 156–166. [CrossRef]

274. De Giovanni, N.; Fucci, N. The Current Status of Sweat Testing For Drugs of Abuse: A Review. *Curr. Med. Chem.* **2013**, *20*, 545–561. [PubMed]

275. Gallardo, E.; Queiroz, J.A. The role of alternative specimens in toxicological analysis. *Biomed. Chromatogr.* **2008**, *22*, 795–821. [CrossRef] [PubMed]

276. Meier, S.I.; Koelzer, S.C.; Schubert-Zsilavecz, M.; Toennes, S.W. Analysis of drugs of abuse in Cerumen—correlation of postmortem analysis results with those for blood, urine and hair. *Drug Test. Anal.* **2017**, *9*, 1572–1585. [CrossRef] [PubMed]

277. Gallardo, E.; Barroso, M.; Queiroz, J.A. LC-MS: A powerful tool in workplace drug testing. *Drug Test. Anal.* **2009**, *1*, 109–115. [CrossRef] [PubMed]

278. Samyn, N.; Van Haeren, C. On-site testing of saliva and sweat with Drugwipe and determination of concentrations of drugs of abuse in saliva, plasma and urine of suspected users. *Int. J. Legal Med.* **2000**, *113*, 150–154. [CrossRef] [PubMed]

279. Queiroz, J.A.; Gallardo, E.; Barroso, M. What are the recent advances in forensic oral fluid bioanalysis? *Bioanalysis* **2013**, *5*, 2077–2079. [CrossRef] [PubMed]

280. Gallardo, E.; Barroso, M.; Queiroz, J.A. Current technologies and considerations for drug bioanalysis in oral fluid. *Bioanalysis* **2009**, *1*, 637–667. [CrossRef] [PubMed]

281. Desrosiers, N.A.; Scheidweiler, K.B.; Huestis, M.A. Quantification of six cannabinoids and metabolites in oral fluid by liquid chromatography-tandem mass spectrometry. *Drug Test. Anal.* **2015**, *7*, 684–694. [CrossRef] [PubMed]

282. Lee, D.; Vandrey, R.; Milman, G.; Bergamaschi, M.; Mendu, D.R.; Murray, J.A.; Barnes, A.J.; Huestis, M.A. Oral fluid/plasma cannabinoid ratios following controlled oral THC and smoked cannabis administration. *Anal. Bioanal. Chem.* **2013**, *405*, 7269–7279. [CrossRef] [PubMed]

283. Lee, D.; Milman, G.; Barnes, A.J.; Goodwin, R.S.; Hirvonen, J.; Huestis, M.A. Oral fluid cannabinoids in chronic, daily cannabis smokers during sustained, monitored abstinence. *Clin. Chem.* **2011**, *57*, 1127–1136. [CrossRef] [PubMed]

284. Niedbala, R.S.; Kardos, K.W.; Fritch, D.F.; Kunsman, K.P.; Blum, K.A.; Newland, G.A.; Waga, J.; Kurtz, L.; Bronsgeest, M.; Cone, E.J. Passive cannabis smoke exposure and oral fluid testing. II. Two studies of extreme cannabis smoke exposure in a motor vehicle. *J. Anal. Toxicol.* **2005**, *29*, 607–615. [CrossRef] [PubMed]

285. Saito, T.; Wtsadik, A.; Scheidweiler, K.B.; Fortner, N.; Takeichi, S.; Huestis, M.A. Validated gas chromatographic-negative ion chemical ionization mass spectrometric method for Δ9-tetrahydrocannabinol in sweat patches. *Clin. Chem.* **2004**, *50*, 2083–2090. [CrossRef] [PubMed]

286. Drummer, O.H. Drug testing in oral fluid. *Clin. Biochem. Rev.* **2006**, *27*, 147–159. [PubMed]

287. Balabanova, S.; Schneider, E. Detection of drugs in sweat. *Beitr. Gerichtl. Med.* **1990**, *48*, 45–49. [PubMed]

288. Samyn, N.; De Boeck, G.; Verstraete, A.G. The use of oral fluid and sweat wipes for the detection of drugs of abuse in drivers. *J. Forensic Sci.* **2002**, *47*, 1380–1387. [CrossRef] [PubMed]

289. De La Torre, R.; Pichini, S. Usefulness of sweat testing for the detection of cannabis smoke. *Clin. Chem.* **2004**, *50*, 1961–1962. [CrossRef] [PubMed]

290. Kieliba, T.; Lerch, O.; Andresen-Streichert, H.; Rothschild, M.A.; Beike, J. Simultaneous quantification of THC-COOH, OH-THC, and further cannabinoids in human hair by gas chromatography–tandem mass spectrometry with electron ionization applying automated sample preparation. *Drug Test. Anal.* **2018**, in press. [CrossRef] [PubMed]

291. Barroso, M.; Gallardo, E. Hair analysis for forensic applications: Is the future bright? *Bioanalysis* **2013**, *6*, 1–3. [CrossRef] [PubMed]

292. Barroso, M.; Gallardo, E.; Vieira, D.N.; López-Rivadulla, M.; Queiroz, J.A. Hair: A complementary source of bioanalytical information in forensic toxicology. *Bioanalysis* **2010**, *3*, 67–79. [CrossRef] [PubMed]

293. Beasley, E.; Francese, S.; Bassindale, T. Detection and Mapping of Cannabinoids in Single Hair Samples through Rapid Derivatization and Matrix-Assisted Laser Desorption Ionization Mass Spectrometry. *Anal. Chem.* **2016**, *88*, 10328–10334. [CrossRef] [PubMed]

294. Aamir, M.; Hafeez, A.; Ijaz, A.; Khan, S.A.; Chaudhry, N.; Ahmed, N. Development and validation of a liquid chromatography–tandem mass spectrometry method for cannabis detection in hair of chronic cannabis users under surveillance. *Pakistan J. Pathol.* **2016**, *27*, 61–70.

295. Pichini, S.; Marchei, E.; Martello, S.; Gottardi, M.; Pellegrini, M.; Svaizer, F.; Lotti, A.; Chiarotti, M.; Pacifici, R. Identification and quantification of 11-nor-Δ9-tetrahydrocannabinol-9-carboxylic acid glucuronide (THC-COOH-glu) in hair by ultra-performance liquid chromatography tandem mass spectrometry as a potential hair biomarker of cannabis use. *Forensic Sci. Int.* **2015**, *249*, 47–51. [CrossRef] [PubMed]

296. Concheiro, M.; Huestis, M.A. Drug exposure during pregnancy: Analytical methods and toxicological findings. *Bioanalysis* **2018**, *10*, 587–606. [CrossRef] [PubMed]

297. Kim, J.; de Castro, A.; Lendoiro, E.; Cruz-Landeira, A.; López-Rivadulla, M.; Concheiro, M. Detection of in utero cannabis exposure by umbilical cord analysis. *Drug Test. Anal.* **2018**, *10*, 636–643. [CrossRef] [PubMed]

298. Lamy, S.; Hennart, B.; Houivet, E.; Dulaurent, S.; Delavenne, H.; Benichou, J.; Allorge, D.; Marret, S.; Thibaut, F. Assessment of tobacco, alcohol and cannabinoid metabolites in 645 meconium samples of newborns compared to maternal self-reports. *J. Psychiatr. Res.* **2017**, *90*, 86–93. [CrossRef] [PubMed]

299. Chittamma, A.; Marin, S.J.; Williams, J.A.; Clark, C.; McMillin, G.A. Detection of in utero marijuana exposure by GC–MS, ultra-sensitive ELISA and LC–TOF–MS using umbilical cord tissue. *J. Anal. Toxicol.* **2013**, *37*, 391–394. [CrossRef] [PubMed]

300. Prego-Meleiro, P.; Lendoiro, E.; Concheiro, M.; Cruz, A.; López-Rivadulla, M.; de Castro, A. Development and validation of a liquid chromatography tandem mass spectrometry method for the determination of cannabinoids and phase I and II metabolites in meconium. *J. Chromatogr. A* **2017**, *1497*, 118–126. [CrossRef] [PubMed]

301. Brighenti, V.; Pellati, F.; Steinbach, M.; Maran, D.; Benvenuti, S. Development of a new extraction technique and HPLC method for the analysis of non-psychoactive cannabinoids in fibre-type *Cannabis sativa* L. (hemp). *J. Pharm. Biomed. Anal.* **2017**, *143*, 228–236. [CrossRef] [PubMed]

302. Pellati, F.; Brighenti, V.; Sperlea, J.; Marchetti, L.; Bertelli, D.; Benvenuti, S. New methods for the comprehensive analysis of bioactive compounds in *Cannabis sativa* L. (hemp). *Molecules* **2018**, *23*, 2639. [CrossRef] [PubMed]

303. Richins, R.D.; Rodriguez-Uribe, L.; Lowe, K.; Ferral, R.; O'Connell, M.A.; Prego-Meleiro, P.; Lendoiro, E.; Concheiro, M.; Cruz, A.; López-Rivadulla, M.; et al. Accumulation of bioactive metabolites in cultivated medical Cannabis. *PLoS ONE* **2018**, *113*, e0201119. [CrossRef] [PubMed]

304. Namdar, D.; Mazuz, M.; Ion, A.; Koltai, H. Variation in the compositions of cannabinoid and terpenoids in *Cannabis sativa* derived from inflorescence position along the stem and extraction methods. *Ind. Crops Prod.* **2018**, *113*, 376–382. [CrossRef]

305. Ciolino, L.A.; Ranieri, T.L.; Taylor, A.M. Commercial cannabis consumer products part 2: HPLC-DAD quantitative analysis of cannabis cannabinoids. *Forensic Sci. Int.* **2018**, *289*, 438–447. [CrossRef] [PubMed]

306. Kabir, A.; Holness, H.; Furton, K.G.; Almirall, J.R. Recent advances in micro-sample preparation with forensic applications. *TrAC Trends Anal. Chem.* **2013**, *45*, 264–279. [CrossRef]

307. Dulaurent, S.; Gaulier, J.M.; Imbert, L.; Morla, A.; Lachâtre, G. Simultaneous determination of δ9-tetrahydrocannabinol, cannabidiol, cannabinol and 11-nor-δ9-tetrahydrocannabinol-9-carboxylic acid in hair using liquid chromatography-tandem mass spectrometry. *Forensic Sci. Int.* **2014**, *236*, 151–156. [CrossRef] [PubMed]

308. Mackuľak, T.; Brandeburová, P.; Grenčíková, A.; Bodík, I.; Staňová, A.V.; Golovko, O.; Koba, O.; Mackuľaková, M.; Špalková, V.; Gál, M.; et al. Music festivals and drugs: Wastewater analysis. *Sci. Total Environ.* **2019**, *659*, 326–334. [CrossRef] [PubMed]

309. González-Mariño, I.; Thomas, K.V.; Reid, M.J. Determination of cannabinoid and synthetic cannabinoid metabolites in wastewater by liquid–liquid extraction and ultra-high performance supercritical fluid chromatography-tandem mass spectrometry. *Drug Test. Anal.* **2018**, *10*, 222–228. [CrossRef] [PubMed]

310. Petrović, M.; Debeljak, Ž.; Kezić, N.; Džidara, P. Relationship between cannabinoids content and composition of fatty acids in hempseed oils. *Food Chem.* **2015**, *170*, 218–225. [CrossRef] [PubMed]

311. Rotolo, M.C.; Pellegrini, M.; Martucci, P.; Giacobbe, R.; De Palma, A.; Pacifici, R.; Pichini, S.; Busardò, F.P.; Bisconti, M. Cannabinoids determination in bronchoalveolar lavages of cannabis smokers with lung disease. *Clin. Chem. Lab. Med.* **2018**, in press. [CrossRef] [PubMed]

312. Ottaviani, G.; Cameriere, R.; Cippitelli, M.; Froldi, R.; Tassoni, G.; Zampi, M.; Cingolani, M. Determination of drugs of abuse in a single sample of human teeth by a gas chromatography-mass spectrometry method. *J. Anal. Toxicol.* **2017**, *41*, 32–36. [CrossRef] [PubMed]

313. Kataoka, H.; Saito, K. Recent advances in SPME techniques in biomedical analysis. *J. Pharm. Biomed. Anal.* **2011**, *54*, 926–950. [CrossRef] [PubMed]

314. Barroso, M.; Gallardo, E.; Queiroz, J.A. The role of liquid-phase microextraction techniques in bioanalysis. *Bioanalysis* **2015**, *7*, 2195–2201. [CrossRef] [PubMed]

315. Barroso, M.; Moreno, I.; da Fonseca, B.; Queiroz, J.A.; Gallardo, E. Role of microextraction sampling procedures in forensic toxicology. *Bioanalysis* **2012**, *4*, 1805–1826. [CrossRef] [PubMed]

316. Hall, B.J.; Satterfield-Doerr, M.; Parikh, A.R.; Brodbelt, J.S. Determination of cannabinoids in water and human saliva by solid-phase microextraction and quadrupole ion trap gas chromatography/mass spectrometry. *Anal. Chem.* **1998**, *70*, 1788–1796. [CrossRef] [PubMed]

317. Strano-Rossi, S.; Chiarotti, M. Solid-phase microextraction for cannabinoids analysis in hair and its possible application to other drugs. *J. Anal. Toxicol.* **1999**, *23*, 7–10. [CrossRef] [PubMed]

318. Musshoff, F.; Junker, H.P.; Lachenmeier, D.W.; Kroener, L.; Madea, B. Fully automated determination of cannabinoids in hair samples using headspace solid-phase microextraction and gas chromatography-mass spectrometry. *J. Anal. Toxicol.* **2002**, *26*, 554–560. [CrossRef] [PubMed]

319. Emídio, E.S.; de Menezes Prata, V.; Dórea, H.S. Validation of an analytical method for analysis of cannabinoids in hair by headspace solid-phase microextraction and gas chromatography–ion trap tandem mass spectrometry. *Anal. Chim. Acta* **2010**, *670*, 63–71. [CrossRef] [PubMed]

320. Lachenmeier, D.W.; Kroener, L.; Musshoff, F.; Madea, B. Determination of cannabinoids in hemp food products by use of headspace solid-phase microextraction and gas chromatography–mass spectrometry. *Anal. Bioanal. Chem.* **2004**, *378*, 183–189. [CrossRef] [PubMed]

321. Racamonde, I.; Villaverde-de-Sáa, E.; Rodil, R.; Quintana, J.B.; Cela, R. Determination of Δ9-tetrahydrocannabinol and 11-nor-9-carboxy-Δ9-tetrahydrocannabinol in water samples by solid-phase microextraction with on-fiber derivatization and gas chromatography–mass spectrometry. *J. Chromatogr. A* **2012**, *1245*, 167–174. [CrossRef] [PubMed]

322. Dizioli Rodrigues de Oliveira, C.; Yonamine, M.; de Moraes Moreau, R.L. Headspace solid-phase microextraction of cannabinoids in human head hair samples. *J. Sep. Sci.* **2007**, *30*, 128–134. [CrossRef] [PubMed]

323. Musshoff, F.; Lachenmeier, D.W.; Kroener, L.; Madea, B. Automated headspace solid-phase dynamic extraction for the determination of cannabinoids in hair samples. *Forensic Sci. Int.* **2003**, *133*, 32–38. [CrossRef]

324. Lachenmeier, D.W.; Kroener, L.; Musshoff, F.; Madea, B. Application of tandem mass spectrometry combined with gas chromatography and headspace solid-phase dynamic extraction for the determination of drugs of abuse in hair samples. *Rapid Commun. Mass Spectrom.* **2003**, *17*, 472–478. [CrossRef] [PubMed]

325. Sergi, M.; Montesano, C.; Odoardi, S.; Rocca, L.M.; Fabrizi, G.; Compagnone, D.; Curini, R. Micro extraction by packed sorbent coupled to liquid chromatography tandem mass spectrometry for the rapid and sensitive determination of cannabinoids in oral fluids. *J. Chromatogr. A* **2013**, *1301*, 139–146. [CrossRef] [PubMed]

326. Rosado, T.; Fernandes, L.; Barroso, M.; Gallardo, E. Sensitive determination of THC and main metabolites in human plasma by means of microextraction in packed sorbent and gas chromatography–tandem mass spectrometry. *J. Chromatogr. B Anal. Technol. Biomed. Life Sci.* **2017**, *1043*, 63–73. [CrossRef] [PubMed]

327. Moradi, M.; Yamini, Y.; Baheri, T. Analysis of abuse drugs in urine using surfactant-assisted dispersive liquid-liquid microextraction. *J. Sep. Sci.* **2011**, *34*, 1722–1729. [CrossRef] [PubMed]

328. Gonçalves, A.; Gallardo, E.; Barroso, M. Variations in headspace microextraction procedures and current applications in bioanalysis. *Bioanalysis* **2015**, *7*, 2235–2240. [CrossRef] [PubMed]

329. Wang, Y.H.; Avula, B.; Elsohly, M.A.; Radwan, M.M.; Wang, M.; Wanas, A.S.; Mehmedic, Z.; Khan, I.A. Quantitative Determination of Δ9-THC, CBG, CBD, Their Acid Precursors and Five Other Neutral Cannabinoids by UHPLC-UV-MS. *Planta Med.* **2018**, *84*, 260–266. [CrossRef] [PubMed]

330. Gul, W.; Gul, S.W.; Radwan, M.M.; Wanas, A.S.; Mehmedic, Z.; Khan, I.I.; Sharaf, M.H.M.; ElSohly, M.A. Determination of 11 cannabinoids in biomass and extracts of different varieties of Cannabis using high-performance liquid chromatography. *J. AOAC Int.* **2015**, *98*, 1523–1528. [CrossRef] [PubMed]

331. Sharma, P.; Murthy, P.; Bharath, M.M.S. Chemistry, metabolism, and toxicology of cannabis: Clinical implications. *Iran. J. Psychiatry* **2012**, *7*, 149. [PubMed]

332. Citti, C.; Ciccarella, G.; Braghiroli, D.; Parenti, C.; Vandelli, M.A.; Cannazza, G. Medicinal cannabis: Principal cannabinoids concentration and their stability evaluated by a high performance liquid chromatography coupled to diode array and quadrupole time of flight mass spectrometry method. *J. Pharm. Biomed. Anal.* **2016**, *128*, 201–209. [CrossRef] [PubMed]

333. Patel, B.; Wene, D.; Fan, Z. (Tina) Qualitative and quantitative measurement of cannabinoids in cannabis using modified HPLC/DAD method. *J. Pharm. Biomed. Anal.* **2017**, *146*, 15–23. [CrossRef] [PubMed]

334. De Backer, B.; Debrus, B.; Lebrun, P.; Theunis, L.; Dubois, N.; Decock, L.; Verstraete, A.; Hubert, P.; Charlier, C. Innovative development and validation of an HPLC/DAD method for the qualitative and quantitative determination of major cannabinoids in cannabis plant material. *J. Chromatogr. B* **2009**, *877*, 4115–4124. [CrossRef] [PubMed]

335. Cardenia, V.; Gallina Toschi, T.; Scappini, S.; Rubino, R.C.; Rodriguez-Estrada, M.T. Development and validation of a Fast gas chromatography/mass spectrometry method for the determination of cannabinoids in *Cannabis sativa* L. *J. Food Drug Anal.* **2018**, *26*, 1283–1292. [CrossRef] [PubMed]

336. Baciu, T.; Borrull, F.; Aguilar, C.; Calull, M. Recent trends in analytical methods and separation techniques for drugs of abuse in hair. *Anal. Chim. Acta* **2015**, *856*, 1–26. [CrossRef] [PubMed]

337. Rosado, T.; Soares, S.; Malaca, S.; Gonçalves, J.; Barroso, M.; Gallardo, E. The role of liquid chromatography in toxicological analysis. In *High-Performance Liquid Chromatography: Types, Parameters and Applications*; Lucero, I., Ed.; Nova Science Publishers: New York, NY, USA, 2018; pp. 1–120. ISBN 978-1-53613-543-5.

338. Calvi, L.; Pentimalli, D.; Panseri, S.; Giupponi, L.; Gelmini, F.; Beretta, G.; Vitali, D.; Bruno, M.; Zilio, E.; Pavlovic, R.; et al. Comprehensive quality evaluation of medical *Cannabis sativa* L. inflorescence and macerated oils based on HS-SPME coupled to GC–MS and LC-HRMS (q-exactive orbitrap®) approach. *J. Pharm. Biomed. Anal.* **2018**, *150*, 208–219. [CrossRef] [PubMed]

Review

Mitragyna speciosa: Clinical, Toxicological Aspects and Analysis in Biological and Non-Biological Samples

Vânia Meireles [1], Tiago Rosado [1], Mário Barroso [2], Sofia Soares [1], Joana Gonçalves [1], Ângelo Luís [1], Débora Caramelo [1], Ana Y. Simão [1], Nicolás Fernández [3], Ana Paula Duarte [1] and Eugenia Gallardo [1,*]

[1] Centro de Investigação em Ciências da Saúde, Faculdade de Ciências da Saúde da Universidade da Beira Interior (CICS-UBI), 6200-506 Covilhã, Portugal; vaniaandbia@hotmail.com (V.M.); tiagorosadofful@hotmail.com (T.R.); sofia_soares_26@hotmail.com (S.S.); janitagoncalves@hotmail.com (J.G.); afluis27@gmail.com (Â.L.); deboracaramela50@gmail.com (D.C.); anaaysa95@gmail.com (A.Y.S.); apduarte@fcsaude.ubi.pt (A.P.D.)
[2] Serviço de Química e Toxicologia Forenses, Instituto de Medicina Legal e Ciências Forenses—Delegação do Sul, 1169-201 Lisboa, Portugal; mario.j.barroso@inmlcf.mj.pt
[3] Universidad de Buenos Aires, Facultad de Farmacia y Bioquímica, Cátedra de Toxicología y Química Legal, Laboratorio de Asesoramiento Toxicológico Analítico (CENATOXA). Junín 956 7mo piso. Ciudad Autónoma de Buenos Aires (CABA), Buenos Aires C1113AAD, Argentina; nfernandez@ffyb.uba.ar
* Correspondence: egallardo@fcsaude.ubi.pt; Tel.: +35-127-532-9002

Received: 31 January 2019; Accepted: 27 February 2019; Published: 4 March 2019

Abstract: The abuse of psychotropic substances is a well-known phenomenon, and many of them are usually associated with ancestral traditions and home remedies. This is the case of *Mitragyna speciosa* (kratom), a tropical tree used to improve work performance and to withstand great heat. According to several published studies, the main reasons for kratom consumption involve improving sexual performance and endurance, but also social and recreational uses for the feeling of happiness and euphoria; it is also used for medical purposes as a pain reliever, and in the treatment of diarrhea, fever, diabetes, and hypertension. However, this plant has gained more popularity amongst young people over the last years. Since it is available on the internet for purchase, its use is now widely as a drug of abuse, namely as a new psychoactive substance, being a cheaper alternative to opioids that does not require medical prescription in most countries. According to internet surveys by the European Monitoring Centre for Drugs and Drug Addiction in 2008 and 2011, kratom was one of the most widely supplied new psychoactive substances. The composition of kratom is complex; in fact, more than 40 different alkaloids have been identified in *Mitragyna speciosa* so far, the major constituent being mitragynine, which is exclusive to this plant. Besides mitragynine, alkaloids such as corynantheidine and 7-hydroxamitragynine also present pharmacological effects, a feature that may be attributed to the remaining constituents as well. The main goal of this review is not only to understand the origin, chemistry, consumption, and analytical methodologies for analysis and mechanism of action, but also the use of secondary metabolites of kratom as therapeutic drugs and the assessment of potential risks associated with its consumption, in order to aid health professionals, toxicologists, and police authorities in cases where this plant is present.

Keywords: *Mitragyna speciosa*; kratom; secondary metabolites; therapeutic uses; toxicology; analysis

1. Introduction

Several botanical products can be used for recreational purposes, and the effects include changes in mood, perception, behavior, and even in physiological parameters [1]. Although consumers usually have the wrong idea that they are completely safe and consumption does not involve any social or health risks, it is important to note that evidence of toxicity of such products has already been reported [2,3]. Commonly, the consumption of certain plants is associated with specific locations where people use them for what it seems to be the "natural effects" of the plant compounds. Regardless, a recurrent problem is the purification of the natural compounds in order to achieve stronger effects. This justifies the importance of early studies on addiction potential and classification of newly emerging psychoactive compounds.

Globally, the figures concerning consumption of new psychoactive substances (NPS) of natural origin are not clear. According to the European Monitoring Centre for Drugs and Drug Addiction (EMCDDA), the proportion of seizures in the category of other NPS (including those of natural origin) was of 12% in 2013 [4].

Mitragyna speciosa, belonging to the *Rubiaceae* family, found in both Asia and Africa, is a good example of such a NPS of natural origin. It is known as kratom, kakuam, kraton, ketum, ithang, or thom in Thailand and biak-biak in Malaysia or krypton when combined with *O*-demethyltramadol [5–9].

In Thailand, kratom's tree can mostly be found in the south of the country, and it is easily obtained from teashops, being used as a substitute for alcohol and opium.

Two types of kratom can be identified based on the color of the leaf vein, which can be either green or red. Locals usually prefer the red vein, characterized for its bitterness and longer effects [5]. Fresh leaves, at a dosage of normally 10 to 30 fresh leaves per day, are mostly used chewed swallowed as a powder, but they can also be dried for smoking or used to make tea [10].

In 1943, kratom was put under regulatory control by the Kratom Act in Thailand which was believed to be an economic move rather than a decision based on the concern for public health. During that time, taxes were involved with the opium trade and, because it was so expensive, people started to use kratom as a substitute, and this had consequences for the Thai government's income. Later in 1979, kratom was classified in Category V of a narcotics classification by the Thai government in the Narcotics Act, the same as cannabis, opium, and hallucinogenic mushrooms (the least restrictive and punitive level) [10–12].

Kratom was originally used mainly for its medicinal value in treating mild medical problems, namely fever, diarrhea, diabetes, pain, as a wound poultice, and to reduce the strain and fatigue of physical labor; however, it became also known and used to suppress opiate withdrawal symptoms given its affordability and availability [11–14]. In recent years, young consumers started to use kratom tea as a base for a cocktail known as "4 × 100", consisting of kratom tea, cough syrup, Coca-Cola, and ice cubes. This eventually became a concern since these consumers were using additives such as benzodiazepines to enhance the effects [10].

Vicknasingam et al. [13] studied the major reasons for kratom consumption and also the socio-demographic characteristics of its users. The study was conducted on 136 active users, of which 76.5% had a previous history of drug use. The presented reasons for kratom's consumption were reduction in addiction to other drugs, improvement of opiate addiction withdrawal symptoms, and its affordability relatively to heroin. A lot of short and long-term users claimed to have felt an increase in their capability for hard work, activeness, and heightened sexual desire [13,15]. An anonymous cross-sectional online survey was conducted in the USA in 2006, where 8049 users were studied through available social media and online resources from the American Kratom Association [16]. This study concluded that kratom is primarily used by middle-aged (31–50 years) and middle-income ($35,000 and above) individuals, the main purposes being to treat pain (68%) and emotional or mental conditions (66%).

Mitragyna speciosa can still be easily found on the internet for purchase, being a rather cheap alternative for opioids that does not require medical prescription [17,18]. In Europe, products labeled as *Mitragyna speciosa* ('kratom acetate' or 'mitragynine acetate') have been available since the early 2000s [19]. In recent years, products containing kratom are sold as 'incense' for their psychoactive effects, but concentrations of these active components vary depending on the variety of kratom used, circumstances, and harvesting time. The United Nations Office on Drugs and Crime questionnaire on NPS also revealed that kratom was one of the top three plant-based substances, along with khat and *Salvia divinorum*. Because kratom was not often under surveillance in national drug abuse surveys, information on its prevalence has been limited. Kratom and its active alkaloids are not listed under the 1961 and 1971 Conventions, but several countries have made policies for its control, also including mitragynine and 7-hydroxymitragynine (7-HMG) [20]. According to the internet surveys by EMCDDA in 2008 and 2011, kratom was one of the most widely supplied NPS [21]. Currently, *Mitragyna speciosa* is not illegal in most European countries or in the USA. In many EU countries, such as Denmark, Latvia, Lithuania, Poland, Romania, and Sweden, *Mitragyna speciosa* and/or mitragynine and 7-HMG are controlled drugs due to their high misuse potential. In other countries they are under control by the narcotic laws, including Australia, Malaysia, Myanmar, and Thailand (which has legalized the use of kratom and cannabis plants for medicinal use on December 2018). In New Zealand, *Mitragyna speciosa* and mitragynine are controlled under the Medicines Amendment Regulations [21].

Different formulations are available, including raw leaves, capsules, tablets, powder, and concentrated extracts. So far, more than 40 alkaloids have been identified in *Mitragyna speciosa*, the major constituent being mitragynine, which is exclusive to this plant [5,22–24]. Their relative amount varies monthly and according to the geographic origin of the plant [25,26]. Other constituents are paynantheine (PAY)–9%, speciogynine (SG)–7%, 7-HMG–2%, and speciociliatine (SC)–1% [25,27]. 7-HMG is a 7-hydroxyindolenine derivative of mitragynine (Figure 1) [28].

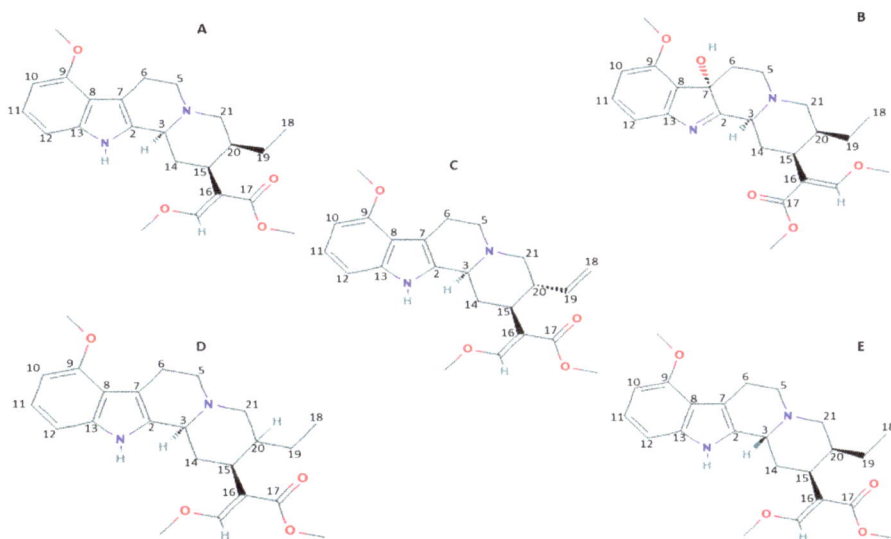

Figure 1. Structures of secondary metabolites: (**A**) mitragynine, (**B**) 7-hydroxymitragynine (7-HMG), (**C**) paynantheine (PAY), (**D**) speciogynine (SG) and (**E**) speciociliatine (SC).

These are indole alkaloids of the corynanthe-type with a monoterpene (iridoid) moiety. Other compounds include raubasine and a few yohimbe alkaloids [26,29]. In general, kratom contains at least one alkaloid that can block calcium channels and reduces *N*-methyl-D-aspartate (NMDA)-induced currents [30]. Other compounds, such as flavonoids, terpenoid saponins, polyphenols, and various glycosides are also present [25]. Veeramohan et al. [31] performed a metabolomics study using the mature leaves of the green variety of *Mitragyna speciosa* in order to obtain a more complete profile of kratom's secondary metabolites.

The alkaloids known to have a pharmacological effect are mitragynine, corynantheidine, and 7-HMG, but the remaining constituents might also provide this effect [25].

2. Research Methodology

The search for this review was conducted online on Pubmed, Google Scholar, and European Monitoring Centre for Drugs and Drug Addiction websites. Research papers, bibliographic reviews and case reports were included, the research done in Portuguese and in English. The search strings used were: "*Mitragyna speciosa*" and "consumption" and "toxicology" and "pharmacokinetics" and "case reports" and "pharmacological effects". The search was performed between December of 2018 and January of 2019. No publishing date restrictions were used. In order to assess their relevance, all papers fulfilling the search strings were screened independently by four of the authors. Only those that were selected by at least two authors were subjected to review and were included in the manuscript.

3. Toxicokinetics and Pharmacodynamics

Kratom's pharmacokinetics in humans has not been well studied so far, and several factors such as metabolic half-life, protein binding properties, elimination rates, and metabolism are not yet known [26,32]. Studies in rats showed that the absorption of *Mitragyna speciosa* after oral administration presents a much smaller AUC compared to intravenous administration, despite the oral dose being higher. The low oral bioavailability may be related to poor aqueous solubility of *Mitragyna speciosa*, which results in a smaller fraction for absorption [33]. Mitragynine is also believed to be a basic drug, becoming highly solubilized and ionized in the stomach, which reduces its absorption and therefore bioavailability [34]. Furthermore, using Caco-2 cells to predict intestinal absorption, mitragynine showed better permeability than 7-HMG [35].

In terms of elimination/half-life, mitragynine demonstrated biphasic elimination from plasma, suggesting distribution into inner tissue compartments. However, given the short half-life (mean half-life of 2.9 ± 2.1 h after injection), it is rapidly eliminated. Still, there are some contradictory reports on this matter, stating a higher half-life for mitragynine [35,36]. A case report of a young kratom user showed that approximately 10–14 days after consumption has stopped kratom metabolites could still be detected in urine. Saturation of enzymatic pathways or high plasma protein binding could account for this situation, but none was proven to be right [35].

Concerning distribution, according to a case report, after conducting high-throughput molecular screening of mitragynine activity at central nervous system receptors, it was shown that it is a mu- and kappa-opioid agonist [37]. Mitragynine and 7-HMG are transported by passive diffusion, presenting reflux ratios of 1 and 1.2 respectively [35]. Also, a complementary pharmacokinetics study was performed, in which the effects of a single intravenous dose of mitragynine (5 mg/kg, mitragynine hydrochloride) were compared to those of either a single oral dose (20 mg/kg, mitragynine hydrochloride), lyophilized kratom tea, or the organic fraction of the lyophilized kratom tea at an equivalent mitragynine dose of 20 mg/kg in rats. After intravenous administration, mitragynine exhibited a decrease in the concentration–time profile, indicating its fast distribution from the systemic circulation or central compartment to peripheral compartments [38]. Another study was performed by Yusof et al. [39], who have evaluated for the first time the rate and the extent of mitragynine and 7-HMG transport across the blood–brain barrier.

Kratom metabolism is mainly hepatic and there is some evidence that it can affect the metabolism and efficiency of other drugs via induction of drug-metabolizing enzymes such as CYP450s and UDP-glucuronosyl transferase (UGT) [40].

An assay evaluated the effect of *Mitragyna speciosa* alkaloid extract on CYP, and has found that kratom was responsible for CYP3A4, CYP2D6, and CYP2C9 inhibition [41], but unfortunately there are no studies that can help finding which particular kratom alkaloid is responsible for this inhibition. Kamble et al. [42] verified that CYP3A4 was mainly responsible for the metabolism, with minor contributions of CYP2D6 and CYP2C9. The same authors have described that mitragynine was extensively metabolized in liver microsomes primarily to *O*-demethylated and mono-oxidated metabolites. Due to these cytochrome-related genetic variations in humans, these enzymes will partly account for inter-individual differences in drug metabolism and toxicity [43].

Additionally, Philipp et al. [44] observed that isomeric compounds found in the kratom users' urine were SG and its metabolites, which can be also used as markers for *Mitragyna speciosa* presence.

Renal excretion of mitragynine is not considered significant, and mitragynine is not expected to be prone to substantial postmortem redistribution [36,45].

There are several studies that evaluate the effects of *Mitragyna speciosa* on human recombinant CYP450 enzyme activities [41]. This leads to implications, especially when mitragynine is co-administered together with herbal or modern drugs which follow the same metabolic pathway, contributing to herb–drug interactions [46].

According to Hanapi et al. [46], mitragynine might inhibit cytochrome P450 enzyme activities, specifically CYP2D6, and the strongest inhibitory effect was observed on CYP2D6, with a half-maximal inhibitory concentration (IC50) value of 0.45 ± 0.33 mM, followed by CYP2C9 and CYP3A4 with IC50 values of 9.70 ± 4.80 and 41.32 ± 6.74 µM respectively. Similar results are presented by Kong et al. [41], with apparent IC50 values of 0.78 µg/mL and 0.636 µg/mL for CYP3A4 and CYP2D6, respectively. Cinosi et al. [47] corroborate the possibility of a drug interaction if mitragynine and 7-hydroxymitragynine are administered together with drugs that are P-glycoprotein substrates. The authors mention, however, that *Mitragyna speciosa* is unlikely to have any significant clinical effects on CYP3A4 activity, but on the other hand might inhibit CYP2D6. Moreover, Lim et al. [48] performed an in vitro evaluation of cytochrome P450 induction and of the inhibition potential of mitragynine, and found that this alkaloid induces mRNA and protein expression of CYP1A2 consistent with the increased CYP1A2 enzymatic activity. Nevertheless, this alkaloid appears as a weak CYP3A4 inducer at the transcriptional level and a weak CYP3A4 enzyme inhibitor, leading to the same conclusion of Cinosi et al. [47], that it is unlikely to cause any significant clinical effects on CYP3A4 activity.

In this sense, the overall opinion is that the concomitantly administered drugs that may modulate these CYP isoenzymes activities will lead to clinically significant drug–drug interactions. Such interactions may result in serious adverse drug reactions, especially regarding drugs with short therapeutic windows such as carbamazepine, theophylline, digoxin warfarin, and phenytoin [49].

According to a review made by Ulbricht et al. [50], *Mitragyna speciosa* is likely to be unsafe if used by patients with neurologic disorders or that are taking either neurologic agents, such as alcohol, sedatives, benzodiazepines, opioids, or opium-containing products, or stimulant substances, such as caffeine, caffeine-containing products, cocaine, yohimbine, or related compounds. Also, the co-administration with monoamine oxidase inhibitors (MAOIs) is not advised. Recently, a case report of a fatality in a 27-year-old man was described by Hughes [51], who found a toxic blood concentration of quetiapine in conjunction with mitragynine.

Concerning the interactions of *Mitragyna speciosa* herb and food, there are some reports on this matter. According to a previous systematic review [50], the concomitant use of MAOIs, ayahuasca (*Banisteriopsis caapi*), syrian rue (*Peganum harmala*), or passion flower (*Passiflora incarnata*) with *Mitragyna speciosa* may potentially cause serious reactions. Moreover, yohimbe (*Pausinystalia yohimbe*) combined with *Mitragyna speciosa* may cause overstimulation and increased blood pressure, as it also occurs with the concomitant use of caffeine [50].

There have been reports on the concomitant use of opioids with *Mitragyna speciosa* causing oversedation or potential respiratory depression [52,53]. *Mitragyna speciosa* has reportedly been used for centuries for its psychoactive properties, opium-like effects, and ability to treat opioid addiction and opioid withdrawal. Reports starting in the mid-1800s give an account of *Mitragyna speciosa* being used as an opium substitute [54].

4. Clinical Effects/Pharmacology

Kratom has been found to have addiction potential in animal models when mitragynine and 7-HMG were given orally for five days [55].

4.1. Analgesic Properties

Mitragynine has a high affinity to mu-opioid receptors [56–58]. These receptors mediate analgesia, respiratory depression, and euphoria. It has been shown that its antinociceptive activity is mostly mediated by the supraspinal mu- and delta-opioid receptor subtypes, therefore making it the alkaloid responsible for the analgesic activity of kratom [57–59]. This also corroborates the claim that kratom can be used as an opium substitute or to diminish opium addiction, reducing the pain from withdrawal symptoms. Its affinity for kappa-receptors is considerably lower [58]. However, Stolt et al. [60] concluded that it exhibits analgesic effects via kappa-receptors and showed as well depressant effects on locomotor activity via presynaptic dopamine effects. The reinforcing effects of 7-HMG are mediated in part by mu- and delta-opiate receptors [61].

It is possible to use kratom as an anesthetic, and Vermaire et al. [62] reported the first case of this application by a patient using kratom for chronic pain.

Stimulation of post-synaptic alpha-2 adrenergic receptors, and/or blockage stimulation of 5-HT2 receptors by *Mitragyna speciosa* is also suggested. It is theorized that the effectiveness of the methanolic extract on alleviating positive and negative symptoms of psychosis may be due to inhibition of D_2 and 5-HT$_2$ receptors [63,64].

7-HMG also demonstrated high opioid receptor potency. In terms of analgesic activity, both mitragynine and 7-HMG were found to be more potent than morphine (mitragynine is about 13 times more effective, while 7-HMG is four times more effective) [13,55]. However, in a more recent study, kratom powder was found to have less affinity for the mu-opioid receptor than morphine [65].

At a cellular level, mitragynine can inhibit neurotransmitter release by reversibly blocking neuronal Ca^{2+} channels. It is proposed by the authors that the decrease in neurotransmitters leads to inhibition of pain transduction [66]. Mitragynine also inhibited adenylyl cyclase in NG108-15 cells through opioid receptors.

Cardiotoxicity was observed by induction of potentially fatal ventricular tachyarrhythmia (Torsade de Pointes). Blockage of the human Ether-a-go-go-Related Gene (hERG) channel in the heart constitutes a major risk of cardiotoxicity, and it is believed that *Mitragyna speciosa* suppresses hERG-mediated K^+ currents and prolongs action duration [67].

Opioid agonistic activities were studied with twitch contraction in guinea pig ileum induced by electrical stimulation. The crude extract inhibited the twitch contraction, which was reversed by naloxone. Also, each extracted alkaloid (7-HMG, mitragynine, SC, PAY, and SG) inhibited the electrically-induced twitch contraction in a concentration-dependent fashion [68].

Both methanolic and the alkaloid extract of *Mitragyna speciosa* leaves were found to prolong the latency of nociceptive response on heat-induced pain in the hot plate test in mice, but not in the tail-flick test [69]. However, when Sabetghadam et al. [70] performed a study comparing the antinociceptive effects of alkaloid (20 mg/kg), methanolic (200 mg/kg), and aqueous extracts (100–400 mg/kg), they concluded that they all prolonged the latency of nociceptive responses in both tests. These analgesic effects were blocked by naloxone, which suggests partial mediation by opioid-receptors, similar to what occurs with morphine. Returning to the tail-flick and hot-plate tests, 7-HMG was again demonstrated to have a more potent antinociceptive activity than morphine. Its higher lipophilicity apparently makes it easier to penetrate the blood–brain barrier [71].

4.2. Anti-Inflammatory Properties

The anti-inflammatory effects of *Mitragyna speciosa* have also been studied [56,72,73]. The cyclooxygenase isoforms, COX-1 and COX-2, are involved in the inflammatory pathway that catalyzes prostaglandin PGE2 formation, which is one of the strongest inflammatory mediators. Mitragynine is capable of inhibiting COX-2 mRNA and protein expression, and therefore inhibits PGE2 formation. At lower concentrations it did not affect COX-1 mRNA and protein expression, but caution is advised at higher doses [72]. Overall, authors suggest that the anti-inflammatory properties of *Mitragyna speciosa* may result from a combination of inhibition of pro-inflammatory mediator release and vascular permeability in addition to enhanced immunity, stimulation of tissue repair, and healing processes [73].

4.3. Gastrointestinal Effects

Kratom also seems to have gastrointestinal effects [56]. The in vivo effect of the methanolic extract of kratom leaves in the gastrointestinal tract of rats reduced defecation frequency and fecal weight in castor oil-induced diarrhea. A single dose of the extract resulted in intestinal transit reduction; however, further decreases were not observed with prolonged intake. Since pre-treatment with naloxone had no impact on defecation frequency, it is believed that kratom may affect other pathways besides opioid-receptors [74].

Centrally injected mitragynine into the fourth ventricle of anesthetized rats resulted in a dose-dependent inhibition of 2-deoxy-D-glucose-stimulated gastric acid secretion; however, this effect was reversed by naloxone, which indicates the involvement of opioid receptors [75]. Mitragynine injected into the lateral cerebroventricle had no influence in acid secretion. Its effects of anorexia and weight loss may be related to the direct inhibition of neurons in the lateral hypothalamus. As for 7-HMG, a subcutaneous injection on mice resulted in gastrointestinal transit inhibition [71].

Mitragyna speciosa both acute and chronic effects include reduction of food and water consumption, and the additionally gained weight had a tendency to be reduced [76].

A study on the modulation of the glucose transport system of L8 muscle cells demonstrated that kratom can increase the rate of glucose uptake as well as protein levels of glucose transport, corroborating anti-diabetic effects [77].

4.4. Anti-Depressant Activity

Furthermore, kratom has also shown anti-depressant activity [78]. The overproduction of corticosterone reflects a hyperactivity of the hypothalamic–pituitary–adrenal axis, which provides a depression indicator. By significantly reducing corticosterone concentration in mice exposed to the forced swim test and tail suspension tests, mitragynine seems to possess anti-depressant effects [79].

Ismail et al. [80] also discovered an impairment between spatial learning and memory processing during chronic administration of kratom, observing learning deficits similar to those induced by chronic morphine or Δ-9-tetrahydrocannabinol treatment. However, an investigation on the acute effects of *Mitragyna speciosa* extract and mitragynine on short-term memory and motor coordination in mice showed that neither of them had a significant effect [81]. In 2018, a study conducted in humans [82] corroborated precisely these results, and apparently high intakes of kratom juice (>3 glasses daily) did not impair motor, memory, attention, nor executive function of regular kratom users.

4.5. Antioxidant and Anti-Bacterial Properties

As for antioxidant and anti-bacterial properties, *Mitragyna speciosa* proved to have both [83]. Nevertheless, there is no sufficient evidence that supports the use of *Mitragyna speciosa* for clinical indications and this becomes even clearer due to the contradictory information existing on this matter.

5. Toxicology

The pharmacologic effects of kratom leaves and their constituents are dose-dependent. Low to moderate dosages (1 to 5 g) can offer light stimulant effects to help workers against fatigue, while moderate to high dosages (5 to 15 g) may have opioid-like effects [13]. However, kratom also presents stimulant effects at high dosages (>15 g) [25,84]. Anxiety, irritability, and enhanced aggression are described, and long-term high dose consumption has been related to several atypical effects [13]. Hyperpigmentation of the cheeks, tremor, anorexia, weight loss, and psychosis have been noted in individuals with long-term addiction [84]. Although the use of kratom in opioid withdrawal situations is discussed in the scientific literature, some authors [85–88] have examined the consequences of withdrawal from kratom. Withdrawal is highly uncomfortable for some users, and as such maintaining abstinence becomes difficult. In fact, clinicians need to be aware of withdrawal symptoms and implement a similar approach as for opioid withdrawal scenarios, with long-term maintenance to prevent relapse. Trakulsrichai et al. [36] performed a study on the pharmacokinetics of mitragynine in 10 male subjects using kratom tea, and no serious adverse effects were found. All subjects have reported developing tongue numbness after drinking the tea and an increase in blood pressure and heart rate. These last symptoms had a delayed onset of 8 hours after tea consumption, which was even later than T_{max} (0.83 ± 0.35 h), and as such further studies are required.

A recent study reported the death of rats after treatment with 200 mg/kg total alkaloid extract [89]. Other assays showed greater toxicity of the alkaloid extract when compared to the methanolic extract, with LD_{50} values of 173.20 mg/kg and 4.90 g/kg, respectively, in mice. In a 14-day period to evaluate acute toxicity, 100, 500, and 1000 mg/kg doses of standardized methanolic extract were administered to rats and did not affect spontaneous behavior, food and water consumption, absolute and relative organ weight, nor hematological parameters. It did however significantly increase blood pressure one hour after administration, and the highest dose of extract also induced acute severe hepatotoxicity and mild nephrotoxicity after single dose administration [90]. Sub-chronic high doses of *Mitragyna speciosa* have also been found to damage the kidneys and lungs, as emphysema, over-inflation of the alveoli, and an increase in serum creatinine and blood urea were observed [91]. Furthermore, both the plant extract and mitragynine showed cytotoxicity to human neuronal cells, but no genotoxicity in the mouse lymphoma gene mutation assay (Saidin). Also, no mutagenic effects were observed in a study performed using the Ames test [92]. The results concerning the benefits and toxicity of kratom are inconclusive; for instance, Fluyau et al. [93] have not determined if the biochemical benefits of the plant outweigh its toxicity and risks. On the contrary, it seems that the potential side effects outweigh the benefits, and severe and real health hazards can, insidiously, lead to death.

Cases involving multiple toxicity and fatal outcomes after mitragynine or kratom use have been reported, but the underlying causes remain unclear. Recently, in 2019, Rusli et al. [94] attempted to correlate the effects of mitragynine with glycoprotein-P, a multidrug transporter which modulates xenobiotic pharmacokinetics and plays a key role in the mediation of drug–drug interactions. Using biomolecular techniques, these authors concluded that mitragynine interacted with important residues at the nucleotide binding domain site of glycoprotein-P's structure, but not with the residues from the substrate binding site. Therefore, mitragynine is likely to be a glycoprotein-P inhibitor in vitro but it is not a substrate. Hence, concurrent administration of mitragynine-containing kratom products with psychoactive drugs which are glycoprotein-P substrates may lead to toxicity, and this can be clinically significant.

6. Case Reports

Some case reports have also been published. In the following section the main case reports found in literature will be discussed, in order to better understand the toxic effects of this plant. A 64-year-old male, who regularly used kratom to self-medicate his chronic pain, was found by his wife unconscious and seizing. A urine concentration of mitragynine of 167 ± 15 ng/mL was detected [95].

Nine unintentional deaths were reported due to consumption of krypton. Both mitragynine (0.02 to 0.18 μg/g) and O-desmethyltramadol (0.4 to 4.3 μg/g) concentrations were determined in postmortem blood samples [96].

A 44-year-old subject with chronic abdominal pain started taking kratom after reading about it on the internet. The increase of dose intake and subsequent attempts to reduce failed due to experiencing withdrawal symptoms. The patient gained 60 pounds, became lethargic and developed myxedematous face. A severe primary hypothyroidism was diagnosed, and the authors have related it to *Mitragyna speciosa* due to the reduction of the thyroid gland response to thyroid-stimulating hormone [97].

Another case report of a 25-year-old man suggested that kratom had induced intrahepatic cholestasis, which was confirmed by liver biopsy. Mitragynine was detected in both urine and serum samples [98].

Furthermore, a 44-year-old man with a history of depression, alcohol dependence, and other substance misuse was admitted for kratom detoxification. Prior to his admission, the patient was consuming approximately 40 g of kratom divided into 4 doses over 24 h. The patient also experienced withdrawal symptoms, even though he was regularly consuming kratom, which suggests the short half-lives of the active substances in kratom and a dependence syndrome primarily via agonist activity at the opioid receptors [99].

Domingo et al. [100] also reported a 22-year-old male with a history of drug addiction who used to mix an unknown amount of herbal substances. Prior to his death he fell from a window before going to bed but did not attend the hospital. A very high blood concentration of mitragynine was detected; however, the cause of death was determined to be aspiration of chyme. It is believed that, although kratom was not the direct cause of death, it had an important role in it. High doses produce sedative effects, and postmortem examination confirmed a humerus fracture of the left arm. It seems that the pain was alleviated by mitragynine, explaining the lack of urgency of the subject to seek medical attention [100].

Kratom's consumption in Southeast Asia is changing. A recent study performed by Singh et al. [101,102] based on self-reported information suggested that prolonged kratom use does not result in serious health risks nor impairs social functioning. Two recent trends have also emerged: the first involves the reported use of kratom to ease withdrawal from opioid dependence in rural settings, while the second is related to adulterated kratom cocktails being consumed by young people to induce euphoria in urban areas.

The presented evidences corroborate the fact that kratom is not only toxic but can also be lethal. The Food and Drug Administration [103] reported 44 deaths associated to kratom use, one of them involving mitragynine alone. These findings have prompted the institution to issue warning letters to numerous businesses that were illegally selling kratom. Nevertheless, it is not always clear which substances may be responsible for the effects, because in many situations kratom is not the only product being consumed, hence further studies are required on this matter.

7. Analytical Methodologies

To date, there are some techniques that have been suggested for the determination of *Mitragyna speciosa*, with special focus on mitragynine [104]. These techniques are imperative, not only for identification and quantification of plant components, but also for metabolic studies, and forensic and clinical toxicology. Therefore, it is important to achieve easy, inexpensive, and efficient ways to identify this plant or its components in biological specimens [104]. An increased focus must be given when kratom is present with other products or when there is adulteration of its chemical composition. Chromatographic methods seem to be the most commonly used, with high-performance liquid chromatography (HPLC) being the most popular [105]. Other methods include gas chromatography and liquid chromatography coupled to mass spectrometry (MS). Genetic methods have inclusively been used to identify the plant [9]. Some of the methods are reviewed in Table 1 (biological samples) and Table 2 (plant material).

Kowalczuk et al. [106] proposed a comprehensive authentication procedure that involves botanical analysis of leaf material and mitragynine identification by thin layer chromatography (TLC) and HPLC. Although microscopic analysis cannot be used by itself for kratom identification due to fragmentation of material and similarities between species, it can help in gathering information on the characteristic elements of the powdered material, especially because of the difficulty of dried plant material analysis due to incomplete removal of chlorophyll.

Lesiak et al. [32] proposed the identification of unique biomarkers for *Mitragyna speciosa* recurring to high resolution (HR)-DART-MS, a robust and fast way for data acquisition, without the need for sample pre-preparation steps. Fresh leaves and leaf extract analysis allowed the identification of *Mitragyna speciosa* following the detection of mitragynine isomers and 7-HMG. However, there was a significant difference in the amount of information provided by each different specimen, with a drop of 56% of the obtained information when the leaf extract was used. The possibility of identifying *Mitragyna speciosa* by comparison of the mass spectral data with those of unknown plant leaves was also approached with the help of linear discriminant analysis (LDA), being successful [32].

Parthasarathy et al. [107] reported a method with HPLC-diode array detection (DAD). DAD may be used for *Mitragyna speciosa* analysis because it stands as a fast and simple method, although it is not specific enough and seems to lack clear definition [105]. Comparison of extracts showed a higher mitragynine concentration in methanol and alkaloid-rich extracts when compared to the water extract. This is explained by the poor mitragynine solubility in water. Acid–base extraction technique also increased mitragynine concentration by converting the compound (and also other alkaloids) into its salt form, which is water soluble, and then back extracting the compound into the organic layer after neutralization, resulting in more concentrated extracts [107].

Ion mobility spectrometry (IMS) has also been used for the detection of mitragynine in 15 commercial samples. Its high sensitivity, at the ng level, and portability makes it attractive for screening. Fuenffinger et al. [108] used IMS and later compared the results with those obtained using liquid chromatography–tandem mass spectrometry (LC–MS/MS). LC–MS/MS detected mitragynine in one additional sample, whose concentration was below the IMS detection limit.

Furthermore, a monoclonal antibody (MAb) against mitragynine was produced and its ability to provide detection in leaf samples was also studied. The immunogens were prepared by means of the glutaraldehyde and carbodiimide methods. Immunogenicity was confirmed by determining the hapten numbers using matrix-assisted laser desorption/ionization time-of-flight mass spectrometry (MALDI-TOF-MS). This method provided a rapid and sensitive way of mitragynine quantification [109].

Gas chromatography (GC) systems are viable and readily accessible due to their high selectivity and relative low maintenance costs. Their coupling to MS provides good determination capabilities for compounds. Still, there are some issues that cannot be ignored. The high temperature required for alkaloid elution combined with the upper temperature limit of the polymeric GC stationary phases impairs the parametric adjustment of resolution of alkaloid mixtures, and derivatization is often deemed necessary [105]. In addition, these systems are not capable of adequately resolving a number of diastereomers, such as mitragynine's. This stands as an even bigger issue given the importance of mitragynine in *Mitragyna speciosa* analysis [105]. A study using GC–MS for urine samples could only detect mitragynine metabolites and some SC, SG, and PAY metabolites, with detection limits of 100 ng/mL for all diastereomers and PAY [110].

A comparison between GC and MS, supercritical fluid chromatography (SFC) and DAD, and UHPLC and MS and DAD for the analysis of mitragynine and other indole and oxindole alkaloids reported the GC method as less satisfactory. It proved to be unable to resolve mitragynine and SC. These diastereomers are only differentiated by the orientation of a single inner hydrogen atom, which makes the separation very hard by GC with a liquid stationary phase. In addition, the use of standard capillary columns may also have contributed to the inadequate resolution of the compounds.

SFC methods stood as a better choice given that they are faster, simpler and do not require as much organic liquids as the HPLC techniques [105]. Both were able to analyze mitragynine and other indole and oxindole alkaloids, but they differ in their effectiveness to identify mitragynine when its stereoisomers SG and SC are also present; indeed, and although mitragynine is the main compound of *Mitragyna speciosa*, it is important to find methods capable of identifying possible interferences from other diastereomers, which highlights the need for chromatographic separation [105].

The extraction technique can influence the yield in raw extracts and the relative alkaloid content of *Mitragyna speciosa* leaves, also highlighting the importance of extraction optimization. Mudge et al. [111] used the HPLC–UV technique to determine mitragynine and 7-HMG, and compared extraction solvents reporting methanol as the best choice; furthermore, they observed better extraction efficiency of mitragynine with 70% methanol with 0.5 M acetic acid. Other factors, such as the extraction method (shaking versus sonicating), solvent volume (10 versus 20 mL), and time (30 versus 60 min) were evaluated. Although results were inconclusive, shaking seemed to improve precision [111]. Other assays [112] compared ultrasound assisted extraction (UAE), microwave-assisted extraction (MAE), and supercritical carbon dioxide extraction (SFE-CO$_2$) (using methanol, ethanol, water, and binary mixtures). Using LC/ESI–MS analysis, MAE (methanol:water, 1:1) gave the highest alkaloid fraction amount, while UAE showed the best yield for mitragynine. The authors concluded that UAE (methanol:water) seemed to be the most effective method to obtain a large quantity of the alkaloid [112].

Scientific literature concerning the determination of the main active compounds of *Mitragyna speciosa* in biological fluids is very scarce, mostly focusing on urine specimens. In these cases, hydrolysis is usually performed with β-glucuronidase and/or arylsulfatase because metabolites are majorly excreted in the conjugate form [110,113–116]. Regarding extraction procedures, some authors use liquid–liquid extraction with methyl tert-butyl ether [113,117], ethyl tert-butyl ether [115], or n-butyl chloride [116].

However, solid phase extraction (SPE) seems promising. It yields clean chromatograms due to its capability of removing interferences from the matrix, leading to increased sensitivity, precision, and accuracy; it also presents short total analysis time and requires smaller sample volumes [33,114,118]. In fact, Mcintyre et al. [45] describe a fatal case report where peripheral blood, central blood, liver, vitreous, gastric content, and urine were used to screen for mitragynine by SPE (C$_{18}$) followed by GC–MS. Using this approach the authors achieved limits of detection and limits of quantitation of 0.03 and 0.05 mg/L, respectively. Holler et al. [116] report the first publication of a death involving propylhexedrine and mitragynine. The authors determined mitragynine presence in urine and blood, after previous hydrolysis with β-glucuronidase and sulfatase. The extraction was performed with 3 mL of n-butyl chloride and the analysis was performed using a LC–MS/MS system. The authors achieved limits of detection and quantitation of 0.25 and 1 ng/mL respectively, and successfully applied the extraction technique to other specimens (liver, vitreous humor, kidney, heart, spleen, lung, and bile) in order to detect mitragynine. Heart was the only specimen in which the compound was not detected.

Bar adsorptive microextraction, using a modified N-vinylpyrrolidone polymer sorbent phase, combined with liquid desorption followed by HPLC–DAD, was used in human urine matrices (BAμE–LD/HPLC–DAD). This technique provided high selectivity for mitragynine, good performance, and it is easy to work-up and environmentally friendly [119].

Although most of these methods proved to be reliable for mitragynine analysis, they require complex sample preparations. They can also be too laborious, expensive, and not so easily accessible; therefore, further studies are required on this matter. One should keep in mind that so far kratom constituents are not detected by conventional drug screening tests (e.g., immunoassay tests).

Tables 1 and 2 review the available literature (PubMed) about the analytical techniques (from 2010 to present) studied in human biological matrices and plant material.

Table 1. Analytical methods for the identification and/or quantification of *Mitragyna speciosa* in biological samples.

Compounds	Biological Sample (amount)	Analytical Technique	Internal Standard	Extraction Process	Linear Range (ng/mL)	LOD (ng/mL)	LOQ (ng/mL)	Recovery (%)	Reference
Mitragynine, 7-hydroxymitragynine, speciogynine, speciociliatine, and paynantheine	Urine (1 mL)	LC-ESI-MS-QTOF	mitragynine-d₃ 7-hydroxymitragynine-d₃	Solid-phase extraction (PolyChrom ClinII cartridges)	2–500	0.25–1	0.5–1	96–63	[120]
Mitragynine, 5-desmethylmitragynine and 17-desmethyldihydro-Mitragynine, and 7-hidroxymitragynine	Urine (0.2 mL)	UHPLC-ESI/MS-MS and LC-ESI/MS-MS	Mitraphylline	Enzymatic hydrolysis and liquid-liquid extraction (*methyl tert-butyl ether*)	1–500	-	1.00	78–94	[113]
Mitragynine	Urine (1 mL)	HPLC-DAD	-	BAμE (N-vinylpyrrolidone polymer) and back-extraction with methanol/acetonitrile (1:1, *v/v*) under sonication	0.6–24	0.1	0.33	103	[119]
Mitragynine	Urine (1 mL)	LC-ESI-MS (QTRAP)	methyltestosterone	Enzymatic hydrolysis and liquid-liquid extraction (ethyl tert-butyl ether)	0.25–1.5	0.2	0.25	83	[115]
Mitragynine	Peripheral blood, central blood, liver, vitreous, gastric content, and urine (1 mL)	GC-MS (EI)	mitragynine-d₃	Solid-phase extraction (Trace-J cartridges)	50–1000	30	50	-	[45]
Mitragynine, paynantheine, speciogynine, speciociliatine, 16-carboxy-mitragynine, 9-O-demethyl-mitragynine, and 9-O-demethyl-16-carboxy-mitragynine	Urine (3 mL)	GC-MS (EI)	-	Enzymatic hydrolysis and solid-phase extraction (HCX cartridge)	-	100	-	-	[110]
Mitragynine	Urine (2 mL)	LC-ESI/MS-MS	Ajmalicine	Liquid extraction; liquid-liquid extraction (*Methyl tert-butyl ether*)	0.01–5	0.02	0.1	81	[117]
Mitragynine	Blood and urine (1 mL), tissues (liver, kidney, heart, spleen, lung – 1g), bile, and vitreous humor	LC-ESI/MS-MS	Proadifen	Enzymatic hydrolysis and liquid-liquid extraction (n-butyl chloride)	1–10	0.25	1	103	[116]
Mitragynine	Rat serum (0.1 mL)	HPLC-UV LC-ESI-MS	Acenaphthene	Liquid–liquid extraction (diethyl ether)	100–10,000	30	100	85–84	[121]
Mitragynine	Rat plasma (0.1 mL)	HPLC-UV	Mefloquine	Solid-phase extraction (MCX Oasis cartridges)	50–1000	25	50	96–98	[33]
Mitragynine	Rat and human urine (1 mL)	HPLC-DAD	-	Solid-phase extraction (Oasis® HLB cartridge)	100–10,000	-	100	93–101	[118]
Mitragynine and metabolites	Rat and human urine (1 mL)	LC-ESI.LIT and LC-ESI.Orbitrap MS	-	Enzymatic hydrolysis and solid-phase extraction (Isolute Confirm HCX and Isolute Confirm C18 cartridges)	-	-	-		[114]

BAμE: Bar adsorptive microextraction; DAD: Diode-array detection; EI: Electron ionization mode; ESI: Electrospray ionization; GC: Gas chromatography; HPLC: High-performance liquid chromatography; HPLC–UV: High-pressure liquid chromatography with ultraviolet detector; LC: Liquid chromatography; LD: Liquid desorption; LIT: Linear ion trap; MS: Mass spectrometry; LOQ: Limit of quantitation; MS/MS: Tandem mass spectrometry; MTBE: Methyl t-butyl ether; RP–HPLC: Reverse-phase high performance liquid chromatography; LOD: Limit of detection; TBME: t-Butyl methyl ether; TOF: Time of flight; UHPLC: Ultra-high-performance liquid chromatography; SIM: Selective ion mode; SPE: Solid-phase extraction.

Table 2. Analytical methods for the identification and/or quantification of *Mitragyna speciosa* in leaves and plant material.

Compounds	Sample (Amount)	Analytical Technique	Extraction	LOD	LOQ	Recovery (%)	Reference
Several secondary metabolites	Mature leaves (100 mg)	LC-ESI-TOF-MS	Ice cold methanol	-	-	-	[31]
Mitragynine	Dried leaves (1.13 kg)	icELISA and HPLC–DAD	Methanol maceration, acid-base extraction, and silica gel column chromatography	32.47 µg/mL	-	-	[109]
Mitragynine	Leaves (5 kg)	HPLC–DAD	Methanol maceration and liquid extraction (chloroform)	0.25 µg/mL	0.5 µg/mL	95–101	[107]
	Ketum drink (1 mL)		Direct injection				
Mitragynine 7-OH mitragynine	Raw materials and powdered extracts (100 mg) and capsules	HPLC–UV	For dry test materials (0.5 M acetic acid in 70% methanol)	0.002% (w/w)	0.006% (w/w)	94–95	[111]
	Liquid finished products and/or beverages			0.2 µg/mL	0.6 µg/mL		
7-hidroxymitragynine	Raw materials, powdered extracts, and capsules		For beverages (dilution with methanol)	0.004% (w/w)	0.011% (w/w)	96–99	
	Liquid finished products and/or beverages			0.4 µg/mL	1.1 µg/mL		
Mitragynine	Ketum cocktail	HPLC–DAD	Freeze drying and reconstitution with methanol:water (80:20, v/v)	1.000 µg/mL	3.000 µg/mL	95	[122]
Mitragynine	Dried plant material (2 g)	TLC and HPLC–UV	Ethanol	1 µg/mL	-	-	[106]
Mitragynine	Kratom (powder or ground leaves material (100 mg); ¼ tea-spoon, liquid: 250 µL, capsule: 1)	IMS and LC–MS/MS	Methanol and ultrasonic bath sonication	0.5 ng/µL 2000 µg/mL	6000 µg/mL	-	[108]
Mitragynine, 7-hydroxymitragynine, and mitraphylline (stereoisomers, mitraciliatine, speciogynine, speciociliatine)	Plant material as fresh leaves (1.0 cm × 0.5 cm)	HR-DART-MS	Ethanol	-	-	-	[32]

DAD: Diode-array detection; DART: Direct analysis in real time; HPLC: High-performance liquid chromatography; HPLC–UV: High-pressure liquid chromatography with ultraviolet detector; HR: High resolution; icELISA: Indirect competitive enzyme-linked immunosorbent assay; IMS: Ion mobility spectrometry; LC: Liquid chromatography; LDA: Linear discriminant analysis; LOD: Limit of detection; LOQ: Limit of quantitation; MS: Mass spectrometry; MS/MS: Tandem mass spectrometry; TLC: Thin layer chromatography; TOF: Time of flight.

8. Conclusions and Future Perspective

It is still very compelling for people to use substances that can enhance their abilities. Several NPS or so-called 'designer drugs' are usually used in non-medical scenarios as synthetic alternatives for illicit drugs of abuse. Kratom is an example of these new trended drugs. Its consumption is traditional in southern Thailand, and it was formerly consumed for the purposes of withstanding great heat and fatigue. Nowadays there are a wide amount of other reasons for consumption, such as opium substitution, to diminish opium addiction, or reduce pain from withdrawal symptoms. Unfortunately, kratom itself seems to cause dependence, therefore leading to withdrawal symptoms whenever people stop using it. It has also been reported to cause an increase in blood pressure, hepatotoxicity, nephrotoxicity, emphysema, over-inflation of the alveoli, and cytotoxicity to human neuronal cells and there are even several reports regarding fatalities after kratom consumption. This alone is a pretty good reason to pay more attention to this plant. It is important to develop simple, inexpensive, and effective methods for *Mitragyna speciosa* analysis so that more information about toxicity, interactions with other drugs, metabolic actions, and pharmacology can be understood. This becomes even clearer due to the ease of acquisition on the internet. The lack of a convenient test for mitragynine detection makes it a lot harder for authorities to detect kratom users, and therefore harder to provide health care for them. A small plant that was originally used traditionally in a particular region in Asia is now used worldwide with no need for medical prescription or supervision and for which a dependence treatment is yet to be known.

Mitragyna speciosa also seems to present interesting effects, namely antinociceptive, anti-inflammatory, gastrointestinal, anti-depressant, antioxidant, and anti-bacterial. Still, there is no sufficient evidence that supports its use for clinical purposes, and therefore further studies are required.

Author Contributions: V.M. was responsible for the article search and writing of the manuscript sections concerning secondary metabolites. T.R. was responsible for the article search and writing of the manuscript sections concerning analytical methodologies. M.B. was responsible for designing the study, writing the section about legal aspects and toxicology, and revising the manuscript. S.S. was responsible for the article search and writing of the manuscript sections concerning toxicology. J.G. was responsible for the article search and writing of the manuscript sections concerning the case reports. Â.L. was responsible for the article search and writing of the manuscript sections concerning clinical effects and pharmacology. D.C. participated in the article search about analytical methods for the identification and/or quantification of *Mitragyna speciosa* in leaves and plant material and in writing of the manuscript. A.Y.S. participated in the article search about analytical methods for the identification and/or quantification of *Mitragyna speciosa* in biological samples and writing of the manuscript. N.F. was responsible for the article search and writing of the manuscript sections concerning pharmacokinetics and pharmacodynamics. A.P.D. was responsible for designing the study and revising the manuscript. E.G. was responsible for designing the study, organization, and revising the manuscript.

Funding: This reseach was funded by FEDER funds through the POCI—COMPETE 2020—Operational Programme Competitiveness and Internationalization in Axis I—Strengthening research, technological development, and innovation (Project POCI-01-0145-FEDER-007491) and National Funds by FCT—Fundação para a Ciência e a Tecnologia (Project UID/Multi /00709/2013). S. Soares and J. Gonçalves acknowledge Program Santander–Totta Universidades in the form of a fellowship (Bolsa BID/UBI–Santander Universidades/2018). Â. Luís acknowledges the contract in the scientific area of microbiology (Scientific Employment) financed by FCT.

Conflicts of Interest: The authors declare that they have no conflict of interest or financial involvement regarding this submission.

References

1.   Dennehy, C.E.; Tsourounis, C.; Miller, A.E. Evaluation of Herbal Dietary Supplements Marketed on the Internet for Recreational Use. *Complement. Altern. Med.* **2014**, *39*, 1634–1639. [CrossRef] [PubMed]
2.   Singh, D.; Müller, C.P.; Vicknasingam, B.K. Kratom (*Mitragyna speciosa*) dependence, withdrawal symptoms and craving in regular users. *Drug Alcohol Depend.* **2014**, *139*, 132–137. [CrossRef] [PubMed]
3.   Singh, D.; Müller, C.P.; Vicknasingam, B.K.; Mansor, S.M. Social Functioning of Kratom (*Mitragyna speciosa*) Users in Malaysia. *J. Psychoact. Drugs* **2015**, *47*, 125–131. [CrossRef] [PubMed]

4. European Monitoring Centre for Drugs and Drug Adiction. New Psychoactive Substances in Europe. Available online: http://www.emcdda.europa.eu/system/files/publications/65/TD0415135ENN.pdf (accessed on 12 January 2019).

5. Adkins, J.E.; Boyer, E.W.; Mccurdy, C.R. *Mitragyna speciosa*, A Psychoactive Tree from Southeast Asia with Opioid Activity. *Curr. Top. Med. Chem.* **2011**, *11*, 1165–1175. [CrossRef] [PubMed]

6. Takayama, H. Chemistry and Pharmacology of Analgesic Indole Alkaloids from the Rubiaceous Plant, *Mitragyna speciosa*. *Chem. Pharm. Bull.* **2004**, *52*, 916–928. [CrossRef] [PubMed]

7. Gong, F.; Gu, H.; Xu, Q.; Kang, W. Genus Mitragyna: Ethnomedicinal uses and pharmacological studies. *Phytopharmacology* **2012**, *3*, 263–272.

8. Davis, G.G. Drug abuse: Newly-Emerging drugs and trends. *Clin. Lab. Med.* **2012**, *32*, 407–417. [CrossRef] [PubMed]

9. Maruyama, T.; Kawamura, M.; Kikura-Hanajiri, R.; Takayama, H.; Goda, Y. The botanical origin of kratom (*Mitragyna speciosa*; Rubiaceae) available as abused drugs in the Japanese markets. *J. Nat. Med.* **2009**, *63*, 340–344. [CrossRef] [PubMed]

10. Tanguay, P. Kratom in Thailand. *Transl. Inst. Legis. Reform Drug Policies* **2011**, *13*, 1–16. [CrossRef]

11. Saingam, D.; Assanangkornchai, S.; Geater, A.F.; Balthip, Q. Pattern and consequences of krathom (*Mitragyna speciosa* Korth.) use among male villagers in southern Thailand: A qualitative study. *Int. J. Drug Policy* **2018**, *24*, 351–358. [CrossRef] [PubMed]

12. Singh, D.; Narayanan, S.; Vicknasingam, B. Traditional and non-traditional uses of Mitragynine (Kratom): A survey of the literature. *Brain Res. Bull.* **2016**, *126*, 41–46. [CrossRef] [PubMed]

13. Vicknasingam, B.; Narayanan, S.; Beng, G.T.; Mansor, S.M. The informal use of ketum (*Mitragyna speciosa*) for opioid withdrawal in the northern states of peninsular Malaysia and implications for drug substitution therapy. *Int. J. Drug Policy* **2010**, *21*, 283–288. [CrossRef] [PubMed]

14. Swogger, M.T.; Hart, E.; Erowid, F.; Erowid, E.; Trabold, N.; Yee, K.; Parkhurst, K.A.; Priddy, B.M.; Walsh, Z. Experiences of Kratom Users: A Qualitative Analysis. *J. Psychoact. Drugs* **2015**, *47*, 360–367. [CrossRef] [PubMed]

15. Assanangkornchai, S.; Muekthong, A. The Use of Mitragynine speciosa ("Krathom"), an Addictive Plant, in Thailand. *Subst. Use Misuse* **2006**, *6084*, 2145–2157.

16. Grundmann, O. Patterns of Kratom use and health impact in the US—Results from an online survey. *Drug Alcohol Depend.* **2017**, *176*, 63–70. [CrossRef] [PubMed]

17. Schmidt, M.M.; Sharma, A.; Schifano, F.; Feinmann, C. "Legal highs" on the net-Evaluation of UK-based Websites, products and product information. *Forensic Sci. Int.* **2011**, *206*, 92–97. [CrossRef] [PubMed]

18. Hillebrand, J.; Olszewski, D.; Sedefov, R. Legal Highs on the Internet. *Subst. Use Misuse* **2010**, *45*, 330–340. [CrossRef] [PubMed]

19. European Monitoring Centre for Drugs and Drug Adiction. Khat Drug Profile. Available online: http://www.emcdda.europa.eu/publications/drug-profiles/khat (accessed on 11 January 2019).

20. United Nations Office on Drugs and Crime (UNODC). UNODC Early Warning Advisory (EWA) on New Psychoactive Substances (NPS). Available online: https://www.unodc.org/LSS/Home/NPS (accessed on 16 January 2019).

21. Kratom (*Mitragyna speciosa*) Drug Profile. Available online: http://www.emcdda.europa.eu/publications/drug-profiles/kratom (accessed on 11 January 2019).

22. Ahmad, K.; Aziz, Z. *Mitragyna speciosa* use in the northern states of Malaysia: A cross-sectional study. *J. Ethnopharmacol.* **2012**, *141*, 446–450. [CrossRef] [PubMed]

23. Jansen, K.; Prast, C. Ethnopharmacology of kratom and mitragyna alkaloids. *J. Ethnopharmacol.* **1988**, *23*, 115–119. [CrossRef]

24. Shellard, E.J. Ethnopharmacology of kratom and the Mitragyna alkaloids. *J. Ethnopharmacol.* **1989**, *25*, 123–124. [CrossRef]

25. Feng, L.-Y.; Battulga, A.; Han, E.; Chung, H.; Li, J.-H. New psychoactive substances of natural origin: A brief review. *J. Food Drug Anal.* **2017**, *25*, 461–471. [CrossRef] [PubMed]

26. Raffa, R.B. *Kratom and Other Mitragynines: The Chemistry and Pharmacology of Opioids from a Non-Opium Source*, 1st ed.; Raffa, R.B., Ed.; CRC Press: Boca Raton, FL, USA, 2014.

27. Schro, S.; Stu, B.; Arndt, T.; Claussen, U.; Gu, B.; Werle, A.; Wolf, G. Kratom alkaloids and O-desmethyltramadol in urine of a "Krypton" herbal mixture consumer. *Forensic Sci. Int.* **2011**, *208*, 47–52.

28. Ponglux, D.; Wongseripipatana, S.; Takayama, H.; Kilcuchi, M.; Kurihara, M. A New Indole Alkaloid, 7a-Hydroxy-7H-mitragynine, from *Mitragyna speciosa* in Thailand. *Planta Med.* **1994**, *60*, 581–582. [CrossRef] [PubMed]

29. Prozialeck, W.C.; Jivan, J.K.; Andurkar, S.V. Pharmacology of Kratom: An Emerging Botanical Agent with Stimulant, Analgesic and Opioid-Like Effects. *J. Am. Osteopath. Assoc.* **2012**, *112*, 792–799. [PubMed]

30. Hendrickson, J.B.; Sims, J.J. Mitragyna alkaloids: The structure of stipulatine. *Tetrahedron Lett.* **1963**, *4*, 929–935. [CrossRef]

31. Veeramohan, R.; Azizan, K.A.; Aizat, W.M.; Goh, H.-H.; Mansor, S.M.; Yusof, N.S.M.; Baharum, S.N.; Ng, C.L. Metabolomics data of *Mitragyna speciosa* leaf using LC-ESI-TOF-MS. *Data Br.* **2018**, *18*, 1212–1216. [CrossRef] [PubMed]

32. Lesiak, A.D.; Cody, R.B.; Dane, A.J.; Musah, R.A. Rapid detection by direct analysis in real time-mass spectrometry (DART-MS) of psychoactive plant drugs of abuse: The case of *Mitragyna speciosa* aka "Kratom". *Forensic Sci. Int.* **2014**, *242*, 210–218. [CrossRef] [PubMed]

33. Parthasarathy, S.; Ramanathan, S.; Ismail, S.; Adenan, M.I.; Mansor, S.M.; Murugaiyah, V. Determination of mitragynine in plasma with solid-phase extraction and rapid HPLC-UV analysis, and its application to a pharmacokinetic study in rat. *Anal. Bioanal. Chem.* **2010**, *397*, 2023–2030. [CrossRef] [PubMed]

34. Ramanathan, S.; Parthasarathy, S.; Murugaiyah, V.; Magosso, E.; Tan, S.C.; Mansor, S.M. Understanding the physicochemical properties of mitragynine, a principal alkaloid of *Mitragyna speciosa*, for preclinical evaluation. *Molecules* **2015**, *20*, 4915–4927. [CrossRef] [PubMed]

35. Manda, V.K.; Avula, B.; Ali, Z.; Khan, I.A.; Walker, L.A.; Khan, S.I. Evaluation of in vitro absorption, distribution, metabolism, and excretion (ADME) properties of mitragynine, 7-hydroxymitragynine, and mitraphylline. *Planta Med.* **2014**, *80*, 568–576. [CrossRef] [PubMed]

36. Trakulsrichai, S.; Sathirakul, K.; Auparakkitanon, S.; Krongvorakul, J.; Sueajai, J.; Noumjad, N.; Sukasem, C.; Wananukul, W. Pharmacokinetics of mitragynine in man. *Drug Des. Dev. Ther.* **2015**, *9*, 2421–2429.

37. Boyer, E.; Babu, K.; Adkins, J.; McCurdy, C.; Harpern, J. Self-treatment of opioid withdrawal using kratom (*Mitragynia speciosa* Korth). *Addiction* **2013**, *103*, 1048–1050. [CrossRef] [PubMed]

38. Avery, B.A.; Boddu, S.P.; Sharma, A.; Furr, E.B.; Leon, F.; Cutler, S.J.; McCurdy, C.R. Comparative Pharmacokinetics of Mitragynine after Oral Administration of *Mitragyna speciosa* (Kratom) Leaf Extracts in Rats. *Planta Med.* **2018**, in press. [CrossRef] [PubMed]

39. Yusof, S.R.; Mohd Uzid, M.; Teh, E.-H.; Hanapi, N.A.; Mohideen, M.; Mohamad Arshad, A.S.; Mordi, M.N.; Loryan, I.; Hammarlund-Udenaes, M. Rate and extent of mitragynine and 7-hydroxymitragynine blood–brain barrier transport and their intra-brain distribution: The missing link in pharmacodynamic studies. *Addict. Biol.* **2018**, in press. [CrossRef] [PubMed]

40. Azizi, J.; Ismail, S.; Mansor, S.M. *Mitragyna speciosa* Korth leaves extracts induced the CYP450 catalyzed aminopyrine-*N*-demethylase (APND) and UDP-glucuronosyl transferase (UGT) activities in male Sprague-Dawley rat livers. *Drug Metab. Drug Interact.* **2013**, *28*, 95–105. [CrossRef] [PubMed]

41. Kong, W.M.; Chik, Z.; Ramachandra, M.; Subramaniam, U.; Raja Aziddin, R.E.; Mohamed, Z. Evaluation of the effects of *Mitragyna speciosa* alkaloid extract on cytochrome P450 enzymes using a high throughput assay. *Molecules* **2011**, *16*, 7344–7356. [CrossRef] [PubMed]

42. Kamble, S.H.; Sharma, A.; King, T.I.; León, F.; McCurdy, C.R.; Avery, B.A. Metabolite profiling and identification of enzymes responsible for the metabolism of mitragynine, the major alkaloid of *Mitragyna speciosa* (kratom). *Xenobiotica* **2018**, *14*, 1–31. [CrossRef] [PubMed]

43. Uno, Y.; Uehara, S.; Murayama, N.; Yamazaki, H. Cytochrome P450 1A1, 2C9, 2C19, and 3A4 Polymorphisms Account for Interindividual Variability of Toxicological Drug Metabolism in Cynomolgus Macaques. *Chem. Res. Toxicol.* **2018**, *31*, 1373–1381. [CrossRef] [PubMed]

44. Philipp, A.A.; Wissenbach, D.K.; Weber, A.A.; Zapp, J.; Maurer, H.H. Metabolism studies of the Kratom alkaloid speciociliatine, a diastereomer of the main alkaloid mitragynine, in rat and human urine using liquid chromatography-linear ion trap mass spectrometry. *Anal. Bioanal. Chem.* **2011**, *399*, 2747–2753. [CrossRef] [PubMed]

45. Mcintyre, I.M.; Trochta, A.; Stolberg, S.; Campman, S.C. Mitragynine 'Kratom' Related Fatality: A Case Report with Postmortem Concentrations. *J. Anal. Toxicol.* **2014**, *39*, 152–155. [CrossRef] [PubMed]

46. Hanapi, N.A.; Ismail, S.; Mansor, S.M. Inhibitory effect of mitragynine on human cytochrome P450 enzyme activities. *Pharmacogn. Res.* **2013**, *5*, 241–246.

47. Cinosi, E.; Martinotti, G.; Simonato, P.; Singh, D.; Demetrovics, Z.; Roman-Urrestarazu, A.; Bersani, F.S.; Vicknasingam, B.; Piazzon, G.; Li, J.H.; et al. Following "the Roots" of Kratom (*Mitragyna speciosa*): The Evolution of an Enhancer from a Traditional Use to Increase Work and Productivity in Southeast Asia to a Recreational Psychoactive Drug in Western Countries. *Biomed. Res. Int.* **2015**, *2015*, 1–11. [CrossRef] [PubMed]

48. Koe, X.F.; Jamil, M.F.A.; Adenan, M.I.; Tan, M.L.; Lim, E.L.; Seah, T.C.; Majid, M.I.A.; Wahab, H.A. In vitro evaluation of cytochrome P450 induction and the inhibition potential of mitragynine, a stimulant alkaloid. *Toxicol. In Vitr.* **2012**, *27*, 812–824.

49. Showande, S.J.; Fakeye, T.O.; Kajula, M.; Hokkanen, J.; Tolonen, A. Potential inhibition of major human cytochrome P450 isoenzymes by selected tropical medicinal herbs—Implication for herb–drug interactions. *Food Sci. Nutr.* **2019**, *7*, 44–55. [CrossRef] [PubMed]

50. Ulbricht, C.; Costa, D.; Dao, J.; Isaac, R.; Leblanc, Y.C.; Rhoades, J.; Windsor, R.C. An evidence-based systematic review of kratom (*Mitragyna speciosa*) by the natural standard research collaboration. *J. Diet. Suppl.* **2013**, *10*, 152–170. [CrossRef] [PubMed]

51. Hughes, R.L. Fatal combination of mitragynine and quetiapine—A case report with discussion of a potential herb-drug interaction. *Forensic Sci. Med. Pathol.* **2018**, *15*, 110–113. [CrossRef] [PubMed]

52. Chan, K.B.; Pakiam, C.; Rahim, R.A. Psychoactive plant abuse: The identification of mitragynine in ketum and in ketum preparations. *Bull. Narc.* **2007**, *249*, 249–256.

53. Roche, K.M.; Hart, K.; Sangalli, B.; Lefberg, J.; Bayer, M. Kratom: A Case of a Legal High. *Clin. Toxicol.* **2008**, *46*, 598.

54. Ward, J.; Rosenbaum, C.; Hernon, C.; McCurdy, C.R.; Boyer, E.W. Herbal Medicines for the Management of Opioid Addiction. *CNS Drugs* **2011**, *25*, 999–1007. [CrossRef] [PubMed]

55. Matsumoto, K.; Horie, S.; Takayama, H.; Ishikawa, H.; Aimi, N.; Ponglux, D.; Murayama, T.; Watanabe, K. Antinociception, tolerance and withdrawal symptoms induced by 7-hydroxymitragynine, an alkaloid from the Thai medicinal herb *Mitragyna speciosa*. *Life Sci.* **2005**, *78*, 2–7. [CrossRef] [PubMed]

56. Hassan, Z.; Muzaimi, M.; Navaratnam, V.; Yusoff, N.H.M.; Suhaimi, F.W.; Vadivelu, R.; Vicknasingam, B.K.; Amato, D.; von Hörsten, S.; Ismail, N.I.W.; et al. From Kratom to mitragynine and its derivatives: Physiological and behavioural effects related to use, abuse, and addiction. *Neurosci. Biobehav. Rev.* **2013**, *37*, 138–151. [CrossRef] [PubMed]

57. Thongpradichote, S.; Matsumoto, K.; Tohda, M.; Takayama, H.; Aimi, N.; Sakai, S.I.; Watanabe, H. Identification of opioid receptor subtypes in antinociceptive actions of supraspinally-administered mitragynine in mice. *Life Sci.* **1998**, *62*, 1371–1378. [CrossRef]

58. Yamamoto, L.T.; Horie, S.; Takayama, H.; Aimi, N.; Sakai, S.I.; Yano, S.; Shan, J.; Pang, P.K.T.; Ponglux, D.; Watanabe, K. Opioid receptor agonistic characteristics of mitragynine pseudoindoxyl in comparison with mitragynine derived from Thai medicinal plant *Mitragyna speciosa*. *Gen. Pharmacol.* **1999**, *33*, 73–81. [CrossRef]

59. White, C.M. Pharmacologic and clinical assessment of kratom. *Bull. Am. Soc. Hosp. Pharm.* **2018**, *75*, 261–267. [CrossRef] [PubMed]

60. Stolt, A.-C.; Schröder, H.; Neurath, H.; Grecksch, G.; Höllt, V.; Meyer, M.R.; Maurer, H.H.; Ziebolz, N.; Havemann-Reinecke, U.; Becker, A. Behavioral and neurochemical characterization of kratom (*Mitragyna speciosa*) extract. *Psychopharmacology* **2014**, *231*, 13–25. [CrossRef] [PubMed]

61. Hemby, S.E.; McIntosh, S.; Leon, F.; Cutler, S.J.; McCurdy, C.R. Abuse liability and therapeutic potential of the *Mitragyna speciosa* (kratom) alkaloids mitragynine and 7-hydroxymitragynine. *Addict. Biol.* **2018**, in press. [CrossRef] [PubMed]

62. Vermaire, D.J.; Skaer, D.; Tippets, W. Kratom and General Anesthesia: A Case Report and Review of the Literature. *A A Pract.* **2019**, *12*, 103–105. [CrossRef] [PubMed]

63. Vijeepallam, K.; Pandy, V.; Kunasegaran, T.; Murugan, D.D.; Naidu, M. *Mitragyna speciosa* leaf extract exhibits antipsychotic-like effect with the potential to alleviate positive and negative symptoms of psychosis in mice. *Front. Pharmacol.* **2016**, *7*, 464. [CrossRef] [PubMed]

64. Watanabe, K.; Yano, S.; Horie, S.; Yamamoto, L. Inhibitory effect of mitragynine, an alkaloid with analgesic effect from Thai medicinal plant *Mitragyna speciosa*, on electrically stimulated contraction of isolated guinea-pig ileum through the opioid receptor. *Life Sci.* **1997**, *60*, 933–942. [CrossRef]

65. Havemann-Reinecke, U. P01-50-Kratom and alcohol dependence: Clinical symptoms, withdrawal treatment and pharmacological mechanisms—A case report. *Eur. Psychiatry* **2011**, *26*, 50. [CrossRef]

66. Matsumoto, K.; Yamamoto, L.T.; Watanabe, K.; Yano, S.; Shan, J.; Pang, P.K.T.; Ponglux, D.; Takayama, H.; Horie, S. Inhibitory effect of mitragynine, an analgesic alkaloid from Thai herbal medicine, on neurogenic contraction of the vas deferens. *Life Sci.* **2005**, *78*, 187–194. [CrossRef] [PubMed]

67. Lu, J.; Wei, H.; Wu, J.; Fadzly, M.; Jamil, A. Evaluation of the Cardiotoxicity of Mitragynine and Its Analogues Using Human Induced Pluripotent Stem Cell- Derived Cardiomyocytes. *PLoS ONE* **2014**, *9*, e115648. [CrossRef] [PubMed]

68. Horie, S.; Koyama, F.; Takayama, H.; Ishikawa, H.; Aimi, N.; Ponglux, D.; Matsumoto, K.; Murayama, T. Indole alkaloids of a Thai medicinal herb, *Mitragyna speciosa*, that has opioid agonistic effect in guinea-pig ileum. *Planta Med.* **2005**, *71*, 231–236. [CrossRef] [PubMed]

69. Reanmongkol, W.; Keawpradub, N.; Sawangjaroen, K. Effects of the extracts from *Mitragyna speciosa* Korth. leaves on analgesic and behavioral activities in experimental animals. *Songklanakarin J. Sci. Technol.* **2017**, *29*, 39–48.

70. Sabetghadam, A.; Ramanathan, S.; Mahsufi Mansor, S. The evaluation of antinociceptive activity of alkaloid, methanolic, and aqueous extracts of Malaysian *Mitragyna speciosa* Korth leaves in rats. *Pharmacogn. Res.* **2010**, *2*, 181–185.

71. Matsumoto, K.; Hatori, Y.; Murayama, T. Involvement of μ-opioid receptors in antinociception and inhibition of gastrointestinal transit induced by 7-hydroxymitragynine, isolated from Thai herbal medicine *Mitragyna speciosa*. *Eur. J. Pharmacol.* **2006**, *549*, 63–70. [CrossRef] [PubMed]

72. Utar, Z.; Majid, M.I.A.; Adenan, M.I.; Jamil, M.F.A.; Lan, T.M. Mitragynine inhibits the COX-2 mRNA expression and prostaglandin E2 production induced by lipopolysaccharide in RAW264.7 macrophage cells. *J. Ethnopharmacol.* **2011**, *136*, 75–82. [CrossRef] [PubMed]

73. Mossadeq, W.M.S.; Sulaiman, M.R.; Mohamad, T.A.T.; Chiong, H.S.; Zakaria, Z.A.; Jabit, M.L.; Baharuldin, M.T.H.; Israf, D.A. Anti-Inflammatory and Antinociceptive Effects of *Mitragyna speciosa* Korth. *Med. Princ. Pract.* **2009**, *18*, 378–384. [CrossRef] [PubMed]

74. Chittrakarn, S.; Sawangjaroen, K.; Prasettho, S.; Janchawee, B.; Keawpradub, N. Inhibitory effects of kratom leaf extract (*Mitragyna speciosa* Korth.) on the rat gastrointestinal tract. *J. Ethnopharmacol.* **2008**, *116*, 173–178. [CrossRef] [PubMed]

75. Tsuchiya, S.; Miyashita, S.; Yamamoto, M.; Horie, S.; Sakai, S. Effect of mitragynine, derived from Thai folk medicine, on gastric acid secretion through opioid receptor in anesthetized rats. *Eur. J. Pharmacol.* **2002**, *443*, 185–188. [CrossRef]

76. Sabetghadam, A.; Ramanathan, S.; Sasidharan, S.; Mansor, S.M. Subchronic exposure to mitragynine, the principal alkaloid of *Mitragyna speciosa*, in rats. *J. Ethnopharmacol.* **2013**, *146*, 815–823. [CrossRef] [PubMed]

77. Purintrapiban, J.; Keawpradub, N. Study on glucose transport in muscle cells by extracts from *Mitragyna speciosa* (Korth) and mitragynine. *Nat. Prod. Res.* **2011**, *25*, 1379–1387. [CrossRef] [PubMed]

78. Kumarnsit, E.; Keawpradub, N.; Nuankaew, W. Effect of *Mitragyna speciosa* aqueous extract on ethanol withdrawal symptoms in mice. *Fitoterapia* **2007**, *78*, 182–185. [CrossRef] [PubMed]

79. Farah Idayu, N.; Taufik Hidayat, M.; Moklas, M.A.M.; Sharida, F.; Nurul Raudzah, A.R.; Shamima, A.R.; Apryani, E. Antidepressant-like effect of mitragynine isolated from *Mitragyna speciosa* Korth in mice model of depression. *Phytomedicine* **2011**, *18*, 402–407. [CrossRef] [PubMed]

80. Ismail, N.I.W.; Jayabalan, N.; Mansor, S.M.; Müller, C.P.; Muzaimi, M. Chronic mitragynine (kratom) enhances punishment resistance in natural reward seeking and impairs place learning in mice. *Addict. Biol.* **2017**, *22*, 967–976. [CrossRef] [PubMed]

81. Hazim, A.I.; Mustapha, M.; Mansor, S.M. The effects on motor behaviour and short-term memory tasks in mice following an acute administration of *Mitragyna speciosa* alkaloid extract and mitragynine. *J. Med. Plants* **2011**, *5*, 5810–5817.

82. Singh, D.; Narayanan, S.; Müller, C.P.; Vicknasingam, B.; Yücel, M.; Ho, E.T.W.; Hassan, Z.; Mahsufi Mansor, S. Long-Term Cognitive Effects of Kratom (*Mitragyna speciosa* Korth.) Use. *J. Psychoact. Drugs* **2018**, *51*, 19–27. [CrossRef] [PubMed]

83. Parthasarathy, S.; Bin Azizi, J.; Ramanathan, S.; Ismail, S.; Sasidharan, S.; Mohd, M.I.; Mansor, S.M. Evaluation of antioxidant and antibacterial activities of aqueous, methanolic and alkaloid extracts from *Mitragyna speciosa* (rubiaceae family) leaves. *Molecules* **2009**, *14*, 3964–3974. [CrossRef] [PubMed]

84. Suwanlert, S. A study of kratom eaters in Thailand. *Bull. Narc.* **1975**, *27*, 21–27. [PubMed]

85. Stanciu, C.N.; Gnanasegaram, S.A.; Ahmed, S.; Penders, T. Kratom Withdrawal: A Systematic Review with Case Series. *J. Psychoact. Drugs* **2019**, *51*, 12–18. [CrossRef] [PubMed]

86. Smid, M.C.; Charles, J.E.; Gordon, A.J.; Wright, T.E. Use of Kratom, an Opioid-like Traditional Herb, in Pregnancy. *Obstet. Gynecol.* **2018**, *132*, 926–928. [CrossRef] [PubMed]

87. Davidson, L.; Rawat, M.; Stojanovski, S.; Chandrasekharan, P. Natural Drugs, Not So Natural Effects: Neonatal Abstinence Syndrome Secondary to 'Kratom'. *J. Neonatal-Perinat. Med.* **2018**, 1–4. [CrossRef] [PubMed]

88. Swogger, M.T.; Walsh, Z. Kratom use and mental health: A systematic review. *Drug Alcohol Depend.* **2018**, *183*, 134–140. [CrossRef] [PubMed]

89. Azizi, J.; Ismail, S.; Mordi, M.N.; Ramanathan, S.; Said, M.I.M.; Mansor, S.M. In vitro and in vivo effects of three different *Mitragyna speciosa* korth leaf extracts on phase II drug metabolizing enzymes-glutathione transferases (GSTs). *Molecules* **2010**, *15*, 432–441. [CrossRef] [PubMed]

90. Harizal, S.N.; Mansor, S.M.; Hasnan, J.; Tharakan, J.K.J.; Abdullah, J. Acute toxicity study of the standardized methanolic extract of *Mitragyna speciosa* Korth in Rodent. *J. Ethnopharmacol.* **2010**, *131*, 404–409. [CrossRef] [PubMed]

91. Ilmie, M.U.; Jaafar, H.; Mansor, S.M.; Abdullah, J.M. Subchronic toxicity study of standardized methanolic extract of *Mitragyna speciosa* Korth in Sprague-Dawley Rats. *Front. Neurosci.* **2015**, *9*, 1–6. [CrossRef] [PubMed]

92. Saidin, N.A.; Randall, T.; Takayama, H.; Holmes, E.; Gooderham, N. Malaysian Kratom, a phyto-pharmaceutical of abuse: Studies on the mechanism of its cytotoxicity. *Toxicology* **2008**, *253*, 19–20. [CrossRef]

93. Fluyau, D.; Revadigar, N. Biochemical benefits, diagnosis, and clinical risks evaluation of kratom. *Front. Psychiatry* **2017**, *8*, 62. [CrossRef] [PubMed]

94. Rusli, N.; Amanah, A.; Kaur, G.; Adenan, M.I.; Sulaiman, S.F.; Wahab, H.A.; Tan, M.L. The inhibitory effects of mitragynine on P-glycoprotein in vitro. *Naunyn-Schmiedebergs Arch. Pharmacol.* **2019**, 1–16. Available online: https://link.springer.com/article/10.1007%2Fs00210-018-01605-y (accessed on 3 March 2019).

95. Nelsen, J.L.; Lapoint, J.; Hodgman, M.J.; Aldous, K.M. Seizure and Coma Following Kratom (*Mitragynina speciosa* Korth) Exposure. *J. Med. Toxicol.* **2010**, *6*, 424–426. [CrossRef] [PubMed]

96. Kronstrand, R.; Roman, M.; Thelander, G.; Eriksson, A. Unintentional Fatal Intoxications with Mitragynine and O-Desmethyltramadol from the Herbal Blend Krypton. *J. Anal. Toxicol.* **2011**, *35*, 242–247. [CrossRef] [PubMed]

97. Hypothyroidism, S.P.; Sheleg, S.V.; Collins, G.B. A Coincidence of Addiction to "kratom" and Severe Primary Hypothyroidism. *Am. Soc. Addict. Med.* **2011**, *5*, 300–301.

98. Kapp, F.G.; Maurer, H.H.; Auwärter, V.; Winkelmann, M. Hermanns-Clausen, M. Intrahepatic Cholestasis Following Abuse of Powdered Kratom (*Mitragyna speciosa*). *J. Med. Toxicol.* **2011**, *7*, 227–231. [CrossRef] [PubMed]

99. McWhirter, L.; Morris, S. A case report of inpatient detoxification after kratom (*Mitragyna speciosa*) dependence. *Eur. Addict. Res.* **2010**, *16*, 229–231. [CrossRef] [PubMed]

100. Domingo, O.; Roider, G.; Stöver, A.; Graw, M.; Musshoff, F.; Sachs, H.; Bicker, W. Mitragynine concentrations in two fatalities. *Forensic Sci. Int.* **2017**, *271*, e1–e7. [CrossRef] [PubMed]

101. Singh, D.; Narayanan, S.; Vicknasingam, B.; Corazza, O.; Santacroce, R.; Roman-Urrestarazu, A. Changing trends in the use of kratom (*Mitragyna speciosa*) in Southeast Asia. *Hum. Psychopharmacol. Clin. Exp.* **2017**, *32*, e2582. [CrossRef] [PubMed]

102. Singh, D.; Narayanan, S.; Müller, C.P.; Swogger, M.T.; Chear, N.J.Y.; Bin Dzulkapli, E.; Yusoff, N.S.M.; Ramachandram, D.S.; León, F.; McCurdy, C.R.; et al. Motives for using Kratom (*Mitragyna speciosa* Korth.) among regular users in Malaysia. *J. Ethnopharmacol.* **2019**, *233*, 34–40. [CrossRef] [PubMed]

103. Food and Drug Administration Statement from FDA Commissioner Scott Gottlieb, M.D., on the Agency's Scientific Evidence on the Presence of Opioid Compounds in Kratom, Underscoring Its Potential for Abuse. Available online: https://www.fda.gov/newsevents/newsroom/pressannouncements/ucm595622.htm (accessed on 18 January 2019).

104. Kikura-Hanajiri, R. Detection of mitragyne and its analogs. In *Kratom and Other Mitragynines: The Chemistry and Pharmacology of Opioids from a Non-Opium Source*; Raffa, R.B., Ed.; CRC Press: Boca Raton, FL, USA, 2014; pp. 153–166.

105. Wang, M.; Carrell, E.J.; Ali, Z.; Avula, B.; Avonto, C.; Parcher, J.F.; Khan, I.A. Comparison of three chromatographic techniques for the detection of mitragynine and other indole and oxindole alkaloids in *Mitragyna speciosa* (kratom) plants. *J. Sep. Sci.* **2014**, *37*, 1411–1418. [CrossRef] [PubMed]

106. Kowalczuk, A.; Losak, A.; Zjawiony, A.L. Comprehensive methodology for identification of Kratom in police laboratories. *Forensic Sci. Int.* **2013**, *233*, 238–243. [CrossRef] [PubMed]

107. Parthasarathy, S.; Ramanathan, S.; Murugaiyah, V. A simple HPLC-DAD method for the detection and quantification of psychotropic mitragynine in *Mitragyna speciosa* (ketum) and its products for the application in forensic investigation. *Forensic Sci. Int.* **2013**, *226*, 183–187. [CrossRef] [PubMed]

108. Fuenffinger, N.; Ritchie, M.; Ruth, A.; Gryniewicz-ruzicka, C. Evaluation of ion mobility spectrometry for the detection of mitragynine in kratom products. *J. Pharm. Biomed. Anal.* **2017**, *134*, 282–286. [CrossRef] [PubMed]

109. Limsuwanchote, S.; Wungsintaweekul, J.; Keawpradub, N.; Putalun, W.; Morimoto, S.; Tanaka, H. Development of indirect competitive ELISA for quantification of mitragynine in Kratom (*Mitragyna speciosa* (Roxb.) Korth.). *Forensic Sci. Int.* **2015**, *244*, 70–77. [CrossRef] [PubMed]

110. Philipp, A.A.; Meyer, M.R.; Wissenbach, D.K.; Weber, A.A.; Zoerntlein, S.W.; Zweipfenning, P.G.M.; Maurer, H.H. Monitoring of kratom or Krypton intake in urine using GC-MS in clinical and forensic toxicology. *Anal. Bioanal. Chem.* **2011**, *400*, 127–135. [CrossRef] [PubMed]

111. Mudge, E.M.; Brown, P.N. Determination of mitragynine in *Mitragyna speciosa* raw materials and finished products by liquid chromatography with UV detection: Single-laboratory validation. *J. AOAC Int.* **2017**, *100*, 18–24. [CrossRef] [PubMed]

112. Orio, L.; Alexandru, L.; Cravotto, G.; Mantegna, S.; Barge, A. UAE, MAE, SFE-CO$_2$ and classical methods for the extraction of *Mitragyna speciosa* leaves. *Ultrason. Sonochem.* **2012**, *19*, 591–595. [CrossRef] [PubMed]

113. Le, D.; Goggin, M.M.; Janis, G.C. Analysis of Mitragynine and Metabolites in Human Urine for Detecting the Use of the Psychoactive Plant Kratom. *J. Anal. Toxicol.* **2012**, *36*, 616–625. [CrossRef] [PubMed]

114. Philipp, A.A.; Wissenbach, D.K.; Zoerntlein, S.W.; Klein, O.N.; Kanogsunthornrat, J.; Maurer, H.H. Studies on the metabolism of mitragynine, the main alkaloid of the herbal drug Kratom, in rat and human urine using liquid chromatography-linear ion trap mass spectrometry. *J. Mass Spectrom.* **2009**, *44*, 1249–1261. [CrossRef] [PubMed]

115. Guddat, S.; Görgens, C.; Steinhart, V.; Schänzer, W.; Thevis, M. Mitragynine (Kratom)—Monitoring in sports drug testing. *Drug Test. Anal.* **2016**, *8*, 1114–1118. [CrossRef] [PubMed]

116. Holler, J.M.; Vorce, S.P.; McDonough-Bender, P.C.; Magluilo, J.; Solomon, C.J.; Levine, B. A drug toxicity death involving propylhexedrine and mitragynine. *J. Anal. Toxicol.* **2011**, *35*, 54–59. [CrossRef] [PubMed]

117. Lu, S.; Tran, B.N.; Nelsen, J.L.; Aldous, K.M. Quantitative analysis of mitragynine in human urine by high performance liquid chromatography-tandem mass spectrometry. *J. Chromatogr. B Anal. Technol. Biomed. Life Sci.* **2009**, *877*, 2499–2505. [CrossRef] [PubMed]

118. Prutipanlai, S.; Botpiboon, O.; Janchawee, B.; Theanchaiwattana, S. Solid phase extraction method for determination of mitragynine in urine and its application to mitragynine excretion study in rats receiving caffeine. *Trop. J. Pharm. Res.* **2017**, *16*, 1675. [CrossRef]

119. Neng, N.R.; Ahmad, S.M.; Gaspar, H.; Nogueira, J.M.F. Determination of mitragynine in urine matrices by bar adsorptive microextraction and HPLC analysis. *Talanta* **2015**, *144*, 105–109. [CrossRef] [PubMed]

120. Basiliere, S.; Bryand, K.; Kerrigan, S. Identification of five Mitragyna alkaloids in urine using liquid chromatography-quadrupole/time of flight mass spectrometry. *J. Chromatogr. B* **2018**, *1080*, 11–19. [CrossRef] [PubMed]

121. Janchawee, B.; Keawpradub, N.; Chittrakarn, S.; Prasettho, S.; Wararatananurak, P.; Sawangjareon, K. A high-performance liquid chromatographic method for determination of mitragynine in serum and its application to a pharmacokinetic study in rats. *Biomed. Chromatogr.* **2007**, *183*, 176–183. [CrossRef] [PubMed]

122. Chittrakarn, S.; Penjamras, P.; Keawpradub, N. Quantitative analysis of mitragynine, codeine, caffeine, chlorpheniramine and phenylephrine in a kratom (*Mitragyna speciosa* Korth.) cocktail using high-performance liquid chromatography. *Forensic Sci. Int.* **2012**, *217*, 81–86. [CrossRef] [PubMed]

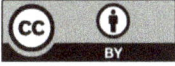

MDPI

Review

The Current Status of the Pharmaceutical Potential of *Juniperus* L. Metabolites

Wilson R. Tavares [1] and Ana M. L. Seca [2,3,*]

1 Faculty of Sciences and Technology, University of Azores, 9501-801 Ponta Delgada, Portugal; wrt-94@hotmail.com
2 Department of Chemistry & QOPNA-Organic Chemistry, Natural Products and Food Stuffs, University of Aveiro, Campus de Santiago, 3810-193 Aveiro, Portugal
3 cE3c—Centre for Ecology, Evolution and Environmental Changes/Azorean Biodiversity Group & Faculty of Sciences and Technology, University of Azores, Rua Mãe de Deus, 9501-321 Ponta Delgada, Portugal
* Correspondence: ana.ml.seca@uac.pt; Tel.: +351-296-650-172

Received: 4 July 2018; Accepted: 20 July 2018; Published: 31 July 2018

Abstract: Background: Plants and their derived natural compounds possess various biological and therapeutic properties, which turns them into an increasing topic of interest and research. *Juniperus* genus is diverse in species, with several traditional medicines reported, and rich in natural compounds with potential for development of new drugs. **Methods:** The research for this review were based in the Scopus and Web of Science databases using terms combining *Juniperus*, secondary metabolites names, and biological activities. This is not an exhaustive review of *Juniperus* compounds with biological activities, but rather a critical selection taking into account the following criteria: (i) studies involving the most recent methodologies for quantitative evaluation of biological activities; and (ii) the compounds with the highest number of studies published in the last four years. **Results:** From *Juniperus* species, several diterpenes, flavonoids, and one lignan were emphasized taking into account their level of activity against several targets. Antitumor activity is by far the most studied, being followed by antibacterial and antiviral activities. Deoxypodophyllotoxin and one dehydroabietic acid derivative appears to be the most promising lead compounds. **Conclusions:** This review demonstrates the *Juniperus* species value as a source of secondary metabolites with relevant pharmaceutical potential.

Keywords: *Juniperus*; secondary metabolites; diterpenes; flavonoids; lignans; cytotoxic; antitumor; antibacterial; amentoflavone; deoxypodophyllotoxin

---

1. Introduction

Plants have been used by humans since the start of mankind thousands of years ago as construction material [1], clothing [2], and obviously, as food and drugs [3]. Although scientific knowledge has permitted the development of medicine to today's standards based on herbal and traditional medicines, the oldest form of medicine known to man, they are still used around the world [4]. The use of plants themselves, their derived natural compounds and their biological and therapeutic properties have become a topic of increasing interest and investigation not only in modern medicine and pharmacology [5], but also in food and cosmetics industries [6].

Juniperus species are a good bet in the development of new drugs with natural compounds, since it is a diverse genus (75 species of *Juniperus* [7]) with several traditional medicinal applications reported. For example, *Juniperus excelsa* M.Bieb. is used to treat abdominal spasm, asthma, diarrhea, fever, gonorrhea, headache, and is also useful as antihypertensive, diuretic, carminative, appetizer, anticonvulsant, and flavoring agent [8]. In Turkey, powdered *Juniperus oxycedrus* subsp. *oxycedrus* L. berries are consumed to lower blood glucose levels [9], while in Mexico, *Juniperus communis* L. is used to treat respiratory problems, gastrointestinal infections, cardiovascular and/or blood disorders, and as astringent [10]. Use of *J. communis* also covers the treatment of urinary problems, migraines, diabetes, gonorrhea, and skin irritations [11].

The extracts and secondary metabolites from *Juniperus* species exhibit also interesting bioactivities [12,13], especially the *Juniperus oxycedrus* L. and *J. communis*, two of the most studied species in terms of their phytochemistry, pharmacological, and therapeutic effects [14,15]. It can be highlighted that extracts and compounds from both plants exhibit antimicrobial, antioxidant, antidiabetic, anti-inflammatory, anticonvulsant, analgesic, and cytotoxic activities [14,15], and additionally *J. communis* also possess antifertility, hepatoprotective, diuretic, neuroprotective, antiparasitic, and anti-ulcer properties [14].

Some of the most relevant studies published in recent years on the bioactivities of *Juniperus* extracts show clearly that *Juniperus* continues to be a hot spot in research on natural products as well as contribute to further highlight the pharmacological potential of this genus and of its chemical constituents. For example, Jung et al. [16] reports the butyrylcholinesterase (BChE) inhibitory activity of the compound valenc-1(10), 3(4), 11(12)-trien-2-one isolated from *Juniperus chinensis* L. with an IC_{50} value of 68.45 µM (IC_{50} = 18.75 µM for berberine). In Lee and colleagues work [17], *Juniperus rigida* Siebold & Zucc. fruit ethanol extract was showed to possess anti-atopic properties in in vivo oxazolone- and 2,4-dinitrochlorobenzene(DNCB), and induced atopic dermatitis in mice models. It was suggested that the therapeutic effect verified by this extract occurs by decreasing the overproduction of interleukin 4 (IL-4) and immunoglobulin E (IgE) and accelerating skin barrier recovery function. Groshi et al. [18] assessed the cytotoxicity of the polar extract (methanol), and non-polar extracts (dichloromethane and *n*-hexane) of *Juniperus phoenicea* L. leaves against four human cancer cell lines concluding that the dichloromethane extract was the most cytotoxic extract against the lung carcinoma cell line A549 (IC_{50} = 13 µg/mL), while *n*-hexane extract exhibits the broadest spectrum of activity with IC_{50} values of 10, 14, 16, and 40 µg/mL against hepatocellular carcinoma cell line HepG2, human breast cancer cell line MCF-7, human lung carcinoma A549, and human bladder carcinoma cell line EJ138, respectively. On the other hand, imbricataloic acid isolated from *Juniperus phoenicea* var. *turbinata* (Guss.) Parl. (syn. *Juniperus turbinata* Guss.) ethanol extract showed the strongest cytotoxic activity (IC_{50} values of 0.06, 0.114, and 0.201 µM on human colon cancer HCT116, human malignant melanoma A375, and human breast adenocarcinoma MDA-MB-231 cell lines, respectively), being several times more potent than the reference compound cisplatin (IC_{50} values of 1.87 to 11.86 µM) [19] indicating that imbricataloic acid make a promising anticancer drug candidate.

The essential oil of *Juniperus* species are also a research target once they exhibit a great diversity of bioactivities. For example, the essential oil of *J. phoenicea* var. *turbinata* (syn. *Juniperus turbinata* Guss.) exhibits cytotoxic effects against HCT116, A375, and MDA-MB-231 human tumor cell lines, in a concentration-dependent inhibitory effect with IC_{50} values of 9.48–33.69 µg/mL [19]. *Juniperus oxycedrus* essential oil exhibited high antitrypanosomal activity (IC_{50} of 0.9 µg/mL) against *Trypanosoma brucei brucei*, with no cytotoxic effects on RAW 267.4 macrophage cell line showing the highest selectivity index (63.4) [20]. The authors of this study suggest that α-pinene would likely be the responsible for the *J. oxycedrus* essential oil antitrypanosomal properties. In another work using male mice [21], *Juniperus virginiana* L. essential oil at 400 and 800 mg/kg showed anxiolytic effect, although it failed to inhibit the anxiety-related behavior by light-dark box.

The interest of the *Juniperus* species is also at the nutritional/functional food level and some studies, including in vivo studies on this subject, have recently been published. Inci and colleagues [22] found that low supplementation levels of *J. communis* berry (0.5% and 1%) in Japanese quails (*Coturnix coturnix japonica*) diets have positive impacts on some body qualities, feed intake, and live weight. *Juniperus* species are also valuable in terms of their wood since it is a viable construction material classified as durable or even very durable, like *J. communis* case [23]. In this context, Ateş et al. [24] suggest that *Juniperus foetidissima* Willd. could be aimed for new natural wood preservatives development since its methanol extract reported antifungal activity against *Pleurotus ostreatus* with an IC_{50} value of 0.30 μg/μL.

Besides all the bioactive activities and other benefit effects of *Juniperus* species mentioned above, it should be noticed that toxicity side effects were found in *Juniperus* species such as the spoonful ingestion of *J. oxycedrus* extract of branches can cause poisoning, leading to fever, hepatotoxicity, renal failure, severe hypotension, and severe cutaneous burns on the face [25]. Adverse effects were also mentioned by Prinsloo and colleagues [3] to *Juniperus sabina* L. that contains thujone, a neurotoxic compound, and to *Juniperus scopulorum* Sarg., which contains safrole, a liver carcinogen substance [3].

Taking into account the abovementioned bioactivities of some *Juniperus* species, their importance as a source of novel natural compounds is well cleared. The increased interest and investigation of these species lead to new discoveries of interesting and promising metabolites. *Juniperus* L. metabolites pharmaceutical potential has been previously well reviewed in 2006 [12] and in 2015 [13], thus this work aims to update the information relative to the recently published studies involving *Juniperus* species secondary metabolites. It is important to highlight that this is not an exhaustive review of all the studies regarding compounds with biological activities form *Juniperus* species, but rather a selection taking into account the compounds whose biological activity and mechanism of action show that they are compounds with high pharmacological potential.

2. Bioactive Secondary Metabolites from *Juniperus* Species

2.1. Terpenoids

2.1.1. Dehydroabietic Acid

The dehydroabietic acid (1) (Figure 1) has a lipophilic abietan-8,11,13-trien structure with only one polar substituent, the equatorial carboxylic group at C-4. This acid is widely distributed in nature, being present in *J. oxycedrus*, *J. phoenicea*, and *Juniperus brevifolia* (Seub.) Antoine [12,13]. This compound has been considered as an interesting starting material for the synthesis of new compounds which means, an excellent leader compound, with important biological properties, having at least two hundred dehydroabietane derivatives described in literature [26]. Dehydroabietic acid (1) and its derivatives display not only antiviral [27] and antitumor [28,29] effects, but also gastroprotective [30], antimicrobial [31], and anti-inflammatory [32] properties.

More recently, new interesting dehydroabietic acid derivatives were studied. Hou and colleagues [33] accessed the in vitro antiproliferative activity of various dehydroabietic acid derivatives possessing a 1,2,3-triazole-tethered nucleus at C-14, against four different human cancer cell lines, showing that the majority of the newly synthesized derivatives displayed effective antiproliferative activities, being the presence of 1,2,3-triazole moiety substituted on C-4 crucial to the high cytotoxic activity. The dehydroabietic acid methyl ester derivative (1a) (Figure 1), with the substituent (2-(4-(3-(*tert*-butoxycarbonylamino)phenyl)-1*H*-1,2,3-triazol-1-yl)acetamido) at C-14, was the most potent derivative tested, exhibiting better IC_{50} values (i.e., 0.7 to 1.2 μM) against the tested cells lines (PC-3, SK-OV-3, MDA-MB-231 and MCF-7 human cell lines) than the clinical anticancer drug fluorouracil (5-Fu) (5.2 to 24.5 μM IC_{50} values). Moreover, it also demonstrated weak cytotoxicity against HL-7702 and HFF-1 normal cells. These results imply that, with proper structure modifications, these types of derivatives could be aimed for development into a new anticancer natural product-like.

In a very recent work [34], the antibacterial activity of various N-sulfonaminoethyloxime derivatives of dehydroabietic acid was assessed against *Staphylococcus aureus* Newman strain and multidrug-resistant *Staphylococcus aureus* strains (NRS-1, NRS-70, NRS-100, NRS-108, and NRS-271). The results showed that these dehydroabietic acid derivatives showed great antibacterial effect with minimum inhibitory concentration (MIC) values ranging from 0.78 to 1.56 μg/mL against the strains tested. With a MIC of 0.39 to 0.78 μg/mL (MIC = 0.63–1.2 μM) against *Staphylococcus aureus* Newman, the meta-CF$_3$ phenyl derivative (1b) (Figure 1) showed the highest antibacterial activity, similar to the positive-control compound vancomycin, that had a MIC of 0.78 to 1.56 µg/mL (MIC = 0.54–1.1 µM) against the same bacteria strain.

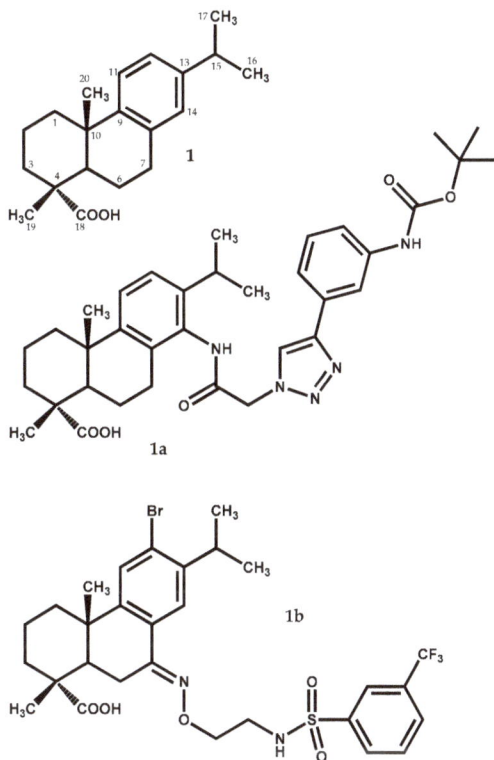

Figure 1. Dehydroabietic acid (**1**) identified in *Juniperus* species and its derivatives (**1a** and **1b**) with significant cytotoxic and antibacterial activities.

2.1.2. Ferruginol

Ferruginol (**2**) (Figure 2) is, like dehydroabietic acid, a tricyclic diterpene with an aromatic ring but without the C-18 carboxylic acid and with a hydroxyl group at C-12. It is widely distributed in *Juniperus* genus [13,35], being particularly abundant in hexane extract of *J. excelsa* berries (32.9% of all the detected compounds) [36]. Several previous reports showed that this compound exhibits a great diversity of bioactivities such as anti-acaricide, antiplasmodial, nematicidal, antibacterial, antileishmanial, antiviral, antifungal, and antitumoral [26,36–41].

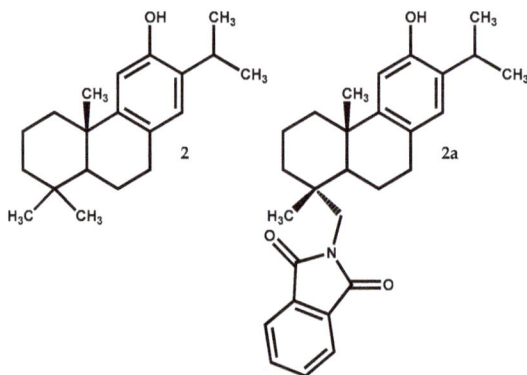

Figure 2. Ferruginol (**2**) from *Juniperus* species and the most active antiviral derivative (**2a**).

A recent study [42] showed that ferruginol (2) has antitumor activity, presenting inhibitory effects on HepG2 (IC_{50} = 11.4 ± 2.9 µg/mL, 39.8 µM) and Hep3B (IC_{50} = 19.4 ± 4.3 µg/mL, 67.7 µM) cell lines, without affecting the normal hepatocyte line L-02 viability (IC_{50} > 100 µg/mL, 349 µM). However, we would like to point out that the results previously mentioned have a standard deviation of around 20% of the value of the mean, which impairs the scientific impact of the results. Since ferruginol (2) exhibited the highest activity against Hep3B and HepG2 cell lines, the authors also assessed the mechanisms of apoptosis caused by compound (2). The results indicated that ferruginol (2) downregulated the expression levels of anti-apoptotic protein Bcl-2 (related to mitochondrial apoptosis pathway) and upregulated pro-apoptotic proteins Bcl-2-associated X (Bax), caspase-3, and caspase-9 [42].

Increased production, accumulation, and aggregation of the neurotoxic peptide amyloid-β (Aβ) within the brain triggers severe molecular changes affecting many signaling pathways associated with neuronal metabolism, signaling, and neuronal communication, leading to spatial memory loss and learning impairment associated with Alzheimer's disease [43]. Amyloid β oligomers induce an imbalance in the calcium signaling kinases (vital for maintaining the integrity and functionality of synapses), which leads to progressive impairment of the synaptic connections, altering the capacity for hippocampal long-term potentiation (LTP) resulting in neuronal apoptosis [44]. A recent study by Zolezzi and colleagues [45] found that ferruginol (2) might have a potential neuroprotective role in neurodegenerative alterations. Their study reports that 10 µM of ferruginol induce an increase in calcium intracellular levels in hippocampal neurons from mice and promote neuroprotection against apoptosis, synaptic protein loss, and LTP inhibition triggered by amyloid β oligomers. The capacity of ferruginol to induce an increase in calcium was correlated with an increase in Ca^{2+}/calmodulin-dependent protein kinase II (CaMKII) and in the active form of protein kinase C (PKC) in hippocampal slices, indicating that the changes in the LTP process and the calcium levels may be intermediated by the activation of calcium-dependent mechanisms involving PKC and CaMKII [46].

Furthermore, ferruginol (2) is the starting material for the synthesis of several compounds with high activity level and less secondary effects. In the work by Roa-Linares and colleagues [47], ferruginol and two analogues, showed relevant antiviral activity against Dengue Virus type 2, human Herpesvirus type 1, and human Herpesvirus type 2. The ferruginol derivative with a phthalimide moiety at C-18 (2a) (Figure 2), was ten times better (EC_{50} = 1.4 µM) than the reference ribavirin (EC_{50} = 13.5 µM) against Dengue Virus type 2 in a post-infection treatment and with a selectivity index value of 57.7, which indicates that this compound presents great potential as a therapeutic agent and should be aimed for further biopharmaceutical and pre-clinical studies [47].

2.1.3. Hinokiol

Hinokiol (3) (Figure 3) is a 3β,12-dihydroxy-abieta-8,11,13-trien present in *Juniperus* species, e.g., *J. brevifolia, J. chinensis, J. excelsa, J. phoenicea, Juniperus procera* Hochst. ex Endl. *Juniperus przewalskii* Kom. and *Juniperus squamata* Buch.-Ham. ex D.Don [12,13], with interest for the scientific community due to its pharmacological potential, since this compound has been reported to inhibit the generation of nitric oxide (NO) and TNF-α, as well as the production of pro-inflammatory enzymes from lipopolysaccharide-stimulated RAW macrophages [48,49]. Antioxidant [50] and hepatoprotective [51] effects have also been reported for hinokiol, as well as antitumor properties against human ovarian carcinoma (HO-8910) and cervical carcinoma (HeLa) cell lines [52].

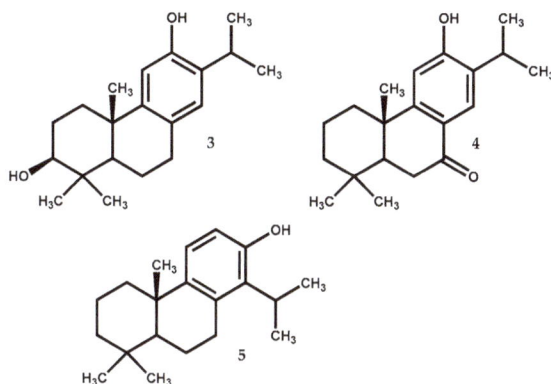

Figure 3. Diterpenes (**3–5**) from *Juniperus* species with significant pharmacological potential.

In a more recent study, Wang and colleagues [53] reported the inhibition of voltage-gated Na^+ channels (VGSCs) by hinokiol at 30 μM, in rat hippocampal CA1 neurons, differentiated NG108-15 cells and neuroblastoma N2A cells; VGSCs are crucial in the excitability of neurons since they permit the influx of Na^+ during the upstroke phase of action potential, which ensures the quality of rapid signal transmission in the nervous system [53]. The VGSC inhibition by hinokiol presented in this work could be interpreted as an anti-anxiety, anaesthetic or anticonvulsant activity, but further research is necessary to clarify this topic and to hypothesize about future pharmacological applications.

2.1.4. Sugiol

Sugiol (4) (Figure 3), 12-hydroxy-abieta-8,11,13-triene-7-one is widely distributed in the Cupressaceae family, being found in *J. brevifolia, J. chinensis, J. communis, Juniperus polycarpos* K.Koch, *J. procera, Juniperus rigida* var. *conferta* (Parl.) Patschke (syn. *J. conferta* Parl.) and *Juniperus formosana* Hayata [12,13,16,54,55]. Sugiol presents hepatoprotective [51] and antioxidant properties [56].

Bajpai and Kang [57] evaluated sugiol for tyrosinase and α-glucosidase inhibitory activity in vitro, in terms of its antimelanogenesis and antidiabetic potential, respectively. The results showed that sugiol at the concentration range of 0.100 to 10 mg/mL presented efficacy on inhibiting α-glucosidase (12.34 to 63.47% of inhibition) similar to acarbose (19.2 to 65.5% of inhibition at same concentration range), while at concentration 0.020 to 0.50 mg/mL, sugiol inhibits 28.2 to 67.4% of tyrosinase activity, only a little less active than kojic acid used as reference (32.4 to 76.5% inhibition at the same concentration range).

The Bajpai research group [58] reports also the potential of sugiol as antiviral once it inhibits the growth of H_1N_1 influenza virus in a cytopathogenic reduction assay using Madin-Darby canine kidney (MDCK) cell line. Severe cytopathic effect occurred in MDCK cells exposed to H_1N_1 influenza virus but in MDCK cells treated with sugiol (500 μg/mL) along with H_1N_1 influenza virus, cytopathic effect was absent. In fact, MDCK cells treated with sugiol showed similar morphology to control MDCK cells that were not exposed to H_1N_1 influenza virus.

Jung et al. [59] showed that sugiol may be useful against human solid tumors as an inhibitor of transketolase (TKT) and of the signal transducer and activator of transcription 3 (STAT3). In fact, the TKT reaction plays a crucial role in the pentose phosphate pathway, and its inhibition interrupts the production of FAD, NAD(P)$^+$, CoA, and ATP, as well as the synthesis of DNA and RNA in cancer cells [60], while STAT3 inhibition plays an important role in the induction of cancer cells apoptosis [61]. In the work by Jung et al. [59], STAT3 activation was 40% inhibited by 20 µM of sugiol in DU145 prostate cancer cells, limiting their proliferation through cell cycle arrest at the G1/S checkpoint. The mechanism of inhibition proposed indicates that inhibition of TKT by sugiol imply ROS-mediated ERK activation and ERK activated phosphorylates STAT3 on Ser727 and recruits a protein tyrosine phosphatase MEG2, which dephosphorylates STAT3 on Tyr705 leading to the inhibition of STAT3 [59].

A very recent study [62] showed that sugiol reduced the cell viability of human pancreatic cancer cells (Mia-PaCa2) in a concentration-dependent manner being the IC_{50} value of 15 µM. The cytotoxic activity of sugiol was found to be caused by reactive oxygen species (ROS)-mediated alterations in mitochondrial membrane potential (MMP), in conjunction with an upregulation of Bax expression (an inducer of apoptosis) and a downregulation of Bcl-2 expression (an antiapoptotic protein). Additionally, the study indicates that sugiol also caused cell cycle arrest in G2/M phase of the cell cycle, ultimately leading to apoptosis. Furthermore, sugiol also inhibited the migratory capacity of Mia-PaCa2 cells at 15 µM concentration. This study suggests that sugiol is a very good candidate to in vivo evaluation against pancreatic cancer. Unfortunately, the authors of this study have not evaluated the compounds cytotoxicity towards a non-tumor cell line under the same conditions and did not use an approved clinical drug as positive control. If they had, they would have increased the impact of their work and its contribution to the field.

2.1.5. Totarol

The compound totarol (5) (Figure 3) is a tricyclic phenolic diterpene with a totarane skeleton. It is found in several *Juniperus* species such as *J. brevifolia*, *J. chinensis*, *J. communis*, *J. conferta*, *J. excelsa*, *J. formosana*, *J. phoenicea*, *J. procera* and *Juniperus drupaceae* Labill. [12,13]. It is the most abundant compound in the hexane extract of *J. brevifolia* bark (11 mg of compound by 100 mg of extract) [54], being also found in species from other genus [63]. This compound seems to be a good bet towards new interesting active drugs development since it displays a range of interesting bioactivities such as antibacterial [64–66], antimycobacterial [38], antileishmanial [36], antimalarial [67,68], antistaphylococcal activity caused by efflux inhibitory properties [69], as well as nematicidal activity and antifouling attributes [36]. Furthermore, totarol could also be used as activity enhancer of some conventional drugs [70].

A promising antimicrobial target is the bacterial cell division machinery and totarol (5), by perturbing the cell division, has the capacity to restrain bacterial growth [71]. A recent study [72] focused on the molecular targets and mechanism of action of totarol in *Bacillus subtilis*. Their quantitative proteome analysis showed that diterpene (5) induced changes in 139 proteins expression levels. The same study also reports that *Bacillus subtilis* major central metabolic dehydrogenases are repressed by totarol (5) at $IC_{50} = 1.5$ µM leading to metabolic shutdown in the bacteria.

Another study [73] reports that totarol (5) has vascular protective effects in vivo, by activating the protein kinase B/heme oxygenase-1 (PKB/HO-1) pathway, further increasing superoxide dismutase (SOD) and antioxidant glutathione (GSH) levels, which leads to ischemia-induced brain injury suppression. An in vitro assay showed totarol as no toxicity on cerebellar granule cells (CGC) at various concentrations (1 to 5 µM), which strengthens its protective properties. In order to simulate the situation of patients with acute stroke, a post-ischemia administration of totarol in rats (1 and 10 µg/kg) was used. The results showed considerable decreases in infarct volume compared with the untreated group. Moreover, totarol treatment (1 and 10 µg/kg) radically enhanced the ischemia-induced neurological deficit. The study also reported notably infarct volume reduction with 10 µg/kg of totarol administration.

2.2. Flavonoids

2.2.1. Amentoflavone

Amentoflavone (6) (Figure 4), is a flavonoid dimer composed by two apigenin units linked by a carbon-carbon bond between C-8 and C-3′, belonging to the biflavonoid family of compounds and is found in several *Juniperus* species, like: *J. oxycedrus*, *J. phoenicea*, *J. rigida*, *J. virginiana*, *J. chinensis*, *J. communis*, *J. drupacea*, *J. foetidissima*, *Juniperus bermudiana* L., *Juniperus indica* Bertol., mboxemphJuniperus macrocarpa Sm., and *Juniperus occidentalis* Hook. [12,13,74].

Amentoflavone (6) possesses a wide variety of bioactivities, such as antiphotoaging [75], antifungal [76], antimicrobial [77], antioxidant [78], anti-inflammatory [79], antidiabetic [80], antipsoriasis [81], diuretic [82] and antitumor [83,84], as well as neuroprotective [85] and osteogenesis effects [86], and it confers cardiovascular injury protection [87]. Although all these bioactivities are well reviewed with great detail by Yu et al. [74] there are still some studies that are worth mentioning that were not included in the review.

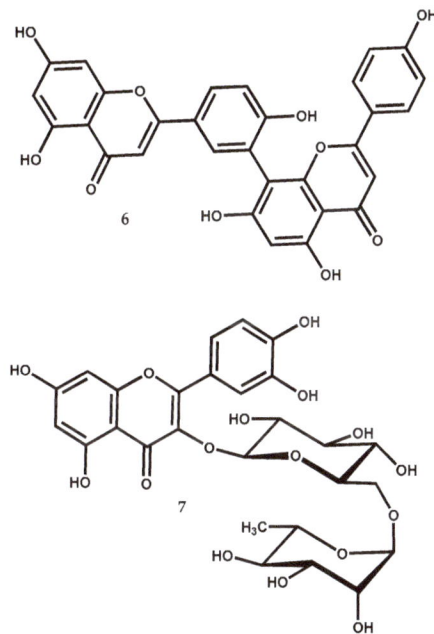

Figure 4. The bioactive flavonoids amentoflavone (**6**) and rutin (**7**) from *Juniperus* species.

Inhibition of prostaglandin D2 (PGD2) has been found as a pharmacological mechanism for the treatment of androgenic alopecia (i.e., pattern hair loss) [88]. A study [89] found that amentoflavone (6) might inhibit PGD2 synthesis and that it has acceptable skin permeability as well as not being irritating or corrosive to skin, suggesting that amentoflavone (6) can be used to develop safe and high-efficacy hair loss treatment.

Estrogens have a crucial role in the initiation and the progression of breast cancers. Aromatase catalyses the rate-limiting step in endogen/estrogen synthesis and its activity is stated to be higher in breast cancer [90]. Tascioglu et al. [91] showed that amentoflavone (6) could act as an aromatase inhibitor being determined the IC_{50} value as 93.6 µM in an in vitro assay.

In a very interesting study [92], the protective effect of amentoflavone (6) against Freund's adjuvant induced arthritis in rats was evaluated. The findings show that treatment with 20 mg/kg and 40 mg/kg doses of amentoflavone (6) has suitable anti-arthritic properties since it demonstrates to positively control inflammation in the adjuvant induced arthritic rat model. Protective effects were also reported in another study [93], where it was demonstrated that amentoflavone (6) protected dopaminergic neurons against MPTP/MPP$^+$-induced neurotoxicity. This neuroprotective activity may have its clinical application in the treatment of some central nervous system (CNS) diseases, such as Parkinson's disease and ischemia.

Another study [94] examined the effects of amentoflavone in human ovarian cancer cell lines OVCAR-3 and SK-OV-3. The results showed that this biflavonoid (6) could considerably suppress cell propagation, block cell cycle progression at the G1/G0 phase and induce cell apoptosis. In both cell lines, amentoflavone (6) displayed dose- and time-dependent inhibition. In SK-OV-3 cells assay, after 48 h of treatment with compound (6) at 20 and 50 µM the cell viability decrease 15% and 20%, respectively, while with incubation time extended to 72 h, the decrease cell viability was 19% and 31% for the respective doses. In OVCAR-3 cells, the results were similar. Also, apoptotic cell population increased after 48 h and 72 h treatment at 20 µM and 50 µM. Furthermore, the results showed that amentoflavone (6) repressed the expression of S-phase kinase protein 2 (Skp2) through ROS/AMPK/mTOR signaling [94], which contributed to amentoflavone antitumor effect against ovarian cancer.

The amentoflavone (6) inhibitory activity on human aldo-keto reductase family 1 member B10 (AKR1B10), which is a detoxification enzyme involved in drug resistance, was studied [95]. The results showed that compound (6) decrease the growth of A549 human lung cancer cells in vitro and in vivo by potently inhibition of human AKR1B10 activity (IC_{50} = 1.54 µM).

A key transcription factor that responds to oxidative stress is nuclear factor erythroid 2-related factor 2 (Nrf2) and its activation is related with prevention of aging, inflammation and cancer [96]. A recent study [97] found that amentoflavone (6) could trigger Nrf2 activation through ROS-mediated activation of the p38-AKT/PKB pathway in HaCaT keratinocytes.

A dipeptidyl peptidase IV (DPP-IV) inhibitors increase the activation of glucagon-like peptide 1 (GLP-1) and glucose-dependent insulinotropic polypeptide (GIP), leading to the inhibition of secretion of glucagon and enhancement of β-cells functionality [98]. Thus the control of DPP-IV activity is an essential factor in management of type 2 diabetes, and amentoflavone (6), with an IC_{50} value of 3.9 ± 0.5 µM, was recognized as a potential DPP-IV inhibitor [99].

2.2.2. Rutin

Rutin, 3,3',4',5,7-pentahydroxyflavone-3-rhamnoglucoside, and also known as quercetin 3-rutinoside (7) (Figure 4), is a flavonol found in many plants including *Juniperus* species like *J. communis*, *J. excelsa*, *J. foetidissima*, and *J. oxycedrus* [12,100].

Recently, two papers [101,102] have exhaustively reviewed the rutin (7) bioactivities and pharmacological potential. They showed that it possesses multiple pharmacological activities, including antioxidant, hepatoprotective, vasoprotective, anticarcinogenic, neuroprotective, cardioprotective and antidiabetic activities [101,102].

A recent work, not included in the mentioned reviews, reported that rutin can provide cardioprotective effect [103]. In this work, rutin at 50 µM was more effective than the cardioprotective agent dexrazoxane (DZR) at same concentration, in preventing pirarubicin-induced toxicity in rat cardiomyoblasts H9c2. The apoptosis rate of rutin (7) treatment after cells exposed to pirarubicin was nearly 20%, while DZR treatment reported an apoptosis rate of about 30% [103]. The authors propose that the protective effect of rutin (7) is related with its ability to scavenge intracellular ROS and inhibit cell apoptosis by modulating the transforming growth factor (TGF)-β1-p38 MAPK signaling pathway.

An interesting work by Parashar et al. [104] found that rutin (7) (100 mg/kg) could alleviate chronic unpredictable stress (CUS) in mice, acting as an antidepressant. Since CUS impairs locomotors abilities of animals [105], the fact that rutin (7) treated animals were more balanced and active than the untreated ones, indicates a strong stimulatory effect on balancing activity, muscle coordination and locomotion. In addition, animals treated with rutin (7) had intact memory and were capable to identify a previously encountered object, thus spending more time discovering a novel object [104]. Stressed animals treated with rutin (7) presented an intact hippocampus with morphology and cell number similar to control animals that were not subjected to CUS [104].

2.3. Lignans

Deoxypodophyllotoxin

Deoxypodophyllotoxin (DPT) (8) (Figure 5) is an aryltetralin cyclolignan having been isolated from several *Juniperus* species like *J. virginiana, J. rigida, J. sabina, J. squamata, J. procera, J. bermudiana, J. chinensis, J. communis, J. phoenicea, Juniperus procumbens* (Siebold ex Endl.) Miq. *Juniperus recurva* Buch.-Ham. ex D.Don, *Juniperus taxifolia* Hook. & Arn. *Juniperus thurifera* L., and *Juniperus* x *media* V.D. Dmitriev [12,13,106,107].

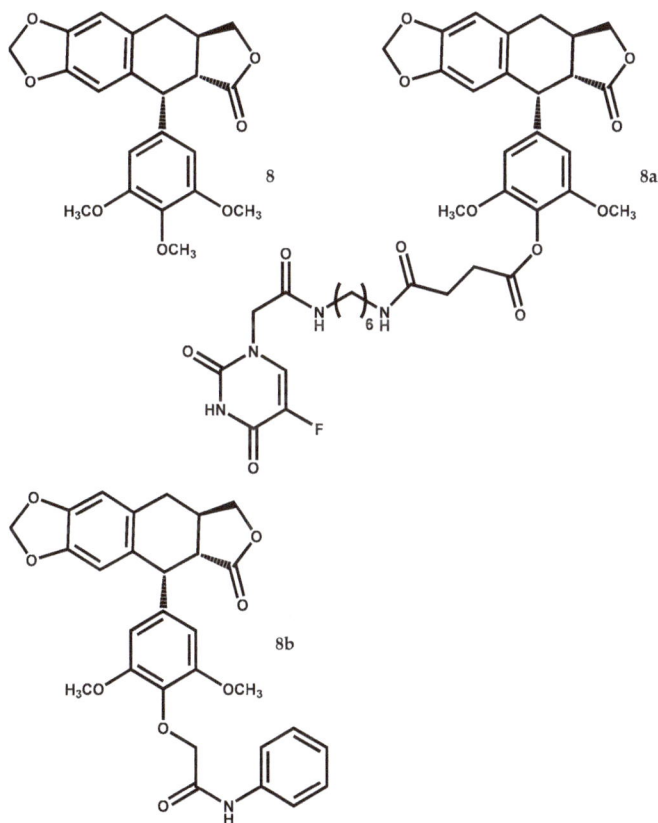

Figure 5. The bioactive lignan deoxypodophyllotoxin (**8**) identified in *Juniperus* species and its cytotoxic derivatives (**8a**) and (**8b**).

The main characteristic of this compound is its great cytotoxic potential as reported in several studies [108–112]. Furthermore, DPT (8) also reported anti-inflammatory [113] and anti-angiogenic [109,111] properties.

A study [114] showed that deoxypodophyllotoxin (8) has a significant cytotoxic activity in vitro since it has inhibited the growth of numerous cancer cell lines (i.e., human glioblastoma-astrocytoma U-87 MG, human glioblastoma SF126, gastric carcinoma SGC-7901, gastric carcinoma BGC-823, ovarian carcinoma HO-8910, human ovarian carcinoma SK-0V-3, human colon carcinoma HT-29, breast carcinoma MDA-MB-231 and human choriocarcinoma JeG-3) with IC_{50} values varying from 13.95 to 26.72 nM, while the clinical anticancer drug etoposide was less efficient ($IC_{50} \geq 73.57$ nM) [114]. Furthermore, the same study [114], also suggests that deoxypodophyllotoxin (8) treatment resulted in a dose- and time-dependent induction of apoptosis via caspase-dependent pathways by decreasing the expression of cyclin-dependent protein kinase 2 (Cdc2), cyclin B1, and cell division cycle 25C protein (Cdc25C), leading to cell cycle arrest in G2/M phase.

A recent study [115] also showed that DPT (8) at 5 nM induced G2/M cell cycle arrest in both human breast cancer cells MCF-7 (MCF-7/S) and their acquired resistant cells (MCF-7/A), while paclitaxel (10 nM) showed no effect on the cell cycle progression of the MCF-7/A cells. Besides that, DPT (8) exhibited antiproliferative activity against the MCF-7/S and MCF-7/A cell lines, with IC_{50} values of 10.61 ± 1.09 nM and 5.86 ± 0.30 nM respectively, with a resistance index (RI) [(IC_{50} of MCF-7/A cell line)/(IC_{50} of MCF-7/S cell line)] of 0.552 [115]. These values were better than the ones obtained by paclitaxel and etoposide [115]. Furthermore, DPT (8) at 12.5 mg/kg, suppressed in vivo the tumor growth in MCF-7/S and in MCF-7/A xenograft mice, exhibiting tumor volume growth inhibition of 49.62% in the MCF-7/S xenografts, approaching the tumor volume growth inhibition of paclitaxel (53.86% at 12.5 mg/kg). In addition, DPT (8) has potential to be a new microtubule inhibitor for breast cancer treatment since its antitubulin polymerization activity showed the absence of the polymerized tubulin, indicating that deoxypodophyllotoxin disrupted microtubule assembly in a different manner than paclitaxel [115]. The results presented by Zang et al. [115] also confirmed that deoxypodophyllotoxin (8) was not a substrate of the P-gp efflux pump and could overcome P-gp-mediated multi-drug resistance, unlike what happens with paclitaxel which is a P-glycoprotein (P-gp) efflux pump substrate [116].

An in vivo study [117] showed the antitumor property of deoxypodophyllotoxin (8) on MDA-MB-231 human breast cancer xenografts in BALB/c nude mice in a concentration-dependent manner. Deoxypodophyllotoxin (8) was combined with hydroxypropyl-β-cyclodextrin (DPT-HP-β-CD) in order to turn it more soluble and facilitate its intravenous administration. The results revealed that DPT (8) exhibited strong inhibitory effect and great antitumor activity, being the treatment with DPT-HP-β-CD (20 mg/kg) in MDA-MB-231 xenograft more efficient than the ones with etoposide (20 mg/kg) and docetaxel (20 mg/kg) [117], two anticancer drugs in clinical therapeutic [118,119]. The authors [117] also point out that, similar to other cancer chemotherapy drugs, DPT-HP-β-CD treatment caused gastrointestinal reactions after intravenous injection, consequential reducing food intake, which led to weight loss in the mice.

An in vitro study from Hu et al. [120] investigated the cytotoxic effect of DPT (8) on human prostate cancer DU-145 cells and its potential action mechanism. The results revealed that DPT (8) induced cell apoptosis and inhibited cell proliferation. Detection of high levels of the caspase-3 expression suggests that caspase-mediated pathways were involved in DPT-induced apoptosis. Moreover, the authors suggest that apoptosis was also induced through downregulation of the levels of phosphorylated Akt and activation of the p53/B-cell lymphoma 2 associated X protein/phosphatase and tensin homolog (i.e., Akt/p53/Bax/PTEN) signaling pathway [120]. Although this work must be emphasized because it exposes a new target involved in the DPT (8) mechanism of action, no control was used nor were IC_{50} values against DU-145 cells line presented, which is a misfortune since it decreases the scientific impact of the study.

Parthanatos is a unique cell-death pathway that is distinctive from necrosis, apoptosis or other recognized forms of cell death. It is a process dependent on the over activation of the nuclear enzyme poly (ADP-ribose) polymerase 1 (PARP-1), causing it to synthesize a massive quantity of PAR polymer until reaching toxic levels, resulting in large-scale chromatin condensation and DNA fragmentation, leading to cell death [121]. A study [122] found that DPT (8) triggered parthanatos in rat C6, human SHG-44 and U87 glioma cell lines via induction of excessive reactive oxygen species (ROS). In addition, alterations of parthanatos-related proteins triggered by DPT (8) occurred in a dose and time dependent manner and involved the induced cytoplasmic accumulation of PAR polymer in SHG-44 and C6 glioma cells as well as the upregulation in the nuclear level of AIF and in the cytoplasmic and nuclear levels of PARP-1 [122].

ROS production plays a crucial role in apoptosis signaling, leading to cancer cell death [123], but it also can trigger autophagy [124]. Since autophagy is a degradation process in intracellular organelles that occurs when cells undergo nutrition deprivation and external stimulus, its activation is essential for preserving intracellular homeostasis and allowing the cell to survive [125]. An interesting study [126], demonstrated that deoxypodophyllotoxin (8) induces both autophagy and apoptosis in osteosarcoma U2OS cells, through modification of mitochondrial membrane potential (MMP), which is related with generation of ROS. Furthermore, DPT (8) suppressed the PI3 K/AKT/mTOR signaling cascades, a pathway that leads the autophagy activation. Hence, these results indicate that deoxypodophyllotoxin (8) triggers simultaneously cytoprotective autophagy and cytotoxic apoptosis.

DPT (8) was used in a recent study [127], to establish a physiologically based pharmacokinetic-pharmacodynamic (PBPK-PD) model that allowed to predict the tumor growth in human lung carcinoma NCI-H460 tumor-bearing mice during deoxypodophyllotoxin (8) multi-dose treatment, as well as in gastric cancer SGC-7901 tumor-bearing mice. Briefly, the PBPK-PD model uses in vitro/in vivo pharmacodynamic correlations and predicts antitumor effectiveness in tumor-bearing mice based on in vitro pharmacodynamics assays results. The authors defend that this PBPK-PD model could be use with other compounds besides DPT, permitting a faster dose regimen design and anticancer candidate screening in drug discovery processes.

Derivative compounds from deoxypodophyllotoxin (8) also present great potential as anticancer drugs, as it is shown in a study from Guan et al. [128]. In their study, cytotoxic activity of various deoxypodophyllotoxin–5-fluorouracil hybrid compounds were evaluated using four human cancer cell lines and the human lung fibroblast non-tumoral cell line WI-38. The majority of the hybrids were more potent in their cytotoxicity to the four tumor cell lines and presented reduced toxicity against the normal cell line than the reference compounds etoposide and 5-FU. The most promising compound was 4′-O-demethyl-4-deoxypodophyllotoxin-4′-yl 4-((6-(2-(5-fluorouracil-yl)acetamido) hexyl) amino)-4-oxobutanoate (8a) (Figure 5) that presented IC_{50} values of 0.27 to 4.03 μM against HeLa, A549, HCT-8 and HepG2 cells, being less toxic (IC_{50} = 113.8 μM) to WI-38 cells than 5-FU and etoposide (IC_{50} values of 78.52 μM and 35.8 μM respectively) [128]. Furthermore, this hybrid compound (8a) can inhibit A549 cell migration by up-regulation TIMP-1 and down-regulation matrix metallopeptidase 9 (MMP-9), as well as cause cell-cycle arrest in the G2/M phase by affecting levels of the cell-cycle regulators p-cdc2, cdc2 and cyclin B1 [128].

The same deoxypodophyllotoxin derivative (8a) (Figure 5), named C069 by Xiang et al. [129], could have antiproliferative effects in human umbilical vein endothelial cells (HUVEC), in a dose- and time-dependent way. C069 (8a) at concentrations of 0.1 and 0.3 μM, showed better antiproliferative activity than etoposide at 1 μM, and low cytotoxicity against human normal lung cells WI-38 [129]. Since HUVEC represent a model cell line used to study angiogenesis processes, its non-proliferation is translated as an anti-angiogenesis property of C069 (8a).

Zhu et al. [130], showed that other DPT derivative (8b) (Figure 5), exhibits the IC_{50} values of 0.22 ± 0.02 μM against MGC-803 cells, being more active than the reference etoposide (IC_{50} values > 10 μM against the same cells line) and it can cause cell cycle arrest in G2/M phase through regulation of cell cycle check point proteins expression, such as p21, cdc25c, CDK1, cyclin A, and cyclin B. The same derivative (8b) at 4 mg/kg was also able to reduce in 45.56% the weights and volumes of HepG2 xenografts in mice in just 14 days [130].

Despise the impressive clinical efficacy of the deoxypodophyllotoxin (8) and its derivatives, their therapeutic use still needs to overcome some difficulties like its poor water solubility [131] and rapid elimination [132].

3. Conclusions

In conclusion, *Juniperus* genus is very rich in species and promising metabolites with pharmaceutical potential, being *J. communis* and *J. oxycedrus* the two most studied species in terms of their phytochemistry, pharmacological and therapeutic effects.

As a summary, the effects of *Juniperus* secondary metabolites and the level of activity/mechanism of action are shown in Table 1.

Table 1. The key points of each secondary metabolite highlighted.

Compound	Biological Activity (Tested Model)	Level of Activity [a] (Control/Mechanism [b])	Ref.
1a	Antitumor (PC-3, SK-OV-3, MDA-MB-231 and MCF-7 cell lines)	IC_{50} = 0.7–1.2 µM (IC_{50} = 5.2–24.5 µM to 5-FU)	[33]
1b	Antibacterial (*Staphylococcus aureus* Newman)	MIC = 0.63–1.2 µM (MIC = 0.54–1.1 µM to vancomycin)	[34]
2	Antitumor (HepG2 cell line)	IC_{50} = 39.8 µM (low cytotoxicity to L-02 cell line)	[42]
	Neuroprotective (hippocampal neurons from mice)	At 10 µM cause ↑ calcium intracellular)	[45]
2a	Antiviral (Dengue Virus type 2)	EC_{50} = 1.4 µM with SI = 57.7 (EC_{50} = 13.5 µM to ribavirin)	[47]
3	Neurons excitability (rat hippocampal CA1 neurons)	At 30 µM cause inhibition of VGSC	[53]
4	Antidiabetic (α–glucosidase inhibition)	At 33.2 mM cause more than 65% of inhibition (at 15.4 mM acarbose cause identical inhibition)	[57]
	Antimelanogenesis (tyrosinase inhibition)	At 1.7 mM cause more than 65% of inhibition (at 3.5 mM kojic acid cause identical inhibition)	[57]
	Antiviral (MDCK cell line exposed to H_1N_1 virus)	At 1.7 mM protect against severe cytopathic effect caused by H_1N_1 virus	[58]
	Antitumor (DU145 cell line)	At 20 µM the STAT3 activation was 40% inhibited	[59]
	Antitumor (Mia-PaCa2 cell line)	IC_{50} = 15 µM (↑ Bax expression, ↑ ROS–mediated alterations, ↓ Bcl–2 expression, ↓ migratory capacity	[62]
5	Antibacterial (*Bacillus subtilis*)	At IC_{50} = 1.5 µM inhibition of metabolic dehydrogenases	[72]
	Vascular-protection (rats)	At 1–10 µg/kg ↓ infarct volume, ↑ ischemia–induced neurological deficit by activation of PKB/HO–1, SOD and GSH	[73]

Table 1. *Cont.*

Compound	Biological Activity (Tested Model)	Level of Activity [a] (Control/Mechanism [b])	Ref.
6	Antitumor (aromatase inhibition)	IC_{50} = 93.6 μM	[91]
	Antitumor (OVCAR-3 and SK-OV-3)	20–50 μM cause ↓ cell propagation, block cell cycle progression at the G1/G0 phase and induce cell apoptosis	[94]
	Antitumor (A549)	IC_{50} = 1.54 μM (inhibition of human AKR1B10 activity)	[95]
	Anti-arthritis (adjuvant induced arthritic rats)	At 20–40 mg/kg cause ↓ inflammation	[92]
	Antidiabetic (DPP-IV inhibition)	IC_{50} = 3.9 μM	[99]
7	Cardioprotective (rat cardiomyoblasts H9c2)	At 50 μM exhibits an apoptosis rate of 20% after pirarubicin–induced toxicity (30% to dexrazoxane)	[103]
	Antidepressant (in mice)	At 100 mg/kg alleviate CUS	[104]
8	Antitumor (U-87 MG, SF126, SGC-7901, BGC-823, HO-8910, SK-0V-3, HT-29, MDA-MB-231, JeG-3)	IC_{50} = 13.95–26.72 nM by ↓ Cdc2 expression, ↓ cyclin B1, ↓ Cdc25C (IC_{50} ≥ 73.57 nM to etoposide)	[114]
	Antitumor (MCF-7/S, MCF-7/A)	IC_{50} = 5.86 nM, RI = 0.552 (paclitaxel and etoposide exhibit higher IC_{50} and RI)	[115]
	Antitumor (MCF-7/S and in MCF-7/A xenograft mice)	At 12.5 mg/kg 49.2% of tumour volume growth inhibition (identical to paclitaxel)	[115]
8a	Antitumor (HeLa, A549, HCT-8 and HepG2 cell lines)	IC_{50} = 0.27–4.03 μM, cell migration inhibition, ↑ TIMP-1 expression, ↓ MMP-9 expression, more selectivity than 5-Fu and etoposide	[128]
	Antitumor (HUVEC cell line)	At 0.1–0.3 μM higher activity and selectivity index than etoposide at 1 μM	[129]
8b	Antitumor (MGC-803 cell line)	IC_{50} = 0.22 μM (IC_{50} values > 10 μM to etoposide)	[130]
	Antitumor (HepG2 xenografts in mice)	At 4 mg/kg ↓ in 45.56% the weights and volumes of tumor	[130]

[a] The activity level presented as half maximal inhibitory concentration; [b] When available, data about activity level of the clinical drug used as positive control and/or action mechanism are given. ↑: increased level; ↓: decrease level.

Regarding bioactivities, antitumor activity is by far the most studied, being followed by antiviral and antibacterial activities, with several works researching compounds found on *Juniperus* species mainly for these properties.

From the compounds mentioned in this review, deoxypodophyllotoxin (8) appears to be the most promising one in terms of development into a pharmaceutical natural drug, since it has reported antitumor effects against breast cancer acquired resistant cells (MCF-7/A), with IC_{50} = 5.86 nM, a very interesting value in the nanomolar level. However, their therapeutic use still needs to overcome obstacles like its poor water solubility. A deoxypodophyllotoxin derivative more soluble could do the trick. The dehydroabietic acid derivative 1a also appears to be a good bet for further studies and development since it has shown IC_{50} values between 0.7–1.2 μM against PC-3, SK-OV-3, MCF-7 and MDA-MB-231 tumor cell lines, an activity higher than the one exhibited by the anticancer agent 5-FU used clinically, and with significant selectivity once dehydroabietic acid derivative 1a displayed very weak cytotoxicity against normal cells.

The majority of the studies addressed in this review were made at the in vitro scale, with only a handful being done in in vivo. In fact, this is only the first step of a long, expensive, and very selective route until it can be declared as a compound with real potential to be a new drug, that is, with therapeutic application or as a new head of series. Thus, while this review work outlines the most promising compounds on which more studies are published in recent years, we are convinced that only the two compounds highlighted in the previous paragraph will be interesting enough to attract the attention of the pharmaceutical industry.

In light of this, the more active and promising compounds presented in *Juniperus* species should be taken to the next step, with future works aiming to in vivo testing assessment of them, particularly the ones with antitumor effects.

On the other hand, studies regarding any bioactivity assay of any compound should always present IC_{50} values of a reference compound in order to increases their scientific impact and facilitate results comparison.

This review hopes to demonstrate the *Juniperus* species value and their importance as a source of metabolites with relevant pharmaceutical potential.

Author Contributions: W.R.T. and A.M.L.S. conceived and wrote the paper.

Funding: This research was funded by Portuguese National Funds, through FCT—Fundação para a Ciência e a Tecnologia, and as applicable co-financed by the FEDER within the PT2020 Partnership Agreement by funding the Organic Chemistry Research Unit (QOPNA) (UID/QUI/00062/2013) and the cE3c centre (UID/BIA/00329/2013).

Acknowledgments: We would like to thank also to University of Azores, University of Aveiro by the Organic Chemistry, Natural Products and Food Stuffs (QOPNA) unit, and Azorean Biodiversity Group (GBA) for technical support.

Conflicts of Interest: The authors declare no conflict of interest.

Abbreviation

5-Fu	Fluorouracil
A375	Human malignant melanoma
A549	Human lung carcinoma
AIF	Apoptosis inducing factor
AKR1B10	Aldo-keto reductase family 1 member B10
AKT/PKB	Protein kinase B
AMPK	Adenosine monophosphate -activated protein kinase
ATP	Adenosine triphosphate
Aβ	Amyloid-β
Bax	Bcl-2-associated X
BChE	Butyrylcholinesterase
BGC-823	Gastric carcinoma
C6	Rat glial tumor
CaMKII	Ca^{2+}/calmodulin-dependent protein kinase II
Cdc2	Cyclin-dependent protein kinase 2
Cdc25C	Cell division cycle 25C protein
CGC	Cerebellar granule cells
CNS	Central nervous system
CoA	Coenzyme A
CUS	Chronic unpredictable stress
DNA	Deoxyribonucleic acid
DNCB	2,4-Dinitrochlorobenzene
DPP-IV	Dipeptidyl peptidase IV
DPT	Deoxypodophyllotoxin
DPT-HP-β-CD	Mixture of deoxypodophyllotoxin with hydroxypropyl-β-cyclodextrin
DU145	Human prostate cancer
DZR	Dexrazoxane
EC$_{50}$	Half maximal effective concentration

EJ138	Human bladder carcinoma
ERK	Extracellular signal-regulated kinase
FAD	Flavin adenine dinucleotide
GIP	Glucose-dependent insulinotropic polypeptide
GLP-1	Glucagon-like peptide 1
GSH	Glutathione
H9c2	Rat cardiomyoblasts
HaCaT	Nontumorigenic human epidermal cells
HCT-8	Human colorectal adenocarcinoma
HCT116	Human colon cancer
HeLa	Human cervical carcinoma
Hep3B	Human hepatoma
HepG2	Human hepatocellular carcinoma
HFF-1	Human normal fibroblast
HL-7702	Human liver normal
HO-8910	Human ovarian carcinoma
HT-29	Human colon carcinoma
HUVEC	Human umbilical vein endothelial cells
IC_{50}	Half maximal inhibitory concentration
IgE	Immunoglobulin E
IL-4	Interleukin 4
JeG-3	Human choriocarcinoma
L-02	Human fetal hepatocyte normal cell line
LTP	Long-term potentiation
MCF-7/A	Acquired resistant human breast cancer
MCF-7/S	Human breast cancer
MCF-7	Human breast cancer
MDA-MB-231	Human breast adenocarcinoma
MDCK	Madin-Darby canine kidney cells
MGC-803	Human gastric cancer
Mia-PaCa2	Human pancreatic carcinoma
MIC	Minimum inhibitory concentration
MMP	Mitochondrial membrane potential
MMP-9	Matrix metallopeptidase 9
MPP^+	1-methyl-4-phenylpyridinium
MPTP	1-methyl-4-phenyl-1,2,3,6-tetrahydropyridine
mTOR	Mammalian target of rapamycin
N2A	Mouse neuroblastoma
$NAD(P)^+$	Nicotinamide adenine dinucleotide phosphate
NCI-H460	Human lung carcinoma
NO	Nitric oxide
Nrf2	Nuclear factor erythroid 2-related factor 2
OVCAR-3	Human ovarian adenocarcinoma
PAR	Poly (ADP-ribose)
PARP-1	Poly (ADP-ribose) synthetase 1
PBPK-PD	Physiologically based pharmacokinetic-pharmacodynamic
PC-3	Human prostate cancer
PGD2	Prostaglandin D2
PKB/HO-1	Protein kinase B/heme oxygenase-1
PKC	Protein kinase C
PTEN	Phosphatase and tensin homolog
RAW 267.4	Macrophage normal cell line
RNA	Ribonucleic acid

ROS	Reactive oxygen species
SF126	Human glioblastoma
SGC-7901	Gastric carcinoma
SHG-44	Human malignant glioma
SI	Selective index
SK-OV-3	Ovarian cancer
Skp2	S-phase kinase protein 2
SOD	Superoxide dismutase
STAT3	Signal transducer and activator of transcription 3
TGF	Transforming growth factor
TIMP-1	TIMP metallopeptidase inhibitor 1
TKT	Transketolase
TNF-α	Tumor necrosis factor α
U-87 MG	Human glioblastoma-astrocytoma
VGSC	Voltage-gated Na^+ channels
WI-38	Human lung fibroblast normal cells

References

1. Youngs, R.L.; Hamza, M.F. Wood: History of use. In *Reference Module in Materials Science and Materials Engineering*, 1st ed.; Hashmi, S., Ed.; Elsevier Inc.: Oxford, UK, 2016; pp. 1–7, ISBN 978-0-12-803581-8.
2. Lukešová, H.; Palau, A.S.; Holst, B. Identifying plant fibre textiles from Norwegian Merovingian period and Viking age graves: The late iron age collection of the University Museum of Bergen. *J. Archaeol. Sci. Rep.* **2017**, *13*, 281–285. [CrossRef]
3. Prinsloo, G.; Nogemane, N.; Street, R. The use of plants containing genotoxic carcinogens as foods and medicine. *Food Chem. Toxicol.* **2018**, *116*, 27–39. [CrossRef] [PubMed]
4. Falzon, C.C.; Balabanova, A. Phytotherapy: An introduction to herbal medicine. *Prim. Care Clin. Off. Pract.* **2017**, *44*, 217–227. [CrossRef] [PubMed]
5. Ghosh, N.; Ghosh, R.C.; Kundu, A.; Mandal, S.C. Herb and drug interaction. In *Natural Products and Drug Discovery*, 1st ed.; Mandal, S.C., Mandal, V., Konishi, T., Eds.; Elsevier Inc.: Oxford, UK, 2018; pp. 467–490, ISBN 978-0-08-102081-4.
6. Rangel, M.L.; Guerrero-Analco, J.A.; Monribot-Villanueva, J.L.; Kiel-Martínez, A.L.; Avendaño-Reyes, S.; Abad, J.P.D.; Bonilla-Landa, I.; Dávalos-Sotelo, R.; Olivares-Romero, J.L.; Angeles, G. Anatomical and chemical characteristics of leaves and branches of *Juniperus deppeana* var. *deppeana* (Cupressaceae): A potential source of raw materials for the perfume and sweet candies industries. *Ind. Crops Prod.* **2018**, *113*, 50–54. [CrossRef]
7. The Plant List. Available online: http://www.theplantlist.org/1.1/browse/G/Cupressaceae/Juniperus (accessed on 28 May 2018).
8. Khan, M.; Khan, A.; Rehman, N.; Gilani, A.H. Pharmacological explanation for the medicinal use of *Juniperus excelsa* in hyperactive gastrointestinal and respiratory disorders. *J. Nat. Med.* **2012**, *66*, 292–301. [CrossRef] [PubMed]
9. Orhan, N.; Aslan, M.; Pekcan, M.; Orhan, D.D.; Bedir, E.; Ergun, F. Identification of hypoglycaemic compounds from berries of *Juniperus oxycedrus* subsp. *oxycedrus through bioactivity guided isolation technique*. *J. Ethnopharmacol.* **2012**, *139*, 110–118. [CrossRef] [PubMed]
10. Sharma, A.; Flores-Vallejo, R.C.; Cardoso-Taketa, A.; Villarreal, M.L. Antibacterial activities of medicinal plants used in Mexican traditional medicine. *J. Ethnopharmacol.* **2017**, *208*, 264–329. [CrossRef] [PubMed]
11. Bais, S.; Gill, N.S.; Rana, N.; Shandil, S. A Phytopharmacological review on a medicinal plant: *Juniperus communis*. *Int. Sch. Res. Not.* **2014**, *2014*, 634723. [CrossRef] [PubMed]
12. Seca, A.M.L.; Silva, A.M.S. The chemical composition of the *Juniperus* genus (1970–2004). In *Recent Progress in Medicinal Plants*; Govil, J.N., Singh, V.K., Bhardwaj, R., Eds.; Studium Press LLC: Houston, TX, USA, 2006; Volume 16, pp. 401–522, ISBN 0-9761849-8-2.

13. Seca, A.M.L.; Pinto, D.C.G.A.; Silva, A.M.S. The current status of bioactive metabolites from the genus *Juniperus*. In *Bioactive Phytochemicals: Perspectives for Modern Medicine*; Gupta, V.K., Ed.; M/S Daya Publishing House: New Delhi, India, 2015; Volume 3, pp. 365–407, ISBN 9789351246749.

14. Al-Snafi, A.E. Medical importance of *Juniperus communis*—A review. *Indo Am. J. Pharm. Sci.* **2018**, *5*, 1779–1792. [CrossRef]

15. Al-Snafi, A.E. Pharmacological and therapeutic effects of *Juniperus oxycedrus*—A review. *Indo Am. J. Pharm. Sci.* **2018**, *5*, 2198–2205. [CrossRef]

16. Jung, H.J.; Min, B.-S.; Jung, H.A.; Choi, J.S. Sesquiterpenoids from the heartwood of *Juniperus chinensis*. *Nat. Prod. Sci.* **2017**, *23*, 208–212. [CrossRef]

17. Lee, S.; Park, N.-J.; Bong, S.-K.; Jegal, J.; Park, S.-A.; Kim, S.-N.; Yang, M.H. Ameliorative effects of *Juniperus rigida* fruit on oxazolone- and 2,4-dinitrochlorobenzene-induced atopic dermatitis in mice. *J. Ethnopharmacol.* **2018**, *214*, 160–167. [CrossRef] [PubMed]

18. Groshi, A.A.; Evans, A.R.; Ismail, F.M.D.; Nahar, L.; Sarker, S.D. Cytotoxicity of Libyan *Juniperus phoenicea* against human cancer cell lines A549, EJ138, HepG2 and MCF7. *Pharm. Sci.* **2018**, *24*, 3–7. [CrossRef]

19. Venditti, A.; Maggi, F.; Quassinti, L.; Bramucci, M.; Lupidi, G.; Ornano, L.; Ballero, M.; Sanna, C.; Bruno, M.; Rosselli, S.; et al. Bioactive constituents of *Juniperus turbinata* Gussone from La Maddalena Archipelago. *Chem. Biodivers.* **2018**, e1800148. [CrossRef] [PubMed]

20. Costa, S.; Cavadas, C.; Cavaleiro, C.; Salgueiro, L.; do Céu Sousa, M. In vitro susceptibility of *Trypanosoma brucei brucei* to selected essential oils and their major components. *Exp. Parasitol.* **2018**, *190*, 34–40. [CrossRef] [PubMed]

21. Zhang, K.; Yao, L. The anxiolytic effect of *Juniperus virginiana* L. essential oil and determination of its active constituents. *Physiol. Behav.* **2018**, *189*, 50–58. [CrossRef] [PubMed]

22. Inci, H.; Ozdemir, G.; Sengul, A.Y.; Sogut, B.; Nursoy, H.; Sengul, T. Using juniper berry (*Juniperus communis*) as a supplement in Japanese quail diets. *Rev. Bras. Zootec.* **2016**, *45*, 230–235. [CrossRef]

23. Brischke, C.; Hesse, C.; Meyer-Veltrup, L.; Humar, M. Studies on the material resistance and moisture dynamics of Common juniper, English yew, Black cherry, and Rowan. *Wood Mater. Sci. Eng.* **2018**, *13*, 222–230. [CrossRef]

24. Ateş, S.; Gür, M.; Özkan, O.E.; Akça, M.; Olgun, Ç.; Güder, A. Chemical contents and antifungal activity of some durable wood extractives vs. *Pleurotus ostreatus*. *Bioresources* **2015**, *10*, 2433–2443.

25. Koruk, S.T.; Ozyilkan, E.; Kava, P.; Colak, D.; Donderici, O.; Cesaretli, Y. Juniper tar poisoning. *Clin. Toxicol.* **2005**, *43*, 47–49. [CrossRef]

26. González, M.A. Aromatic abietane diterpenoids: Their biological activity and synthesis. *Nat. Prod. Rep.* **2015**, *32*, 684–704. [CrossRef] [PubMed]

27. Agudelo-Gómez, L.S.; Betancur-Galvis, L.A.; González, M.A. Anti HHV-1 and HHV-2 activity in vitro of abietic and dehydroabietic acid derivatives. *Pharmacologyonline* **2012**, *1*, 36–42.

28. Zaidi, S.F.H.; Awale, S.; Kalauni, S.K.; Tezuka, Y.; Esumi, H.; Kadota, S. Diterpenes from "Pini Resina" and their preferential cytotoxic activity under nutrient-deprived condition. *Planta Med.* **2006**, *72*, 1231–1234. [CrossRef] [PubMed]

29. Tanaka, R.; Tokuda, H.; Ezaki, Y. Cancer chemopreventive activity of "rosin" constituents of *Pinus* spez. and their derivatives in two-stage mouse skin carcinogenesis test. *Phytomedicine* **2008**, *15*, 985–992. [CrossRef] [PubMed]

30. Sepúlveda, B.; Astudillo, L.; Rodríguez, J.A.; Yáñez, T.; Theoduloz, C.; Schmeda-Hirschmann, G. Gastroprotective and cytotoxic effect of dehydroabietic acid derivatives. *Pharmacol. Res.* **2005**, *52*, 429–437. [CrossRef] [PubMed]

31. Fallarero, A.; Skogman, M.; Kujala, J.; Rajaratnam, M.; Moreira, V.M.; Yli-Kauhaluoma, J.; Vuorela, P. (+)-Dehydroabietic Acid, an Abietane-Type Diterpene, Inhibits *Staphylococcus aureus* Biofilms in vitro. *Int. J. Mol. Sci.* **2013**, *14*, 12054–12072. [CrossRef] [PubMed]

32. Jang, H.J.; Yang, K.-S. Inhibition of nitric oxide production in RAW 264.7 macrophages by diterpenoids from *Phellinus pini*. *Arch. Pharm. Res.* **2011**, *34*, 913–917. [CrossRef] [PubMed]

33. Hou, W.; Luo, Z.; Zhang, G.; Cao, D.; Li, D.; Ruan, H.; Ruan, B.H.; Su, L.; Xu, H. Click chemistry-based synthesis and anticancer activity evaluation of novel C-14 1,2,3-triazole dehydroabietic acid hybrids. *Eur. J. Med. Chem.* **2017**, *138*, 1042–1052. [CrossRef] [PubMed]

34. Zhang, W.-M.; Yao, Y.; Yang, T.; Wang, X.-Y.; Zhu, Z.-Y.; Xu, W.-T.; Lin, H.-X.; Gao, Z.-B.; Zhou, H.; Yang, C.-G.; et al. The synthesis and antistaphylococcal activity of *N*-sulfonaminoethyloxime derivatives of dehydroabietic acid. *Bioorg. Med. Chem. Lett.* **2018**, *28*, 1943–1948. [CrossRef] [PubMed]

35. Han, J.-W.; Shim, D.-W.; Shin, W.-Y.; Kim, M.-K.; Shim, E.-J.; Sun, X.; Koppula, S.; Kim, T.-J.; Kang, T.-B.; Lee, K.-H. *Juniperus rigida* Sieb. extract inhibits inflammatory responses via attenuation of TRIF-dependent signaling and inflammasome activation. *J. Ethnopharmacol.* **2016**, *190*, 91–99. [CrossRef] [PubMed]

36. Samoylenko, V.; Dunbar, D.C.; Gafur, M.A.; Khan, S.I.; Ross, S.A.; Mossa, J.S.; El-Feraly, F.S.; Tekwani, B.L.; Bosselaers, J.; Muhammad, I. Antiparasitic, nematicidal and antifouling constituents from *Juniperus* berries. *Phytother. Res.* **2008**, *22*, 1570–1576. [CrossRef] [PubMed]

37. Becerra, J.; Flores, C.; Mena, J.; Aqueveque, P.; Alarcón, J.; Bittner, M.; Hernández, V.; Hoeneisen, M.; Ruiz, E.; Silva, M. Antifungal and antibacterial activity of diterpenes isolated from wood extractables of Chilean Podocarpaceae. *Bol. Soc. Chil. Quim.* **2002**, *47*, 151–157. [CrossRef]

38. Mossa, J.S.; El-Feraly, F.S.; Muhammad, I. Antimycobacterial constituents from *Juniperus procera*, *Ferula communis* and *Plumbago zeylanica* and their in vitro synergistic activity with isonicotinic acid hydrazide. *Phytother. Res.* **2004**, *18*, 934–937. [CrossRef] [PubMed]

39. Smith, E.C.J.; Williamson, E.M.; Wareham, N.; Kaatz, G.W.; Gibbons, S. Antibacterials and modulators of bacterial resistance from the immature cones of *Chamaecyparis lawsoniana*. *Phytochemistry* **2007**, *68*, 210–217. [CrossRef] [PubMed]

40. Smith, E.C.J.; Wareham, N.; Zloh, M.; Gibbons, S. 2b-Acetoxyferruginol—A new antibacterial abietane diterpene from the bark of *Prumnopitys andina*. *Phytochem. Lett.* **2008**, *1*, 49–53. [CrossRef]

41. Ryu, Y.B.; Jeong, H.J.; Kim, J.H.; Kim, Y.M.; Park, J.-Y.; Kim, D.; Naguyen, T.T.H.; Park, S.-J.; Chang, J.S.; Park, K.H.; et al. Biflavonoids from *Torreya nucifera* displaying SARS-CoV 3CL[pro] inhibition. *Bioorg. Med. Chem.* **2010**, *18*, 7940–7947. [CrossRef] [PubMed]

42. Yang, J.; Xu, C.; Chen, H.; Huang, M.; Ma, X.; Deng, S.; Huang, Y.; Wen, Y.; Yang, X.; Song, P. In vitro and in vivo antitumor effects of the diterpene-enriched extract from *Taxodium ascendens* through the mitochondrial-dependent apoptosis pathway. *Biomed. Pharmacother.* **2017**, *96*, 1199–1208. [CrossRef] [PubMed]

43. Shankar, G.M.; Li, S.; Mehta, T.H.; Garcia-Munoz, A.; Shepardson, N.E.; Smith, I.; Brett, F.M.; Farrell, M.A.; Rowan, M.J.; Lemere, C.A.; et al. Amyloid β-protein dimers isolated directly from Alzheimer brains impair synaptic plasticity and memory. *Nat. Med.* **2008**, *14*, 837–842. [CrossRef] [PubMed]

44. Kuchibhotla, K.V.; Goldman, S.T.; Lattarulo, C.R.; Wu, H.-Y.; Hyman, B.T.; Bacskai, B.J. Aβ plaques lead to aberrant regulation of calcium homeostasis in vivo resulting in structural and functional disruption of neuronal networks. *Neuron* **2008**, *59*, 214–225. [CrossRef] [PubMed]

45. Zolezzi, J.M.; Lindsay, C.B.; Serrano, F.G.; Ureta, R.C.; Theoduloz, C.; Schmeda-Hirschmann, G.; Inestrosa, N.C. Neuroprotective effects of ferruginol, jatrophone, and junicedric acid against amyloid-β injury in hippocampal neurons. *J. Alzheimer's Dis.* **2018**, *63*, 705–723. [CrossRef] [PubMed]

46. Yang, H.-W.; Hu, X.-D.; Zhang, H.-M.; Xin, W.-J.; Li, M.-T.; Zhang, T.; Zhou, L.-J.; Liu, X.-G. Roles of CaMKII, PKA, and PKC in the induction and maintenance of LTP of C-fiber-evoked field potentials in rat spinal dorsal horn. *J. Neurophysiol.* **2004**, *91*, 1122–1133. [CrossRef] [PubMed]

47. Roa-Linares, V.C.; Brand, Y.M.; Agudelo-Gomez, L.S.; Tangarife-Castaño, V.; Betancur-Galvis, L.A.; Gallego-Gomez, J.C.; González, M.A. Anti-herpetic and anti-dengue activity of abietane ferruginol analogues synthesized from (+)-dehydroabietylamine. *Eur. J. Med. Chem.* **2016**, *108*, 79–88. [CrossRef] [PubMed]

48. Fan, S.-Y.; Zeng, H.-W.; Pei, Y.-H.; Li, L.; Ye, J.; Pan, Y.-X.; Zhang, J.-G.; Yuan, X.; Zhang, W.-D. The anti-inflammatory activities of an extract and compounds isolated from *Platycladus orientalis* (Linnaeus) Franco in vitro and ex vivo. *J. Ethnopharmacol.* **2012**, *141*, 647–652. [CrossRef] [PubMed]

49. Chen, Y.-C.; Li, Y.-C.; You, B.-J.; Chang, W.-T.; Chao, L.K.; Lo, L.-C.; Wang, S.-Y.; Huang, G.-J.; Kuo, Y.-H. Diterpenoids with anti-inflammatory activity from the wood of *Cunninghamia konishii*. *Molecules* **2013**, *18*, 682–689. [CrossRef] [PubMed]

50. Gaspar-Marques, C.; Simões, M.F.; Valdeira, M.L.; Rodríguez, B. Terpenoids and phenolics from *Plectranthus strigosus*. *Nat. Prod. Res.* **2008**, *22*, 167–177. [CrossRef] [PubMed]

51. Alqasoumi, S.I.; Abdel-Kader, M.S. Terpenoids from *Juniperus procera* with hepatoprotective activity. *Pak. J. Pharm. Sci.* **2012**, *25*, 315–322. [PubMed]

52. Wang, W.-S.; Li, E.-W.; Jia, Z.-J. Terpenes from *Juniperus przewalskii* and their antitumor activities. *Pharmazie* **2002**, *57*, 343–345. [CrossRef] [PubMed]

53. Wang, Y.-W.; Yang, C.-T.; Gong, C.-L.; Chen, Y.-H.; Chen, Y.-W.; Wu, K.-C.; Cheng, T.-H.; Kuo, Y.-H.; Chen, Y.-F.; Leung, Y.-M. Inhibition of voltage-gated Na$^+$ channels by hinokiol in neuronal cells. *Pharmacol. Rep.* **2015**, *67*, 1049–1054. [CrossRef] [PubMed]

54. Seca, A.M.L.; Silva, A.M.S. The chemical composition of hexane extract from bark of *Juniperus brevifolia*. *Nat. Prod. Res.* **2008**, *22*, 975–983. [CrossRef] [PubMed]

55. Seca, A.M.L.; Silva, A.M.S.; Bazzocchi, I.L.; Jimenez, I.A. Diterpene constituents of leaves from *Juniperus brevifolia*. *Phytochemistry* **2008**, *69*, 498–505. [CrossRef] [PubMed]

56. Bajpai, V.K.; Sharma, A.; Kang, S.C.; Baek, K.-H. Antioxidant, lipid peroxidation inhibition and free radical scavenging efficacy of a diterpenoid compound sugiol isolated from *Metasequoia glyptostroboides*. *Asian Pac. J. Trop. Med.* **2014**, *7*, 9–15. [CrossRef]

57. Bajpai, V.K.; Kang, S.C. A diterpenoid sugiol from *Metasequoia glyptostroboides* with α-glucosidase and tyrosinase inhibitory potential. *Bangladesh J. Pharmacol.* **2014**, *9*, 312–316. [CrossRef]

58. Bajpai, V.K.; Kim, N.-H.; Kim, K.; Kang, S.C. Antiviral potential of a diterpenoid compound sugiol from *Metasequoia glyptostroboides*. *Pak. J. Pharm. Sci.* **2016**, *29*, 1077–1080. [PubMed]

59. Jung, S.-N.; Shin, D.-S.; Kim, H.-N.; Jeon, Y.J.; Yun, J.; Lee, Y.-J.; Kang, J.S.; Han, D.C.; Kwon, B.-M. Sugiol inhibits STAT3 activity via regulation of transketolase and ROS-mediated ERK activation in DU145 prostate carcinoma cells. *Biochem. Pharmacol.* **2015**, *97*, 38–50. [CrossRef] [PubMed]

60. Wang, J.; Zhang, X.; Ma, D.; Lee, W.-N.; Xiao, J.; Zhao, Y.; Go, V.L.; Wang, Q.; Yen, Y.; Recker, R.; et al. Inhibition of transketolase by oxythiamine altered dynamics of protein signals in pancreatic cancer cells. *Exp. Hematol. Oncol.* **2013**, *2*, 18. [CrossRef] [PubMed]

61. Aggarwal, B.B.; Kunnumakkara, A.B.; Harikumar, K.B.; Gupta, S.R.; Tharakan, S.T.; Koca, C.; Dey, S.; Sung, B. Signal transducer and activator of transcription-3, inflammation, and cancer: How intimate is the relationship? *Ann. N. Y. Acad. Sci.* **2009**, *1171*, 59–76. [CrossRef] [PubMed]

62. Hao, C.; Zhang, X.; Zhang, H.; Shang, H.; Bao, J.; Wang, H.; Li, Z. Sugiol (12-hydroxyabieta-8,11, 13-trien-7-one) targets human pancreatic carcinoma cells (Mia-PaCa2) by inducing apoptosis, G2/M cell cycle arrest, ROS production and inhibition of cancer cell migration. *J. BUON* **2018**, *23*, 205–210. [PubMed]

63. Cox, R.E.; Yamamoto, S.; Otto, A.; Simoneit, B.R.T. Oxygenated di- and tricyclic diterpenoids of southern hemisphere conifers. *Biochem. Syst. Ecol.* **2007**, *35*, 342–362. [CrossRef]

64. Jaiswal, R.; Beuria, T.K.; Mohan, R.; Mahajan, S.K.; Panda, D. Totarol inhibits bacterial cytokinesis by perturbing the assembly dynamics of FtsZ. *Biochemistry* **2007**, *46*, 4211–4220. [CrossRef] [PubMed]

65. Kim, M.B.; O'Brien, T.E.; Moore, J.T.; Anderson, D.E.; Foss, M.H.; Weibel, D.B.; Ames, J.B.; Shaw, J.T. The synthesis and antimicrobial activity of heterocyclic derivatives of totarol. *ACS Med. Chem. Lett.* **2012**, *3*, 818–822. [CrossRef] [PubMed]

66. Foss, M.H.; Eun, Y.-J.; Grove, C.I.; Pauw, D.A.; Sorto, N.A.; Rensvold, J.W.; Pagliarini, D.J.; Shaw, J.T.; Weibel, D.B. Inhibitors of bacterial tubulin target bacterial membranes in vivo. *Med. Chem. Commun.* **2013**, *4*, 112–119. [CrossRef] [PubMed]

67. Clarkson, C.; Musonda, C.C.; Chibale, K.; Campbell, W.E.; Smith, P. Synthesis of totarol amino alcohol derivatives and their antiplasmodial activity and cytotoxicity. *Bioorg. Med. Chem.* **2003**, *11*, 4417–4422. [CrossRef]

68. Tacon, C.; Guantai, E.M.; Smith, P.J.; Chibale, K. Synthesis, biological evaluation and mechanistic studies of totarol amino alcohol derivatives as potential antimalarial agents. *Bioorg. Med. Chem.* **2012**, *20*, 893–902. [CrossRef] [PubMed]

69. Smith, E.C.J.; Kaatz, G.W.; Seo, S.M.; Wareham, N.; Williamson, E.M.; Gibbons, S. The phenolic diterpene totarol inhibits multidrug efflux pump activity in *Staphylococcus aureus*. *Antimicrob. Agents Chemother.* **2007**, *51*, 4480–4483. [CrossRef] [PubMed]

70. Gordien, A.Y.; Gray, A.I.; Franzblau, S.G.; Seidel, V. Antimycobacterial terpenoids from *Juniperus communis* L. (Cuppressaceae). *J. Ethnopharmacol.* **2009**, *126*, 500–505. [CrossRef] [PubMed]

71. Evans, G.B.; Furneaux, R.H.; Gainsford, G.J.; Murphy, M.P. The synthesis and antibacterial activity of totarol derivatives. Part 3: Modification of ring-B. *Bioorg. Med. Chem.* **2000**, *8*, 1663–1675. [CrossRef]

72. Reddy, P.J.; Ray, S.; Sathe, G.J.; Gajbhiye, A.; Prasad, T.S.K.; Rapole, S.; Panda, D.; Srivastava, S. A comprehensive proteomic analysis of totarol induced alterations in *Bacillus subtilis* by multipronged quantitative proteomics. *J. Proteom.* **2015**, *114*, 247–262. [CrossRef] [PubMed]

73. Gao, Y.; Xu, X.; Chang, S.; Wang, Y.; Xu, Y.; Ran, S.; Huang, Z.; Li, P.; Li, J.; Zhang, L.; et al. Totarol prevents neuronal injury in vitro and ameliorates brain ischemic stroke: Potential roles of Akt activation and HO-1 induction. *Toxicol. Appl. Pharmacol.* **2015**, *289*, 142–154. [CrossRef] [PubMed]

74. Yu, S.; Yan, H.; Zhang, L.; Shan, M.; Chen, P.; Ding, A.; Li, S.F.Y. A review on the phytochemistry, pharmacology, and pharmacokinetics of amentoflavone, a naturally-occurring biflavonoid. *Molecules* **2017**, *22*, 299. [CrossRef] [PubMed]

75. Lee, C.-W.; Na, Y.; Park, N.-H.; Kim, H.-S.; Ahn, S.M.; Kim, J.W.; Kim, H.-K.; Jang, Y.P. Amentoflavone inhibits UVB-induced matrix metalloproteinase-1 expression through the modulation of AP-1 components in normal human fibroblasts. *Appl. Biochem. Biotechnol.* **2012**, *166*, 1137–1147. [CrossRef] [PubMed]

76. Hwang, I.-S.; Lee, J.; Jin, H.-G.; Woo, E.-R.; Lee, D.G. Amentoflavone stimulates mitochondrial dysfunction and induces apoptotic cell death in *Candida albicans*. *Mycopathologia* **2012**, *173*, 207–218. [CrossRef] [PubMed]

77. Coulerie, P.; Nour, M.; Maciuk, A.; Eydoux, C.; Guillemot, J.-C.; Lebouvier, N.; Hnawia, E.; Leblanc, K.; Lewin, G.; Canard, B.; et al. Structure-activity relationship study of biflavonoids on the Dengue virus polymerase DENV-NS5 RdRp. *Planta Med.* **2013**, *79*, 1313–1318. [CrossRef] [PubMed]

78. Li, X.; Wang, L.; Han, W.; Mai, W.; Han, L.; Chen, D. Amentoflavone protects against hydroxyl radical-induced DNA damage via antioxidant mechanism. *Turk. J. Biochem.* **2014**, *39*, 30–36. [CrossRef]

79. Abdallah, H.M.; Almowallad, F.M.; Esmat, A.; Shehata, I.A.; Abdel-Sattar, E.A. Anti-inflammatory activity of flavonoids from *Chrozophora tinctoria*. *Phytochem. Lett.* **2015**, *13*, 74–80. [CrossRef]

80. Laishram, S.; Sheikh, Y.; Moirangthem, D.S.; Deb, L.; Pal, B.C.; Talukdar, N.C.; Borah, J.C. Anti-diabetic molecules from *Cycas pectinata* Griff. traditionally used by the Maiba-Maibi. *Phytomedicine* **2015**, *22*, 23–26. [CrossRef] [PubMed]

81. An, J.; Li, Z.; Dong, Y.; Ren, J.; Huo, J. Amentoflavone protects against psoriasis-like skin lesion through suppression of NF-κB-mediated inflammation and keratinocyte proliferation. *Mol. Cell. Biochem.* **2016**, *413*, 87–95. [CrossRef] [PubMed]

82. Aguilar, M.I.; Benítez, W.V.; Colín, A.; Bye, R.; Ríos-Gómez, R.; Calzada, F. Evaluation of the diuretic activity in two Mexican medicinal species: *Selaginella nothohybrida* and *S. lepidophylla* and its effects with ciclooxigenases inhibitors. *J. Ethnopharmacol.* **2015**, *163*, 167–172. [CrossRef] [PubMed]

83. Chen, J.-H.; Chen, W.-L.; Liu, Y.-C. Amentoflavone induces anti-angiogenic and anti-metastatic effects through suppression of NF-κB activation in MCF-7 cells. *Anticancer Res.* **2015**, *35*, 6685–6694. [PubMed]

84. Ndongo, J.T.; Issa, M.E.; Messi, A.N.; Mbing, J.N.; Cuendet, M.; Pegnyemb, D.E.; Bochet, C.G. Cytotoxic flavonoids and other constituents from the stem bark of *Ochna schweinfurthiana*. *Nat. Prod. Res.* **2015**, *29*, 1684–1687. [CrossRef] [PubMed]

85. Jeong, E.J.; Hwang, L.; Lee, M.; Lee, K.Y.; Ahn, M.-J.; Sung, S.H. Neuroprotective biflavonoids of *Chamaecyparis obtusa* leaves against glutamate-induced oxidative stress in HT22 hippocampal cells. *Food Chem. Toxicol.* **2014**, *64*, 397–402. [CrossRef] [PubMed]

86. Zha, X.; Xu, Z.; Liu, Y.; Xu, L.; Huang, H.; Zhang, J.; Cui, L.; Zhou, C.; Xu, D. Amentoflavone enhances osteogenesis of human mesenchymal stem cells through JNK and p38 MAPK pathways. *J. Nat. Med.* **2016**, *70*, 634–644. [CrossRef] [PubMed]

87. Zheng, X.-K.; Liu, C.-X.; Zhai, Y.-Y.; Li, L.-L.; Wang, X.-L.; Feng, W.-S. Protection effect of amentoflavone in *Selaginella tamariscina* against TNF-α-induced vascular injure of endothelial cells. *Acta Pharm. Sin.* **2013**, *48*, 1503–1509.

88. Garza, L.A.; Liu, Y.; Yang, Z.; Alagesan, B.; Lawson, J.A.; Norberg, S.M.; Loy, D.E.; Zhao, T.; Blatt, H.B.; Stanton, D.C.; et al. Prostaglandin D$_2$ inhibits hair growth and is elevated in bald scalp of men with androgenetic alopecia. *Sci. Transl. Med.* **2012**, *4*, 126ra34. [CrossRef] [PubMed]

89. Fong, P.; Tong, H.H.Y.; Ng, K.H.; Lao, C.K.; Chong, C.I.; Chao, C.M. In silico prediction of prostaglandin D2 synthase inhibitors from herbal constituents for the treatment of hair loss. *J. Ethnopharmacol.* **2015**, *175*, 470–480. [CrossRef] [PubMed]

90. Brodie, A.; Sabnis, G.; Jelovac, D. Aromatase and breast cancer. *J. Steroid Biochem. Mol. Biol.* **2006**, *102*, 97–102. [CrossRef] [PubMed]

91. Tascioglu, A.; Ozcan, S.; Akdemir, A.; Orhan, H.G. In vitro and in silico evaluation of aromatase inhibitory activity of apigenin and amentoflavone; dual benefit of St. John's Wort in postmenopausal women. *Toxicol. Lett.* **2016**, *258*, S125. [CrossRef]

92. Bais, S.; Abrol, N.; Prashar, Y.; Kumari, R. Modulatory effect of standardised amentoflavone isolated from *Juniperus communis* L. against Freund's adjuvant induced arthritis in rats (histopathological and X Ray analysis). *Biomed. Pharmacother.* **2017**, *86*, 381–392. [CrossRef] [PubMed]

93. Cao, Q.; Qin, L.; Huang, F.; Wang, X.; Yang, L.; Shi, H.; Wu, H.; Zhang, B.; Chen, Z.; Wu, X. Amentoflavone protects dopaminergic neurons in MPTP-induced Parkinson's disease model mice through PI3K/Akt and ERK signaling pathways. *Toxicol. Appl. Pharmacol.* **2017**, *319*, 80–90. [CrossRef] [PubMed]

94. Liu, H.; Yue, Q.; He, S. Amentoflavone suppresses tumor growth in ovarian cancer by modulating Skp2. *Life Sci.* **2017**, *189*, 96–105. [CrossRef] [PubMed]

95. Jung, Y.-J.; Lee, E.H.; Lee, C.G.; Rhee, K.-J.; Jung, W.-S.; Choi, Y.; Pan, C.-H.; Kang, K. AKR1B10-inhibitory *Selaginella tamariscina* extract and amentoflavone decrease the growth of A549 human lung cancer cells in vitro and in vivo. *J. Ethnopharmacol.* **2017**, *202*, 78–84. [CrossRef] [PubMed]

96. Chun, K.-S.; Kundu, J.; Kundu, J.K.; Surh, Y.-J. Targeting Nrf2-Keap1 signaling for chemoprevention of skin carcinogenesis with bioactive phytochemicals. *Toxicol. Lett.* **2014**, *229*, 73–84. [CrossRef] [PubMed]

97. Wahyudi, L.D.; Jeong, J.; Yang, H.; Kim, J.-H. Amentoflavone-induced oxidative stress activates NF-E2-related factor 2 via the p38 MAP kinase-AKT pathway in human keratinocytes. *Int. J. Biochem. Cell Biol.* **2018**, *99*, 100–108. [CrossRef] [PubMed]

98. Liao, W.-L.; Lee, W.-J.; Chen, C.-C.; Lu, C.H.; Chen, C.-H.; Chou, Y.-C.; Lee, I.-T.; Sheu, W.H.-H.; Wu, J.-Y.; Yang, C.-F.; et al. Pharmacogenetics of dipeptidyl peptidase 4 inhibitors in a Taiwanese population with type 2 diabetes. *Oncotarget* **2017**, *8*, 18050–18058. [CrossRef] [PubMed]

99. Beidokhti, M.N.; Lobbens, E.S.; Rasoavaivo, P.; Staerk, D.; Jäger, A.K. Investigation of medicinal plants from Madagascar against DPP-IV linked to type 2 diabetes. *S. Afr. J. Bot.* **2018**, *115*, 113–119. [CrossRef]

100. Yaglioglu, A.S.; Eser, F. Screening of some *Juniperus* extracts for the phenolic compounds and their antiproliferative activities. *S. Afr. J. Bot.* **2017**, *113*, 29–33. [CrossRef]

101. Ganeshpurkar, A.; Saluja, A.K. The pharmacological potential of rutin. *Saudi Pharm. J.* **2017**, *25*, 149–164. [CrossRef] [PubMed]

102. Gullón, B.; Lú-Chau, T.A.; Moreira, M.T.; Lema, J.M.; Eibes, G. Rutin: A review on extraction, identification and purification methods, biological activities and approaches to enhance its bioavailability. *Trends Food Sci. Technol.* **2017**, *67*, 220–235. [CrossRef]

103. Wang, Y.; Zhang, Y.; Sun, B.; Tong, Q.; Ren, L. Rutin protects against pirarubicin-induced cardiotoxicity through TGF-β1-p38 MAPK signaling pathway. *Evid. Based Complement. Altern. Med.* **2017**, *2017*, 1759385. [CrossRef] [PubMed]

104. Parashar, A.; Mehta, V.; Udayabanu, M. Rutin alleviates chronic unpredictable stress-induced behavioral alterations and hippocampal damage in mice. *Neurosci. Lett.* **2017**, *656*, 65–71. [CrossRef] [PubMed]

105. Chakravarty, S.; Reddy, B.R.; Sudhakar, S.R.; Saxena, S.; Das, T.; Meghah, V.; Swamy, C.V.B.; Kumar, A.; Idris, M.M. Chronic unpredictable stress (CUS)-induced anxiety and related mood disorders in a zebrafish model: Altered brain proteome profile implicates mitochondrial dysfunction. *PLoS ONE* **2013**, *8*, e63302. [CrossRef] [PubMed]

106. Renouard, S.; Lopez, T.; Hendrawati, O.; Dupre, P.; Doussot, J.; Falguieres, A.; Ferroud, C.; Hagege, D.; Lamblin, F.; Laine, E.; et al. Podophyllotoxin and deoxypodophyllotoxin in *Juniperus bermudiana* and 12 other *Juniperus* species: Optimization of extraction, method validation, and quantification. *J. Agric. Food Chem.* **2011**, *59*, 8101–8107. [CrossRef] [PubMed]

107. Zhao, Y.; Yang, Y.; Chen, Q.; Kasimu, R.; Aisa, H.A. Isolation of deoxypodophyllotoxin and podophyllotoxin from *Juniperus sabina* by high speed counter current chromatography. *Afinidad* **2016**, *73*, 236–239.

108. Muto, N.; Tomokuni, T.; Haramoto, M.; Tatemoto, H.; Nakanishi, T.; Inatomi, Y.; Murata, H.; Inada, A. Isolation of apoptosis and differentiation inducing substances toward human promyelocytic leukemia HL-60 cells from leaves of *Juniperus taxifolia*. *Biosci. Biotechnol. Biochem.* **2008**, *72*, 477–484. [CrossRef] [PubMed]

109. Jiang, Z.; Wu, M.; Miao, J.; Duan, H.; Zhang, S.; Chen, M.; Sun, L.; Wang, Y.; Zhang, X.; Zhu, X.; et al. Deoxypodophyllotoxin exerts both anti-angiogenic and vascular disrupting effects. *Int. J. Biochem. Cell Biol.* **2013**, *45*, 1710–1719. [CrossRef] [PubMed]

110. Wu, M.; Jiang, Z.; Duan, H.; Sun, L.; Zhang, S.; Chen, M.; Wang, Y.; Gao, Q.; Song, Y.; Zhu, X.; et al. Deoxypodophyllotoxin triggers necroptosis in human non-small cell lung cancer NCI-H460 cells. *Biomed. Pharmacother.* **2013**, *67*, 701–706. [CrossRef] [PubMed]

111. Wang, Y.-R.; Xu, Y.; Jiang, Z.-Z.; Guerram, M.; Wang, B.; Zhu, X.; Zhang, L.-Y. Deoxypodophyllotoxin induces G2/M cell cycle arrest and apoptosis in SGC-7901 cells and inhibits tumor growth in vivo. *Molecules* **2015**, *20*, 1661–1675. [CrossRef] [PubMed]

112. Wang, Y.; Wang, B.; Guerram, M.; Sun, L.; Shi, W.; Tian, C.; Zhu, X.; Jiang, Z.; Zhang, L. Deoxypodophyllotoxin suppresses tumor vasculature in HUVECs by promoting cytoskeleton remodeling through LKB1-AMPK dependent Rho A activation. *Oncotarget* **2015**, *6*, 29497–29512. [CrossRef] [PubMed]

113. Jin, M.; Moon, T.C.; Quan, Z.; Lee, E.; Kim, Y.K.; Yang, J.H.; Suh, S.-J.; Jeong, T.C.; Lee, S.H.; Kim, C.-H.; et al. The naturally occurring flavolignan, deoxypodophyllotoxin, inhibits lipopolysaccharide-induced iNOS expression through the NF-κB activation in RAW264.7 macrophage cells. *Biol. Pharm. Bull.* **2008**, *31*, 1312–1315. [CrossRef] [PubMed]

114. Guerram, M.; Jiang, Z.-Z.; Sun, L.; Zhu, X.; Zhang, L.-Y. Antineoplastic effects of deoxypodophyllotoxin, a potent cytotoxic agent of plant origin, on glioblastoma U-87 MG and SF126 cells. *Pharmacol. Rep.* **2015**, *67*, 245–252. [CrossRef] [PubMed]

115. Zang, X.; Wang, G.; Cai, Q.; Zheng, X.; Zhang, J.; Chen, Q.; Wu, B.; Zhu, X.; Hao, H.; Zhou, F. A promising microtubule inhibitor deoxypodophyllotoxin exhibits better efficacy to multidrug-resistant breast cancer than paclitaxel via avoiding efflux transport. *Drug Metab. Dispos.* **2018**, *46*, 542–551. [CrossRef] [PubMed]

116. Dumontet, C.; Jordan, M.A. Microtubule-binding agents: A dynamic field of cancer therapeutics. *Nat. Rev. Drug Discov.* **2010**, *9*, 790–803. [CrossRef] [PubMed]

117. Khaled, M.; Belaaloui, G.; Jiang, Z.-Z.; Zhu, X.; Zhang, L.-Y. Antitumor effect of deoxypodophyllotoxin on human breast cancer xenograft transplanted in BALB/c nude mice model. *J. Infect. Chemother.* **2016**, *22*, 692–696. [CrossRef] [PubMed]

118. Montecucco, A.; Zanetta, F.; Biamonti, G. Molecular mechanisms of etoposide. *EXCLI J.* **2015**, *14*, 95–108. [CrossRef] [PubMed]

119. Seca, A.M.L.; Pinto, D.C.G.A. Plant secondary metabolites as anticancer agents: Successes in clinical trials and therapeutic application. *Int. J. Mol. Sci.* **2018**, *19*, 263. [CrossRef] [PubMed]

120. Hu, S.; Zhou, Q.; Wu, W.-R.; Duan, Y.-X.; Gao, Z.-Y.; Li, Y.-W.; Lu, Q. Anticancer effect of deoxypodophyllotoxin induces apoptosis of human prostate cancer cells. *Oncol. Lett.* **2016**, *12*, 2918–2923. [CrossRef] [PubMed]

121. Fatokun, A.A.; Dawson, V.L.; Dawson, T.M. Parthanatos: Mitochondrial-linked mechanisms and therapeutic opportunities. *Br. J. Pharmacol.* **2014**, *171*, 2000–2016. [CrossRef] [PubMed]

122. Ma, D.; Lu, B.; Feng, C.; Wang, C.; Wang, Y.; Luo, T.; Feng, J.; Jia, H.; Chi, G.; Luo, Y.; et al. Deoxypodophyllotoxin triggers parthanatos in glioma cells via induction of excessive ROS. *Cancer Lett.* **2016**, *371*, 194–204. [CrossRef] [PubMed]

123. Ouyang, L.; Shi, Z.; Zhao, S.; Wang, F.-T.; Zhou, T.-T.; Liu, B.; Bao, J.-K. Programmed cell death pathways in cancer: A review of apoptosis, autophagy and programmed necrosis. *Cell Prolif.* **2012**, *45*, 487–498. [CrossRef] [PubMed]

124. Xu, J.; Wu, Y.; Lu, G.; Xie, S.; Ma, Z.; Chen, Z.; Shen, H.-M.; Xia, D. Importance of ROS-mediated autophagy in determining apoptotic cell death induced by physapubescin B. *Redox Biol.* **2017**, *12*, 198–207. [CrossRef] [PubMed]

125. Kenific, C.M.; Debnath, J. Cellular and metabolic functions for autophagy in cancer cells. *Trends Cell Biol.* **2015**, *25*, 37–45. [CrossRef] [PubMed]

126. Kim, S.-H.; Son, K.-M.; Kim, K.-Y.; Yu, S.-N.; Park, S.-G.; Kim, Y.-W.; Nam, H.-W.; Suh, J.-T.; Ji, J.-H.; Ahn, S.-C. Deoxypodophyllotoxin induces cytoprotective autophagy against apoptosis via inhibition of PI3K/AKT/mTOR pathway in osteosarcoma U2OS cells. *Pharmacol. Rep.* **2017**, *69*, 878–884. [CrossRef] [PubMed]

127. Chen, Y.; Zhao, K.; Liu, F.; Li, Y.; Zhong, Z.; Hong, S.; Liu, X.; Liu, L. Predicting antitumor effect of deoxypodophyllotoxin in NCI-H460 tumor-bearing mice on the basis of in vitro pharmacodynamics and a physiologically based pharmacokinetic-pharmacodynamic model. *Drug Metab. Dispos.* **2018**, *46*, 897–907. [CrossRef] [PubMed]

128. Guan, X.-W.; Xu, X.-H.; Feng, S.-L.; Tang, Z.-B.; Chen, S.-W.; Hui, L. Synthesis of hybrid 4-deoxypodophyllotoxin-5-fluorouracil compounds that inhibit cellular migration and induce cell cycle arrest. *Bioorg. Med. Chem. Lett.* **2016**, *26*, 1561–1566. [CrossRef] [PubMed]

129. Xiang, R.; Guan, X.-W.; Hui, L.; Jin, Y.-X.; Chen, S.-W. Investigation of the anti-angiogenesis effects induced by deoxypodophyllotoxin-5-FU conjugate C069 against HUVE cells. *Bioorg. Med. Chem. Lett.* **2017**, *27*, 713–717. [CrossRef] [PubMed]

130. Zhu, X.; Fu, J.; Tang, Y.; Gao, Y.; Zhang, S.; Guo, Q. Design and synthesis of novel 4'-demethyl-4-deoxypodophyllotoxin derivatives as potential anticancer agents. *Bioorg. Med. Chem. Lett.* **2016**, *26*, 1360–1364. [CrossRef] [PubMed]

131. Khaled, M.; Jiang, Z.-Z.; Zhang, L.-Y. Deoxypodophyllotoxin: A promising therapeutic agent from herbal medicine. *J. Ethnopharmacol.* **2013**, *149*, 24–34. [CrossRef] [PubMed]

132. Yang, Y.; Chen, Y.; Zhong, Z.-Y.; Zhang, J.; Li, F.; Jia, L.-L.; Liu, L.; Zhu, X.; Liu, X.-D. Validated LC–MS/MS assay for quantitative determination of deoxypodophyllotoxin in rat plasma and its application in pharmacokinetic study. *J. Pharm. Biomed. Anal.* **2014**, *88*, 410–415. [CrossRef] [PubMed]

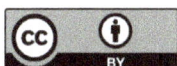

medicines

MDPI

Review

Scabiosa Genus: A Rich Source of Bioactive Metabolites

Diana C. G. A. Pinto [1],*, Naima Rahmouni [1,2], Noureddine Beghidja [2] and Artur M. S. Silva [1]

[1] Department of Chemistry and QOPNA, University of Aveiro, Campus de Santiago, 3810193 Aveiro, Portugal; rahmouni_na@yahoo.fr (N.R.); artur.silva@ua.pt (A.M.S.S.)

[2] Unité de Recherche et Valorisation des Ressources Naturelles, Molécules Bioactives et Analyse Physico-Chimiques et Biologiques, Université des Frères Mentouri Constantine 1, Constantine, Algérie; nourbeghidja@yahoo.fr

* Correspondence: diana@ua.pt; Tel.: +351-234-401-407

Received: 17 September 2018; Accepted: 6 October 2018; Published: 9 October 2018

Abstract: The genus *Scabiosa* (family Caprifoliaceae) is considered large (618 scientific plant names of species) although only 62 have accepted Latin binominal names. The majority of the *Scabiosa* species are widely distributed in the Mediterranean region and some *Scabiosa* species are used in traditional medicine systems. For instance, *Scabiosa columbaria* L. is used traditionally against diphtheria while *S. comosa* Fisch. Ex Roem. and Schult. is used in Mongolian and Tibetan traditional medical settings to treat liver diseases. The richness of *Scabiosa* species in secondary metabolites such as iridoids, flavonoids and pentacyclic triterpenoids may contribute to its use in folk medicine. Details on the most recent and relevant pharmacological in vivo studies on the bioactive secondary metabolites isolated from *Scabiosa* species will be summarized and thoroughly discussed.

Keywords: *Scabiosa*; flavonoids; iridoids; pentacyclic triterpenoids; antioxidant; anti-inflammatory; antibacterial; anticancer

---

1. Introduction

From the pharmacological perspective, plants are a treasure. In fact, the plant itself or its secondary metabolites are the source of useful drugs. They still are the main source of bioactive compounds that can be used directly in remedies, or can inspire the synthesis of more active derivatives [1]. Accordingly, the scientific community has renewed its interest in pharmacologically active natural compounds trying to find cures for many diseases. Moreover, herbal remedies are also enjoying a revival in developed countries, and in many countries, traditional medicine is the first option, or the only one, for health maintenance and disease prevention or treatment. In this context, *Scabiosa* species are significant due their applications in traditional medicine systems but also due to their richness in bioactive compounds.

Some authors indicate that there are 100 species of *Scabiosa* [2]. However, from the 618 scientific plant names listed, only 62 are accepted species names, with the others being synonyms and/or unresolved names [3]. Currently, genus *Scabiosa* belongs to the family of Caprifoliaceae, although in previous reports appears included in the Dipsacaceae family. However, due to morphological and molecular phylogenetic analyses, Dipsacaceae is no longer recognised as a family and their species are currently placed in the family Caprifoliaceae [4]. These changes in the species taxonomy, although understandable, may lead to several confusions in the literature and consequently increase difficulties to the phytochemical researchers (usually chemists).

All the botanic names referred herein were confirmed in "The Plant List" database [3] and the full-accepted binominal Latin scientific name will be displayed in the first citation while in subsequent citations *Scabiosa* will be indicated by the first capital letter and the authors' names will be omitted.

The genus *Scabiosa* L. is considered a large taxonomically complex genus with several species distributed in the Mediterranean Basin, Asia and southern Africa [5,6]. *Scabiosa* species are annual plants with basal leaf rosettes and leafy stems. They are mostly shrubs with variation in size from 10 cm, such as in *Scabiosa stellata* L. case [7], to 60 cm, in the case of *Scabiosa atropurpurea* L. [8]. Their flowers have crowded small heads with colours ranging from white to purple, which is why some are used as ornamental plants. *Scabiosa* species are also used as medicinal plants, and phytochemical studies revealed that they are able to produce interesting secondary metabolites some of which have proved to be promising therapeutic agents. Thus, herein we report and discuss the information on traditional medicine applications, bioactive natural compounds isolated from *Scabiosa* species, highlighting the more relevant metabolites and/or bioactivities.

2. *Scabiosa* Genus: Traditional and Pharmacological Applications

There are a few reports indicating that species from the genus *Scabiosa* are used in traditional medicine. However, it should be highlighted that several species need some taxonomic confirmations. For example, *Scabiosa succisa* L., which is reported to be used in the treatment of bronchitis, influenza and asthma [9], is also considered a synonym of *Succisa pratensis* Moench., the current accepted name for the species [10]. Besides, several publications still use the former family name Dipsacaceae. Despite the mentioned drawbacks, the use of *Scabiosa* species in traditional medicine systems is happening, particularly in China [11]. For instance, *Scabiosa atropurpurea* L. is used in Catalonia to treat measles and furuncles [12] and it is also a recognized medicinal plant in France [13]. Another species with several references is *Scabiosa columbaria* L. which is used to treat diphtheria [14] and respiratory infections, high blood pressure and uterine disorders [15,16], among others. Three other species are also reported to have medicinal uses, *Scabiosa stellata* L. is used to treat heel cracks [17] and both *Scabiosa tschilliensis* Grüning and *Scabiosa comosa* Fisch. Ex Roem. and Schult. are used to treat liver diseases [11]. Recently, the natural medicine Gurigumu-7, used in traditional Mongolian medicine and including in its composition the flowers of *S. comosa*, was evaluated for its hepatoprotective effect. Moreover, not only the beneficial effect and consequently clinical efficacy was proved but also that the more active fraction is the methanolic one, suggesting that the active compounds are the polar ones [18].

Studies to confirm the medicinal use and/or to find the pharmacological properties of *Scabiosa* species are reduced and mainly concerned with extracts activities. Moreover, the studied species are also restricted and toxicological evaluations were not accomplished. An overview of the evaluations carried out revealed that the majority are in vitro assessments of the antimicrobial and the antioxidant activities. Some in vitro cytotoxic evaluations were also reported, as well as the less common activities, such as anti-HCV [19], anti-tyrosinase [2] and acetylcholinesterase inhibition [20].

Although the biological assessments are scarce, some can be mentioned; for example, the ethanolic extract of *S. atropurpurea*, plant is used in Peru as an antibacterial remedy and its capacity to inhibit *Staphylococcus aureus* was evaluated. The minimum inhibitory concentration (MIC) obtained (32 mg/mL) indicates that the extract activity is not strong (only values below 5 mg/mL are considered strong) but it is an indication that it might have active metabolites [21]. As far as we are aware, the only in vivo study was performed with *S. atropurpurea* ethanolic extract, which demonstrated antihyperglycaemic, hepatoprotective and antioxidant activities [22].

Scabiosa hymettia Boiss. and Spruner: although not a medicinal plant it was evaluated to establish its antimicrobial value. The methanolic and chloroform extracts were evaluated against Gram-(+) and Gram-(−) bacteria and human pathogenic fungi. Both extracts showed moderate activity against the microorganisms used [23]. *Scabiosa columbaria* was also investigated for its antimicrobial activity and, therefore, this validated its use in traditional medicine [24]. Other medicinal plants such as *S. comosa* and *S. tschilliensis* were demonstrated to have in their chemical composition metabolites with antioxidant and anti-HCV activities. These results also validate their traditional use in several medicine systems [19]. Furthermore, the antioxidant capacity of *S. tschilliensis* was recently proved by other authors [25]. In the beginning of this year, another medicinal plant, *S. stellata*, was investigated in order to find its antioxidant, antibacterial and anti-tyrosinase power. Although the extracts exhibit some activity, it is clear that the pure compounds are more active [2]. Our final examples are the cases of *Scabiosa prolifera* L., for which in vitro antioxidant and cytotoxic activities were demonstrated [26], and *Scabiosa arenaria* Forssk., for which acetylcholinesterase inhibition, antioxidant activity [20] and antimicrobial activity [27] were reported. The problem with these results is in the species identification, both *S. prolifera* and *S. arenaria* are unresolved names [3].

3. Structural Pattern of the Secondary Metabolites Isolated from *Scabiosa* Species

To understand the pharmacological activity of the genus *Scabiosa* it is essential to perform detailed and extensive phytochemical investigations. In fact, the isolation of secondary metabolites and evaluation of their biological activities including the study of their mechanisms of action are important to validate (or not) the traditional medicine based in this species and, ultimately, to find new drugs. Up to date, only a few *Scabiosa* species were subjected to phytochemical studies, however, a wide spectrum of secondary metabolites has been identified and allowed to confirm that this genus species is rich in flavonoids and terpenoids. Herein, profiling analysis, although valuable research works, will not be discussed; this manuscript will be focused in the isolated secondary metabolites, emphasizing the flavonoid, iridoid and triterpenoid derivatives. The names of these constituents and the plants from which they were isolated are listed in Table 1 and their structures are depicted in Figures 1–4.

Table 1. Secondary metabolites isolated from *Scabiosa* species.

N°	Name [1]	Plant Part (Solvent)	Species
		Flavonoid Derivatives	
1	Apigenin [a]	Whole plant (MeOH) [28] Whole plant (EtOH) [29]	*S. tenuis* [28] *S. stellata* [29]
2	Astragallin [b]	Flowering plants (CH$_2$Cl$_2$/MeOH) [23]	*S. hymettia* [23]
3	Cynaroside [b]	Whole plant (MeOH or ButOH) [28] Aerial (leaves and stems) parts (EtOH) [22] Epigeal part (MeOH) [30]	*S. atropurpurea* [22] *S. olgae* [30] *S. tenuis* [28] *S. argentea* [28]
4	Diosmetin-7-*O*-β-glucoside [b]	Whole plant (ButOH) [28]	*S. argentea* [28]
5	Hyperin [3,b]	Whole plant (EtOH) [2]	*S. stellata* [2]
6	Isoorientin [b]	Whole plant (EtOH) [2,29] Whole plant (ButOH) [28]	*S. argentea* [28] *S. stellata* [2,29]
7	Isovitexin [b]	Whole plant (MeOH) [28]	*S. tenuis* [28]
8	Kaempferol-3-*O*-[3-*O*-acetyl-6-*O*-(*E*)-*p*-coumaroyl]-β-D-glucoside [b]	Flowering plants (CH$_2$Cl$_2$/MeOH) [23] Whole plant (EtOH) [31]	*S. hymettia* [23] *S. stellata* [31]
9	Lucenin [2,b]	Whole plant (EtOH) [29]	*S. stellata* [29]
10	Luteolin [a]	Aerial (leaves and stems) parts (EtOH) [22] Whole plant (EtOH) [29] Whole plant (MeOH) [28]	*S. atropurpurea* [22] *S. tenuis* [28] *S. stellata* [29]
11	Luteolin-7-*O*-β-gentiobioside [c]	Whole plant (MeOH or ButOH) [28]	*S. argentea* [28] *S. tenuis* [28]
12	Luteolin-7-*O*-rutinoside [c]	Aerial (leaves and stems) parts (EtOH) [22]	*S. atropurpurea* [22]
13	Quercetin [a]	Whole plant (ButOH) [28]	*S. argentea* [28]
14	Quercetin-3-*O*-arabinoside [b]	Whole plant (ButOH) [28]	*S. argentea* [28]
15	Quercetin-3-*O*-galactoside [b]	Whole plant (ButOH) [28]	*S. argentea* [28]

Table 1. *Cont.*

N°	Name [1]	Plant Part (Solvent)	Species
16	Swertiajaponin [b]	Whole plant (EtOH) [2]	*S. stellata* [2]
17	Tamarixetin 3-β-L-rhamnosyl-(1→2)[β-L-rhamnosyl-(1→6)]β-D-glucoside] [d]	Whole plant (EtOH) [29]	*S. stellata* [29]
18	Tiliroside [b]	Whole plant (EtOH) [29]	*S. stellata* [29]
19	Vitexin [b]	Whole plant (MeOH) [28]	*S. tenuis* [28]
	Terpenoid derivatives		
20	7-O-(E-Caffeoyl)sylvestroside I [c]	Whole plant (EtOH) [2]	*S. stellata* [2]
21	7-O-(E-p-Coumaroyl)sylvestroside I [c]	Whole plant (EtOH) [2]	*S. stellata* [2]
22	Cantleyoside [c]	Flowers (MeOH) [32] Whole plant (MeOH) [33]	*S. atropurpurea* [32] *S. variifolia* [33]
23	Eustomoruside [b]	Whole plant (EtOH) [2]	*S. stellata* [2]
24	Eustomoside [b]	Whole plant (EtOH) [2]	*S. stellata* [2]
25,26	Hookeroside A [g] and B [h]	Whole plant (MeOH) [34]	*S. tschilliensis* [34]
27	Loganic acid [b]	Flowering plants (CH₂Cl₂/MeOH) [23] Flowers (MeOH) [32] Whole plant (MeOH) [33]	*S. hymettia* [23] *S. atropurpurea* [32] *S. variifolia* [33]
28	Loganin [b]	Flowering plants (CH₂Cl₂/MeOH) [23] Flowers (MeOH) [32] Whole plant (MeOH) [33]	*S. hymettia* [23] *S. atropurpurea* [32] *S. variifolia* [33]
29	Palustroside III [d]	Whole plant (EtOH) [31]	*S. stellata* [31]
30 to 40	Scabiosaponin A [g], B [h], C [h], D [f], E [f], F [f], G [g], H [g], I [f], J [f] and K [g]	Whole plant (MeOH) [34]	*S. tschilliensis* [34]
41 to 48	Scabiostellatosides A [g], B [g], C [h], D [h], E [h], F [h], G [e] and H [d]	Whole plant (EtOH) [31]	*S. stellata* [31]
49 to 52	Scabrioside A [d], B [e], C [e], and D [f]	Roots (MeOH) [35]	*S. rotata* [35]
53	Septemfidoside [c]	Whole plant (EtOH) [2]	*S. stellata* [2]
54 to 60	Songoroside A [b], C [c], E [d], G [e], I [f], M [g] and O [h]	Roots (EtOH) [36]	*S. songarica* [2] [36]
61	Stigmasterol [a]	Whole plant (hexane) [37]	*S. stellata* [37]
62	Sweroside [b]	Whole plant (EtOH) [2] Flowers (MeOH) [32] Whole plant (MeOH) [33]	*S. atropurpurea* [32] *S. variifolia* [33] *S. stellata* [2]
63	Swertiamarin [b]	Flowering plants (CH₂Cl₂/MeOH) [23] Flowers (MeOH) [32] Whole plant (MeOH) [33]	*S. hymettia* [23] *S. atropurpurea* [32] *S. variifolia* [33]
64	Sylvestroside I [c]	Whole plant (EtOH) [2]	*S. stellata* [2]
65	Ursolic acid [a]	Whole plant (EtOH) [31] Whole plant (hexane) [37]	*S. stellata* [32,37]
66	β-Sitosterol-β-D-glucoside [b]	Whole plant (hexane) [37]	*S. stellata* [37]

[1] Compounds are presented in alphabetic order; [2] Although the authors indicate that they study the species *Scabiosa soongorica* Schrenk, we think that the current name is *Scabiosa songarica* Schrenk; [3] This name is a synonym of hyperoside, herein is indicated the name adopted by the authors [2]; [a] isolated as aglycones; [b] isolated as monoglycosides; [c] isolated as diglycosides; [d] isolated as triglycosides; [e] isolated as tetraglycosides; [f] isolated as pentaglycosides; [g] isolated as hexaglycosides; [h] isolated as heptaglycosides.

It should be also pointed out that only the phytochemical studies involving accepted *Scabiosa* species will be presented. In fact, this option may cause the elimination of some phytochemical studies but it is also a fact that ambiguous identifications automatically invalidate the reported results.

Important biological properties, such as anticancer [38], anti-inflammatory [39] and antioxidant [40] activities, just to mention a few [41] are the reason why flavone derivatives are included amongst the most important secondary metabolites. Subsequently the occurrence of these metabolites both as aglycones and glycosides in *Scabiosa* genus (Figure 1; Table 1) can explain and/or confirm the claimed medicinal properties. The structures analysis (Figure 1) demonstrates that the flavone derivatives isolated from species of the genus *Scabiosa* are mostly derivatives of apigenin, diosmetin and luteolin, which are polyhydroxylated flavones. The other derivatives reported are flavonol types such as kaempferol and quercetin derivatives, also polyhydroxylated compounds.

The occurrence of flavonoids in the *Scabiosa* genus is also important from the taxonomical point of view as has been shown by Perdetzoglou et al. [28], where the flavonoid types of compounds were used to establish that *Scabiosa argentea* L. and *Scabiosa tenuis* Spruner ex Boiss. are taxonomically independent species [28].

In other cases, such as the species *S. hymettia* were isolated two interesting kaempferol derivatives, astragallin (kaempferol 3-*O*-β-D-glucoside) **2** and the new natural compound kaempferol-3-*O*-[3-*O*-acetyl-6-*O*-(*E*)-*p*-coumaroyl]-β-D-glucoside **8** (Figure 1; Table 1), which may explain the plant antimicrobial activity [23]. Most recently several flavonoids were isolated from *S. stellata* [2,29], not only are found for the first time in the genus, but also confirm its richness in these metabolites. Interesting derivatives, such as compounds **5**, **9**, **16**, **17** and **18** (Figure 1; Table 1) may be responsible for the plant antioxidant activity [2,29]. Biological activities found in *S. atropurpurea* [22] could also be related to its flavonoid content, mostly luteolin derivatives, from which luteolin-7-*O*-rutinoside **12** (Figure 1; Table 1) can be highlighted because it was found for the first time in the genus [22].

Conversely, the recent work of Al-Qudah et al. [26], where the species identification is not properly presented, cannot be highlighted here, although the authors claimed the isolation of flavonoids that might explain the plant antioxidant activity.

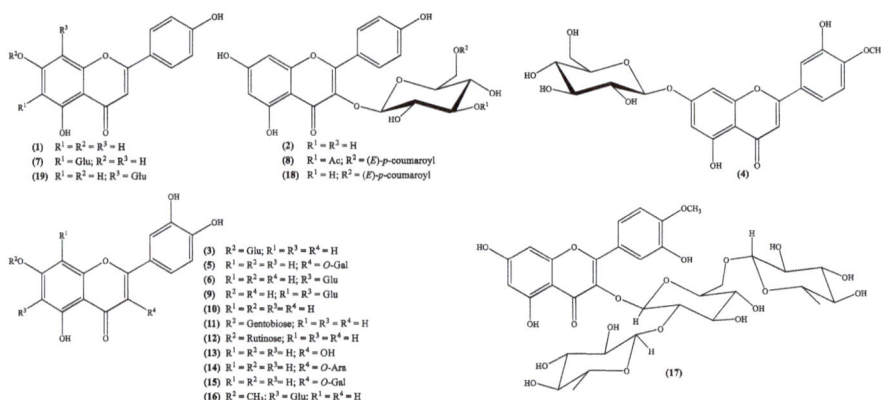

Figure 1. Flavonoids isolated from the genus *Scabiosa* (Ara = arabinose; Gal = galactose; Glu = glucose).

As far as we are aware only stigmasterol **61** and β-sitosterol-β-D-glucoside **66** (Figure 2) were isolated from *S. stellata* [37]. Lipophilic profiles could show the presence of steroid derivatives, but those works are not included in this review because herein are just referred the isolated and fully characterized metabolites. Nevertheless, the presence of β-sitosterol derivatives seems to be important due to their recognised biological properties and potential use in treatment of various illnesses [42], but also stigmasterol seems to be a potential therapeutic agent for neurodegenerative diseases [43]. Therefore, *S. stellata* can be a source of these important secondary metabolites.

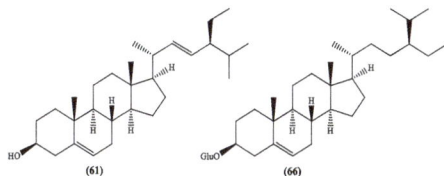

Figure 2. Steroids isolated from the genus *Scabiosa* (Glu = glucose).

Several biological activities are also attributed to iridoids [44,45] and this fact improves the value of *Scabiosa* species, which are recognized to produce several iridoid derivatives (Figure 3 and Table 1). The works that reported these metabolites are recent and the plants are well identified allowing their recommendation for further studies, in particular the species *S. hymettia* [23] and *Scabiosa variifolia* Boiss. [33], which are not reported as medicinal plants, but certainly can be a source of important bioactive compounds. In the cases of *S. atropurpurea* [32] and *S. stellata* [2] we are in the presence of medicinal plants, thus these studies are always recommended to validate their medicinal use. The recent reported new natural sylvestroside I 64 and derivatives, 7-*O*-(*E*-caffeoyl)sylvestroside I **20** and 7-*O*-(*E*-*p*-coumaroyl)sylvestroside I **21** (Figure 3) [2] can be highlighted, not only because they are new compounds but also due to the presence of a cinnamic acid moiety. This moiety is an important fragment of chlorogenic acids, which are known natural compounds and recognized for their important biological activities [46]. In fact, the chlorogenic derivatives 3,5-*O*-dicaffeoylquinic acid and 4,5-*O*-dicaffeoylquinic acid were recently isolated from *S. stellata* [2,29] and, to find reports about the isolation of these metabolites we have to go back to the work of Zemtsova et al. where they claimed the isolation of chlorogenic acid from *Scabiosa olgae* Albov [30] and from *Scabiosa bipinnata* C. Koch [47]. Another relevance of the sylvestroside I **64** and derivatives isolated is the moderate cytotoxic activity (IC$_{50}$ 35.9 µg/mL) against brosarcoma cell lines (HT1080) shown by 7-*O*-(*E*-caffeoyl) sylvestroside I **20** [2], result that once again point out the *S. stellata* value as source of interesting secondary metabolites.

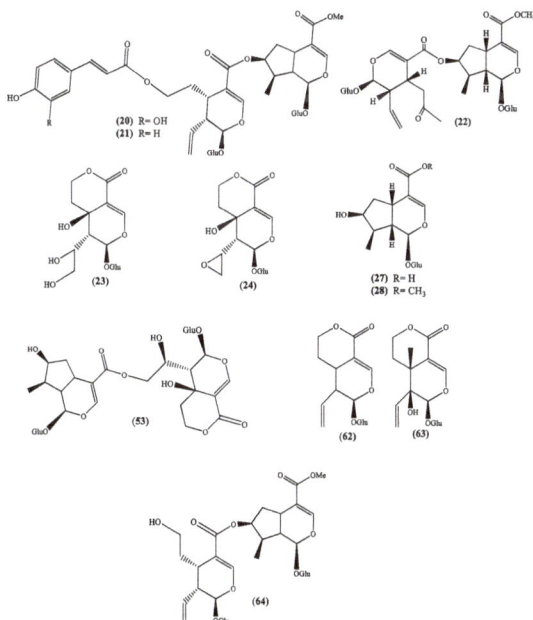

Figure 3. Iridoids isolated from the genus *Scabiosa* (Glu = glucose).

Although the number of *Sacabiosa* species studied from the phytochemical point of view is scarce, one thing is clear; this genus species produces terpenoids such as the above mentioned but also pentacyclic triterpenoids. Terpenoids is one of the largest and most diverse classes of secondary metabolites produced by plants where they play several functions [48], but they are also used by humans in the pharmaceutical industry [49]. From the biological perspective, pentacyclic triterpenoids can be highlighted due to their anti-inflammatory [50] and the antitumor [51,52] activities, but their natural occurrence is also extensive [53].

The richness of the *Scabiosa* species in pentacyclic triterpenoids seems to be obvious (Figure 4 and Table 1) and it is evident that almost all the isolated pentacyclic triterpenoids are saponins. This seems to be a characteristic of the genus *Scabiosa*, being the main aglycones oleanolic and pomolic acids, with glucose, xylose, rhamnose and arabinose as sugars (Figure 4). It should be stressed that, among the several biological activities reported for oleanolic acid [54], its potential as a cancer therapy drug [55] is the most significant. Pomolic acid, is a less studied pentacyclic triterpenoid, but nevertheless showed anti-HIV activity [54].

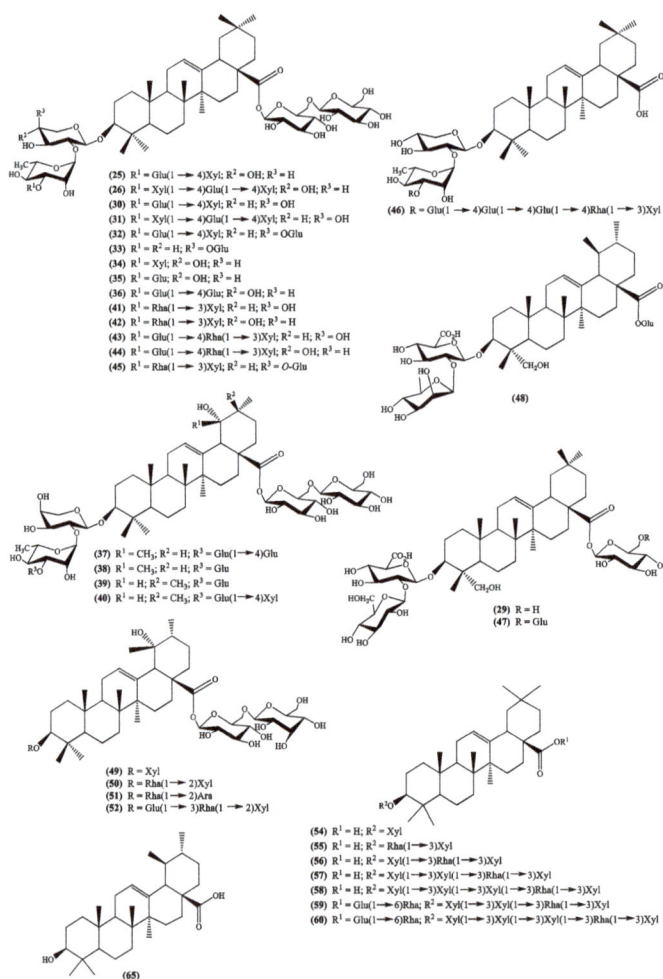

(25) R¹ = Glu(1 → 4)Xyl; R² = OH; R³ = H
(26) R¹ = Xyl(1 → 4)Glu(1 → 4)Xyl; R² = OH; R³ = H
(30) R¹ = Glu(1 → 4)Xyl; R² = H; R³ = OH
(31) R¹ = Xyl(1 → 4)Glu(1 → 4)Xyl; R² = H; R³ = OH
(32) R¹ = Glu(1 → 4)Xyl; R² = H; R³ = OGlu
(33) R¹ = R² = H; R³ = OGlu
(34) R¹ = Xyl; R² = OH; R³ = H
(35) R¹ = Glu; R² = OH; R³ = H
(36) R¹ = Glu(1 → 4)Glu; R² = OH; R³ = H
(41) R¹ = Rha(1 → 3)Xyl; R² = H; R³ = OH
(42) R¹ = Rha(1 → 3)Xyl; R² = OH; R³ = H
(43) R¹ = Glu(1 → 4)Rha(1 → 3)Xyl; R² = H; R³ = OH
(44) R¹ = Glu(1 → 4)Rha(1 → 3)Xyl; R² = OH; R³ = H
(45) R¹ = Rha(1 → 3)Xyl; R² = H; R³ = O-Glu

(46) R = Glu(1 → 4)Glu(1 → 4)Glu(1 → 4)Rha(1 → 3)Xyl

(48)

(37) R¹ = CH₃; R² = H; R³ = Glu(1→4)Glu
(38) R¹ = CH₃; R² = H; R³ = Glu
(39) R¹ = H; R² = CH₃; R³ = Glu
(40) R¹ = H; R² = CH₃; R³ = Glu(1→4)Xyl

(29) R = H
(47) R = Glu

(49) R = Xyl
(50) R = Rha(1 → 2)Xyl
(51) R = Rha(1 → 2)Ara
(52) R = Glu(1 → 3)Rha(1 → 2)Xyl

(54) R¹ = H; R² = Xyl
(55) R¹ = H; R² = Rha(1→3)Xyl
(56) R¹ = H; R² = Xyl(1→3)Rha(1→3)Xyl
(57) R¹ = H; R² = Xyl(1→3)Xyl(1→3)Rha(1→3)Xyl
(58) R¹ = H; R² = Xyl(1→3)Xyl(1→3)Rha(1→3)Xyl
(59) R¹ = Glu(1→6)Rha; R² = Xyl(1→3)Xyl(1→3)Rha(1→3)Xyl
(60) R¹ = Glu(1→6)Rha; R² = Xyl(1→3)Xyl(1→3)Xyl(1→3)Rha(1→3)Xyl

(65)

Figure 4. Pentacyclic triterpenoids isolated from the genus *Scabiosa* (Ara = arabinose; Gal = galactose; Glu = glucose; Rha = rhamnose; Xyl = xylose).

The literature survey demonstrates that *S. tschilliensis* can be a good source of pentacyclic triterpenoids acids, such as oleanolic and pomolic (Figure 4 and Table 1), through a cleavage of the sugar moieties. Moreover, the presence of these secondary metabolites may explain the plant medicinal use.

Scabiosa rotata M.Bieb., as far as we are aware, is not used in folk medicine but is also a good source of pomolic acid (Figure 4 and Table 1). On the other hand, *S. songarica* Schrenk and the medicinal plant *S. stellata* can be regarded as good sources of oleanolic acid (Figure 4 and Table 1).

To the extent that we could investigate, *S. stellata* seems to be the species presenting more diversity in the saponins aglycones. Along with oleanolic acid, ursolic acid and hederagenin derivatives were isolated (Figure 4 and Table 1).

4. In Vivo Assessments of Nominated Metabolites

The aim of this review is an update on the information about *Scabiosa* species secondary metabolites as well as their biological potential. In fact, from the above-mentioned secondary metabolites, some (e.g., iridoids, flavonoids and pentacyclic triterpenoids) can be highlighted, due to their recognized activities. Unfortunately, many studies involve extracts or are in vitro assessments. Herein, we select the most interesting secondary metabolites or their aglycones for which in vivo assessments were reported. Consequently, the activities mentioned herein will be also limited to the ones that were evaluated in vivo.

4.1. Flavonoid-Type Metabolites

The analysis of the flavonoids isolated from *Scabiosa* genus (Figure 1 and Table 1) point toward that their occurrence is in the glycoside form. However, the main aglycones (apigenin, diosmetin, kaempferol, luteolin and quercetin) biological potential is well known. Tamarixetin, the aglycone of compound **17**, may be the less known one and consequently less studied. Nevertheless, its in vitro ability to inhibit the proliferation of leukemia cells [56] and enhancement of the Ca^{2+} transients, both in vitro and in vivo [57], have been demonstrated. Moreover, the 3-O-β-D-glucopyranoside derivative reveals ability to, in vivo, inhibit the matrix metalloproteinase-9, that can be regarded as potential drug to treat gastric ulceration [58].

Tiliroside **18** (Figure 1) is a kaempferol glycoside derivative whose structure was elucidated in 1964 [59] and was found first in *Tilia* species but nowadays is present in several plants. Through the years, this flavonol type compound gathered the scientific community's interest and interesting in vitro activities were reported. These include antidiabetic activity [60,61], inhibition of neuroinflammation in murine cultured microglial cells BV2 (cells immortalized after infection with a recombinant retrovirus) [62] and antiproliferative properties on human breast cancer cell lines (T47D and MCF7) [63]. The in vivo studies are less, nonetheless some can be emphasized. For example, Barbosa et al. [64] in their efforts to validate the use of medicinal plants to treat diarrhea, performed some in vivo antiprotozoal assessments, against the protozoa *Giardia lamblia*. Among the tested flavonoids is tiliroside **18**, for which an ED_{50} value of 1.429 μmol/kg was obtained, a value that is similar to the one obtained with metronidazole (ED_{50} 1.134 μmol/kg), one of the positive controls used in the study. Nevertheless, is less active than the other positive control, emetine (ED_{50} 0.351 μmol/kg) [64]. The tiliroside **18** anti-inflammatory potential was also evaluated and an in vivo study showed that it can inhibit the mouse paw oedema (ED_{50} = 35.6 mg/kg) and the mouse ear inflammation (ED_{50} = 357 Ag/ear) [65]. The inhibition of the enzymatic and non-enzymatic lipid peroxidation (IC_{50} = 12.6 and 28 μM, respectively) and the scavenger properties, both in the superoxide radical (IC_{50} = 21.3 μM) and in the DPPH assay (IC_{50} = 6 μM), suggest that tiliroside **18** anti-inflammatory activity is related to its antioxidant activity [65]. More recently, Jin et al. [66] proposed that tiliroside **18** anti-inflammatory activity can be explained through its involvement in the downregulation of the inducible nitric oxide synthase (iNOS) and cyclooxygenase-2 (COX-2) protein expression levels and in the inactivation of mitogen-activated protein kinase (MAPK) signaling pathway [66].

Finally, the in vivo antihypertensive and vasorelaxant effects of tiliroside **18** were also evaluated and the mechanism of action studied [67]. The findings suggest that tiliroside **18** induces a decrease in blood pressure and through the blockage blockade of Ca^{2+} channels (Ca_V 1.2) in vascular smooth muscle cells (VSMCs) promotes the vasorelaxant effect [67].

As far as we could find, vitexin **19** (Figure 1) was the first C-glycoside flavonoid isolated from natural sources [68], and accordingly to the publication, was isolated from *Vitex littoralis*, which is a synonym of *Vitex parviflora* A.Juss. [3]. Vitexin **19**, an apiginin glycoside, is among the flavonoid derivatives found in *Scabiosa* species, the most studied one. It is included in structure activity relationships [69] or even used as inspiration to develop new active compounds [70].

Although, herein we are disclosing the more recent in vivo studies, it is a surprise that this metabolite's in vivo evaluation started in 1995 with a study of its antithyroid effects, concluding that can be used to prevent goiter [71]. The more recent studies include antimicrobial activity against *Pseudomonas aeruginosa*, for which the vitexin **19** activity was moderated [72], cardioprotective effects, which demonstrated that vitexin **19** mitigated myocardial ischemia reperfusion injury and suppressed apoptosis and autophagy in myocardium cells [73], and its protection of dopaminergic neurons, which suggests its use in Parkinson's disease therapy [74].

As expected, anti-inflammatory in vivo studies were also recently reported; from those we emphasize the Rosa et al. work [75] due to the detailed analysis that included the cytotoxicity evaluation. The authors tested several doses and confirm that vitexin **19** was not cytotoxic towards macrophage normal cell line (RAW 264.7) and established that its anti-inflammatory action was due to the inactivation of pro-inflammatory pathways [75]. In fact, the anti-inflammatory activity of vitexin **19** seems to be the related with its possible use to alleviate epilepsy [76].

As a final point, the anticancer evaluations suggest that vitexin **19** antitumor efficacy can be related to its ability to activate the c-Jun NH_2-terminal kinase-signaling pathway. Consequently, vitexin **19** can be regarded as a possible drug to treat hepatocellular carcinoma [77] or colorectal cancer [78,79]. Moreover, a recent detailed review [80] disclosed the potential of this flavonoid towards is use in cancer therapy.

Taken together, the above-mentioned findings seem to clearly state that *Scabiosa* species produce important bioactive flavonoids that can explain their medicinal use but also can incentive more investigations.

4.2. Iridoid Type Metabolites

Likewise, the flavonoids, the iridoids isolated from *Scabiosa* genus (Figure 3 and Table 1) are glycosylated. Actually, a recent study showed that these glycosides can be considered responsible for the hepatoprotective effect of the Gentianaceae herbs extracts [81], extracts that are commonly used as food additives. An in vitro assay established that a fraction of the *Pterocephalus hookeri* (C.B. Clarke) Höeck ethanolic extract presents analgesic and anti-inflammatory activities, and these activities were attributed to the fraction of the main constituents, the bis-iridoid type compounds [82].

From the analysis of some reviews involving iridoids activity, it can be noticed that a few examples, from which logonin **28** and swertiamarin **63** (Figure 3) can be highlighted, are being evaluated in vivo studies. Anti-inflammatory [83] and antidiabetic [84] evaluations of both the above-mentioned iridoids and the anti-advanced glycation end products formation potential of logon in **28** [85] are important examples, moreover if we consider the fact that these iridoids can be found in *Scabiosa* species.

Swertiamarin **63** is an interesting compound for which several in vivo studies were reported. The first example reports on its ability to reduce the sensitivity to painful stimuli [86], which is similar to the one showed by paracetamol. In the three in vivo studied models, swertiamarin **63** was shown to be active in a dose-dependent manner, but also shown to be safe up to 2000 mg/kg bw [86]. Later on, it was confirmed that swertiamarin 63 can be used to treat type II diabetes mellitus because it can regulate the peroxisome proliferator-activated receptor gamma (PPAR-γ) and increases insulin sensitivity [87]. Recently Mir and coworkers [88] demonstrated, in vivo, that swertiamarin **63** can inhibit both α-amylase and α-glucosidase which are enzymes involved in carbohydrate metabolism. This study accentuates the antidiabetic therapeutic potential of this iridoid glucoside.

In 2014, two interesting and complementary works of the Ignacimuthu research group [89,90], aiming to validated the medicinal properties of a plant used in Indian traditional medicine, evaluated the in vivo anti-inflammatory activity of swertiamarin **63**. The first aspect to be highlighted is the fact that no adverse effects were detected with a dose up to 500 mg/kg bw [89], however, the dosages used in the studies were much lower and also had beneficial effects. The combined assays (in vivo, in vitro and in silico) suggest that swertiamarin **63** anti-inflammatory effect is accomplished through the suppressing of pro-inflammatory mediators and inducing anti-inflammatory mediators such as helper T cells cytokines (Th2) [89]. Furthermore, the authors showed that swertiamarin **63** decreases the levels of nuclear factor kappa-light-chain-enhancer of activated B cells (NF-κB) and phospho-IκB alpha (p-IκBα), attenuates the release of both phospho-signal transducer and activator of transcription 3 (p-STAT3) and phospho-Janus kinase 2 (p-JAK2) levels [90]. Thus, swertiamarin **63** and/or its derivatives can become interesting therapeutics to treat rheumatoid arthritis.

Recently, this research group added more information about the swertiamarin 63 effects on and/or prevention of rheumatoid arthritis [91]. Again, the authors joined several methodologies to assess the biological activity, including an in vivo model (Freund's complete adjuvant), which is the type of assessment that is discussed herein. Receptor activator of nuclear factor κB ligand (RANKL) and its receptor RANK, osteoprotegerin (OPG) and tartrate resistant acid phosphatase (TRAP) are recognized osteoclastogenis markers, a reason why their levels were measured in this study. The in vivo results showed that a treatment with swertiamarin **63** decreases the expression of the markers RANKL/RANK and TRAP and increases the OPG levels and these good results suggest that the anti-osteoclastogenic activity of swertiamarin **63** raises its potential use in rheumatoid arthritis treatment [91].

The antimicrobial activity of swertiamarin **63** was also reported [92]; however, the in vivo studies, as far as we could find, are limited. An interesting in vivo study was recently reported by Bodakhe and coworkers [93] where they disclose the synergistic effect of swertiamarin **63** against *Plasmodium berghei*. The results showed that the use of this iridoid improves the activity; however, its use to treat malaria should be investigated further.

Sweroside **62**, similar in structure (Figure 3 and Table 1) and in natural occurrence to swertiamarin **63** is, however, less evaluated in in vivo models. As far as we are aware, two in vivo studies were recently published, the evaluation of sweroside **62** ability to inhibit the body pigmentation and the tyrosinase activity, using zebrafish in vivo model [94], and inhibit human leukemia cell lines (HL-60) growth in xenograft mouse models [95]. Both studies are recent and preliminary, nevertheless are a confirmation that sweroside **62** biological properties may also be as remarkable as the ones found for swertiamarin **63**.

Naturally, our last example is logonin **28** (Figure 3 and Table 1), the other iridoid found in *Scabiosa* species that has been the focus of several in vivo studies. The first in vivo study that we could find involves the interesting antiamnesic activity [96] through the inhibition of acetylcholinesterase, result that indicates the potential therapeutic use of logonin **28** in Alzheimer's disease treatment. This neuroprotective potential was observed by other research group [97] and later on was also detected in diabetic male rats [98]. More recently, was demonstrated the logonin **28** potential to be used in the treatment of neuromuscular diseases [99] through the increase of the survival motor neuron (SMN) protein level.

The logonin **28** beneficial effect on in vivo studies involving mice with induced diabetes was also observed in the diabetic nephropathy control [100,101]. Both works suggest that logonin **28** can be a good remedy to treat this disease, through the inhibition of connective tissue growth factor (CTGF) expression [100], or the inhibition of advanced glycation end-product (AGE) pathways [101]. In our opinion, the beneficial effects are evident but the medicinal implementation needs at least toxicological studies.

Our final examples are two, very recent works, that demonstrate the potential of logonin **28** to control inflammations. One article shows that this iridoid inhibits the substance P neurokinin-1 receptor and in doing so prevents the bladder hyperactivity [102]. Moreover, the mechanism of action seems to be through the downregulation of inflammatory leukocytes, decrease of induce intercellular adhesion molecule-1 (ICAM-1) expression and decrease of reactive oxygen species (ROS) production. All these aspects suggest an anti-inflammatory potential of logonin **28** [102]. The other example is a combination of in vitro and in vivo assays where the authors demonstrated that logonin **28** can relieve the inflammation stress [103].

The above mention findings for the chosen iridoids indicate that *Scabiosa* species medicinal use maybe due to these important bioactive secondary metabolites.

4.3. Pentacyclic Triterpenoid Type Metabolites

As can be seen in Figure 4, *Scabiosa* genus is rich in saponins where the main aglycones are oleanolic and pomolic acids, nonetheless, ursolic acid and hederagenin derivatives can also be found. These saponins in vivo assessments are scarce and the only aglycone until now isolated is the ursolic acid **65** (Figure 4), however, for the above mentioned aglycones, several in vivo studies reporting interesting results were published. For example, pomolic acid anti-inflammatory and apoptotic activities [104] and the antitumor activity of hederagenin [105] or macranthoside B, a natural hederagenin glycoside, [106] or hederagenin synthetic derivatives [107].

Nevertheless, ursolic and oleanolic acids are the most studied ones due to their recognized biological properties. If ursolic acid or its derivatives are not abundant in *Scabiosa* genus the same cannot be said about oleanolic acid and its glycoside derivatives, which are ubiquitous in this genus. Therefore, it is obvious that this genus can be an important source of this pentacyclic triterpenoid, reason why it is interesting to notice that recent biological assays involve oleanolic acid in vivo studies. In fact, the therapeutic potential of oleanolic acid was recently reviewed [108] and from that detailed work it is possible to conclude that indeed this natural compound is a good candidate to become a medicine. Due to this biological potential, the in vivo evaluations are increasing and in the last three years several publications involving the usual activities, such as antitumor [109–111], antidiabetic [112–115], anti-malarial [116] and anti-atherosclerosis [117] or the less common such as its beneficial effect on wound healing and regeneration [118] and the inhibition of matrix metalloproteinase-3 (MMP-3) production [119] have been published. It should be highlighted that this enzyme is involved in the articular cartilage destruction, thus oleanolic acid may be a potential drug to be used in the prevention of osteoarthritis cartilage damage [119].

Oleanolic acid has, however, a problem that might prevent its use in medicine; its low solubility in water and consequently its low bioavailability. Recent works have been devoted to solving this vital aspect [120–123] and some attention is being given to the use of nanoparticles [122,123]. Although, as was referred above, the genus *Scabiosa* is richer in this acid saponins, it cannot be ignored that the species can deliver oleanolic acid if used in the diet or be a source to isolate it.

5. Conclusions

At the end of this survey, it is possible to recognize the richness of *Scabiosa* genus in bioactive secondary metabolites. From which flavonoids and iridoids can be highlighted both from the biological properties previously revealed, but also for the in vivo assays already performed. In fact, from the secondary metabolites found in *Scabiosa* species these are the most evaluated ones. Moreover, these metabolites can validate some traditional uses but also can encourage other uses; in fact, these metabolites suggest that *Scabiosa* species can have interesting effects such as anti-inflammatory and anti-cancer activities, just to mention a few. Not only can these metabolites enlarge the traditional use of *Scabiosa* species but also can inspire the development of new drugs with therapeutic improvements.

Saponins are also abundant in the *Scabiosa* genus and are important secondary metabolites. However, their biological evaluations in vivo are restricted to their aglycones. This prompted us to suggest that these saponis should be evaluated to find out their biological potential and maybe find new drugs. These secondary metabolites can also be evaluated from the nutritional value and maybe prompt the use of *Scabiosa* species in food preparations.

It is also important to highlight the fact that, in the last few years, several new natural compounds were isolated from the *Scabiosa* species. Furthermore, the survey herein presented also demonstrates that several species are, from the phytochemical point of view, neglected. These findings should encourage further studies that can reveal the medicinal potential of this genus species. Indeed, *Scabiosa* species may be a good source of new bioactive natural compounds.

Author Contributions: N.R., N.B. and D.C.G.A.P. performed the literature survey; D.C.G.A.P. and A.M.S.S. conceived and wrote the paper.

Funding: This research was funded by Portuguese National Funds, through FCT—Fundação para a Ciência e a Tecnologia, and as applicable co-financed by the FEDER within the PT2020 Partnership Agreement by funding the Organic Chemistry Research Unit (QOPNA) (UID/QUI/00062/2013). Also by the Algerian MESRS (Ministère de l'Enseignement Supérieure et la Recherche Scientifique) via PNE (Programme National Exceptionnel) for financial support, namely the NR displacement.

Acknowledgments: Thanks are due to the University of Aveiro, to the FCT/MEC and POPH/FSE for the financial support of the QOPNA research Unit. Thanks are also due to the Algerian MESRS (Ministère de l'Enseignement Supérieure et la Recherche Scientifique) for financial support.

Conflicts of Interest: The authors declare no conflict of interest.

References

1. Cragg, G.M.; Newman, D.J. Natural products: A continuing source of novel drug leads. *Biochim. Biophys. Acta* **2013**, *1847*, 3670–3695. [CrossRef] [PubMed]
2. Lehbili, M.; Magid, A.A.; Hubert, J.; Kabouche, A.; Voutquenne-Nazabadioko, L.; Renault, J.-H.; Nuzillard, J.-M.; Morjani, H.; Abedini, A.; Gangloff, S.C.; et al. Two new bis-iridoids isolated from *Scabiosa stellata* and their antibacterial, antioxidant, anti-tyrosinase and cytotoxic activities. *Fitoterapia* **2018**, *125*, 41–48. [CrossRef] [PubMed]
3. The Plant List Database. Available online: http://www.theplantlist.org/tpl1.1/search?q=Scabiosa (accessed on 10 September 2018).
4. George, E.B.; Ronald, J.T. *Toxic Plants of North America*; John Wiley and Sons: Oxford, UK, 2013; pp. 319–322.
5. Carlson, S.E.; Linder, P.H.; Donoghue, M.J. The historical biogeography of *Scabiosa* (dipsacaceae): Implications for Old World plant disjunctions. *J. Biogeogr.* **2012**, *39*, 1086–1100. [CrossRef]
6. Mostafa, E.-N.; Sedigheh, N.-S. Palynological study of some Iranian species of *Scabiosa* L. (Caprifoliaceae). *Bangladesh J. Plant Taxon.* **2016**, *23*, 215–222. [CrossRef]
7. Quezel, P.; Santa, S. *Nouvelle Flore de l'Algérie et des Régions Désertiques Méridionales*; du CNRS: Paris, France, 1963; pp. 890–893.
8. Erarslan, Z.B.; Yeşil, Y. The anatomical properties of *Scabiosa atropurpurea* L. (Caprifoliaceae). *Istanbul J. Pharm.* **2018**, *48*, 1–5.
9. Girre, L. Connaître et Reconnaître Les Plantes Médicinales in Bulletin des Bibliothèques de France (BBF). Available online: http://bbf.enssib.fr/consulter/bbf-1980-07-0373-023 (accessed on 6 October 2018).
10. Ferrer-Gallego, P.P. Lectotypification of Linnaean names in the genus *Scabiosa* (Dipsacaceae). *Taxon* **2014**, *63*, 1353–1357. [CrossRef]
11. Chinese Pharmacopoeia Committee. *Drug Standards of Ministry of Public Health of China (Mongolian medicine Fascicule)*; Chemical Industry Press: Beijing, China, 1998.
12. Bonet, M.À.; Parada, M.; Selga, A.; Vallès, J. Studies on pharmaceutical ethnobotany in the regions of L'Alt Empordà and Les Guilleries (Catalonia, Iberian Peninsula). *J. Ethnopharmacol.* **1999**, *68*, 145–168. [CrossRef]
13. Gras, A.; Garnatje, T.; Ibáñez, N.; López-Pujol, J.; Nualart, N.; Vallès, J. Medicinal plant uses and names from the herbarium of Francesc Bolòs (1773–1844). *J. Ethnopharmacol.* **2017**, *204*, 142–168. [CrossRef] [PubMed]
14. Rigat, M.; Bonet, M.À.; Garcia, S.; Garnatje, T.; Vallès, J. Studies on pharmaceutical ethnobotany in the high river Ter valley (Pyrenees, Catalonia, Iberian Peninsula). *J. Ethnopharmacol.* **2007**, *113*, 267–277. [CrossRef] [PubMed]

15. Kose, L.S.; Moteetee, A.; Vuuren, S.V. Ethnobotanical survey of medicinal plants used in the Maseru district of Lesotho. *J. Ethnopharmacol.* **2015**, *170*, 184–200. [CrossRef] [PubMed]

16. Moteetee, A.; Kose, L.S. Medicinal plants used in Lesotho for treatment of reproductive and post reproductive problems. *J. Ethnopharmacol.* **2016**, *194*, 827–849. [CrossRef] [PubMed]

17. Bammi, J.; Douira, A. Les plantes médicinales dans la forêt de L'Achach (Plateau Central, Maroc). *Acta Bot. Malacit.* **2002**, *27*, 131–145.

18. Xu, H.; Ma, Q.; Ma, J.; Wu, Z.; Wang, Y.; Ma, C. Hepato-protective effects and chemical constituents of a bioactive fraction of the traditional compound medicine-Gurigumu-7. *BMC Complement. Altern. Med.* **2016**, *16*, 179. [CrossRef] [PubMed]

19. Ma, J.N.; Bolraa, S.; Ji, M.; He, Q.Q.; Ma, C.M. Quantification and antioxidant and anti-HCV activities of the constituents from the inflorescences of *Scabiosa comosa* and *S. tschilliensis*. *Nat. Prod. Res.* **2016**, *30*, 590–594. [CrossRef] [PubMed]

20. Hlila, M.B.; Mosbah, H.; Mssada, K.; Jannet, H.B.; Aouni, M.; Selmi, B. Acetylcholinesterase inhibitory and antioxidante properties of roots extracts from the Tunisian *Scabiosa arenaria* Forssk. *Ind. Crop. Prod.* **2015**, *67*, 62–69. [CrossRef]

21. Bussmann, R.W.; Malca-García, G.; Glenn, A.; Sharon, D.; Chait, G.; Díaz, D.; Pourmand, K.; Jonat, B.; Somogy, S.; Guardado, G.; et al. Minimum inhibitory concentrations of medicinal plants used in Northern Peru as antibacterial remedies. *J. Ethnopharmacol.* **2010**, *132*, 101–108. [CrossRef] [PubMed]

22. Elhawary, S.S.; Eltantawy, M.E.; Sleem, A.A.; Abdallah, H.M.; Mohamed, N.M. Investigation of phenolic content and biological activities of *Scabiosa atropurpurea* L. *World Appl. Sci. J.* **2011**, *15*, 311–317.

23. Christopoulou, C.; Graikou, K.; Chinou, I. Chemosystematic value of chemical constituents from *Scabiosa hymettia* (Dipsacaceae). *Chem. Biodivers.* **2008**, *5*, 318–323. [CrossRef] [PubMed]

24. Vuuren, S.F.v.; Naidoo, D. An antimicrobial investigation of plants used traditionally in southern Africa to treat sexually transmitted infections. *J. Ethnopharmacol.* **2010**, *130*, 552–558. [CrossRef] [PubMed]

25. Wang, J.; Liu, K.; Li, X.; Bi, K.; Zhang, Y.; Huang, J.; Zhang, R. Variation of active constituents and antioxidant activity in *Scabiosa tschiliensis* Grüning from different stages. *J. Food Sci. Technol.* **2017**, *54*, 2288–2295. [CrossRef] [PubMed]

26. Al-Qudah, M.A.; Otoom, N.K.; Al-Jaber, H.; Saleh, A.M.; Zarga, M.H.A.; Afifi, F.U.; Orabi, S.T.A. New flavonol glycoside from *Scabiosa prolifera* L. aerial parts with in vitro antioxidant and cytotoxic activities. *Nat. Prod. Res.* **2017**, *31*, 2865–2874. [CrossRef] [PubMed]

27. Hlila, B.M.; Mosbah, H.; Majouli, K.; Nejma, A.B.; Jannet, H.B.; Mastouri, M.; Aouni, M.; Selmi, B. Antimicrobial activity of *Scabiosa arenaria* Forssk. extracts and pure compounds using bioguided fractionation. *Chem. Biodivers.* **2016**, *13*, 1262–1272. [CrossRef] [PubMed]

28. Perdetzoglou, D.; Skaltsa, H.; Tzakou, O.; Harval, C. Comparative phytochemical and morphological study of two species of the *Scabiosa* L. genus. *Feddes Repert.* **1994**, *105*, 157–165. [CrossRef]

29. Rahmouni, N.; Pinto, D.C.G.A.; Beghidja, N.; Benayache, S.; Silva, A.M.S. *Scabiosa stellata* L. phenolic content clarifies its antioxidant activity. *Molecules* **2018**, *23*, 1285. [CrossRef] [PubMed]

30. Zemtsova, G.N.; Bandyukova, V.A.; Dzhumyrko, S.F. Flavones and phenolic acids of *Scabiosa olgae. Chem. Nat. Compd.* **1972**, *8*, 662. [CrossRef]

31. Lehbili, M.; Magid, A.A.; Kabouche, A.; Voutquenne-Nazabadioko, L.; Morjani, H.; Harakat, D.; Kabouche, Z. Triterpenoid saponins from *Scabiosa stellata* collected in North-eastern Algeria. *Phytochemistry* **2018**, *150*, 40–49. [CrossRef] [PubMed]

32. Polat, E.; Alankus-Caliskan, O.; Karayildirim, T.; Bedir, E. Iridoids from *Scabiosa atropurpurea* L. subsp. *maritima* Arc. (L.). *Biochem. Syst. Ecol.* **2010**, *38*, 253–255. [CrossRef]

33. Papalexandrou, A.; Magiatis, P.; Perdetzoglou, D.; Skaltsounis, A.L.; Chinou, I.B.; Harvala, C. Iridoids from *Scabiosa variifolia* (Dipsacaceae) growing in Greece. *Biochem. Syst. Ecol.* **2003**, *31*, 91–93. [CrossRef]

34. Zheng, Q.; Koike, K.; Han, L.K.; Okuda, H.; Nikaido, T. New biologically active triterpenoid saponins from *Scabiosa tschiliensis. J. Nat. Prod.* **2004**, *67*, 604–613. [CrossRef] [PubMed]

35. Baykal, T.; Panayir, T.; Tasdemir, D.; Sticher, O.; Çalis, I. Triterpene saponins from *Scabiosa rotata. Phytochemistry* **1998**, *48*, 867–873. [CrossRef]

36. Akimailiev, S.A.; Putieva, Z.M.; Alimbaeva, P.K.; Abubakirov, N.K. Triterpene glycosides of Scabiosa soogorica. V. β-Sitosterol β-D-glucopyranoside and songoroside A. *Khim. Pir. Soedin.* **1988**, *1988*, 885–886.

37. Rahmouni, N.; Pinto, D.C.G.A.; Santos, S.A.O.; Beghidja, N.; Silva, A.M.S. Lipophilic composition of *Scabiosa stellata* L.: An underexploited plant from Batna (Algeria). *Chem. Pap.* **2018**, *72*, 753–762. [CrossRef]

38. Cárdenas, M.; Marder, M.; Blank, V.C.; Roguin, L.P. Antitumor of some natural flavonoids and synthetic derivatives on various human and murine cancer cell lines. *Bioorg. Med. Chem.* **2006**, *14*, 2966–2971. [CrossRef] [PubMed]

39. Moscatelli, V.; Hnatyszyn, O.; Acevedo, C.; Megías, J.; Alcaraz, M.J.; Ferraro, G. Flavonoids from *Artemisia copa* with anti-inflammatory activity. *Planta Med.* **2006**, *72*, 72–74. [CrossRef] [PubMed]

40. Beyer, G.; Melzig, M.F. Effects of selected flavonoids and caffeic acid derivatives on hypoxanthine-xanthine oxidase-induced toxicity in cultivated Human cells. *Planta Med.* **2003**, *69*, 1125–1129. [PubMed]

41. Verma, A.K.; Pratap, R. The biological potential of flavones. *Nat. Prod. Rep.* **2010**, *27*, 1571–1593. [CrossRef] [PubMed]

42. Saeidnia, S.; Manayi, A.; Gohari, A.R.; Abdollahi, M. The story of beta-sitosterol: A review. *Eur. J. Med. Plants* **2014**, *4*, 590–609. [CrossRef]

43. Haque, M.N.; Bhuiyan, M.M.H.; Moon, I.S. Stigmasterol activates Cdc42-Arp2 and Erk1/2-Creb pathways to enrich glutamatergic synapses in cultures of brain neurons. *Nutr. Res.* **2018**, *56*, 71–78. [CrossRef] [PubMed]

44. Ghisalberti, E.L. Biological and pharmacological activity of naturally occurring iridoids and secoiridoids. *Phytomedicine* **1998**, *5*, 147–163. [CrossRef]

45. Tundis, R.; Loizzo, M.R.; Menichini, F.; Statti, G.A.; Menichini, F. Biological and Pharmacological activities of iridoids: Recent developments. *Mini-Rev. Med. Chem.* **2008**, *8*, 399–420. [CrossRef] [PubMed]

46. Marques, V.; Farah, A. Chlorogenic acids and related compounds in medicinal plants and infusions. *Food Chem.* **2009**, *113*, 1370–1376. [CrossRef]

47. Kuril'chenko, V.A.; Zemtsova, G.N.; Bandyukova, V.Y. A chemical study of *Scabiosa bipinnata*. *Khim. Prir. Soedin.* **1971**, 534–535. [CrossRef]

48. Pichersky, E.; Raguso, R.A. Why do plants produce so many terpenoid componds? *New Phytol.* **2016**, *2016*. [CrossRef]

49. Singh, B.; Sharma, R.A. Plant terpenes: Defense responses, phylogenetic analysis, regulation and clinical applications. *3 Biotech* **2015**, *5*, 129–151. [CrossRef] [PubMed]

50. Yadav, V.R.; Prasad, S.; Sung, B.; Kannappan, R.; Aggarwal, B.B. Targeting inflammatory pathways by triterpenoids for prevention and treatment of cancer. *Toxins* **2010**, *2*, 2428–2466. [CrossRef] [PubMed]

51. Kamble, S.M.; Goyal, S.N.; Patil, C.R. Multifunctional pentacyclic triterpenoids as adjuvants in cancer chemotherapy: A review. *RSC Adv.* **2014**, *4*, 33370–33382. [CrossRef]

52. Chudzik, M.; Korzonek-Szlacheta, I.; Król, W. Triterpenes as potentially cytotoxic compounds. *Molecules* **2015**, *20*, 1610–1625. [CrossRef] [PubMed]

53. Jäger, S.; Trojan, H.; Kopp, T.; Laszczyk, M.N.; Scheffler, A. Pentacyclic triterpene distribution in various plants-rich sources for a new group of multi-potent plant extracts. *Molecules* **2009**, *14*, 2016–2031. [CrossRef] [PubMed]

54. Sultana, N.; Ata, A. Oleanolic acid and related derivatives as medicinally important compounds. *J. Enzym. Inhib. Med. Chem.* **2008**, *23*, 739–756. [CrossRef] [PubMed]

55. Shanmugam, M.K.; Dai, X.; Kumar, A.P.; Tan, B.K.H.; Sethi, G.; Bishayee, A. Oleanolic acid and its synthetic derivatives for the prevention and therapy of cancer: Preclinical and clinical evidence. *Cancer Lett.* **2014**, *346*, 206–216. [CrossRef] [PubMed]

56. Nicolini, F.; Burmistrova, O.; Marrero, M.T.; Torres, F.; Hernández, C.; Quintana, J.; Estévez, F. Induction of G_2/M phase arrest and apoptosis by the flavonoid tamarixetin on Human leukemia cells. *Mol. Carcinog.* **2014**, *53*, 939–950. [PubMed]

57. Hayamizu, K.; Morimoto, S.; Nonaka, M.; Hoka, S.; Sasaguri, T. Cardiotonic actions of quercetin and its metabolite tamarixetin through a digitalis-like enhancement of Ca^{2+} transients. *Arch Biochem. Biophys.* **2018**, *637*, 40–47. [CrossRef] [PubMed]

58. Yadav, D.K.; Bharitkar, Y.P.; Hazra, A.; Pal, U.; Verma, S.; Jana, S.; Singh, U.P.; Maiti, N.C.; Mondal, N.B.; Swarnakar, S. Tamarixetin 3-*O*-β-D-glucopyranoside from *Azadirachta indica* leaves: Gastroprotective role through inhibition of matrix metalloproteinase-9 activity in mice. *J. Nat. Prod.* **2017**, *80*, 1347–1353. [CrossRef] [PubMed]

59. Harborne, J.B. Plant polyphenols—XI: The structure of acylated anthocyanins. *Phytochemistry* **1964**, *3*, 151–160. [CrossRef]

60. Zhu, Y.; Zhang, Y.; Liu, Y.; Chu, H.; Duan, H. Synthesis and biological activity of trans-tiliroside derivatives as potent anti-diabetic agents. *Molecules* **2010**, *15*, 9174–9183. [CrossRef] [PubMed]

61. Qin, N.; Li, C.-B.; Jin, M.-N.; Shi, L.-H.; Duan, H.-Q.; Niu, W.-Y. Synthesis and biological activity of novel tiliroside derivants. *Eur. J. Med. Chem.* **2011**, *46*, 5189–5195. [CrossRef] [PubMed]

62. Velagapudi, R.; Aderogba, M.; Olajide, O.A. Tiliroside, a dietary glycosidic flavonoid, inhibits TRAF-6/NF-kB/p38-mediated neuroinflammation in activated BV2 microglia. *Biochim. Biophys. Acta* **2014**, *1840*, 3311–3319. [CrossRef] [PubMed]

63. Da'i, M.; Wikantyasning, E.R.; Wahyuni, A.S.; Kusumawati, I.T.D.; Saifudin, A.; Suhendi, A. Antiproliferative properties of tiliroside from *Guazuma ulmifolia* lamk on T47D and MCF7 cancer cell lines. *Natl. J. Physiol. Pharm. Pharmacol.* **2016**, *6*, 627–633. [CrossRef]

64. Barbosa, E.; Calzada, F.; Campos, R. In vivo antigiardial activity of three flavonoids isolated of some medicinal plants used in Mexican tradicional medicine for the treatment of diarrhea. *J. Ethnopharmacol.* **2007**, *109*, 552–554. [CrossRef] [PubMed]

65. Sala, A.; Recio, M.C.; Schinella, G.R.; Máñez, S.; Giner, R.M.; Cerdá-Nicolás, M.; Ríos, J.-L. Assessment of the anti-inflammatory activity and free radical scavenger activity of tiliroside. *Eur. J. Pharmacol.* **2003**, *461*, 53–61. [CrossRef]

66. Jin, X.; Song, S.; Wang, J.; Zhang, Q.; Qiu, F.; Zhao, F. Tiliroside, the major component of Agrimonia pilosa Ledeb ethanol extract, inhibits MAPK/JNK/p38-mediated inflammation in lipopolysaccharide-activated RAW 264.7 macrophages. *Exp. Ther. Med.* **2016**, *12*, 499–505. [CrossRef] [PubMed]

67. Silva, G.C.; Pereira, A.C.; Rezende, B.A.; da Silva, J.F.P.; Cruz, J.S.; de Souza, M.F.V.; Gomes, R.A.; Teles, Y.C.F.; Cortes, S.F.; Lemos, V.S. Mechanism of the antihypertensive and vasorelaxant effects of the flavonoif tiliroside in resistance arteries. *Planta Med.* **2013**, *79*, 1003–1008. [PubMed]

68. Perkin, A.G. CI.-Colouring matters of the New Zealand dyewood puriri, Vitex littoralis. Part I. *J. Chem. Soc. Trans.* **1898**, *73*, 1019–1031. [CrossRef]

69. Baldim, J.L.; Alcântara, B.G.V.; Domingos, O.S.; Soares, M.G.; Caldas, I.S.; Novaes, R.D.; Oliveira, T.B.; Lago, J.H.G.; Chagas-Paula, D.A. The correlation between chemical structures and antioxidant, prooxidant, and antitrypanosomatid properties of flavonoids. *Oxid. Med. Cell. Longev.* **2017**, *2017*. [CrossRef] [PubMed]

70. Ling, T.; Lang, W.; Feng, X.; Das, S.; Maier, J.; Jeffries, C.; Shelat, A.; Rivas, F. Novel vitexin-inspired scaffold against leukemia. *Eur. J. Med. Chem.* **2018**, *146*, 501–510. [CrossRef] [PubMed]

71. Gaitan, E.; Cooksey, R.C.; Legan, J.; Lindsay, R.H. Antithyroid effects in vivo and in vitro of vitexin: A C-glucosylflavone in millet. *J. Clin. Endocrinol. Metab.* **1995**, *80*, 1144–1147. [PubMed]

72. Das, M.C.; Sandhu, P.; Gupta, P.; Rudrapaul, P.; De, U.C.; Tribedi, P.; Akhter, Y.; Bhattacharjee, S. Attenuation of Pseudomonas aeruginosa biofilm formation by vitexin: A combinatorial study with azithromycin and gentamicin. *Sci. Rep.* **2016**, *6*, 23347. [CrossRef] [PubMed]

73. Tang, Z.; Yang, L.; Zhang, X. Vitexin mitigates myocardial ischemia reperfusion-induced damage by inhibiting excessive autophagy to suppress apoptosis via the PI3K/Akt/mTOR signaling cascade. *RSC Adv.* **2017**, *7*, 56406–56416. [CrossRef]

74. Hu, M.; Li, F.; Wang, W. Vitexin protects dopaminergic neurons in MPTP-induced Parkinson's disease through PI3K/Akt signaling pathway. *Drug Des. Dev. Ther.* **2018**, *12*, 565–573. [CrossRef] [PubMed]

75. Rosa, S.I.G.; Rios-Santos, F.; Balogun, S.O.; Martins, D.T.O. Vitexin reduces neutrophil migration to inflammatory focus by down-regulating pro-inflammatory mediators via inhibition of p38, ERK1/2 and JNK pathway. *Phytomedicine* **2016**, *23*, 9–17. [CrossRef] [PubMed]

76. Luo, W.; Min, J.; Huang, W.-X.; Wang, X.; Peng, Y.; Han, S.; Yin, J.; Liu, W.-H.; He, X.-H.; Peng, B.-W. Vitexin reduces epilepsy after hypoxic ischemia in the neonatal brain via inhibition of NKCC1. *J. Neuroinflamm.* **2018**, *15*, 186. [CrossRef] [PubMed]

77. He, J.-D.; Wang, Z.; Li, S.-P.; Xu, Y.-J.; Yu, Y.; Ding, Y.-J.; Yu, W.-L.; Zhang, R.-X.; Zhang, H.-M.; Du, H.-Y. Vitexin suppresses autophagy to induce apoptosis in hepatocellular carcinoma via activation of the JNK signaling pathway. *Oncotarget* **2016**, *7*, 84520–84532. [PubMed]

78. Bhardwaj, M.; Paul, S.; Jakhar, R.; Khan, I.; Kang, J.I.; Kim, H.M.; Yun, J.W.; Lee, S.-J.; Cho, H.J.; Lee, H.G.; et al. Vitexin confers HSF-1 mediated autophagic cell death by activating JNK and ApoL1 in colorectal carcinoma cells. *Oncotarget* **2017**, *8*, 112426–112441. [CrossRef] [PubMed]

79. Bhardwaj, M.; Cho, H.J.; Paul, S.; Jakhar, R.; Khan, I.; Lee, S.-J.; Kim, B.-Y.; Krishnan, M.; Khaket, T.P.; Lee, H.G.; et al. Vitexin induces apoptosis by suppressing autophagy in multi-drug resistant colorectal cancer cells. *Oncotarget* **2018**, *9*, 3278–3291. [CrossRef] [PubMed]

80. Ganesan, K.; Xu, B. Molecular targets of vitexin and isovitexin in cancer therapy: A critical review. *Ann. N. Y. Acad. Sci.* **2017**, *1401*, 102–113. [CrossRef] [PubMed]

81. Dai, K.; Yi, X.-J.; Huang, X.-J.; Li, M.; Li, J.; Yang, G.-Z.; Gao, Y.; Muhammad, A. Hepatoprotective activity of iridoids, seco-iridoids and analogs glycosides from Gentianaceae on HepG2 cells via CYP3A4 induction and mitochondrial pathway. *Food Funct.* **2018**, *9*, 2673–2683. [CrossRef] [PubMed]

82. Chen, Y.; Yu, H.; Guo, F.; Wu, Y.; Li, Y. Antinociceptive and anti-inflammatory activities of a standardizedextractract of bis-iridoids from Pterocephalus hookeri. *J. Ethnopharmacol.* **2018**, *216*, 233–238. [CrossRef] [PubMed]

83. Viljoen, A.; Mncwangi, N.; Vermaak, I. Anti-inflammatory iridoids of botanical origin. *Curr. Med. Chem.* **2012**, *19*, 2104–2127. [CrossRef] [PubMed]

84. Habtemariam, S. Antidiabetic potential of monoterpenes: A case of small molecules punching above their weight. *Int. J. Mol. Sci.* **2018**, *19*, 4. [CrossRef] [PubMed]

85. West, B.J.; Deng, S.; Uwaya, A.; Isami, F.; Abe, Y.; Yamagishi, S.-I.; Jensen, C.J. Iridoids are natural glycation inhibitors. *Glycoconj. J.* **2016**, *33*, 671–681. [CrossRef] [PubMed]

86. Jaishree, V.; Badami, S.; Kumar, M.R.; Tamizhmani, T. Antinociceptive activity of swertiamarin isolated from *Enicostemma axillare*. *Phytomedicine* **2009**, *16*, 227–232. [CrossRef] [PubMed]

87. Patel, T.P.; Soni, S.; Parikh, P.; Gosai, J.; Chruvattil, R.; Gupta, S. Swertiamarin: An active lead from *Enicostemma littorale* regulates hepatic and adipose tissue gene expression by targeting PPAR-γ and improves insulin sensitivity in experimental NIDDM rat model. *Evid.-Based Complement. Altern. Med.* **2013**, *2013*. [CrossRef] [PubMed]

88. Ahamad, J.; Hassan, N.; Amin, S.; Mir, S.R. Swertiamarin contributes to glucose homeostasis via inhibition of carbohydrate metabolizing enzymes. *J. Nat. Remed.* **2016**, *4*, 125–130. [CrossRef]

89. Saravanan, S.; Pandikumar, P.; Babu, N.P.; Islam, V.I.H.; Thirugnanasambantham, K.; Paulraj, M.G.; Balakrishna, K.; Ignacimuthu, S. In vivo and in vitro immunomodulatory potential of swertiamarin isolated from *Enicostema axillare* (Lam.) A. Raynal that acts as an anti-inflammatory agent. *Inflammation* **2014**, *37*, 1374–1388. [CrossRef] [PubMed]

90. Saravanan, S.; Islam, V.I.H.; Babu, N.P.; Pandikumar, P.; Thirugnanasambantham, K.; Chellappandian, M.; Raj, C.S.D.; Paulraj, M.G.; Ignacimuthu, S. Swertiamarin attenuates inflammation mediators via modulating NF-κB/I κB and JAK2/STAT3 transcription factors in adjuvant induced arthritis. *Eur. J. Pharm. Sci.* **2014**, *56*, 70–86. [CrossRef] [PubMed]

91. Hairul-Islam, M.I.; Saravanan, S.; Thirugnanasambantham, K.; Chellappandian, M.; Raj, C.S.D.; Karikalan, K.; Paulraj, M.G.; Ignacimuthu, S. Swertiamarin, a natural steroid, prevent bone erosion by modulating RANKL/RANK/OPG signaling. *Int. Immunopharmacol.* **2017**, *53*, 114–124. [CrossRef] [PubMed]

92. Šiler, B.; Mišić, D.; Nestorović, J.; Banjanac, T.; Glamočlija, J.; Soković, M.; Ćirić, A. Antibacterial and antifungal screening of Centaurium pulchellum crude extracts and main secoiridoid compounds. *Nat. Prod. Commun.* **2010**, *5*, 1525–1530. [PubMed]

93. Shitlani, D.; Choudhary, R.; Pandey, D.P.; Bodakhe, S.H. Ameliorative antimalarial effects of the combination of rutin and swertiamarin on malarial parasites. *Asian Pac. J. Trop. Dis.* **2016**, *6*, 453–459. [CrossRef]

94. Jeong, Y.T.; Jeong, S.C.; Hwang, J.S.; Kim, J.H. Modulation effects of sweroside isolated from the *Lonicera japonica* on melanin synthesis. *Chem. Biol. Interac.* **2015**, *238*, 33–39. [CrossRef] [PubMed]

95. Han, X.-L.; Li, J.-D.; Wang, W.-L.; Yang, C.; Li, Z.-Y. Sweroside eradicated leukemia cells and attenuated pathogenic processes in mice by inducing apoptosis. *Biomed. Pharm.* **2017**, *95*, 477–486. [CrossRef] [PubMed]

96. Lee, K.Y.; Sung, S.H.; Kim, S.H.; Jang, Y.P.; Oh, T.H.; Kim, Y.C. Cognitive-enhancing activity of loganin isolated from Cornus officinalis in scopolamine-induced amnesic mice. *Arch Pharm. Res.* **2009**, *32*, 677–683. [CrossRef] [PubMed]

97. Kwon, S.-H.; Kim, H.-C.; Lee, S.-Y.; Jang, C.-G. Loganin improves learning and memory impairments induced by scopolamine in mice. *Eur. J. Pharm.* **2009**, *619*, 44–49. [CrossRef] [PubMed]

98. Babri, S.; Azami, S.H.; Mohaddes, G. Effect of acute administration of loganin on special memory in diabetic male rats. *Adv. Pharm. Bull.* **2013**, *3*, 91–95. [PubMed]

99. Tseng, Y.-T.; Chen, C.-S.; Jong, Y.-J.; Chang, F.-R.; Lo, Y.-C. Loganin possesses neuroprotective properties, restores SMN protein and activates protein synthesis positive regulator Akt/mTOR in experimental models of spinal muscular atrophy. *Pharm. Res.* **2016**, *111*, 58–75. [CrossRef] [PubMed]

100. Jiang, W.-L.; Zhang, S.-P.; Hou, J.; Zhu, H.-B. Effect of loganin on experimental diabetic nephropathy. *Phytomedicine* **2012**, *19*, 217–222. [CrossRef] [PubMed]

101. Liu, K.; Xu, H.; Lv, G.; Liu, B.; Lee, M.K.K.; Lu, C.; Lv, X.; Wu, Y. Loganin attenuates diabetic nephropathy in C57BL/6J mice with diabetes induced by streptozotocin and fed with diets containing high level of advanced glycation end products. *Life Sci.* **2015**, *123*, 78–85. [CrossRef] [PubMed]

102. Tsai, W.-H.; Wu, C.-H.; Cheng, C.-H.; Chien, C.-T. Ba-Wei-Di-Huang-Wan through its active ingredient loganin counteracts substance P-enhanced NF-κB/ICAM-1 signaling in rats with bladder hyperactivity. *Neurourol. Urodynam.* **2016**, *35*, 771–779. [CrossRef] [PubMed]

103. Li, Y.; Li, Z.; Shi, L.; Zhao, C.; Shen, B.; Tian, Y.; Feng, H. Loganin inhibits the inflammatory response in mouse 3T3L1 adipocytes and mouse model. *Int. Immunopharm.* **2016**, *36*, 173–179. [CrossRef] [PubMed]

104. Schinella, G.; Aquila, S.; Dade, M.; Giner, R.; Recio, M.C.; Spegazzini, E.; Buschiazzo, P.; Tournier, H.; Rios, J.L. Anti-inflammatory and apoptotic activities of pomolic acid isolated from *Cecropia pachystachya*. *Planta Med.* **2008**, *74*, 215–220. [CrossRef] [PubMed]

105. Kim, E.H.; Baek, S.; Shin, D.; Lee, J.; Roh, J.-L. Hederagenin induces apoptosis in cisplatin-resistant head and neck cancer cells by inhibiting the Nrf2-ARE antioxidant pathway. *Oxid. Med. Cell. Longev.* **2017**, *2017*. [CrossRef] [PubMed]

106. Wang, J.; Zhao, X.-Z.; Qi, Q.; Tao, L.; Zhao, Q.; Mu, R.; Gu, H.-Y.; Wang, M.; Feng, X.; Guo, Q.-L. Macranthoside B, a hederagenin saponin extracted from *Lonicera macranthoides* and its anti-tumor activities in vitro and in vivo. *Food Chem. Toxicol.* **2009**, *47*, 1716–1721. [CrossRef] [PubMed]

107. Rodríguez-Hernández, D.; Demuner, A.J.; Barbosa, L.C.A.; Csuk, R.; Heller, L. Hederagenin as a triterpene template for the development of new antitumor compounds. *Eur. J. Med. Chem.* **2015**, *105*, 57–62. [CrossRef] [PubMed]

108. Ayeleso, T.B.; Matumba, M.G.; Mukwevho, E. Oleanolic acid and its derivatives: Biological activities and therapeutic potential in chronic diseases. *Molecules* **2017**, *22*, 1915. [CrossRef] [PubMed]

109. Gao, Y.S.; Yuan, Y.; Song, G.; Lin, S.Q. Inhibitory effect of ursolic acid and oleanolic acid from *Eriobotrya fragrans* on A549 cell viability in vivo. *Genet. Mol. Res.* **2016**, *15*. [CrossRef] [PubMed]

110. Abdelmageed, N.; Morad, S.A.S.; Elghoneimy, A.A.; Syrovets, T.; Simmet, T.; El-zorba, H.; El-Banna, H.A.; Cabot, M.; Abdel-Aziz, M.I. Oleanolic acid methyl ester, a novel cytotoxic mitocan, induces cell cycle arrest and ROS-mediated cell death in castration-resistant prostate cancer PC-3 cells. *Biomed. Pharm.* **2017**, *96*, 417–425. [CrossRef] [PubMed]

111. Caunii, A.; Oprean, C.; Cristea, M.; Ivan, A.; Danciu, C.; Tatu, C.; Paunescu, V.; Marti, D.; Tzanakakis, G.; Spandidos, D.A.; et al. Effects of ursolic and oleanolic on SK-MEL-2 melanoma cells: In vitro and in vivo assays. *Int. J. Oncol.* **2017**, *51*, 1651–1660. [CrossRef] [PubMed]

112. Xue, S.; Yin, J.; Shao, J.; Yu, Y.; Yang, L.; Wang, Y.; Xie, M.; Fussenegger, M.; Ye, H. A synthetic-biology-inspired therapeutic strategy for targeting and treating hepatogenous diabetes. *Mol. Ther.* **2017**, *25*, 443–455. [CrossRef] [PubMed]

113. Gajęcka, M.; Przybylska-Gornowicz, B.; Zakłos-Szyda, M.; Dąbrowski, M.; Michalczuk, L.; Koziołkiewicz, M.; Babuchowski, A.; Zielonka, Ł.; Lewczuk, B.; Gajęcki, M.T. The influence of a natural triterpene preparation on the gastrointestinal tract of gilts streptozocin-induced diabetes and on cell metabolic activity. *J. Funct. Foods* **2017**, *33*, 11–20. [CrossRef]

114. Munhoz, A.C.M.; Fröde, T.S. Isolated compounds from natural products with potential antidiabetic activity —A systematic review. *Curr. Diabetes Rev.* **2018**, *14*, 36–106. [CrossRef] [PubMed]

115. Su, S.; Wu, G.; Cheng, X.; Fan, J.; Peng, J.; Su, H.; Xu, Z.; Cao, M.; Long, Z.; Hao, Y.; et al. Oleanolic acid attenuates PCBs-induced adiposity and insulin resistance via HNF1b-mediated regulation of redox and PPAR γ signaling. *Free Radic. Biol. Med.* **2018**, *124*, 122–134. [CrossRef] [PubMed]

116. Beaufay, C.; Hérent, M.-F.; Quetin-Leclercq, J.; Bero, J. In vivo anti-malarial activity and toxicity studies of triterpenic esters isolated from *Keetia leucantha* and crude extracts. *Malar. J.* **2017**, *16*, 406. [CrossRef] [PubMed]

117. Pan, Y.; Zhou, F.; Song, Z.; Huang, H.; Chen, Y.; Shen, Y.; Jia, Y.; Chen, J. Oleanolic acid protects against pathogenesis of atherosclerosis, possibly via FXR-mediated angiotensin (Ang)-(1-7) upregulation. *Biomed. Pharmacol.* **2018**, *97*, 1694–1700. [CrossRef] [PubMed]

118. Bernabé-García, A.; Armero-Barranco, D.; Liarte, S.; Ruzafa-Martínez, M.; Ramos-morcillo, A.J.; Nicolás, F.J. Oleanolic acid induces migration in Mv1Lu and MDA-MB-231 epithelial cells involving EGF receptor and MAP kinases activation. *PLoS ONE* **2017**, *12*, e0172574. [CrossRef] [PubMed]

119. Kang, D.-G.; Lee, H.J.; Kim, K.T.; Hwang, S.-C.; Lee, C.J.; Park, J.S. Effect of oleanolic acid on the activity, secretion and gene expression of matrix metalloproteinase-3 in articular chondrocytes in vitro and the production of matrix metalloproteinase-3 in vivo. *Korean J. Physiol. Pharmacol.* **2017**, *21*, 197–204. [CrossRef] [PubMed]

120. Gao, N.; Guo, M.; Fu, Q.; He, Z. Application of hot melt extrusión to enhance the dissolution and oral bioavailability of oleanolic acid. *Asian J. Pharm. Sci.* **2017**, *12*, 66–72. [CrossRef]

121. Liu, Y.; Luo, X.; Xu, X.; Gao, N.; Liu, X. Preparation, characterization and in vivo pharmacokinetic study of PVP-modified oleanolic acid liposomes. *Int. J. Pharm.* **2017**, *517*, 1–7. [CrossRef] [PubMed]

122. Zhang, W.; Liang, C.; Liu, H.; Li, Z.; Chen, R.; Zhou, M.; Li, D.; Ye, Q.; Luo, C.; Sun, J. Polymeric nanoparticles developed by vitamin E-modified aliphatic polycarbonate polymer to promote oral absorption of oleanolic acid. *Asian J. Pharm. Sci.* **2017**, *12*, 586–593. [CrossRef]

123. Xia, X.; Liu, H.; Lv, H.; Zhang, J.; Zhou, J.; Zhao, Z. Preparation, characterization, and in vitro/vivo studies of oleanolic acid-loaded lactoferrin nanoparticles. *Drug Des. Dev. Ther.* **2017**, *11*, 1417–1427. [CrossRef] [PubMed]

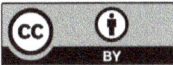

![medicines logo] **medicines**

MDPI

Review

Nanoemulsions of Essential Oils: New Tool for Control of Vector-Borne Diseases and In Vitro Effects on Some Parasitic Agents

Javier Echeverría [1],* and Ricardo Diego Duarte Galhardo de Albuquerque [2],*

[1]   Facultad de Química y Biología, Universidad de Santiago de Chile, Casilla 40, Correo 33,
      Santiago 9170022, Chile
[2]   Laboratório de Tecnologia em Produtos Naturais, Universidade Federal Fluminense,
      Niterói 24241-002, Brazil
*   Correspondence: javier.echeverriam@usach.cl (J.E.); ricardo-diego-cf@hotmail.com (R.D.D.G.d.A.);
      Tel.: +56-2-2718-1154 (J.E.); +55-21-9-7525-2662 (R.D.D.G.d.A.)

Received: 31 January 2019; Accepted: 19 March 2019; Published: 27 March 2019

Abstract: The control of infectious/parasitic diseases is a continuing challenge for global health, which in turn requires new methods of action and the development of innovative agents to be used in its prevention and/or treatment. In this context, the control of vectors and intermediate hosts of etiological agents is an efficient method in the prevention of human and veterinary diseases. In later stages, it is necessary to have bioactive compounds that act efficiently on the agents that produce the disease. However, several synthetic agents have strong residual effects in humans and other animals and cause environmental toxicity, affecting fauna, flora and unbalancing the local ecosystem. Many studies have reported the dual activity of the essential oils (EOs): (i) control of vectors that are important in the cycle of disease transmission, and (ii) relevant activity against pathogens. In general, EOs have an easier degradation and cause less extension of environmental contamination. However, problems related to solubility and stability lead to the development of efficient vehicles for formulations containing EOs, such as nanoemulsions. Therefore, this systematic review describes several studies performed with nanoemulsions as carriers of EOs that have larvicidal, insecticidal, repellent, acaricidal and antiparasitic activities, and thus can be considered as alternatives in the vector control of infectious and parasitic diseases, as well as in the combat against etiological agents of parasitic origin.

Keywords: nanoemulsion; essential oils; vector control; infectious diseases

1. Introduction

1.1. Essential Oils and Biological Activity

In recent years, the use of essential oils (EOs) from aromatic plants as low-risk insecticides, antifungals, antifeedants, antivector growth regulators, oviposition deterrents and repellents [1–4] has increased due to its popularity among organic farmers and environmentally conscious consumers.

The production of EOs is mainly carried out through procedures of hydrodistillation, steam distillation, dry distillation, or mechanical cold pressing of plants [5]. The most widely used preparation method is based on the Clevenger steam distillation apparatus, which has been adapted and expanded for industrial scale production. Recently, modern EO extraction methods have begun to be used, including microwave-assisted processing and supercritical fluid extraction [6].

A typical EO can contain, on average, between 20 and 80 different compounds. The constituents of EOs mainly belong to two phytochemical groups: terpenoids (monoterpenes and sesquiterpenes of low molecular weight) and, to a lesser extent, phenylpropanoids (volatile phenolic compounds).

The terpenoids are the main constituents of the EOs. The monoterpenes present in the EOs may contain terpenes which are hydrocarbons (α-pinene and D-limonene), alcohols (cadinol), aldehydes (cinnamaldehyde and citronellal), ketones (thujone), ethers (1,8-cineol) and lactones (artemisin). The sesquiterpenes have a wide variety of structures, more than 100 skeletons, since the lengthening of the chain to 15 carbons increases the number of possible cyclizations. Aromatic compounds are less common and include phenylpropanoids (*p*-allylanisole) and phenolic compounds (thymol).

The composition of EOs is very diverse in different plant species. An example of this is the eucalyptus (*Eucalyptus globulus*), whose main constituent of the EO is monoterpene 1,8-cineol, while in coriander (*Coriandrum sativum*), the sesquiterpene linalool is the most abundant. In turn, within the same species of plants, the existence of chemotypes is very common. For example, thyme (*Thymus vulgaris*) has numerous chemotypes named after the main compound, for example, thymol, carvacrol, terpineol and linalool.

In botanical terms, EOs are produced in approximately 17,500 species of higher aromatic plants, belonging mainly to a few families, including *Myrtaceae*, *Lauraceae*, *Lamiaceae* and *Asteraceae*. The synthesis and accumulation of EOs in plants are associated with the presence of complex specific and highly specialized secretory structures, such as glandular trichomes (*Lamiaceae*), secretory cavities (*Myrtaceae*, *Rutaceae*) and resin ducts (*Asteraceae*, *Apiaceae*). Depending on the species taxonomically considered, the EOs can be stored in various plant organs, for example, in flowers, leaves, wood, roots, rhizomes, fruits and seeds [7].

At the biological level, the EOs have important effects as repellents, insecticides and growth reducers in a great variety of insects. They have been used effectively to control phytophagous insects pre- and post-harvest, as insect repellents with vectors of diseases and for the control of domestic and/or garden insects. The mechanism of action of the compounds present in EOs on insects is mainly through neurotoxic effects, involving several modes of actions, in particular, through the inhibition of acetylcholinesterase (AChE) [8], functionality disruption of gamma-aminobutyric acid (GABA) receptors [9], and as agonist of octopaminergic system [10].

Although the biological effects of the individual chemical components of the EOs are generally known, the toxicology of their combinations or mixtures is a much more difficult aspect to evaluate. However, one of the most outstanding and attractive characteristics of the EOs is that they are, in general, low-risk products on animals, and their environmental persistence is short. Their toxicity for mammals is low, having values of oral LD_{50} that varies from 1000 to 2000 mg kg^{-1} in rats. In addition, due to their use as medicines, some EOs are relatively well studied experimentally and clinically.

The toxicity of EO components has been divided into three structural classes based on the toxicological potential [11]: Class I (low functionality, low oral toxicity, e.g., limonene), Class II (some functionality, intermediate toxicity, e.g., menthofuran) and Class III (reactive functionality, high potential toxicity, e.g., elemicin). Based on this classification and other toxicological criteria, different procedures have been developed to evaluate the safety of the use of EOs [12].

Moreover, the EOs also could be promising antiprotozoal agents, opening perspectives to the discovery of more effective drugs of vegetal origin for the treatment of related diseases by targeting the etiological agents. In several species with antiprotozoal activity, the compounds camphor, carvacrol, eugenol, terpinen-4-ol, or thymol were the main oil constituents, which denotes a supposed variety in its mechanisms of action, since these substances belong to different structural groups [13,14].

1.2. Nanotechnology and Nanoemulsions

Nanotechnology is a transdisciplinary and promising field of science for its diverse potential of application, ranging from the field of electronic and mechanical engineering, telecommunications, civil construction, industrial chemistry, to practical use in the health area, as the development of nanostructured drugs, biological carriers and sensors for diagnosis [15,16]. With the advancement of technologies in electron microscopy in the 1980s, it became possible to observe, study, manipulate and develop nanostructured systems, which led a technological revolution in several fields of science [17].

Nanometric materials have a size in the range of 0.1 to 200 nm and present particular physicochemical properties in relation to structured materials on a macroscopic scale [18]. In the field of biological and health sciences, nanotechnology has provided a promising alternative for research and development of drug delivery systems, as allow better delivery of the drug to its place of action, a factor that provides a series of patient benefits such as increased therapeutic efficacy, dose reduction, lower number of administrations, and a decrease in side effects. Still, regarding technical stability, nanosystems have the advantage of protecting active substances against mechanisms of inactivation and degradation, besides providing the incorporation of substances with very different polarity in relation to the matrix, to promote prolonged release and/or targeting of drug action in a certain tissue. These events occur due to different factors, such as the larger contact surface, which promotes greater absorption, distribution and tissue uptake of the drug, in addition to the physicochemical properties of the coating or matrix polymers, which may provide greater affinity with the target tissue or greater protection against physiological barriers in the organism [15,19,20].

An emulsion is a liquid dispersion of two different immiscible liquids. The macroscopic separation of the two different phases is controlled by the addition of the surfactant. When this emulsion system tends to reach nanometric size from 20 to 200 nm, it is called "nanoemulsion". Nanoemulsions can be formed through the dispersion of the oil in water or water in oil and allow the placement of different active substances. They have some individual characteristics, such as transparency when viewed by the naked eye, and a bluish reflection may be observed, due to the diffusion of light between the nanoparticles, which is known as the Tyndall effect [21]. The extremely small size of the particles also confers greater resistance to the effects of cremation and sedimentation, because the effect of gravity is smaller on them [22].

The surfactant has a vital role in the formation of these nanoemulsion systems. The interfacial tension generated due to the immiscibility of two different liquid systems is reduced through the use of surfactant. This property of lowering the interfacial tension between the phases tends to make the surfactant an essential part of the nanoemulsion system. This formulation process for the nanoemulsion is carried out through the low or high energy emulsification method. The low energy method includes the phase inversion method, while the high energy method includes ultrasound and high-pressure homogenization. In addition, the system displays low interfacial tension, which facilitates easier dispersion of different substances. This fact is a major advantage when the incorporation of highly lipophilic materials, such as EOs, into aqueous systems is necessary [22,23]. Thus, the nanoemulsions have diverse applications in several fields, such as, for example, pharmaceuticals, cosmetics, agriculture, etc. [24]. In the current scenario, different approaches are being carried out in the development of nanoemulsion with an efficient insect repellent, larvicidal and insecticidal activity using EOs.

1.3. Essential Oil Nanoemulsion

In recent years, several scientific works have reported the use of nanoemulsions as suitable carriers of active EOs. The easy preparation, simple composition, higher thermodynamic stability, low cost of production and the possibility of production on an industrial scale provide a substantial advantage to this technology through the biological and pharmacological use of EOs [25,26].

Nanoemulsions of EOs are promising tools for combating vector-borne diseases through population control of transmitting agents. This is possible due to the inherent physicochemical properties of the nanometric emulsion system [27]. The nanometer size of the nanoemulsion improves its specificity and delivery target, resulting in greater effectiveness than bulk pesticides. Furthermore, nanoemulsions pesticides have a lower surfactant concentration than microemulsions, and surfactants are considerably more environmentally friendly and are cost-effective and economically viable. EOs dispersed in different nanoformulations can act through several mechanisms of action, such as the deregulation of the growth hormone that tends to stop the insect shedding, which leads to its mortality, as well as enzymatic inhibition, among others [28–30]. Finally, recent studies have also reported the biological activity of nanoemulsified essential oils on etiological agents of parasitic origin, which potentially increases the diversification of the use of these nanoemulsions in the control of infectious/parasitic diseases.

2. Biological Activities of Essential Oil Nanoemulsions

2.1. Larvicidal Activity

Culex quinquefasciatus is a mosquito species acting as cyclic vector for *Wuchereria bancrofti*, a human filarial nematode, that causes filariasis. This disease mainly causes lymphedema, which in turn leads to patient morbidity and is potentially fatal. In 2014, Sugumar et al. [31] developed a eucalyptus EO-based nanoemulsion that showed larvicidal activity against *C. quinquefasciatus*. The treated larvae exhibited lower protein levels, as well as significant reduction in the levels of acetylcholinesterase and acid/basic phosphatase. In this way, the developed nanoemulsions can be used as a safe and effective alternative in the control of vector-borne filariasis.

Ghosh et al. [32] demonstrated the activity of the nanoemulsionated EO from *Ocimum basilicum* L. against third instar larvae from *Aedes aegypti*, one of the main dengue-transmitting mosquitoes. The EO composition was shown to be 88% of methyl chavicol (estragole), a phenylpropanoid with insecticidal property [33]. Thus, in this work, the hundred-fold dilution of nanoemulsion caused larval mortality of 60 and 70% after exposure periods of 60 and 75 min, respectively. Complete loss of larval viability in this concentration was observed after an exposure period of 90 min. However, the ten-fold diluted nanoemulsion induced 100% larval mortality of *A. aegypti* in 15 min [32].

In 2015, Brazilian researchers developed a nanoemulsion with *Rosmarinus officinalis* EO as an active constituent against 4th instar larvae of *A. aegypti*. The mortality ratio was evaluated after 24 h and 48 h of contact with the nanoemulsion at 250 ppm, which induced 80 and 90% mortality, respectively [34]. 1,8-cineol is the main constituent of this EO and showed potent larvicidal activity [35,36]. Previously in 2005, Prajapati et al. [37] demonstrated that the non-emulsified *R. officinalis* EO exhibited a DL_{95} of 408 ppm after 24 h of contact, which, in comparison, denotes the greater larvicidal effectiveness of the nanoemulsion.

Volpato et al. [38], in 2016, evaluated the effect of *Cinnamomum zelanycum* EO on mealworm (*Alphitobius diaperinus*), an insect of Coleoptera order that causes poultry diseases by transmitting pathogenic bacteria and viruses. In the chemical analysis, the EO presented cinnamaldehyde as the major constituent. The nanoemulsions at a concentration of 5% caused 70% mortality of the larvae at the L8 stage after two days, and had a three-fold more pronounced effect when compared to treatment with unemulsified EO within 3 days. Moreover, the nanoemulsions showed no deleterious effects on survival and reproduction tests of springtails (*Folsomia candida*), evidencing that nanoencapsulation of cinnamon oil significantly reduced its toxic effects without altering the effectiveness in controlling *A. diaperinus*.

More recently, in 2017, larvicidal activity against *A. aegypti* was also demonstrated by the work of Botas et al. [39]. They produced nanoemulsions based on EO of *Baccharis reticulata*, as well as D-limonene, its major component (25%). The two nanoemulsions caused mortality of the larvae of *A. aegypti*, with LC_{50} values of 118.94 µg/mL and 81.19 µg/mL, respectively. These results reinforce the importance of D-limonene as the main active agent of the EO composition, probably by inhibition of acetylcholinesterase, an activity also demonstrated through this study. In the same year, Balasubramani et al. [40] described a similar effect on *A. aegypti* larvae. In this work, the nanoemulsion of leaf EO from *Vitex negundo* L. was active against 2nd and 3rd instar larvae, after 12 and 24 h exposure periods. After a 12 h exposure period, the LC_{50} values of 2nd and 3rd instar larvae were 64.54 and 70.31 ppm, respectively. In comparison, the values of the non-emulsioned EO were 118.15 and 92.63, respectively. Likewise, after a 24 h exposure period, the nanoemulsion LC_{50} values were 28.84 and 43.29 ppm, whereas the non-emulsioned EO values were 77.35 and 56.13 ppm, respectively.

Still more recently, researchers from Iran published a work about inhibition of *Anopheles stephensi*, a major vector of malaria in their country, by the action of the nanoemulsion-based in EO from *Artemisia dracunculus* (Asteraceae). A bioassay of nanoemulsion on 3rd and 4th instar larvae was performed, with LC_{50} or LC_{90} of 11.36 or 17.54 ppm, respectively. The major EO constituent was *p*-allylanisole [41]. Similarly, one year later, some of these authors also evaluated the larvicidal effect on *A. stephensi* by the action of nanoemulsionated EO from *Anethum graveolens* (Umbelliferae), which presented *p*-cymene and α-phellandrene as main compounds. After 1 h of contact, larvicidal activities of 50 and 90% were found at 38.8 and 65 ppm, respectively, against 3rd and 4th instar larvae of *A. stephensi*. The authors considered it to be a preparation with appropriate activity against larvae of *A. stephensi* with no minimum environmental effect [42]. Moreover, in comparison with a similar study with *A. graveolens* non-emulsified EO, the nanoemulsion showed more effectiveness, since the oil LD_{50} without nanoemulsification was 100 ppm after the same contact time [43].

In late 2018, Sundararajan et al. [44] showed the activity of the nanoemulsionated leaf EO from *Ocimum basilicum* on 2nd and 3rd instar larvae of *C. quinquefasciatus*. *Trans*-β-Guaiene (16.89%) and α-Cadinol (15.66%) were the major compounds of this EO. The larvicidal activity was observed after a 24 h exposure period, and significant mortality was observed after the treatments with nanoemulsion, in which the 2nd and 3rd instar larvae exhibited maximum mortality at 100 ppm (96.87 ± 0.55% and 93.89 ± 0.55%, respectively). All studies described in this section are shown in Table 1.

Table 1. Larvicidal activity of essential oil nanoemulsions.

Specie	Common Name	Main Essential Oil Compound(s)	Emulsificant	Insect	References
Anethum graveolens	Dill	*p*–Cymene and α-phellandrene	Tween 20	*Anopheles stephensi*	[42]
Artemisia dracunculus	Tarragon	*p*-Allylanisole	Tween 20	*Anopheles stephensi*	[41]
Baccharis reticularia	Sand-Rosemary	D-limonene	Tween 80	*Aedes aegypti*	[39]
Cinnamomum zeylanicum	True cinnamon tree	Cinnamaldehyde	Tween 80	*Alphitobius diaperinus*	[38]
Eucalyptus globulus	Eucalyptus	1,8-cineole	Tween 80	*Culex quinquefasciatus*	[31]
Ocimum basilicum	Basil	Methyl-chavicol	Tween 20	*Aedes aegypti*	[32]
Ocimum basilicum	Basil	*trans*-β-Guaiene and α-Cadinol	Tween 80	*Culex quinquefasciatus*	[44]
Rosmarinus officinalis	Rosemary	1,8-cineole	Tween 20	*Aedes aegypti*	[34]
Vitex negundo	Chinese chaste tree	2(*R*)-acetoxymethyl-1,3,3-trimethyl-4t-(3-methyl-2-buten-1-yl)-1t-cyclohexanol	Tween 80	*Aedes aegypti*	[40]

2.2. Insecticidal and Repellent Activity

Other scientific groups also have conducted studies on adult insects, as well as on other insect development stages. In 2017, Ramar et al. [45] evaluated the effect of different nanoformulations of EO from *Ocimum sanctum* on *A. aegypti* and *C. quinquefasciatus* adult species. Through the filter paper impregnation method, the formulation containing 30% of EO caused 98% (*A. aegypti*) and 100% (*C. quinquefasciatus*) of knock down activity when diluted to a concentration of 50 mg/cm^2.

In 2008, Sakulku et al. [46] showed the repellent effect of a citronella EO nanoemulsion against *A. aegypti*, using the human-bait technique, based on standard test of World Health Organization (WHO). The nanoemulsion containing 20% oil and 1:1 glycerol-water ratio resulted in a high protection time (2.8 h), which can be considered high in comparison with EO diluted to 10% in olive oil, which, in turn, showed a protection time of only 54.75 min. D-limonene and citronellal were the principal substances of the EO (40% each) and have repellent activity [47].

One year later, Nuchuchua et al. [48] reported the repellent effect of nanoemulsions from different EOs on *A. aegypti* adults. In this study, seven formulations were made using different proportions of oils from *Cymbopogon nardus* (citronella oil), *Ocimum americanum* (hairy basil) and *Vetiveria zizanioides* (vetiver). Using the human-bait technique, the formulation with percentage concentration of 10:5:5 (citronella, hairy basil and vetiver) produced a protection time of 4.7 h. Limonene and citronellal (citronella), 3-carene and caryophyllene (hairy basil) and vetiveric acid (vetiver) were the major compounds in the EOs, and probably acted through synergic mechanisms. All nanoemulsions described in this section are shown in Table 2.

Table 2. Insecticidal, repellent and acaricidal activity of essential oil nanoemulsions.

Specie	Common Name	Main Essential Oil Compound(s)	Emulsificant	Insect/Parasite	References
Cinnamomum verum	Cinnamomum	Cinnamaldehyde	Tween 80	*Rhipicephalus microplus* (Acaricidal activity)	[49]
Cymbopogon nardus	Citronella	D-limonene and citronellal	Montanov 82	*Aedes aegypti* (Repellent activity)	[46]
Cymbopogon nardus, Ocimum americanum and *Vetiveria zizanioides*	Citronella, Hairy Basil and Vetiver	D-limonene and citronellal (*C. nardus*), 3-carene and caryophyllene (*O. americanum*), vetiveric acid (*V. zizanioides*)	Montanov 82	*Aedes aegypti* (Repellent activity)	[48]
Eucalyptus globulus	Eucalyptus	1,8-cineole	Tween 80	*Rhipicephalus microplus* (Acaricidal activity)	[50]
Ocimum sanctum	Holy Basil	Not described	Not described	*Culex quinquefasciatus* and *Aedes aegypti* (Inseticide activity)	[45]

2.3. Acaricidal Activity

Rhipicephalus microplus is an Ixodidae tick that causes severe economic losses on livestock, and it is the main vector of tick-transmitted agents such as *Babesia bigemina*, *B. bovis* and *Anaplasma marginale*. Some groups of researchers have reported the acaricidal activity of EO nanoemulsions against this species. Santos et al. [49] demonstrated the activity of the nanoemulsion-based in 5% *Cinnamomum verum* EO that caused 97% and 63.5% of oviposition inhibition, in vitro and in vivo, respectively. In comparison, other study made by Monteiro et al. [51] showed that the non-emulsioned EO did not caused oviposition inhibition. Moreover, after 20 days, the cows that were previously infested and treated with the nanoemulsion were free of the parasites [49]. Similar work done by Galli et al. [50] and contributors with *Eucalyptus globulus* nanoemulsion showed that the formulations at 1% and 5% inhibited parasite reproduction by 50% and 61.2%, respectively. All oil nanoemulsions with acaricidal activity are shown in Table 2.

2.4. Antiparasitic Activity on Etiological Agents

Trypanosoma evansi is a flagellate parasite and the etiological agent of the disease known as "Surra" and "Mal das Cadeiras" in Brazilian horses and rarely affects humans. In 2013, Baldissera et al. [52] evaluated the in vitro trypanocidal activity of the nanoemulsified *Schinus molle* EO. The nanoemulsion at 0.5% and 1% were able to reduce the number of living parasites in 81% and 100%, respectively. When these results were compared with the non-emulsified EO, this one showed a lower mortality rate, with 63% and 68%, respectively. In 2017, Ziaei et al. [53] observed the in vitro effect of *Lavandula officinalis* EO nanoemulsion on *Trichomonas vaginalis*, a flagellated parasite that causes trichomoniasis. At the concentration of 100 µg/mL, the nanoemulsion showed 81.9% of growth inhibition and exhibited low toxicity and macrophages (90.9% viability).

In 2017, Shokri et al. [54] also investigated the antiparasitic activity of nanoemulsionated EO of a *Lavanudula* species. The nanoemulsion of *L. angustifolia*, as well as of *R. officinalis*, showed an antileishmanial effect against *Leishmania major*, one of the etiological agents of cutaneous leishmaniasis in Iran. 1,8-cineol (22.29%) and linalool (11.22%) were the major compounds of *L. angustifolia* EO. The nanoemulsions of *L. angustifolia* and *R. officinalis* EOs showed antileishmania activity on promastigote with IC_{50} = 0.11 µL/mL and IC_{50} = 0.08 µL/mL, respectively. Compared to a similar study with the non-emulsioned EO of *R. officinalis*, this one showed IC_{50} = 2.6 µL/mL [55], which demonstrates a greater potency of the nanoemulsion to cause the mortality of the parasite. During the amastigote assay, both nanoemulsions were effective at least in concentration of 0.12 µL/mL and

0.06 µL/mL respectively, on mean infected macrophages (MIR) and amastigotes in macrophages [54]. In the same year, Moazeni et al. [56] evaluated the effect of *Zataria multiflora* EO on *Echinococcus granulosus sensu lato*, which causes cystic echinococcosis, a zoonotic infection with economic and public health importance in worldwide. The effect was observed on the protoscoleces form, originated in liver hydatid cysts collected from naturally infected sheep. The in vivo results showed that the scolicidal power of the nanoemulsion at concentration of 1 mg/mL was 88.01% and 100% after 10 and 20 min, respectively, while at a concentration of 2 mg/mL, the formulation showed 100% of scolicidal power after 10 min. When compared with a study made by Mahmoudvand et al. [57] in 2017, with non-emulsified oil, the nanoemulsion showed a more pronounced effect, since the EO alone at a concentration of 3125 µL/mL caused only 43.3% and 78.6% mortality after 10 and 20 min of exposure time, respectively. The in vivo studies revealed that the sizes of the largest cysts, as well as the total number of the cysts, were significantly lower in the mice treated with nanoemulsion [56]. It has been previously reported that thymol is the main compound of *Z. multiflora* EO [58] and is involved with the scolicidal activity [57,59,60] and destructive effect on the germinal layer of hydatid cysts [61]. All studies described in this section are shown in Table 3.

Table 3. Antiparasitic activity of essential oil nanoemulsions.

Species	Common Name	Main Essential Oil Compound(s)	Emulsificant	Parasite	References
Lavandula angustifolia and *Rosmarinus officinalis*	Lavander and Rosemary	1,8-cineole and linalool	Tween 80	*Leishmania major*	[54]
Lavandula officinalis	Lavender	1,8-cineole	Tween 80	*Trichomonas vaginalis*	[53]
Schinus molle	Peruvian peppertree	Not Described	Tween 20	*Trypanosoma evansi*	[52]
Zataria multiflora	Avishan Shirazi	Thymol	Tween 80	Protoscoleces of the hydatid cysts	[56]

In general, recent works on the use of nanoemulsions with EOs as active agents in the control of diseases caused by different agents have reported the diversity of targets and efficiency when compared to other agents already used, as well as their simplicity of production [62,63]. The technology of nanoemulsion production provides several advantages with respect to the dispersed active principle and formulation stability, such as (i) better protection of the active against chemical or biological degradation, (ii) lower probability of creaming or sedimentation of droplets, (iii) greater contact surface of the target with the droplets that contains the active agent, (iv) possibility of dispersion of immiscible substances in a certain solvent, which in the case of EOs is usually water, besides the simplicity of production, (v) low cost of reagents, and (vi) less residual damage to the environment when compared to synthetic products, widely used in modern times [22,27,63].

Regarding the potentialization of the action of the dispersed active in the formulation, this is the main advantage provided by the nanoformulations, since the EOs have serious problems of dispersion in aqueous vehicles and that mainly, in the case of contact with insects and other vectors, who have a large part of their cycle or living environment in contact with water, this is a limiting factor for the effectiveness of the action [24,25]. These facts can be observed when some results showed in the present review are compared with similar studies made with non-emulsified oils in which the EOs alone were not able to equalize the activity extension of the nanoformulations.

The diversity of the constituents of the EOs, mainly monoterpenes, sesquiterpenes and phenylpropanoids, contributes to the variety of mechanisms of action in the control of vectors and etiological agents of infectious/parasitic diseases, increasing the possibility of synergistic effect [64–66]. Some studies have described the probable toxicological or pharmacological effects of nanoemulsified EOs, such as eucalyptus oil, which decreased protein levels and caused inhibition of enzymes such as acetylcholinesterase and acid phosphatase in *C. quinquefasciatus* larvae [31], as well as the probably anticholinesterasic effect of *B. reticulata* EO on *A. aegypti* larvae [32]. In both cases, terpenes were the major components of the EOs, whereas in other works that showed phenols and phenylpropanoids as major constituents, the mechanisms of actions presented other specificities, as for example in the works of Ghosh et al. [32] (methyl-chavicol) and Moazeni et al. [58] (thymol). Finally, the nanoemulsion process of EOs benefits the performance of the action of its active components by several physical, chemical and biological factors, making real the potential application of these vegetal metabolites in the control of infectious/parasitic diseases.

3. Conclusions

The nanomodification of EOs, which are hydro-immiscible in nature, significantly improves life utility and effectiveness as a pesticide or antiparasitic. Nanoformulation requires a smaller quantity of EO to develop a formulation, and the use of bio-surfactants and water also makes these nanopesticides conducive and friendly to the environment. The removal of the volatile organic solvent from the pesticide formulation improves its bio-security property and makes it a "greener" strategy for the control of vectors of pathogenic diseases. A higher degree of delivery to the target of action, stability of formulation, water dispersion, low cost, and lower ecological toxicity make these essential oil nanoformulations very efficient and highly ecological. Based on the works incorporated in this study, it can be concluded that the nanopesticides can be an efficient tool with an eco-safe property and can be applied safely to the control of vectors of diseases in humans and animals. Moreover, other studies with EO nanoemulsions have also shown its antiparasitic activity on etiological agents, which considers the possible use of these formulations in the treatment of infections, as well as their prevention.

Author Contributions: Conceptualization, J.E. and R.D.D.G.d.A.; methodology, J.E. and R.D.D.G.d.A.; validation, J.E.; formal analysis, J.E. and R.D.D.G.d.A.; investigation, J.E. and R.D.D.G.d.A.; resources, J.E.; data curation, J.E. and R.D.D.G.d.A.; writing—original draft preparation, J.E. and R.D.D.G.d.A.; writing—review and editing, J.E. and R.D.D.G.d.A.; visualization, J.E. and R.D.D.G.d.A.; supervision, J.E. and R.D.D.G.d.A.; project administration, J.E.; funding acquisition, J.E.

Funding: This research was funded by CONICYT PAI/ACADEMIA No. 79160109.

Acknowledgments: The authors would like to thank a postdoctoral FONDECYT grant No. 3130327 and CONICYT PAI/ACADEMIA No. 79160109 (awarded to J.E.).

Conflicts of Interest: The authors declare no conflict of interest.

References

1. Urzúa, A.; Santander, R.; Echeverría, J.; Cabezas, N.; Palacios, S.M.; Rossi, Y. Insecticide properties of the essential oils from *Haplopappus foliosus* and *Bahia ambrosoides* against the house fly, *Musca domestica* L. *J. Chil. Chem. Soc.* **2010**, *55*, 392–395. [CrossRef]
2. Urzúa, A.; Santander, R.; Echeverría, J.; Villalobos, C.; Palacios, S.M.; Rossi, Y. Insecticidal properties of *Peumus boldus* Mol. essential oil on the house fly, *Musca domestica* L. *Bol. Latinoam Caribe Plantas Med. Aromat.* **2010**, *9*, 465–469.
3. Urzúa, A.; di Cosmo, D.; Echeverría, J.; Santander, R.; Palacios, S.M.; Rossi, Y. Insecticidal effect of *Schinus latifolius* essential oil on the housefly, *Musca domestica* L. *Bol. Latinoam Caribe Plantas Med. Aromat.* **2011**, *10*, 470–475.
4. Espinoza, J.; Urzúa, A.; Bardehle, L.; Quiroz, A.; Echeverría, J.; González-Teuber, M. Antifeedant effects of essential oil, extracts, and isolated sesquiterpenes from *Pilgerodendron uviferum* (D. Don) Florin heartwood on red clover borer *Hylastinus obscurus* (Coleoptera: Curculionidae). *Molecules* **2018**, *23*, 1282. [CrossRef]
5. Ferhat, M.A.; Meklati, B.Y.; Chemat, F. Comparison of different isolation methods of essential oil from *Citrus* fruits: Cold pressing, hydrodistillation and microwave 'dry'distillation. *Flavour Fragr. J.* **2007**, *22*, 494–504. [CrossRef]
6. Kaufmann, B.; Christen, P. Recent extraction techniques for natural products: Microwave-assisted extraction and pressurised solvent extraction. *Phytochem. Anal.* **2002**, *13*, 105–113. [CrossRef]
7. Figueiredo, A.C.; Barroso, J.G.; Pedro, L.G.; Scheffer, J.J.C. Factors affecting secondary metabolite production in plants: Volatile components and essential oils. *Flavour Fragr. J.* **2008**, *23*, 213–226. [CrossRef]
8. Mills, C.; Cleary, B.V.; Walsh, J.J.; Gilmer, J.F. Inhibition of acetylcholinesterase by tea tree oil. *J. Pharm. Pharmacol.* **2004**, *56*, 375–379. [CrossRef]

9. Priestley, C.M.; Williamson, E.M.; Wafford, K.A.; Sattelle, D.B. Thymol, a constituent of thyme essential oil, is a positive allosteric modulator of human GABAA receptors and a homo-oligomeric GABA receptor from *Drosophila melanogaster*. *Br. J. Pharmacol.* **2003**, *140*, 1363–1372. [CrossRef]

10. Enan, E.E. Molecular response of *Drosophila melanogaster* tyramine receptor cascade to plant essential oils. *Insect Biochem. Mol. Biol.* **2005**, *35*, 309–321. [CrossRef]

11. Munro, I.C.; Ford, R.A.; Kennepohl, E.; Sprenger, J.G. Correlation of structural class with no-observed-effect levels: A proposal for establishing a threshold of concern. *Food Chem. Toxicol.* **1996**, *34*, 829–867. [CrossRef]

12. Smith, R.L.; Cohen, S.M.; Doull, J.; Feron, V.J.; Goodman, J.I.; Marnett, L.J.; Portoghese, P.S.; Waddell, W.J.; Wagner, B.M.; Hall, R.L. A procedure for the safety evaluation of natural flavor complexes used as ingredients in food: Essential oils. *Food Chem. Toxicol.* **2005**, *43*, 345–363. [CrossRef] [PubMed]

13. Monzote, L.; Alarcón, O.; Setzer, W.N. Antiprotozoal activity of essential oils. *Agric. Conspec. Sci.* **2012**, *77*, 167–175.

14. Ramos-Lopez, M.A.; Sanchez-Mir, E.; Fresan-Orozco, M.C.; Perez-Ramos, J. Antiprotozoa activity of some essential oils. *J. Med. Plants Res.* **2012**, *6*, 2901–2908. [CrossRef]

15. Rossi-Bergmann, B. A nanotecnologia: Da saúde para além do determinismo tecnológico. *Ciênc. Cult.* **2008**, *60*, 54–57.

16. De Souza Marcone, G.P. Nanotecnologia e nanociência: Aspectos gerais, aplicações e perspectivas no contexto do Brasil. *Rev. Eletrôn. Perspect. Ciênc. Tecnol.* **2016**, *7*, 1–24.

17. De Melo, C.P.; Pimenta, M. Nanociências e nanotecnologia. *Parcerias Estratég.* **2010**, *9*, 9–22.

18. Dúran, N. *Nanotecnologia: Introdução, Preparação e Caracterização de Nanomateriais e Exemplos de Aplicação*; Artliber: São Paulo, Brazil, 2006; ISBN 8588098334.

19. Pimentel, L.F.; Jácome Júnior, A.T.; Mosqueira, V.C.F.; Santos-Magalhães, N.S. Nanotecnologia farmacêutica aplicada ao tratamento da malária. *Rev. Bras. Ciênc. Farm.* **2007**, *43*, 503–514. [CrossRef]

20. Craparo, E.F.; Bondì, M.L.; Pitarresi, G.; Cavallaro, G. Nanoparticulate systems for drug delivery and targeting to the central nervous system. *CNS Neurosci. Ther.* **2011**, *17*, 670–677. [CrossRef]

21. Salager, J.-L.; Antón, R.E.; Andérez, J.M.; Aubry, J.M. Formulation des micro-émulsions par la méthode HLD. In *Techniques de l'Ingénieur*, 1st ed.; Editions T.I.: Paris, France, 2001; pp. 1–20.

22. Solans, C.; Izquierdo, P.; Nolla, J.; Azemar, N.; Garcia-Celma, M.J. Nano-emulsions. *Curr. Opin. Colloid Interface Sci.* **2005**, *10*, 102–110. [CrossRef]

23. Forgiarini, A.; Esquena, J.; González, C.; Solans, C. Studies of the relation between phase behavior and emulsification methods with nanoemulsion formation. In *Trends in Colloid and Interface Science XIV*; Springer: Berlin/Heidelberg, Germany, 2000; pp. 36–39. [CrossRef]

24. Chime, S.A.; Kenechukwu, F.C.; Attama, A.A. Nanoemulsions—advances in formulation, characterization and applications in drug delivery. In *Application of Nanotechnology in Drug Delivery*; InTechOpen: London, UK, 2014.

25. De Campos, V.E.B.; Ricci-Júnior, E.; Mansur, C.R.E. Nanoemulsions as delivery systems for lipophilic drugs. *J. Nanosci. Nanotechnol.* **2012**, *12*, 2881–2890. [CrossRef] [PubMed]

26. Trommer, H.; Neubert, R.H.H. Overcoming the stratum corneum: The modulation of skin penetration. *Skin Pharmacol. Physiol.* **2006**, *19*, 106–121. [CrossRef] [PubMed]

27. Wang, L.; Li, X.; Zhang, G.; Dong, J.; Eastoe, J. Oil-in-water nanoemulsions for pesticide formulations. *J. Colloid Interface Sci.* **2007**, *314*, 230–235. [CrossRef] [PubMed]

28. Hazra, D.K. Nano-formulations: High definition liquid engineering of pesticides for nano-formulations: High definition liquid engineering of pesticides for advanced crop protection in agriculture. *Adv. Plant. Agric. Res.* **2017**, *6*, 1–2. [CrossRef]

29. Mishra, P.; Balaji, A.P.B.; Tyagi, B.K.; Mukherjee, A.; Chandrasekaran, N. Nanopesticides: A boon towards the control of dreadful vectors of lymphatic filariasis. In *Lymphatic Filariasis*; Springer: Singapore, 2018; pp. 247–257.

30. Mishra, P.; Balaji, A.P.B.; Mukherjee, A.; Chandrasekaran, N. Bio-based nanoemulsions: An eco-safe approach towards the eco-toxicity problem. In *Handbook of Ecomaterials*; Springer: Singapore, 2018; pp. 1–23.

31. Sugumar, S.; Clarke, S.K.; Nirmala, M.J.; Tyagi, B.K.; Mukherjee, A.; Chandrasekaran, N. Nanoemulsion of *Eucalyptus* oil and its larvicidal activity against *Culex quinquefasciatus*. *Bull. Entomol. Res.* **2014**, *104*, 393–402. [CrossRef]

32. Ghosh, V.; Sugumar, S.; Mukherjee, A.; Chandrasekaran, N. Cinnamon oil nanoemulsion formulation by ultrasonic emulsification: Investigation of Its bactericidal activity. *J. Nanosci. Nanotechnol.* **2013**, *13*, 114–122. [CrossRef]

33. Chang, C.L.; Kyu Cho, I.; Li, Q.X. Insecticidal activity of basil oil, trans-anethole, estragole, and linalool to adult fruit flies of *Ceratitis capitata*, *Bactrocera dorsalis*, and *Bactrocera cucurbitae*. *J. Econ. Entomol.* **2009**, *102*, 203–209. [CrossRef]

34. Duarte, J.L.; Amado, J.R.R.; Oliveira, A.E.M.F.M.; Cruz, R.A.S.; Ferreira, A.M.; Souto, R.N.P.; Falcão, D.Q.; Carvalho, J.C.T.; Fernandes, C.P. Evaluation of larvicidal activity of a nanoemulsion of *Rosmarinus officinalis* essential oil. *Rev. Bras. Farmacogn.* **2015**, *25*, 189–192. [CrossRef]

35. Conti, B.; Canale, A.; Bertoli, A.; Gozzini, F.; Pistelli, L. Essential oil composition and larvicidal activity of six Mediterranean aromatic plants against the mosquito *Aedes albopictus* (Diptera: Culicidae). *Parasitol. Res.* **2010**, *107*, 1455–1461. [CrossRef] [PubMed]

36. Conti, B.; Canale, A.; Cioni, P.L.; Flamini, G. Repellence of essential oils from tropical and mediterranean lamiaceae against *Sitophilus zeamais*. *Bull. Insectol.* **2010**, *63*, 197–202.

37. Prajapati, V.; Tripathi, A.K.; Aggarwal, K.K.; Khanuja, S.P.S. Insecticidal, repellent and oviposition-deterrent activity of selected essential oils against *Anopheles stephensi*, *Aedes aegypti* and *Culex quinquefasciatus*. *Bioresour. Technol.* **2005**, *96*, 1749–1757. [CrossRef] [PubMed]

38. Volpato, A.; Baretta, D.; Zortéa, T.; Campigotto, G.; Galli, G.M.; Glombowsky, P.; Santos, R.C.V.; Quatrin, P.M.; Ourique, A.F.; Baldissera, M.D. Larvicidal and insecticidal effect of *Cinnamomum zeylanicum* oil (pure and nanostructured) against mealworm (*Alphitobius diaperinus*) and its possible environmental effects. *J. Asia Pac. Entomol.* **2016**, *19*, 1159–1165. [CrossRef]

39. Botas, G.d.S.; Cruz, R.A.S.; de Almeida, F.B.; Duarte, J.L.; Araújo, R.S.; Souto, R.N.P.; Ferreira, R.; Carvalho, J.C.T.; Santos, M.G.; Rocha, L.; et al. *Baccharis reticularia* DC. and limonene nanoemulsions: Promising larvicidal agents for *Aedes aegypti* (Diptera: Culicidae) control. *Molecules* **2017**, *22*, 1990. [CrossRef]

40. Balasubramani, S.; Rajendhiran, T.; Moola, A.; Kumari, B. Development of nanoemulsion from *Vitex negundo* L. essential oil and their efficacy of antioxidant, antimicrobial and larvicidal activities (*Aedes aegypti* L.). *Environ. Sci. Pollut. Res.* **2017**, *24*, 15125–15133. [CrossRef]

41. Osanloo, M.; Amani, A.; Sereshti, H.; Abai, M.R.; Esmaeili, F.; Sedaghat, M.M. Preparation and optimization nanoemulsion of tarragon (*Artemisia dracunculus*) essential oil as effective herbal larvicide against *Anopheles stephensi*. *Ind. Crops Prod.* **2017**, *109*, 214–219. [CrossRef]

42. Osanloo, M.; Sereshti, H.; Sedaghat, M.M.; Amani, A. Nanoemulsion of dill essential oil as a green and potent larvicide against *Anopheles stephensi*. *Environ. Sci. Pollut. Res.* **2018**, *25*, 6466–6473. [CrossRef]

43. Amer, A.; Mehlhorn, H. Larvicidal effects of various essential oils against *Aedes*, *Anopheles*, and *Culex* larvae (Diptera, Culicidae). *Parasitol. Res.* **2006**, *99*, 466–472. [CrossRef] [PubMed]

44. Sundararajan, B.; Moola, A.K.; Vivek, K.; Kumari, B.D.R. Formulation of nanoemulsion from leaves essential oil of *Ocimum basilicum* L. and its antibacterial, antioxidant and larvicidal activities (*Culex quinquefasciatus*). *Microb. Pathog.* **2018**, *125*, 475–485. [CrossRef]

45. Ramar, M.; Manonmani, P.; Arumugam, P.; Kannam, S.K.; Erusan, R.R.; Baskaran, N.; Murugan, K. Nano-insecticidal formulations from essential oil (*Ocimum sanctum*) and fabricated in filter paper on adult of *Aedes aegypti* and *Culex quinquefasciatus*. *J. Entomol. Zool. Stud.* **2017**, *5*, 1769–1774.

46. Sakulku, U.; Nuchuchua, O.; Uawongyart, N.; Puttipipatkhachorn, S.; Soottitantawat, A.; Ruktanonchai, U. Characterization and mosquito repellent activity of citronella oil nanoemulsion. *Int. J. Pharm.* **2009**, *372*, 105–111. [CrossRef]

47. Sritabutra, D.; Soonwera, M.; Waltanachanobon, S.; Poungjai, S. Evaluation of herbal essential oil as repellents against *Aedes aegypti* (L.) and *Anopheles dirus* Peyton & Harrion. *Asian Pac. J. Trop. Biomed.* **2011**, *1*, S124–S128. [CrossRef]

48. Nuchuchua, O.; Sakulku, U.; Uawongyart, N.; Puttipipatkhachorn, S.; Soottitantawat, A.; Ruktanonchai, U. In vitro characterization and mosquito (*Aedes aegypti*) repellent activity of essential-oils-loaded nanoemulsions. *Aaps Pharmscitech.* **2009**, *10*, 1234. [CrossRef] [PubMed]

49. Santos, D.S.; Boito, J.P.; Santos, R.C.V.; Quatrin, P.M.; Ourique, A.F.; dos Reis, J.H.; Gebert, R.R.; Glombowsky, P.; Klauck, V.; Boligon, A.A. Nanostructured cinnamon oil has the potential to control *Rhipicephalus microplus* ticks on cattle. *Exp. Appl. Acarol.* **2017**, *73*, 129–138. [CrossRef] [PubMed]

50. Galli, G.M.; Volpato, V.; Santos, R.C.V.; Gebert, R.R.; Quatrin, P.; Ourique, A.F.; Klein, B.; Wagner, R.; Tonin, A.A.; Baldissera, M.D. Effects of essential oil of Eucalyptus globulus loaded in nanoemulsions and in nanocapsules on reproduction of cattle tick (Rhipicephalus microplus). *Arch. Zootec.* **2018**, *67*, 494–498. [CrossRef]

51. Monteiro, I.N.; dos Santos Monteiro, O.; Costa-Junior, L.M.; da Silva Lima, A.; de Aguiar Andrade, E.H.; Maia, J.G.S.; Mouchrek Filho, V.E. Chemical composition and acaricide activity of an essential oil from a rare chemotype of *Cinnamomum verum* Presl on *Rhipicephalus microplus* (Acari: Ixodidae). *Vet. Parasitol.* **2017**, *238*, 54–57. [CrossRef]

52. Baldissera, M.D.; Da Silva, A.S.; Oliveira, C.B.; Zimmermann, C.E.P.; Vaucher, R.A.; Santos, R.C.V.; Rech, V.C.; Tonin, A.A.; Giongo, J.L.; Mattos, C.B. Trypanocidal activity of the essential oils in their conventional and nanoemulsion forms: In vitro tests. *Exp. Parasitol.* **2013**, *134*, 356–361. [CrossRef]

53. Ziaei Hezarjaribi, H.; Nadeali, N.; Saeedi, M.; Soosaraei, M.; Jorjani, O.N.; Momeni, Z.; Fakhar, M. The effect of lavender essential oil and nanoemulsion on *Trichomonas vaginalis* in vitro. *Feyz J. Kashan Univ. Med. Sci.* **2017**, *21*, 326–334.

54. Shokri, A.; Saeedi, M.; Fakhar, M.; Morteza-Semnani, K.; Keighobadi, M.; Teshnizi, S.H.; Kelidari, H.R.; Sadjadi, S. Antileishmanial activity of *Lavandula angustifolia* and *Rosmarinus officinalis* essential oils and nano-emulsions on *Leishmania major* (MRHO/IR/75/ER). *Iran. J. Parasitol.* **2017**, *12*, 622–631.

55. Bouyahya, A.; Et-Touys, A.; Bakri, Y.; Talbaui, A.; Fellah, H.; Abrini, J.; Dakka, N. Chemical composition of *Mentha pulegium* and *Rosmarinus officinalis* essential oils and their antileishmanial, antibacterial and antioxidant activities. *Microb. Pathog.* **2017**, *111*, 41–49. [CrossRef]

56. Moazeni, M.; Borji, H.; Darbandi, M.S.; Saharkhiz, M.J. In vitro and in vivo antihydatid activity of a nano emulsion of *Zataria multiflora* essential oil. *Res. Vet. Sci.* **2017**, *114*, 308–312. [CrossRef] [PubMed]

57. Mahmoudvand, H.; Mirbadie, S.R.; Sadooghian, S.; Harandi, M.F.; Jahanbakhsh, S.; Saedi Dezaki, E. Chemical composition and scolicidal activity of *Zataria multiflora* Boiss essential oil. *J. Essent. Oil Res.* **2017**, *29*, 42–47. [CrossRef]

58. Moazeni, M.; Larki, S.; Saharkhiz, M.J.; Oryan, A.; Lari, M.A.; Alavi, A.M. Efficacy of the aromatic water of *Zataria multiflora* on hydatid cysts: An In vivo study. *Antimicrob. Agents Chemother.* **2014**, *58*, 6003–6008. [CrossRef] [PubMed]

59. Elissondo, M.C.; Albani, C.M.; Gende, L.; Eguaras, M.; Denegri, G. Efficacy of thymol against *Echinococcus granulosus* protoscoleces. *Parasitol. Int.* **2008**, *57*, 185–190. [CrossRef]

60. Yones, D.A.; Taher, G.A.; Ibraheim, Z.Z. In vitro effects of some herbs used in Egyptian traditional medicine on viability of protoscolices of hydatid cysts. *Korean J. Parasitol.* **2011**, *49*, 255. [CrossRef]

61. Elissondo, M.C.; Pensel, P.E.; Denegri, G.M. Could thymol have effectiveness on scolices and germinal layer of hydatid cysts? *Acta Trop.* **2013**, *125*, 251–257. [CrossRef]

62. Schummer, J. Multidisciplinarity, interdisciplinarity, and patterns of research collaboration in nanoscience and nanotechnology. *Scientometrics* **2004**, *59*, 425–465. [CrossRef]

63. Choi, H.; Mody, C.C.M. The long history of molecular electronics: Microelectronics origins of nanotechnology. *Soc. Stud. Sci.* **2009**, *39*, 11–50. [CrossRef]

64. Tripathi, A.K.; Upadhyay, S.; Bhuiyan, M.; Bhattacharya, P.R. A review on prospects of essential oils as biopesticide in insect-pest management. *J. Pharmacogn. Phyther.* **2009**, *1*, 52–63.

65. Meira, C.S.; Menezes, L.R.A.; dos Santos, T.B.; Macedo, T.S.; Fontes, J.E.N.; Costa, E.V.; Pinheiro, M.L.B.; da Silva, T.B.; Teixeira Guimarães, E.; Soares, M.B.P. Chemical composition and antiparasitic activity of essential oils from leaves of *Guatteria friesiana* and *Guatteria pogonopus* (Annonaceae). *J. Essent. Oil Res.* **2017**, *29*, 156–162. [CrossRef]

66. Dos Santos Sales, V.; Monteiro, Á.B.; de Araújo Delmondes, G.; do Nascimento, E.P. Antiparasitic activity and essential oil chemical analysis of the *Piper tuberculatum* Jacq fruit. *Iran. J. Pharm. Res. IJPR* **2018**, *17*, 268–275.

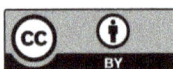

medicines

MDPI

Review

New Approaches to Detect Biosynthetic Gene Clusters in the Environment

Ray Chen [1,2], Hon Lun Wong [1,2] and Brendan Paul Burns [1,2,*]

[1] School of Biotechnology and Biomolecular Sciences, The University of New South Wales, Sydney 2052, Australia; ray.chen@student.unsw.edu.au (R.C.); h.l.wong@unsw.edu.au (H.L.W.)

[2] Australian Centre for Astrobiology, The University of New South Wales, Sydney 2052, Australia

* Correspondence: Brendan.burns@unsw.edu.au; Tel.: +61-2-9385-3659

Received: 26 January 2019; Accepted: 22 February 2019; Published: 25 February 2019

Abstract: Microorganisms in the environment can produce a diverse range of secondary metabolites (SM), which are also known as natural products. Bioactive SMs have been crucial in the development of antibiotics and can also act as useful compounds in the biotechnology industry. These natural products are encoded by an extensive range of biosynthetic gene clusters (BGCs). The developments in omics technologies and bioinformatic tools are contributing to a paradigm shift from traditional culturing and screening methods to bioinformatic tools and genomics to uncover BGCs that were previously unknown or transcriptionally silent. Natural product discovery using bioinformatics and omics workflow in the environment has demonstrated an extensive distribution of BGCs in various environments, such as soil, aquatic ecosystems and host microbiome environments. Computational tools provide a feasible and culture-independent route to find new secondary metabolites where traditional approaches cannot. This review will highlight some of the advances in the approaches, primarily bioinformatic, in identifying new BGCs, especially in environments where microorganisms are rarely cultured. This has allowed us to tap into the huge potential of microbial dark matter.

Keywords: natural products; biosynthetic gene clusters; secondary metabolites; antiSMASH

1. Introduction

Microorganisms in the environment can produce a wide range of secondary metabolites (SM). SMs are natural products with diverse chemical structures. This diversity in chemical structures enables these natural products to carry out a variety of functions. SMs can act as antibiotics, antitumor agents, cholesterol-lowering agents and so on [1]. These natural products have been critical in the development of therapeutics in medicine as it has been reported that approximately 70% of the anti-infective drugs are derived from natural products in the environment [2]. Without their discoveries, many of the therapeutics used to treat bacterial infections and diseases would not be available today.

Antimicrobial resistance is an emerging global challenge threatening future public health. Previous reports have predicted a worst-case scenario whereby the global economic impact of antimicrobial resistance will result in more than 10 million annual deaths, which is a loss of 2.0–3.5% of the world gross domestic product that is worth approximately 60–100 trillion USD by 2050 [3,4]. This growing problem emphasizes the importance of natural product discovery, particularly the search for new antimicrobials as an alternative to currently overused antibiotics. The synthesis and complexity of a natural product relies on many clustered genes playing various roles from assembly and regulation of expression [5].

Biosynthetic gene clusters (BGCs) are a physical grouping of all the genes responsible for the assembly of a SM [6]. BGCs contain genes encoding all enzymes that are required to produce a SM as well as pathway-specific regulatory genes [5]. Polyketide synthases (PKS) and non-ribosomal peptide synthases (NRPS) are two major biosynthetic systems containing multiple modules and enzymes [7]. PKS and NRPS synthesize the two major classes of SMs, which are namely polyketides and non-ribosomal peptides, respectively. PKS and NRPS are popular targets in genome mining for natural products and are well-known to synthesize a diverse range of products with beneficial applications in medicine and research, such as antibiotics, antifungals and immunosuppressants [8].

The developments in sequencing technology and readily available bioinformatic pipelines have enabled large quantities of BGCs to be mined from environmental microorganisms without having to culture them and test their bioactivity [9]. These tools also provide an incredible opportunity to elucidate the secondary metabolism properties of microbial dark matter, which is the uncultured majority of microbial diversity. Computational tools offer a feasible route to study SMs and BGCs in bacteria and are useful in generating and processing large amounts of data as seen in metagenomic studies. An extensive list of bioinformatics pipelines has been previously reviewed [10,11]. This review will highlight some notable examples, such as antiSMASH, ClustScan, NAPDOS and ClusterFinder.

Although computational tools have been useful for studying secondary metabolism from metagenomic datasets, the analysis of metagenomic data is challenging as the software requires high quality genome-resolved genomes or binned metagenomes [12]. Computational tools themselves have their own limitations, such as the reliance of databases and rules from previous knowledge, which may hinder the identification of novel BGCs as current algorithms cannot detect them. These limitations make it difficult to unlock the full chemical diversity of the environment [12].

To date, studies have screened for SMs in environments hosting large bacterial diversity and presumably large chemical diversity, such as aquatic ecosystems, soils and host microbiomes [13–15]. The purpose of this review is to highlight various methods used to identify BGCs in the environment and provide examples of how recent studies have explored the genetic basis for novel natural product synthesis, which have wide ranging medical and industrial applications.

2. Traditional Approaches in Natural Product Discovery

Prior to the advent of DNA sequencing and genomics, the search for natural products from microorganisms was conducted primarily using culture-dependent techniques in the laboratory [16]. The discovery of natural products typically involved sampling from the environment, culturing these samples and finally screening extracted products. However, it is very difficult to culture environmental microorganisms in the laboratory. The number of bacterial species that can be grown in the laboratory comprise only a small fraction of the total diversity that exists in nature [17]. Culturing microbes under different conditions was commonly used to produce and subsequently identify SMs without any knowledge of the genes and enzymes involved [18].

Biochemical assays are used primarily to screen for SMs or characterize function. Recently, the development of high throughput biochemical assays has helped to uncover more SMs. A study used thymol blue and bromothymol blue indicators to detect the pH drop in relation to sugar fermentation in *Vibrio cholerae* cultures. After screening 39,000 crude extracts, 49 were found to block fermentation and three were characterized as novel broad-spectrum antibiotics [19]. However, not all SMs can be detected and characterized using biochemical assays as some are produced at undetectable levels. Therefore, these approaches are more effective at identifying SMs that are secreted in relatively large amounts in nature and under laboratory conditions [18].

3. Omics Approaches for Natural Product Discovery

Traditional approaches have led to the discovery of many therapeutics that are now used today. However, natural product discovery efforts have since declined largely due to the increasing rediscovery rates of known compounds [20]. In addition, many microorganisms in the environment cannot be cultured in the laboratory, hence deterring research efforts for many years until the introduction of genomics and other omics technologies. Natural product discovery is undergoing an extensive paradigm shift, which is driven by technological developments in genomics, bioinformatics, analytical chemistry and synthetic biology [10]. Genome mining has been established as an important approach to complement bioprospecting efforts as they allow researchers to survey large datasets to determine whether the genomes of interest harbor BGCs of interest. This can be achieved before undertaking a more costly and laborious chemistry-driven approach to extract the natural product encoded by the BGC in a bacterial host. It has become possible to computationally identify thousands of BGCs in genome sequences and to systematically explore BGCs of interest for experimental characterization.

3.1. Metagenome Screening for BGCs Using Degenerate Primers

Degenerate primers are oligonucleotide sequences, with some positions containing more than one possible nucleotide base. This property can be used to target and amplify areas in the genome that are very similar but have slight variations [21]. This is especially useful when the same gene is to be amplified in different microbes as the same gene can vary slightly between species [8]. Degenerate primers can amplify genes of interest from the genomes of unculturable bacteria. A previous study reported that the NRPS genes associated with adenylation and thiolation domains are well-conserved in the genome, enabling degenerate primers to better target NRPS clusters in a variety of bacterial species as opposed to designing different primer sets for each species [22].

Customized primer sets were used to screen for NRPS and type I PKS (PKS-I) systems in Actinomycetes [8]. NRPS and PKS-I are known to produce a diverse range of SMs. Actinomycetes are gram-positive bacteria from the actinobacteria phylum and have been the focus for natural product discovery in previous decades due to the discovery of several antimicrobials, such as streptomycin and actinomycin, from the Actinomycetes phylum [16]. Primer sets were tested on 210 reference strains that covered the major families and 33 different genera in actinomycetes. PCR amplification of primers targeting NRPS was observed in 79.5% of strains while PCR amplification of primers targeting PKS-I was seen in 56.7% of strains [8]. The results of this study demonstrate the richness of NRPS and PKS-I-like sequences in actinomycetes, which is reflected in the diversity of antibiotics and other natural products that were previously reported in actinomycetes. Although degenerate primers can help to quantify biosynthetic capacity, they cannot be used to identify and characterize the structures of SM, which is one of the current major challenges for natural product discovery.

In a recent study, degenerate primers derived from conserved biosynthetic motifs were used to survey the ketosynthase domains from 185 soil microbiome samples [23]. BGCs encoding epoxyketone proteasome inhibitors were detected and a further analysis led to the isolation and characterization of seven epoxyketone natural products, including compounds with a unique warhead structure. Degenerate primers are useful in amplifying BGCs of interest but cannot be used to characterize a natural product. They must be used in conjunction with bioinformatic approaches with defined metagenomic tools so that natural products can be derived from metagenomic data in the environment.

3.2. BGC Detection and Analyses via Bioinformatic Pipelines

Many bioinformatics tools have now been developed to detect known BGCs in regular genome sequences and genome-resolved metagenomes [7]. There are also emerging tools aiming to detect novel BGCs hidden in cultured bacterial genomes and especially in environmental genome-resolved metagenomes [24].

antiSMASH, NAPDOS and ClustScan are examples of bioinformatics software that provide low novelty but high confidence in its analysis [25,26] and thus, are suitable for users looking for gene clusters of a known biosynthetic class or for surveying all detectable BGCs in single or multiple genomes for annotation purposes.

Although many bioinformatic tools can identify biosynthetic genes with high accuracy, it implies that only biosynthetic pathways with rules implemented in the software can be detected. Therefore, any pathway that may use unknown or unrelated alternative enzymes will be missed [12]. In addition, computational tools rely heavily on high quality genome-resolved metagenomes for effective and reliable outputs [12]. The quality of the sequencing data or resolved genomes from metagenomes can influence the reliability of results. Further complications regarding the analysis of metagenomic sequencing data for BGCs have been previously reviewed in more detail [10,27].

To address the limitations of identifying novel BGCs, the ClusterFinder algorithm is a recently developed software providing low confidence but high novelty analysis [24]. Predicting gene clusters from novel classes is valuable as they have the possibility of encoding molecules with new chemical scaffolds. ClusterFinder uses a hidden Markov model that switches between BGC and non-BGC analysis to look for patterns of broad gene functions encoded in a genomic region rather than searching for the presence of specific individual signature genes. This method enabled ClusterFinder to identify a large, previously unrecognized family of gene clusters that encode the biosynthesis of aryl polyenes in a wide range of bacteria from various phyla [24].

3.3. Expression of Transcriptionally Silent BGCs in Host Bacteria

One of the major challenges in natural product discovery is that the vast majority of BGCs are either transcriptionally silent or expressed at very low levels under standard laboratory conditions [28]. To address this issue, silent BGCs can be switched on by manipulating genetic elements embedded within BGCs [9]. Triggering BGC expression in a native host may involve artificially knocking-in a strong promoter that is located upstream of the target BGC [28]. For example, a CRISPR-Cas9 system-based promoter knock-in strategy was used to activate multiple silent BGCs in five different Streptomyces species, which led to the discovery of a novel pentangular polyketide from *Streptomyces viridochromogenes*. Activating silent BGCs in native hosts demonstrates great potential for high throughput discovery of natural products [29].

The advances in synthetic biology techniques have resulted in silent BGCs being activated in heterologous hosts [30]. Heterologous hosts can provide a significant growth advantage over native hosts and can bypass the regulatory system in the latter. This is especially useful as BGCs can be activated in unculturable microorganisms. However, one of the major problems associated with direct cloning is the low yield of positive clones, which is caused by the nonspecific targeting of random genomic fragments. Further refinement in the direct capture of gene clusters led to the discovery of taromycin A in *Streptomyces coelicolor* [31]. Moore et al. successfully extended this method to the heterologous expression of BGCs in *Bacillus subtilis* and *Escherichia coli*, which subsequently led to the discovery of a distinct group of thiotetronic acid natural products by combining this approach with targeted genome mining [32,33].

The use of chemical elicitors provide an alternative route to enhance the expression of silent BGCs [34]. This approach aims to increase the recovery of novel SMs that were previously hidden in silent BGCs both in culturable bacteria and in the unculturable majority of bacterial groups. Nodwell et al. demonstrated the use of chemical elicitor 'CI-ARC' to increase the yield of SM production in a collection of Actinomycetes strains [34]. The study also successfully identified a SM with activity against both bacteria and eukaryotes. This approach provides a mechanism to distinguish between SMs without knowing their biological activity, against a background of other material that is present.

3.4. Emerging Bioinformatic Approaches in Natural Product Discovery

The following section describes several computational perspectives that have demonstrated potential in uncovering new BGCs that encode novel bioactive SMs.

The EvoMining approach has been recently proposed as a strategy to identify new BGC classes [35]. EvoMining assumes that the genes encoding for SM enzymes have evolved from genes in primary metabolic enzymes due to duplication and divergence over time. The EvoMining software has been developed to detect divergences in the phylogenetic trees of enzymes in core pathways shared between bacterial species. This enables the software to identify enzymes that have likely been repurposed for SM biosynthesis. Using this approach, Cruz-Morales et al. identified arseno-organic metabolites in *S. coelicolor* and *Streptomyces lividans* [35]. These arseno-organic metabolites were derived from BGCs, which code for previously unknown compounds and enzymes [35]. The EvoMining approach provides a promising insight for uncovering hidden chemical diversity by incorporating evolutionary principles into genome mining.

Large-scale comparative genomic alignment has been proposed to identify new types of biosynthetic pathways. This strategy involves detecting syntenic blocks of multiple orthologous genes that are not part of the core genome of a taxon and occur in different genomic contexts in different strains and species [10]. A study using this approach successfully identified the kojic acid and oxylipin gene clusters from the accessory genome of Aspergillus species [36]. Kojic acid and oxylipin do not have any signature genes that are specific to known pathways and hence, this approach may provide users with a way to identify novel SM genes that were previously undiscovered in well-studied microorganisms.

4. BGC and Natural Product Mining in Different Environments

The following sections, while not exhaustive, are designed to provide some examples of work carried out in BGC 'mining' from different environments, specifically providing examples from soil, aquatic and host microbiomes. Noticeably, numerous studies have demonstrated that a combination of existing laboratory approaches along with the use of computational tools have provided new insights in the bioprospecting field. This is particularly crucial for studies looking to identify new natural products from microbial dark matter.

4.1. Natural Product Discoveries in Soil Environments

Soil environments have been reported to hold a highly diverse range of microorganisms and are known sources for antibiotics, antifungals and other natural products that are involved in bacterial communication and interaction within a given ecosystem [37–39]. However, many bacteria are unculturable and therefore, a vast majority of them remain understudied [40]. A global study conducted by Charlop-Powers in 2015 compared biosynthetic diversity and NRPS/PKS diversity in soil microbiomes across the globe [13]. Soil samples were collected from five continents covering different biomes. Degenerate primers that are specific to adenylation and ketosynthase domains were used for large-scale PCR. The observation of large differences in domain abundance from all except the most proximal and biome-similar samples suggests that different soil microbiomes can encode largely distinct collections of SMs.

The iChip method developed in 2010 offered a new way to isolate and cultivate unculturable bacteria in situ from many environments [41]. The miniature diffusion chambers from the iChip device allow bacterial species to be exposed to natural growth factors in the environment, hence enabling their growth and survival. Five years later, a study applying the iChip technology on soil samples led to the discovery of 'teixobactin', a new antibiotic that can inhibit cell wall synthesis while having undetectable antibiotic resistance in the infectious pathogens *Staphloccous aureus* and *Mycobacterium tuberculosis* [42]. The BGC giving rise to teixobactin is composed of two large NRPS-encoding genes and was identified using a homology search tool. This study demonstrates the importance for integrating novel laboratory techniques alongside computational tools as this will enable new microorganisms to be isolated, with the potential to extract new natural products and reconstruct their metabolic pathways.

A recently published study recovered hundreds of near-complete genomes from the Northern Californian grassland soil and analyzed them using antiSMASH [43]. These genomes contained newly identified members from Acidobacteria, Verrucomicobia and Gemmatimonadetes as well as the candidate phylum Rokubacteria. These members are abundant in soils but are under-represented in culture [40,43]. Members from these phyla were also previously not known to be linked to SM production but were found to encode diverse PK and NRP BGCs that were thought to have diverged from well-studied gene clusters [43]. The study demonstrates that the biosynthetic potential for phylogenetically diverse microorganisms in soils has previously been underestimated [43]. In addition, the knowledge gained in this study may provide a framework for future studies to target novel but abundant microorganisms in soils, which may represent a source for new pharmaceutical compounds.

4.2. Natural Product Discoveries in Aquatic Ecosystems

Aquatic ecosystems are relatively unexplored but have been reported to harbor a high diversity of microorganisms, which may reflect the biosynthetic potential of these ecosystems [14,44]. A previous study observed marine Actinomycetes as a robust source for beneficial SMs [45]. This study determined that 85% of marine bioactive compounds identified and described from 1997 to 2008 came from Streptomyces (57%) and Salinispora (28%), both of which are members of the Actinomycetes phylum. An example of a beneficial SM isolated from Actinomycetes is marizomib (salinosporamide A). Marizomib is an anticancer drug that was first isolated from *Salinispora tropica* and is currently undergoing clinical trials as it has demonstrated high cytotoxicity against breast cancer, human colon carcinoma and non-small lung cancer [46,47].

Early and recent studies have observed specific marine microorganisms, such as Roseobacter and Pseudovibrio having potential for SM production [48,49]. Members of Roseobacter have been reported to be widespread and abundant in marine environments with diverse metabolism, thus providing an opportunity to mine their genomes for potential natural products. The work from Martens et al. used degenerate primers that were specific with conserved sequence motifs to screen the strains of Roseobacter [49]. PCR products were cloned, sequenced and compared with genes of known function, revealing genes that show similarity with PKS and NRPS. Some strains also demonstrated antagonistic activity and acetylated homoserine lactone (AHL) production, which suggests that the Roseobacter clade is a potential and largely untapped source of SM.

Pseudovibrio-related bacteria have previously been isolated from marine sources as free-living and host-associated bacteria [50,51]. They have been shown to proliferate under extreme oligotrophic conditions, tolerate high heavy-metal concentrations and metabolize potentially toxic compounds [52–54]. The data from studies described by Romano suggest that apart from nutrient cycling, members of host-associated Pseudovibrio can provide their host with both vitamins/cofactors and protection from potential pathogens via the synthesis of antimicrobial SMs [48]. Marine environments provide an incentive for researchers to target marine microorganisms with potentially large and useful biosynthetic capacities as seen in Actinomycetes, Pseudovibrio and Roseobacter.

In a recent study, antiSMASH and NAPDOS were used to screen for SMs in recovered genome bins from Lake Stechlin, north-east Germany [14]. Of the 243 BGCs identified, 125 were classified as terpenes and represent the most abundant cluster type. Terpene products are commonly found in plants and fungi genomes but it has been recently reported that bacterial terpene synthases are distributed widely in the environment [14]. The second most abundant cluster type are bacteriocins with 35 clusters [14]. Bacteriocins are SMs belonging to a group of antimicrobial peptides, which can target closely related or unrelated strains to the bacteriocin producing bacteria [55]. Bacteriocins have been implicated as a possible alternative to currently overused antibiotics due to their diverse structure and function [55]. In addition, bacteriocins have been observed in probiotics to inhibit gastrointestinal microorganisms or pathogens [56]. A further analysis of BGCs in individual genome bins has revealed an unclassified bacterium with a PKS cluster and three associated domains belonging to the enediynes polyketides pathway. Enediynes polyketides are SMs that have been reported to demonstrate potent anticancer and antibiotic activity largely due to an enediyne core providing cytotoxic properties [57]. Their biosynthesis is also of interest as many unique chemical features were identified, providing a potent opportunity to decipher how the biosynthetic machinery can give rise to complex and unique molecules.

4.3. Exploring BGCs in Host Microbiome Environments

Host microbiome environments house an enormous range of bacteria that have adapted and thrived in the host's environment. In the past few years, studies have focused on natural product discovery in the human microbiome and have provided new insight into the search for novel SMs in different environments [15,58]. Another notable example includes the microbiome in marine sponges.

The microbiome of three deep sea sponges was screened for secondary metabolite potential by using 454 pyrosequencing and degenerate primers to target sequences associated with ketosynthase domains and adenylation domains [59]. Ketosynthase and adenylation fragments were revealed to be distinct from reference sequences in the database. This demonstrates the potential for the microbiome of these marine sponges to possess a diverse range of novel SMs. The sequence analysis of the sponges studied also determined that they have genes involved in the synthesis of streptogramin, lipopeptides and glycopeptides. These bioactive compounds are known classes of antibiotics. The study also indicates that variations in the gene sequences associated with SMs may potentially lead to the identification of natural products, which may serve beneficial roles in human health [59].

A recent study utilized a combination of chemistry, metagenomics and metatranscriptomics techniques to examine how microorganisms play a key role in human health. Using 752 metagenomic samples from the National Institute of Health Human Microbiome Project, the study found human-associated bacteria housing 3,118 BGCs that encode small molecules [15]. Many of these molecules are presumably associated with beneficial properties. Among these BGCs are thiopeptide clusters encoding antibiotics, some of which have a similar structure with molecules already in clinical trials.

5. Conclusions

SMs have played an important role in pharmaceuticals, research and the industry. There are numerous possibilities for expanding our understanding of chemical diversity and how these metabolites function. Various studies have found an abundance of BGCs encoding known SMs and potentially undiscovered ones, which reinforces the notion that high biodiversity can lead to high chemical diversity. In the future, we should see a continuing development of bioinformatics software to address the current limitations of genome mining, analyzing metagenomic data and compound characterization. We may also see new or improved culturing and screening techniques to better explore the vastness of SMs. Many of the discoveries to date have been attributed to many omics and metaomics approaches. However, the limitations of technology and methods still need to be addressed in order to fully exploit the genome mining process and optimize the workflow from the identification of BGC to the expression of the corresponding natural product.

There is growing interest to uncover biosynthetic pathways and new natural products in the environment, particularly environments hosting a rich diversity in microorganisms, such as soils, marine ecosystems and host microbiomes. In addition, other unique microbial ecosystems that occur in often extreme environments, such as microbialites, may also be a new source of novel SM [60]. The identification of a wide range of SMs will help to provide a better understanding of how novel SMs are assembled and detected. The increasing trends and updates in bioinformatics and refinement of the metaomics workflow will complement natural product discovery efforts in the environment and may ultimately lead to an influx of novel compounds with potential applications in medicine and industries.

Author Contributions: R.C. was involved in writing—original draft preparation; H.L.W. was involved in writing—review and editing, B.P.B was involved in supervision, funding acquisition and writing—review and editing.

Funding: This research received no external funding.

References

1. Chávez, A.; Forero, A.; García-Huante, Y.; Romero, A.; Sánchez, M.; Rocha, D.; Sánchez, B.; Rodríguez-Sanoja, R.; Sánchez, S.; Langley, E. Production of microbial secondary metabolites: Regulation by the carbon source AU—Ruiz, Beatriz. *Crit. Rev. Microbiol.* **2010**, *36*, 146–167. [CrossRef]
2. Newman, D.J.; Cragg, G.M. Natural Products as Sources of New Drugs from 1981 to 2014. *J. Nat. Prod.* **2016**, *79*, 629–661. [CrossRef] [PubMed]
3. Taylor, J.; Hafner, M.; Yerushalmi, E.; Smith, R.; Bellasio, J.; Vardavas, R.; Bienkowska-Gibbs, T.; Rubin, J. Estimating the Economic Costs of Antimicrobial Resistance. Available online: https://www.rand.org/content/dam/rand/pubs/research_reports/RR900/RR911/RAND_RR911.pdf (accessed on 25 February 2019).
4. Antimicrobial Resistance: Tackling a Crisis for the Health and Wealth of Nations. Available online: https://amr-review.org/sites/default/files/AMR%20Review%20Paper%20-%20Tackling%20a%20crisis%20for%20the%20health%20and%20wealth%20of%20nations_1.pdf (accessed on 25 February 2019).
5. Keller, N.P.; Turner, G.; Bennett, J.W. Fungal secondary metabolism—From biochemistry to genomics. *Nat. Rev. Microbiol.* **2005**, *3*, 937. [CrossRef] [PubMed]
6. Medema, M.H.; Kottmann, R.; Yilmaz, P.; Cummings, M.; Biggins, J.B.; Blin, K.; de Bruijn, I.; Chooi, Y.H.; Claesen, J.; Coates, R.C.; et al. Minimum Information about a Biosynthetic Gene cluster. *Nat. Chem. Biol.* **2015**, *11*, 625. [CrossRef] [PubMed]
7. Weber, T.; Kim, H.U. The secondary metabolite bioinformatics portal: Computational tools to facilitate synthetic biology of secondary metabolite production. *Synth. Syst. Biotechnol.* **2016**, *1*, 69–79. [CrossRef] [PubMed]
8. Ayuso-Sacido, A.; Genilloud, O. New PCR primers for the screening of NRPS and PKS-I systems in actinomycetes: Detection and distribution of these biosynthetic gene sequences in major taxonomic groups. *Microb. Ecol.* **2005**, *49*, 10–24. [CrossRef] [PubMed]
9. Palazzotto, E.; Weber, T. Omics and multi-omics approaches to study the biosynthesis of secondary metabolites in microorganisms. *Curr. Opin. Microbiol.* **2018**, *45*, 109–116. [CrossRef] [PubMed]
10. Medema, M.H.; Fischbach, M.A. Computational approaches to natural product discovery. *Nat. Chem. Biol.* **2015**, *11*, 639–648. [CrossRef] [PubMed]
11. Chavali, A.K.; Rhee, S.Y. Bioinformatics tools for the identification of gene clusters that biosynthesize specialized metabolites. *Brief. Bioinform.* **2017**, *19*, 1022–1034. [CrossRef] [PubMed]
12. Blin, K.; Kim, H.U.; Medema, M.H.; Weber, T. Recent development of antiSMASH and other computational approaches to mine secondary metabolite biosynthetic gene clusters. *Brief. Bioinform.* **2017**. [CrossRef] [PubMed]
13. Charlop-Powers, Z.; Owen, J.G.; Reddy, B.V.B.; Ternei, M.A.; Guimarães, D.O.; de Frias, U.A.; Pupo, M.T.; Seepe, P.; Feng, Z.; Brady, S.F. Global biogeographic sampling of bacterial secondary metabolism. *eLife* **2015**, *4*, e05048. [CrossRef] [PubMed]
14. Cuadrat, R.R.C.; Ionescu, D.; Dávila, A.M.R.; Grossart, H.-P. Recovering Genomics Clusters of Secondary Metabolites from Lakes Using Genome-Resolved Metagenomics. *Front. Microbiol.* **2018**, *9*, 251. [CrossRef] [PubMed]
15. Donia, M.S.; Cimermancic, P.; Schulze Christopher, J.; Wieland, B.; Laura, C.; Martin, J.; Mitreva, M.; Clardy, J.; Linington Roger, G.; Fischbach Michael, A. A Systematic Analysis of Biosynthetic Gene Clusters in the Human Microbiome Reveals a Common Family of Antibiotics. *Cell* **2014**, *158*, 1402–1414. [CrossRef] [PubMed]
16. Katz, L.; Baltz, R.H. Natural product discovery: Past, present and future. *J. Ind. Microbiol. Biotechnol.* **2016**, *43*, 155–176. [CrossRef] [PubMed]
17. Stewart, E.J. Growing Unculturable Bacteria. *J. Bacteriol.* **2012**, *194*, 4151–4160. [CrossRef] [PubMed]
18. Luo, Y.; Cobb, R.E.; Zhao, H. Recent advances in natural product discovery. *Curr. Opin. Biotechnol.* **2014**, *30*, 230–237. [CrossRef] [PubMed]
19. Ymele-Leki, P.; Cao, S.; Sharp, J.; Lambert, K.G.; McAdam, A.J.; Husson, R.N.; Tamayo, G.; Clardy, J.; Watnick, P.I. A High-Throughput Screen Identifies a New Natural Product with Broad-Spectrum Antibacterial Activity. *PLoS ONE* **2012**, *7*, e31307. [CrossRef]

20. Li, J.W.-H.; Vederas, J.C. Drug Discovery and Natural Products: End of an Era or an Endless Frontier? *Science* **2009**, *325*, 161–165. [CrossRef] [PubMed]

21. Linhart, C.; Shamir, R. The degenerate primer design problem: Theory and applications. *J. Comput. Biol. A J. Comput. Mol. Cell Biol.* **2005**, *12*, 431–456. [CrossRef] [PubMed]

22. Khosla, C.; Gokhale, R.S.; Jacobsen, J.R.; Cane, D.E. Tolerance and Specificity of Polyketide Synthases. *Annu. Rev. Biochem.* **1999**, *68*, 219–253. [CrossRef] [PubMed]

23. Owen, J.G.; Charlop-Powers, Z.; Smith, A.G.; Ternei, M.A.; Calle, P.Y.; Reddy, B.V.B.; Montiel, D.; Brady, S.F. Multiplexed metagenome mining using short DNA sequence tags facilitates targeted discovery of epoxyketone proteasome inhibitors. *Proc. Natl. Acad. Sci. USA* **2015**, *112*, 4221–4226. [CrossRef] [PubMed]

24. Cimermancic, P.; Medema, M.H.; Claesen, J.; Kurita, K.; Brown, L.C.; Mavrommatis, K.; Pati, A.; Godfrey, P.A.; Koehrsen, M.; Clardy, J.; et al. Insights into Secondary Metabolism from a Global Analysis of Prokaryotic Biosynthetic Gene Clusters. *Cell* **2014**, *158*, 412–421. [CrossRef] [PubMed]

25. Blin, K.; Wolf, T.; Chevrette, M.G.; Lu, X.; Schwalen, C.J.; Kautsar, S.A.; Suarez Duran, H.G.; de los Santos, E.L.C.; Kim, H.U.; Nave, M.; et al. antiSMASH 4.0—Improvements in chemistry prediction and gene cluster boundary identification. *Nucleic Acids Res.* **2017**, *45*, W36–W41. [CrossRef] [PubMed]

26. Starcevic, A.; Zucko, J.; Simunkovic, J.; Long, P.F.; Cullum, J.; Hranueli, D. ClustScan: An integrated program package for the semi-automatic annotation of modular biosynthetic gene clusters and in silico prediction of novel chemical structures. *Nucleic Acids Res.* **2008**, *36*, 6882–6892. [CrossRef] [PubMed]

27. Wilson, M.C.; Piel, J. Metagenomic Approaches for Exploiting Uncultivated Bacteria as a Resource for Novel Biosynthetic Enzymology. *Chem. Biol.* **2013**, *20*, 636–647. [CrossRef] [PubMed]

28. Ren, H.; Wang, B.; Zhao, H. Breaking the silence: New strategies for discovering novel natural products. *Curr. Opin. Biotechnol.* **2017**, *48*, 21–27. [CrossRef] [PubMed]

29. Zhang, M.M.; Wong, F.T.; Wang, Y.; Luo, S.; Lim, Y.H.; Heng, E.; Yeo, W.L.; Cobb, R.E.; Enghiad, B.; Ang, E.L.; et al. CRISPR–Cas9 strategy for activation of silent Streptomyces biosynthetic gene clusters. *Nat. Chem. Biol.* **2017**, *13*, 607. [CrossRef] [PubMed]

30. Kouprina, N.; Larionov, V. Selective isolation of genomic loci from complex genomes by transformation-associated recombination cloning in the yeast Saccharomyces cerevisiae. *Nat. Protoc.* **2008**, *3*, 371. [CrossRef] [PubMed]

31. Yamanaka, K.; Reynolds, K.A.; Kersten, R.D.; Ryan, K.S.; Gonzalez, D.J.; Nizet, V.; Dorrestein, P.C.; Moore, B.S. Direct cloning and refactoring of a silent lipopeptide biosynthetic gene cluster yields the antibiotic taromycin A. *Proc. Natl. Acad. Sci. USA* **2014**, *111*, 1957–1962. [CrossRef] [PubMed]

32. Li, Y.; Li, Z.; Yamanaka, K.; Xu, Y.; Zhang, W.; Vlamakis, H.; Kolter, R.; Moore, B.S.; Qian, P.-Y. Directed natural product biosynthesis gene cluster capture and expression in the model bacterium Bacillus subtilis. *Sci. Rep.* **2015**, *5*, 9383. [CrossRef] [PubMed]

33. Ross, A.C.; Gulland, L.E.S.; Dorrestein, P.C.; Moore, B.S. Targeted Capture and Heterologous Expression of the Pseudoalteromonas Alterochromide Gene Cluster in Escherichia coli Represents a Promising Natural Product Exploratory Platform. *Acs Synth. Biol.* **2015**, *4*, 414–420. [CrossRef] [PubMed]

34. Pimentel-Elardo, S.M.; Sørensen, D.; Ho, L.; Ziko, M.; Bueler, S.A.; Lu, S.; Tao, J.; Moser, A.; Lee, R.; Agard, D.; et al. Activity-Independent Discovery of Secondary Metabolites Using Chemical Elicitation and Cheminformatic Inference. *Acs Chem. Biol.* **2015**, *10*, 2616–2623. [CrossRef] [PubMed]

35. Cruz-Morales, P.; Kopp, J.F.; Martínez-Guerrero, C.; Yáñez-Guerra, L.A.; Selem-Mojica, N.; Ramos-Aboites, H.; Feldmann, J.; Barona-Gómez, F. Phylogenomic Analysis of Natural Products Biosynthetic Gene Clusters Allows Discovery of Arseno-Organic Metabolites in Model Streptomycetes. *Genome Biol. Evol.* **2016**, *8*, 1906–1916. [CrossRef] [PubMed]

36. Takeda, I.; Machida, M.; Koike, H.; Umemura, M.; Asai, K. Motif-Independent Prediction of a Secondary Metabolism Gene Cluster Using Comparative Genomics: Application to Sequenced Genomes of Aspergillus and Ten Other Filamentous Fungal Species. *DNA Res.* **2014**, *21*, 447–457. [CrossRef] [PubMed]

37. Torsvik, V.; Goksøyr, J.; Daae, F.L. High diversity in DNA of soil bacteria. *Appl. Environ. Microbiol.* **1990**, *56*, 782–787. [PubMed]

38. Hibbing, M.E.; Fuqua, C.; Parsek, M.R.; Peterson, S.B. Bacterial competition: Surviving and thriving in the microbial jungle. *Nat. Rev. Microbiol.* **2010**, *8*, 15–25. [CrossRef] [PubMed]

39. Daniel, R. The soil metagenome—A rich resource for the discovery of novel natural products. *Curr. Opin. Biotechnol.* **2004**, *15*, 199–204. [CrossRef] [PubMed]

40. Rappe, M.S.; Giovannoni, S.J. The Uncultured Microbial Majority. *Annu. Rev. Microbiol.* **2003**, *57*, 369–394. [CrossRef] [PubMed]

41. Nichols, D.; Cahoon, N.; Trakhtenberg, E.M.; Pham, L.; Mehta, A.; Belanger, A.; Kanigan, T.; Lewis, K.; Epstein, S.S. Use of ichip for high-throughput in situ cultivation of "uncultivable" microbial species. *Appl. Environ. Microbiol.* **2010**, *76*, 2445–2450. [CrossRef] [PubMed]

42. Ling, L.L.; Schneider, T.; Peoples, A.J.; Spoering, A.L.; Engels, I.; Conlon, B.P.; Mueller, A.; Schäberle, T.F.; Hughes, D.E.; Epstein, S.; et al. A new antibiotic kills pathogens without detectable resistance. *Nature* **2015**, *517*, 455. [CrossRef] [PubMed]

43. Crits-Christoph, A.; Diamond, S.; Butterfield, C.N.; Thomas, B.C.; Banfield, J.F. Novel soil bacteria possess diverse genes for secondary metabolite biosynthesis. *Nature* **2018**, *558*, 440–444. [CrossRef] [PubMed]

44. Adnan, M.; Alshammari, E.; Patel, M.; Amir Ashraf, S.; Khan, S.; Hadi, S. Significance and potential of marine microbial natural bioactive compounds against biofilms/biofouling: Necessity for green chemistry. *PeerJ* **2018**, *6*, e5049. [CrossRef] [PubMed]

45. Williams, P.G. Panning for chemical gold: Marine bacteria as a source of new therapeutics. *Trends Biotechnol.* **2009**, *27*, 45–52. [CrossRef] [PubMed]

46. Ahn, K.S.; Sethi, G.; Chao, T.-H.; Neuteboom, S.T.; Chaturvedi, M.M.; Palladino, M.A.; Younes, A.; Aggarwal, B.B. Salinosporamide A (NPI-0052) potentiates apoptosis, suppresses osteoclastogenesis and inhibits invasion through down-modulation of NF-κB–regulated gene products. *Blood* **2007**, *110*, 2286–2295. [CrossRef] [PubMed]

47. Feling, R.H.; Buchanan, G.O.; Mincer, T.J.; Kauffman, C.A.; Jensen, P.R.; Fenical, W.; Salinosporamide, A. A Highly Cytotoxic Proteasome Inhibitor from a Novel Microbial Source, a Marine Bacterium of the New Genus Salinospora. *Angew. Chem. Int. Ed.* **2003**, *42*, 355–357. [CrossRef] [PubMed]

48. Romano, S. Ecology and biotechnological potential of bacteria belonging to the genus Pseudovibrio. *Appl. Environ. Microbiol.* **2018**, *84*, e02516–e02517. [CrossRef] [PubMed]

49. Martens, T.; Gram, L.; Grossart, H.P.; Kessler, D.; Muller, R.; Simon, M.; Wenzel, S.C.; Brinkhoff, T. Bacteria of the Roseobacter clade show potential for secondary metabolite production. *Microb. Ecol.* **2007**, *54*, 31–42. [CrossRef] [PubMed]

50. O'Halloran, J.A.; Barbosa, T.M.; Morrissey, J.P.; Kennedy, J.; Dobson, A.D.; O'Gara, F. Pseudovibrio axinellae sp. nov., isolated from an Irish marine sponge. *Int. J. Syst. Evol. Microbiol.* **2013**, *63*, 141–145. [CrossRef]

51. Hosoya, S.; Yokota, A. Pseudovibrio japonicus sp. nov., isolated from coastal seawater in Japan. *Int. J. Syst. Evol. Microbiol.* **2007**, *57*, 1952–1955. [CrossRef] [PubMed]

52. Bauvais, C.; Zirah, S.; Piette, L.; Chaspoul, F.; Domart-Coulon, I.; Chapon, V.; Gallice, P.; Rebuffat, S.; Pérez, T.; Bourguet-Kondracki, M.-L. Sponging up metals: Bacteria associated with the marine sponge Spongia officinalis. *Mar. Environ. Res.* **2015**, *104*, 20–30. [CrossRef] [PubMed]

53. Schwedt, A.; Seidel, M.; Dittmar, T.; Simon, M.; Bondarev, V.; Romano, S.; Lavik, G.; Schulz-Vogt, H.N. Substrate use of Pseudovibrio sp. growing in ultra-oligotrophic seawater. *PLoS ONE* **2015**, *10*, e0121675. [CrossRef] [PubMed]

54. Nies, D.H. Microbial heavy-metal resistance. *Appl. Microbiol. Biotechnol.* **1999**, *51*, 730–750. [CrossRef] [PubMed]

55. Yang, S.-C.; Lin, C.-H.; Sung, C.T.; Fang, J.-Y. Antibacterial activities of bacteriocins: Application in foods and pharmaceuticals. *Front. Microbiol.* **2014**, *5*, 241. [CrossRef] [PubMed]

56. Dobson, A.; Cotter, P.D.; Ross, R.P.; Hill, C. Bacteriocin production: A probiotic trait? *Appl. Environ. Microbiol.* **2012**, *78*, 1–6. [CrossRef] [PubMed]

57. Van Lanen, S.G.; Shen, B. Biosynthesis of enediyne antitumor antibiotics. *Curr. Top. Med. Chem.* **2008**, *8*, 448–459. [CrossRef] [PubMed]

58. Luber, J.M.; Kostic, A.D. Gut Microbiota: Small Molecules Modulate Host Cellular Functions. *Curr. Biol.* **2017**, *27*, R307–R310. [CrossRef] [PubMed]

59. Borchert, E.; Jackson, S.A.; O'Gara, F.; Dobson, A.D.W. Diversity of Natural Product Biosynthetic Genes in the Microbiome of the Deep Sea Sponges Inflatella pellicula, Poecillastra compressa and Stelletta normani. *Front. Microbiol.* **2016**, *7*, 1027. [CrossRef] [PubMed]

60. Burns, B.P.; Seifert, A.; Goh, F.; Pomati, F.; Neilan, B.A. Genetic potential for secondary metabolite production in stromatolite communities. *FEMS Micro Lett.* **2005**, *243*, 293–301. [CrossRef] [PubMed]

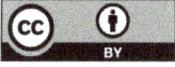

MDPI
St. Alban-Anlage 66
4052 Basel
Switzerland
Tel. +41 61 683 77 34
Fax +41 61 302 89 18
www.mdpi.com

Medicines Editorial Office
E-mail: medicines@mdpi.com
www.mdpi.com/journal/medicines